METHODS IN MOLECULAR BIOLOGY™

Series Editor
John M. Walker
School of Life Sciences
University of Hertfordshire
Hatfield, Hertfordshire, AL10 9AB, UK

For further volumes:
http://www.springer.com/series/7651

Molecular Diagnostics for Melanoma

Methods and Protocols

Edited by

Magdalena Thurin

Cancer Diagnosis Program, National Cancer Institute, National Institutes of Health, Bethesda, MD, USA

Francesco M. Marincola

Sidra Medical and Research Center, Qatar Foundation, Doha, Qatar

Humana Press

Editors
Magdalena Thurin
Cancer Diagnosis Program
National Cancer Institute
National Institutes of Health
Bethesda, MD, USA

Francesco M. Marincola
Sidra Medical and Research Center
Qatar Foundation, Doha, Qatar

ISSN 1064-3745 ISSN 1940-6029 (electronic)
ISBN 978-1-4939-6038-5 ISBN 978-1-62703-727-3 (eBook)
DOI 10.1007/978-1-62703-727-3
Springer New York Heidelberg Dordrecht London

Printed on acid-free paper

Humana Press is a brand of Springer
Springer is part of Springer Science+Business Media (www.springer.com)

Preface

Abstract

A new taxonomy of cancers defined by molecular signatures with prognostic and therapeutic implications is emerging. Pathological assessment of melanoma that is the current standard method to determine diagnosis is improving due to additional criteria evolving from understanding of biology of melanoma. Genomics, epigenomics, and proteomics approaches have already led to molecular reclassification of melanoma in the context with pathological findings. Moreover, discovery of genetic alterations that drive melanoma progression provide the basis for the development of targeted therapies for patients with metastatic disease. Following these discoveries, the U.S. Food and Drug Administration (FDA) approved in 2011 and 2013 small molecular compounds vemurafenib and dabrafenib, respectively, that provide novel treatment options for melanoma patients. Vemurafenib and dabrafenib target mutated V600 codon of BRAF signaling molecule that is a key effector of RAS/RAF/MEK/ERK pathway. Mutations in this gene occur in over half of melanoma tumors and BRAF V600E mutations are the most common. Additional agent targeting downstream MAPK kinases including MEK1/2 inhibitor, trametinib was also approved by the FDA in 2013. Concomitantly with these drugs, companion diagnostic tests for detection of BRAF V600 mutations were also approved. These tests can identify specific subpopulations of melanoma patients with BRAF V600 codon mutations who most likely will benefit from the therapy. These examples are a prototype of a broad category of personalized treatment that uses a companion test to select patients for specific treatment.

Recent, promising approaches to improve responses in melanoma by blocking negative regulators of T cell activity, i.e., cytotoxic T lymphocyte-associated protein 4 (CTLA-4) and programmed cell death 1 (PD-1) receptors were demonstrated and anti-CTLA drug ipilimumab was approved by the FDA in 2011. While there are no approved diagnostics for immunotherapy, promising markers associated with response to ipilimumab and anti-PD1 therapy were identified. Given that the majority of patients do not respond to these drugs and drugs are highly toxic, predictive markers could potentially improve therapeutic ratio of these drugs.

The primary purpose of this volume is to provide updated information on well-characterized diagnostic and prognostic assays and assays predicting response to treatment for routine testing. The focus is also on a few emerging biomarkers categories with potential clinical validity rather than on early discovery stage. Most of chapters provide detailed protocols for markers' detection and novel technologies with potential for clinical application. Several review chapters provide an overview of the current status in diagnosis and therapy of melanoma and discuss the need to incorporate biomarkers to impact patient care. Important issues related to marker development and validation such as statistical approaches and specimen requirements are also discussed.

Introduction

The incidence of melanoma has more than doubled over the last 20 years in the United States and worldwide, accounting for the majority of skin cancer-related deaths. Traditionally, the prognosis and treatment decisions regarding surgical and adjuvant therapy for a patient with cutaneous melanoma have been based on the current AJCC/UICC (American Joint Committee on Cancer/Union for International Cancer Control) criteria, which include histological and morphologic analysis of the tumor tissue, the anatomic site of origin, and assessment of local spread using TNM staging procedures (Chapter 17). Although high mitotic rate and ulceration are considered strong negative prognostic factors in melanoma as outlined by the AJCC/IUCC, these histopathological characteristics cannot always accurately predict who will relapse and who will remain disease free. While most cutaneous melanomas classified as early stage are cured by surgical resection, a subgroup of patients will relapse. Conversely, a subset of thick melanomas will not recur after surgical excision of the primary tumor. These observations suggest the utility of additional prognostic and predictive markers to determine the potential for metastatic relapse at the time of diagnosis and to guide therapeutic decisions in adjuvant settings even in early stage melanoma patients.

Advances in cancer biology and powerful technologies provide increased opportunities for the identification of aberrations in genes, proteins, and molecular profiles. Novel technologies including next generation (NGS) sequencing, gene expression arrays, epigenetics, and proteomics-based methods facilitate molecular discoveries and provide critical information regarding melanoma biology and the mechanism of progression. These approaches identify transcriptional changes, germline and somatic mutations, nucleic acid aberrations, and gene expression that may constitute the basis for development of molecular diagnostics. Consequently, a new molecular classification of melanoma is evolving based on chromosomal aberrations, gene mutations and signaling pathways activation that underlie biologically distinct subsets of tumors that require different clinical management. While novel approaches are increasingly explored for routine testing and evaluation of markers for diagnosis, classification, and prognosis, not many novel tests have been validated for their clinical utility and are available for routine use in melanoma. Thus traditional cancer diagnostics approaches including histopathology and immunohistochemistry (IHC) will likely remain standard tools for the future. Upcoming molecular analyses and novel technologies might be incorporated in the context of these established methods when, for example, the definite diagnosis cannot be reached (Chapters 12–16). They potentially might be systematically incorporated and lead to improvement of the AJCC/IUCC system.

When the treatment is developed for a specific biological target that characterizes only some patients, the test could be developed to identify patients with this target. Novel approaches including NGS offer more precise characterization of biologically distinct subtypes of melanoma and become utilized for personalized treatments. Determination of specific therapy target is becoming increasingly important to select melanoma patients most likely to benefit from targeted treatment, or to avoid treating patients likely to have serious adverse reactions (Chapters 1–3).

The recent approval by the FDA of several drugs for the treatment of metastatic melanoma, including vemurafenib and dabrafenib that target the BRAF V600 codon mutated kinase, provide examples of a parallel development of therapeutic treatment and diagnostic tests that both must be approved. The example of targeted drug design includes in vitro companion diagnostic codeveloped with the drug to determine patient eligibility for specific targeted therapy include cobas® 4800V600 Mutation test (Roche Molecular Diagnostics). Cobas test detects V600E mutated form of BRAF kinase to identify patients with this mutation for treatment with BRAF inhibitors. Alongside the recent approval of trametininb targeting downstream MAPK kinases including MEK1/2 the agency also approved a companion genetic test, the THxID BRAF V600 (Biomerieux) that will help determine whether a patient's melanoma cells have the V600E or V600K mutation in the BRAF gene and are eligible for treatment with trametinib and BRAF inhibitors. Many other mutation analysis of genes relevant for melanoma (e.g., NRAS, KIT, MEK) and other genomic aberrations (e.g., PTEN loss, AKT amplification) are becoming important part of routine pathological assessment available to clinicians for guiding melanoma patients for specific targeted therapy (Chapters 8 and 9).

As molecular mechanisms underlying disease biology are increasingly understood, companion diagnostics are more likely to be developed in tandem with drug, and this principle will be used for a broader category of "personalized" treatments. This approach strongly relies on the accurate stratification of patients based on mutational analysis and potentially immune response profiling to guide drug efficacy and/or resistance using predictive markers.

Novel Technologies for Melanoma Diagnostics

Significant advancements in high-resolution genome-wide molecular techniques have greatly increased an ability to examine and understand genomic changes in melanoma and to identify new genes involved in etiology of this disease. Recent developments in technologies for whole-exome and whole-genome sequencing have already allowed for comprehensive mutation analysis and have led to the identification of a number of new genes and families of genes potentially involved in metastatic melanoma including GRIN2A, MAP3K5, ERBB4, NEDD9, BAP1, RAC1, PREX2, STK19, and others. These approaches enable identification of spectrum of mutations throughout the entire gene including suppressor genes and non-hot spot mutations and will further contribute to the identification of yet unknown rare aberrations. As they offer therapeutic insights for targetable mutations in tumor facilitating biomarker-informed therapies they are likely to be developed into companion diagnostics determining the eligibility criteria for specific targeted therapy. NGS sequencing technologies, however, might not be suitable for identification of genes that are not likely to represent targets for direct therapeutic intervention even in those tumors with identifiable mutations (e.g., 20–30 % of BRAF mutant patients do not respond to vemurafenib). Although NGS-based methods are still mainly used in experimental settings, they are exploited for their clinical utility and rapidly entering the clinical arena as predictive tests for selection of patients for appropriate therapies. High-throughput sequencing approaches to analyze a panel of specific mutations in oncogenes, suppressor genes, and signaling molecules that enable clinicians to match the most appropriate genetic tests to the patient's tumor are currently offered at specialist oncology clinics to identify therapeutic response and emerging resistance in melanoma patients' samples.

Platforms capable of measuring global changes in gene expression levels, high-resolution chromosomal copy number, changes in allelic balance through detection of single-nucleotide polymorphism (SNP), as well as quantitative protein expression, e.g., mass spectrometry or reverse phase protein array (RPPA) are more amenable to impact molecular classification, diagnosis, and prognosis of melanoma. Future pathology assessment will likely include genomic-based approaches such as Comparative genomic hybridization (CGH) and SNP-based platforms. These high-throughput platforms are already available for routine testing to determine prognosis. In addition, technical modifications including automatization, computer-assisted imaging, high-resolution multispectral imaging (Chapter 32), and introduction of multimarker and quantitative IHC-based approaches (Chapters 13 and 14) discussed in this volume support the strengths of these methods to serve the growing prognostic and predictive needs in the clinical management of melanoma.

Validation of Diagnostics

While many of these new tools and approaches proved to be useful for discovering candidate markers, validating cancer biomarkers continues to pose serious challenges. Proper validation of a biomarker is extremely important since the marker is to be used in a clinical setting for the classification of patients into subgroups within morphologically similar tumors and providing prognostic criteria as well as predictive relevance for therapeutic intervention. Marker and assay validation is critical to their clinical application, and several steps including analytical performance and evaluation of clinical validity and utility are needed to successfully demonstrate marker usefulness prior to clinical laboratory implementation. Rapid development of technologies creates specific biases that need to be considered, since strict adherence to protocols developed for each platform is required by the Clinical Laboratory Improvement Amendments (CLIA) certification for each clinical test and clinical laboratory. These technical aspects must be considered in addition to the challenges of clinical validation for the implementation of any marker within the clinical setting.

As part of analytical validation of the assay, the technical and analytical performance characteristics (e.g., stability, accuracy, and reproducibility) of the assay for a marker need to be established. Secondly, determining clinical validity of a molecular diagnostic, i.e., evidence that the marker can separate two subgroups of patients with different outcomes within a large population requires correlation of laboratory test results with clinical parameters. The limited availability of fresh frozen specimens restricted in the past the chance of identifying meaningful clinical association of diagnostics in patient cohorts of sufficient size. However, the advent of technological advances for the analysis of formalin-fixed archival specimens (FFPE) has not only made the discovery of novel markers possible but also facilitated their clinical validation in large cohorts of clinically annotated samples.

Validation studies require a sufficient sample size and independent validation sets to demonstrate prognostic and/or predictive power of molecular factors to warrant patient stratification according to risk for tumor recurrence or for specific therapies. Access to clinically annotated specimens collected from well-controlled clinical studies is an important consideration for establishing the clinical utility of the marker. Specimens collected within multisite clinical trials are especially suitable for retrospective and prospective analyses of associations between outcomes and molecular characteristics. Archived specimens from a large population of untreated patients should be adequate to estimate recurrence in marker-defined subgroups of patients. Specimens from randomized trials with a survival or progression-free survival endpoints are required to establish the clinical validity of markers deemed to be predictive of response to specific treatments. Despite these stringent requirements, it is encouraging to see that many laboratories and new technologies generate potentially clinically applicable tests to guide the treatment of melanoma patients as demonstrated in this volume.

Diagnostics for Precision Care

Historically, systemic therapy for metastatic melanoma provided very low response rates and little to no benefit in overall survival. Recently, several melanoma therapies, including targeted therapies and immunotherapy, have provided alternative treatment options to melanoma patients. Signaling pathway inhibitors such as vemurafenib and dabrafenib, which target mutated BRAF, have conferred improved progression-free survival in patients with advanced melanoma compared to standard therapy. BRAF inhibitors are indicated only in those patients whose tumors harbor the mutated BRAF as wild-type BRAF melanoma are not likely to respond and because of the potential risk of tumor promotion (Chapters 1–3).

The BRAF gene encodes a serine/threonine kinase that is a key effector of the RAF/MEK/ERK pathway. BRAF is a member of the RAF family of kinases (ARAF, BRAF, and CRAF) and transmits intracellular signal from upstream receptor tyrosine kinases to the downstream serine/threonine kinases MEK and ERK. Activating mutations of BRAF are detected at all stages of melanocytic lesions including nevi, primary, and metastatic melanoma. The most common mutation occurs in exon 15 and results in a valine to glutamate substitution at codon 600 (BRAF V600E) in 85 % of tumors harboring mutated BRAF. Other less-frequent mutations observed in the codon 600 such as V600K and D were identified in 15–20 % of melanoma patients. The cobas® 4800 BRAF V600® molecular test detecting V600E mutation is an example of the companion diagnostic test used to determine patients' eligibility for treatment with vemurafenib in cutaneous melanoma. Another test THxID BRAF companion diagnostic will help determine whether a patient's melanoma cells have the V600E or V600K mutations in the BRAF gene and are eligible for treatment with vemurafenib and dabrafenib as well as trametinib.

Other tests that use different platforms and detect variant mutations at codon 600 including IHC-based test are being performed in diagnostic laboratories for treatment with BRAF targeting agents. However, it is important to consider that the outcome of the assay might differ depending on the platform requirements and specimen analyzed. Ultimately, clinicians must decide which test and in which circumstances should be used reliably to identify patients with BRAF mutation as discussed in Chapters 3 and 8.

The mutation frequency of NRAS in cutaneous melanoma is approximately 20 %, whereas mutations of the other RAS genes such as HRAS and KRAS are rare. The most common NRAS mutations affect residues in exon 1 (codon 12) or 2 (codon 60 and 61) and they are mutually exclusive with activating V600E mutations. Attempts to directly target NRAS have not been successful but RAS activates both the PI3K and MAPK pathways, which demonstrates the importance of RAS mutation testing in melanoma as a biomarker in predicting clinical response to inhibitors of both pathways.

Additional agents targeting downstream MAPK kinases including MEK1/2 (MAP2K1 and MAP2K2) inhibitors show promise both as single agents and in combination with BRAF inhibitors. MEK mutations are thought to be rare but approximately 10 % of melanomas harbor somatic mutations in either MEK1 or 2 which might render MEK mutated tumors for the therapy regimens including MEK inhibitors. Most common mutations that are not associated with resistance in MEK1/2 in melanoma involve exon 3 (P124S and I111S) can be tested using PCR or sequencing based methods. Recently FDA approved drug trametinib targeting downstream MAPK kinases including MEK1/2 provides therapeutic options for patients with tumors harboring MAPK pathway activating mutations including BRAF V600 mutations. Although, MEK inhibitors are designed to target BRAF mutant disease, they could also be effective in melanoma harboring activating mutations in MEK1/2 and RAS mutations.

Genomic alterations in PI3K-AKT signaling pathway are considerably less prevalent than MAPK pathway alterations in melanoma but large genetic diversity affects this pathway.

Although activating mutations in PI3K are rare, downstream effectors including PTEN and AKT are altered in majority of melanomas. AKT is a well known oncogene and AKT3 activation due point mutations or overexpression resulting from increased gene copy number may be common in melanoma. The PTEN tumor suppressor gene encodes a lipid phosphatase that regulates cell survival through PI3K/AKT signaling. Allelic loss or altered expression through epigenetic silencing or mutations of PTEN comprises 20 % and 40 % of melanomas, respectively. PTEN loss leads to activation of AKT and increase in activity of another downstream effector mTOR, and inhibitors of AKT and mTOR are explored for clinical application. Molecular profiling to identify patients whose tumors harbor alterations in PI3K-AKT pathways could provide rationale for developing diagnostics to select patients for treatments targeting this pathway.

While activating BRAF and RAS activating mutations are common in cutaneous melanoma, a much smaller subset of melanomas originating from mucosal, acral and chronic sun damage (CSD) skin demonstrate alterations in the KIT receptor tyrosine which do not coincide with BRAF and NRAS mutations. The vast majority of KIT activating point mutations is in exon 11 and they are sensitive to imatinib and other KIT inhibitors such as sunitinib and desatinib. Use of KIT inhibitors for patients with melanoma harboring KIT mutations represents another successful example of a personalized approach with the use of tumor mutational status to direct therapeutic decisions. KIT expression is also observed in nearly 80 % of cases of uveal melanoma (UM). Although amplification and over-expression of the KIT gene have also been identified in patients with melanoma using fluorescence in situ hybridization (FISH) method its mutational status correlates much better with response to imatinib. Sequencing approach to identify rare melanomas with KIT-mutation and the necessity of this particular molecular testing approach is discussed in Chapter 9.

Furthermore, kinome sequencing analysis has identified a high frequency of activating somatic mutations occurring in the receptor tyrosine kinase ERBB4 gene that is a member of the epidermal growth factor receptor (EGFR) superfamily in cutaneous melanoma. Several of these ERBB4 mutations were shown to increase kinase activity. Given the success of small molecule inhibitors of EGFR specific inhibitors of ERBB4 (e.g., gefitnib, erlotnib and lapatinib) could improve existing melanoma treatments in patients with mutated ERBB4 (Chapter 24).

Uveal melanomas also have frequent mutations in α subunit of the G-proteins GNAQ (35 %) and GNA11 (45 %) each (Chapter 21). These mutations are essentially absent from cutaneous and mucosal melanomas and involve the hot spot residues on exon 5. Mutations in GNAQ and GNA11 activate the MEK–ERK pathway and MEK targeting drugs (e.g., selumetinib) are currently in clinical trials for this disease in patients with GNAQ and GNA11 mutations. Genetic testing and gene expression testing in UM can also identify patients at high risk for development of aggressive tumors (type 2) and those with less aggressive tumors (type 1) and these tests became recently available (Chapters 22 and 23). UM tumors also harbor inactivating somatic mutations in BAP1 gene encoding BRCA1 associated protein that is associated with 84 % of type 2 uveal melanomas. This finding implicates BAP1 pathway as a potential target for therapy in these patients.

Although molecular subtypes of cancer patients selected for treatment by the presence of specific molecular targets often experience impressive responses to molecularly targeted therapy, most will suffer from subsequent recurrence and disease progression. Molecularly characterizing tumors to determine acquired alterations such as new mutations or gene copy number changes that lead to the development of drug resistance are critical for the prediction of drug responsiveness and for the combination of treatment strategies. The discovery of multiple new genetic events that occur after patients develop resistance to BRAF inhibitors, many of which have implications for rational therapeutic approaches (MAP3K8/COT-1, PDGFRB, IGF1R, amplification or alternative splicing of BRAF) provide future treatment options for patients with these alterations. The upcoming evidence regarding these mechanisms strongly supports the testing of metastases and validating as diagnostics for clinical use (Chapter 10).

Several susceptibility genes have been identified in melanomas and screening for them can be recommended for patients with a family history of melanoma. Several tests identifying germline mutations in melanoma-associated genes, particularly CDKN2A and CDK4 are available (Chapter 20).

Diagnosis and Prognosis

There is a great need to accurately establish diagnosis, prognosis and to define the outcome of individual melanoma patients but the existing clinicopathologic prognostic factors are not always adequate. The pathologic diagnosis of melanoma remains challenging which creates an unmet need not only for the molecular diagnostics but also for improved histopathology and immunohistopathology approaches (Chapters 16 and 17). Better methods to determine melanoma progression would allow further improvements in the prognostic assessment of melanoma patients. Importantly, the accurate prognosis will benefit proper risk stratification of the early stage melanoma patients for adjuvant treatment.

Multiparameter-based approaches for prognostic biomarkers are beginning to emerge that offer a prognostic algorithms based on the combination of several individual biomarkers with the potential for translation into the clinic. Novel quantitative immunostaining platforms enable measurement of protein markers expression in different cell populations including tumors cells and immune cells as well as cellular and subcellular compartments distribution (Chapter 13). Prognostic impact in primary cutaneous melanoma using immunohistochemical assay based on expression levels of three markers was demonstrated across different tissue platforms and different scoring analysis (Chapter 14). Furthermore, emerging methods use integrated approach that includes quantitative multiplex immune phenotyping. Automated image capture integrate fully quantitative measures of protein expression and spacial relationship within the tumor enabling objective and reproducible analysis to define risk of recurrence or to guide therapeutic decision making (Chapter 32).

As patterns of genomic alterations and genomic mutational status for classification of clinical subgroups of melanoma with a high degree of accuracy emerge the methods to detect these molecular features could further advance differential diagnosis in melanoma (Chapter 12). For example, a study of gene copy number alterations in primary melanomas by array CGH has identified distinct subclasses of melanoma on the basis of anatomic site, extent of UV exposure, and mutational status of several genes, including NRAS and BRAF. Using array CGH to compare DNA copy numbers across progression of disease and in cases with challenging histology (e.g., Spitz nevi) consistent chromosomal aberrations can be characterized. High throughput methods such as gene expression arrays, SNP array and microsatellite instability (MSI) are also used as diagnostics to define risk for metastasis in UM (Chapters 22 and 23). These tests also could be useful to distinguish benign lesions from a potentially malignant one or melanoma of unknown origin when traditional pathological and immunohistochemical methods do not provide definite answers (Chapter 12).

Several studies also identified BRAF and NRAS mutations as prognostic markers and association with worse outcome in patients with melanoma. BRAF mutations are more frequent in cutaneous superficial spreading melanomas (SSM) developing in areas of the body with intermittent sun exposure (50 % of tumors), while the rate of BRAF mutations is lower in acral, mucosal, and cutaneous melanomas with evidence of CSD, and they are essentially absent in uveal melanomas. Melanomas associated with CSD commonly have NRAS (15–20 %) and sometimes KIT (2 %) oncogenic mutations.

In vivo imaging of melanoma is also of great importance to improving therapy. Molecular probes targeting tumor specific biomarkers that are capable of greatly improved melanoma detection and accurate melanoma assessment are being developed, contributing to the improvement of personalized management of melanoma (Chapter 30).

Immune Response Markers

Immunotherapy with immunological drugs such as interferon alpha (IFN-α) 2b and interleukin (IL)-2 is characterized by response rates in the range 10–20 %, with approximately 5 % of the patients exhibiting long-term durable responses (Chapter 4). Alongside the recent success of molecularly based targeted drugs therapeutic blockade of immunologic checkpoints demonstrated better efficacy in inducing responses in melanoma patients than nonspecific immune activators. Anti CTLA-4 antibody ipilimumab showed improvement in clinical outcome in patients with metastatic melanoma compared with control therapy (Chapter 6). More recently inhibition of another checkpoint pathway using PD-1 specific antibody entered clinical trials in melanoma patients. As complete responses are achieved with this treatment in a subgroup of patients and it is associated with relatively high toxicity immune profiling as an approach to individualized treatment would greatly improve its clinical utility (Chapter 6).

Promising markers associated with response to ipilimumab were identified. Expression of FOXP3, ICOS^{hi} T cells and indoleamine 2, 3-dioxygenase (IDO) on tumor infiltrating T cells as well as high titers of anti- melanoma associated antigen NY-ESO-1 antibodies in blood, respectively, can predict response to ipilimumab. Tumor cells and stromal cells express PD-1 ligands (PD-L1 or B7-H1 and PD-L2 or B7-DC). The expression of PD-L1 correlates with response to treatment suggesting that it could be a critical component of successful therapy with anti PD-1 and it could serve as predictive marker for individualized treatment with this agent (Chapters 1 and 2). The prognostic significance of tumor infiltrating lymphocytes (TILs) in melanoma was in detail discussed in Chapter 16. More, recently combination of targeted therapy and immunotherapy as well as sequential treatment with different immunotherapy agents are tested (Chapter 7). Combination therapies might provide synergistic effect but there is a need to define an algorithm based on serological markers and tumor profiling to optimally sequence these treatment modalities. Given that treatment with individual agents is associated with toxicity identification of patients who will respond to combination therapy is of high importance. Considering limitations of the tests for individual markers, novel multiparametric system approaches could be best suited for the assessment of the complex system such as immunological function especially in combination treatment setting (Chapter 31).

The significance of the host genetic background needs to be considered as a critical factor for determining melanoma patient survival as well. Polymorphisms in immune response genes in melanoma, such as INFγ and certain chemokines and cytokines, are established prognostic factors and are closely associated with a melanoma outcome. Specific haplotypes of human leukocyte antigen (HLA) class I and II or costimulatory molecules such as B7-H can determine melanoma prognosis and treatment response (Chapters 18 and 19). Sequence analysis also suggests that specific haplotypes associated with the CTLA-4 gene predict effectiveness of anti CTLA-4 immunotherapy.

Another approach that is showing promising results in patients with metastatic melanoma is adoptive cell therapy with use of tumor infiltrating lymphocytes (TIL). In this approach T cell receptors (TCRs) directed against tumor antigens have been genetically engineered to recognize the specific epitope (e.g., NY-ESO-1). Chimeric antigen receptors (CARs) in which antibody-combining site has been genetically linked to TCR-signaling domain have also been used to target T cells to the tumor via recognition of the specific antigen. The efficacy of these multiple immunotherapy approaches critically depends on the presence in the tumor of the antigenic target for immunotherapy. Patient inclusion criteria in the specific treatment approach include tumor that expressed melanoma-specific antigens such as MAGE proteins, MART-1/MelanA, NY-ESO-1, gp100, HMB-45 and tyrosinase or the mutated form of the antigen. Protein-based approaches or genomic tools including RT-PCR or sequencing of the tumor tissue are used to determine the antigen expression or mutational signature of the tumor and to generate or identify specific TILs.

The advances in basic understanding of the immune system and the host–tumor interactions should ultimately lead to more effective and tailor-made immunotherapy. With promising new drugs modulating immune response such as ipilimumab or anti PD-1 and PD-L1 directed therapy, it is essential to further validate the existing markers and search for new diagnostics to identify patient populations that would benefit from these treatments.

Aims and Approach

The primary goal of this volume is to provide an overview of criteria and methods currently used to determine diagnosis, prognosis and predict the response to treatment of patients' with melanoma. Protocol-based chapters focusing on well-established assays that are currently used in clinical laboratories include a sufficient amount of technical detail so that the informed reader can understand the technology to establish the assay for clinical use. We discuss mutational testing as well as promising serologic markers with a potential to impact patient care via stratification of patients for targeted therapies and immunotherapy. Companion diagnostics have shown their clinical utility (e.g., BRAF and KIT) to determine therapeutic eligibility for the melanoma patients. Other markers show their utility to improve diagnosis and prognosis (e.g., CGH, Gene expression profiling, SNPs and MSI). Several assays to detect lymphatic invasion (Chapter 15), tumor infiltrating lymphocytes (Chapter 16) or quantitative measurements of marker expression using IHC-based approaches (Chapters 13, 14 and 32) that improve standard histopathology methods are discussed. Several novel markers with a potential to be included in standard testing are also described (Chapters 28 and 29). In addition, several chapters address novel technologies with the potential to improve mutation detection (Chapter 33) or identify novel approaches for marker detection (Chapters 26, 27, 31, 33, 34 and 35). Review chapters provide an overview of current strategies in clinical practice (Chapters 1–4) and challenges in clinical management of melanoma patients including the role of markers. The significance of these chapters is to provide background information and the context for the chapters describing specific assays for marker detection. Important issues of specimen collection and statistical design of marker study are addressed (Chapters 36 and 37).

We have tried to include examples of the established methods which represent the major technologies in the field with sufficient technical information and the extensive background information so the reader can both understand the technology and the context of the test. The target audiences are clinical laboratory-based investigators and laboratory scientists who are developers of application of the technologies but other target groups are the users including pathologists and oncologists. We hope that provided examples represent the state of the art in melanoma diagnostics and the review chapters enhance an understanding of the status and challenges in melanoma diagnostics and treatment. As such, hopefully this volume will lead to improvement of the melanoma diagnostic and overall management of patients with this disease.

Acknowledgements

We are truly indebted to our colleagues from Australia, Canada, Germany, Greece, Israel, Italy, Norway, Sweden and the United States of America for contributing chapters to this volume. We would like to thank John M. Jessup and Barbara A. Conley at the Cancer Diagnosis Program, NCI for support during this project. We also thank Kristina Thurin for editorial assistance.

Bethesda, MD, USA *Magdalena Thurin*
Doha, Qatar *Francesco M. Marincola*

Contents

Part III Biomarkers for Classification, Diagnosis, and Prognosis

Part IV Uveal Melanoma

Part V Emerging Markers/Targets in Melanoma

Part VI Emerging Technologies for Marker Validation

Contributors

EMILIA ANDERSSON • *Department of Oncology-Pathology, Karolinska Institute, Karolinska University Hospital, Stockholm, Sweden*

CRISTINA R. ANTONESCU • *Department of Pathology, Memorial Sloan-Kettering Cancer Center, New York, NY, USA*

PAOLO A. ASCIERTO • *Melanoma, Cancer Immunotherapy and Innovative Therapy, Istituto Nazionale Tumori Fondazione "G. Pascale", Naples, Italy*

MICHAEL B. ATKINS • *Georgetown-Lombardi Comprehensive Cancer Center, Washington, DC, USA*

BORIS C. BASTIAN • *Departments of Dermatology and Pathology, University of California San Francisco, San Francisco, CA, USA*

KIM R.M. BLENMAN • *Cancer Immunotherapeutics & Tumor Immunology, Beckman Research Institute, City of Hope Comprehensive Cancer Center, Duarte, CA, USA*

BRIAN A. BOONE • *Department of Surgery, Hillman Cancer Center, University of Pittsburgh Cancer Institute, Pittsburgh, PA, USA*

KENNETH M. BOUCHER • *Huntsman Cancer Institute, University of Utah, Salt Lake City, UT, USA*

MARY JO BUFFO • *University of Pittsburgh Cancer Institute, University of Pittsburgh School of Medicine, Pittsburgh, PA, USA*

LISA BUTTERFIELD • *University of Pittsburgh Cancer Institute, University of Pittsburgh School of Medicine, Pittsburgh, PA, USA*

TIFFANY L. CALDERONE • *Department of Surgical Oncology, The University of Texas MD Anderson Cancer Center, Houston, TX, USA*

RICHARD D. CARVAJAL • *Melanoma/Sarcoma Medical Oncology Service, Department of Medicine, Memorial Sloan-Kettering Cancer Center, New York, NY, USA*

PAMELA B. CASSIDY • *Department of Dermatology, Oregon Health & Science University, Portland, OR, USA*

ELENA CASTELLANOS-RIZALDOS • *Division of DNA Repair and Genome Stability, Department of Radiation Oncology, Dana-Farber Cancer Institute, Harvard Medical School, Boston, MA, USA*

ALESSANDRA CESANO • *Nodality, Inc., South San Francisco, CA, USA*

SANDRA CORAL • *Cancer Bioimmunotherapy Unit, Centro di Riferimento Oncologico, Istituto di Ricovero e Cura a Carattere Scientifico, Aviano, Italy*

JONATHAN L. CURRY • *Department of Pathology, The University of Texas MD Anderson Cancer Center, Houston, TX, USA*

DIWAKAR DAVAR • *Department of Medicine, University of Pittsburgh Medical Center, Pittsburgh, PA, USA*

MICHAEL A. DAVIES • *Department of Melanoma Medical Oncology, The University of Texas MD Anderson Cancer Center, Houston, TX, USA*

KEVIN K. DOBBIN • *Department of Epidemiology and Biostatistics, College of Public Health, University of Georgia, Athens, GA, USA*
DAVID E. ELDER • *Department of Pathology and Laboratory Medicine, Hospital of the University of Pennsylvania, Philadelphia, PA, USA*
KATHRYN G. EWENS • *Department of Genetics, Perelman School of Medicine, University of Pennsylvania, Philadelphia, PA, USA*
SOLDANO FERRONE • *Department of Surgery and Orthopaedic Surgery, Massachusetts General Hospital, Harvard Medical School, Boston, MA, USA*
DAVID E. FISHER • *Department of Dermatology, Massachusetts General Hospital, Boston, MA, USA*
ELISABETTA FRATTA • *Cancer Bioimmunotherapy Unit, Centro di Riferimento Oncologico, Istituto di Ricovero e Cura a Carattere Scientifico, Aviano, Italy*
ARUPA GANGULY • *Department of Genetics, Perelman School of Medicine, University of Pennsylvania, Philadelphia, PA, USA*
JEFFREY E. GERSHENWALD • *Department of Surgical Oncology, The University of Texas MD Anderson Cancer Center, Houston, TX, USA*
GEOFFREY GIBNEY • *Department of Cutaneous Oncology, Moffitt Cancer Center, Tampa, FL, USA*
PHYLLIS A. GIMOTTY • *Department of Biostatistics and Epidemiology, University of Pennsylvania School of Medicine, Philadelphia, PA, USA*
HELEN GOGAS • *First Department of Medicine, University of Athens Medical School, Athens, Greece*
BONNIE E. GOULD ROTHBERG • *Department of Internal Medicine, Yale Cancer Center, New Haven, CT, USA; Department of Epidemiology and Public Health, Yale Cancer Center, New Haven, CT, USA*
ANTONIO M. GRIMALDI • *Unit of Melanoma, Cancer Immunotherapy and Innovative Therapy, Istituto Nazionale Tumori Fondazione "G. Pascale", Naples, Italy*
HANS E. GROSSNIKLAUS • *Emory University School of Medicine, Atlanta, GA, USA*
DUPONT GUERRY • *Department of Medicine, University of Pennsylvania School of Medicine, Philadelphia, PA, USA*
MINAKSHI GUHA • *Divisions of DNA Repair and Genome Stability and Medical Physics and Biophysics, Department of Radiation Oncology, Dana-Farber Cancer Institute, Harvard Medical School, Boston, MA, USA*
OMID HAMID • *The Angeles Clinic and Research Institute, Los Angeles, CA, USA*
J. WILIAM HARBOUR • *Bascom Palmer Eye Institute, Sylvester Comprehensive Cancer Center, University of Miami Miller School of Medicine, Miami, FL, USA*
KEISUKE HATA • *Department of Molecular Oncology, John Wayne Cancer Institute at Saint John's Health Center, Santa Monica, CA, USA*
JASON E. HAWKES • *Department of Dermatology, University of Utah, Salt Lake City, UT, USA*
MEENHARD HERLYN • *Wistar Institute, Philadelphia, PA, USA*
DAVE S.B. HOON • *Department of Molecular Oncology, John Wayne Cancer Institute at Saint John's Health Center, Santa Monica, CA, USA*
ANDREI H. IAGARU • *Radiology-Nuclear Medicine, Stanford University Medical Center, Stanford, CA, USA*
M. JACOBS GABREE • *Massachusetts General Hospital, Center for Cancer Risk Assessment, Boston, MA, USA*

Giorgos Karakousis • *Department of Surgery, University of Pennsylvania School of Medicine, Philadelphia, PA, USA*
Mohammed Kashani-Sabet • *Center for Melanoma Research and Treatment, California Pacific Medical Center Research Institute, San Francisco, CA, USA*
Khun Visith Keu • *Département de Radiobiologie et de Médecine Nucléaire, Université de Sherbrooke, Sherbrooke, Québec, Canada*
Keith J. Killian • *Clinical Genetics Branch, Center for Cancer Research, NCI, NIH, Bethesda, MD, USA*
John M. Kirkwood • *Division of Hematology-Oncology, Department of Medicine, University of Pittsburgh Medical Center, Pittsburgh, PA, USA*
Shigehisa Kitano • *Department of Medicine, Memorial Sloan-Kettering Cancer Center, New York, NY, USA*
Eiji Kiyohara • *Department of Molecular Oncology, John Wayne Cancer Institute at Saint John's Health Center, Santa Monica, CA, USA*
Levy Kopelovich • *Division of Cancer Prevention, National Cancer Institute, Rockville, MD, USA*
Ragini Kudchadkar • *Department of Cutaneous Oncology, Moffitt Cancer Center, Tampa, FL, USA*
Stella Lam • *Department of Molecular Oncology, John Wayne Cancer Institute at Saint John's Health Center, Santa Monica, CA, USA*
Christopher Lau • *Clinical Genetics Branch, Center for Cancer Research, NCI, NIH, Bethesda, MD, USA*
Sancy A. Leachman • *Department of Dermatology, Oregon Health & Science University, Portland, OR, USA*
Peter P. Lee • *Cancer Immunotherapeutics & Tumor Immunology, Beckman Research Institute, City of Hope Comprehensive Cancer Center, Duarte, CA, USA*
Alexander M. Lesokhin • *Department of Medicine, Memorial Sloan-Kettering Cancer Center, New York, NY, USA*
Danielle Levine • *Department of Dermatology, Massachusetts General Hospital, Boston, MA, USA*
Roger S. Lo • *Department of Medicine, Jonsson Comprehensive Cancer Center, David Geffen School of Medicine, University of California, Los Angeles, CA, USA*
Michael T. Lotze • *Department of Surgery, Hillman Cancer Center, University of Pittsburgh Cancer Institute, Pittsburgh, PA, USA*
Michele Maio • *Division of Medical Oncology and Immunotherapy, Department of Oncology, Istituto Toscano Tumori, University Hospital of Siena, Siena, Italy*
G. Mike Makrigiorgos • *Department of Radiation Oncology, Dana-Farber Cancer Institute, Harvard Medical School, Boston, MA, USA*
Maddalena Marchesi • *Department of Oncology-Pathology, Karolinska Institute, Karolinska University Hospital, Stockholm, Sweden*
Francesco M. Marincola • *Sidra Medical and Research Center, Qatar Foundation, Doha, Qatar*
Alexander Marzuka-Alcalá • *Yale School of Medicine, New Haven, CT, USA*
Giuseppe V. Masucci • *Department of Oncology-Pathology, Karolinska Institute, Karolinska University Hospital, Stockholm, Sweden*
James W. Mier • *Beth Israel Deaconess Medical Center, Boston, MA, USA*
Martin C. Mihm Jr. • *Department of Dermatology, Brigham and Women's Hospital, Harvard Medical School, Boston, MA, USA*

COREN A. MILBURY • *Department of Radiation Oncology, Dana-Farber Cancer Institute, Harvard Medical School, Boston, MA, USA*
KATHERINE NATHANSON • *Department of Medicine, Perelman School of Medicine, University of Pennsylvania, Philadelphia, PA, USA*
JEFFREY P. NORTH • *Department of Dermatology, University of California San Francisco, San Francisco, CA, USA; Department of Pathology, University of California San Francisco, San Francisco, CA, USA*
MEHDI NOSRATI • *Center for Melanoma Research and Treatment, California Pacific Medical Center Research Institute, San Francisco, CA, USA*
DAVID J. PANKA • *Beth Israel Deaconess Medical Center, Boston, MA, USA*
GIULIA PARISI • *Division of Medical Oncology and Immunotherapy, Department of Oncology, University Hospital of Siena, Istituto Toscano Tumori, Siena, Italy*
LAWRENCE M. PFEFFER • *Department of Pathology, University of Tennessee Health Science Center, Memphis, TN, USA*
SUSAN R. PFEFFER • *Department of Pathology, University of Tennessee Health Science Center, Memphis, TN, USA*
MICHAEL A. POSTOW • *Department of Medicine, Memorial Sloan-Kettering Cancer Center, New York, NY, USA*
VICTOR G. PRIETO • *Department of Pathology, The University of Texas MD Anderson Cancer Center, Houston, TX, USA*
JOHN F. QUACKENBUSH • *Huntsman Cancer Institute, University of Utah, Salt Lake City, UT, USA*
ALIA B. RASHID • *David G. Cogan Ophthalmic Pathology Laboratory, Massachusetts Eye and Ear Infirmary, Harvard Medical School, Boston, MA, USA*
ANTONI RIBAS • *Division of Hematology-Oncology, Department of Medicine, Jonsson Comprehensive Cancer Center, University of California, Los Angeles, CA, USA*
JENNIFER RICHARDS-YUTZ • *Department of Genetics, Perelman School of Medicine, University of Pennsylvania, Philadelphia, PA, USA*
DAVID L. RIMM • *Department of Pathology, Yale School of MedicineNew Haven, CT, USA*
UDO RUDLOFF • *Surgery Branch, Center for Cancer Research, NCI, NIH, Bethesda, MD, USA*
FRANCESCO SABBATINO • *Department of Surgery, Massachusetts General Hospital, Harvard Medical School, Boston, MA, USA*
YARDENA SAMUELS • *Department of Molecular Cell Biology, Weizmann Institute of Science, Rehovot, Israel*
TOBIAS SCHATTON • *Department of Dermatology, Brigham and Women's Hospital and Transplantation Research Center, Children's Hospital Boston, Harvard Medical School, Boston, MA, USA*
RICHARD A. SCOLYER • *Royal Prince Alfred Hospital, Melanoma Institute Australia and Sydney Medical School, The University of Sydney, Sydney, NSW, Australia*
BARBARA SELIGER • *Institute of Medical Immunology, Martin Luther University Halle-Wittenberg, Halle, Germany*
HUBING SHI • *Department of Medicine, Jonsson Comprehensive Cancer Center, David Geffen School of Medicine, University of California, Los Angeles, CA, USA*
LUCA SIGALOTTI • *Cancer Bioimmunotherapy Unit, Centro di Riferimento Oncologico, Istituto di Ricovero e Cura a Carattere Scientifico, Aviano, Italy*
ESTER SIMEONE • *Unit of Melanoma, Cancer Immunotherapy and Innovative Therapy, Istituto Nazionale Tumori Fondazione "G. Pascale", Naples, Italy*

Ana Slipicevic • *The Wistar Institute, Philadelphia, PA, USA; Department of Pathology, The Norwegian Radium Hospital, Oslo University Hospital, Oslo, Norway*
Rajasekharan Somasundaram • *The Wistar Institute, Philadelphia, PA, USA*
Vernon K. Sondak • *Department of Cutaneous Oncology, Moffitt Cancer Center, Tampa, FL, USA*
David Spellmeyer • *Nodality, Inc., South San Francisco, CA, USA*
Katrin Sproesser • *The Wistar Institute, Philadelphia, PA, USA*
Ryan J. Sullivan • *Center for Melanoma, Massachusetts General Hospital Cancer Center, Boston, MA, USA*
Ahmad A. Tarhini • *Division of Hematology-Oncology, Department of Medicine, University of Pittsburgh Medical Center, Pittsburgh, PA, USA*
John F. Thompson • *Royal Prince Alfred Hospital, Melanoma Institute Australia and Sydney Medical School, The University of Sydney, Sydney, NSW, Australia*
Magdalena Thurin • *Cancer Diagnosis Program, National Cancer Institute, National Institutes of Health, Bethesda, MD, USA*
Hensin Tsao • *Department of Dermatology and Massachusetts General Hospital Cancer Center, Massachusetts General Hospital, Boston, MA, USA*
Swapna S. Vemula • *Departments of Dermatology and Pathology, University of California San Francisco, San Francisco, CA, USA*
John A. Viator • *Department of Biological Engineering, University of Missouri-Columbia, Columbia, MO, USA*
Lisa Villabona • *Department of Oncology-Pathology, Karolinska Institute, Karolinska University Hospital, Stockholm, Sweden*
Xinhui Wang • *Department of Surgery, Massachusetts General Hospital, Harvard Medical School, Boston, MA, USA*
Yangyang Wang • *Department of Surgery, Massachusetts General Hospital, Harvard Medical School, Boston, MA, USA*
Ryan M. Weight • *Drexel University College of Medicine, Hahnemann University Hospital, Philadelphia, PA, USA*
Jedd D. Wolchok • *Department of Medicine, Memorial Sloan-Kettering Cancer Center, New York, NY, USA*
Xiaowei Xu • *Department of Pathology and Laboratory Medicine, Hospital of University of Pennsylvania, Philadelphia, PA, USA*
Jianda Yuan • *Department of Medicine, Memorial Sloan-Kettering Cancer Center, New York, NY, USA*

Part I

Clinical Challenges and Current Status of Treatment of Melanoma

Chapter 1

Novel Insights/Translational Implication from the Emerging Biology of Melanoma

Antoni Ribas

Abstract

Melanoma is a main example of how applying advances in basic biology, pharmacology, and molecular diagnostics into the clinic results in unprecedented benefits to patients. After many years of lack of advances in the treatment of patients with metastatic melanoma, the advent of new therapies that block driver oncogenic signaling and modulate immune responses to cancer provided the first studies with a positive impact in overall survival (OS) of patients with advanced melanoma. The pace of progress in the treatment of this disease has been greatly accelerated by these initial breakthroughs, and it continues with new generation agents and combinatorial approaches.

Key words BRAF, CTLA4, PD-1, Immunotherapy, Targeted therapy

1 Introduction

In a short period of time melanoma has become a poster child of how science can be translated into better patient care. This is a big change in this disease where treatment for advanced disease had shown very little progress since the advent of modern oncology. In fact, until 2010 there had never been a therapy that had demonstrated improvement in overall survival in patients with metastatic melanoma. The lack of insight into the biology of this cancer and how it interacts with the host had precluded advances in treatments. Nonspecific genotoxins like chemotherapy and radiotherapy had provided marginal benefits, with occasional patients having tumor responses without an ability to understand what guided response or resistance. Melanoma has a remarkable ability to correct DNA damage by chemotherapy, which is likely endowed from its cell of origin, the melanocyte, which is a pigmented skin cell designed by Nature to withstand DNA damage from ultraviolet light and protect the surrounding skin cells. Furthermore, a series of immunotherapy strategies had repeatedly provided evidence of

Magdalena Thurin and Francesco M. Marincola (eds.), *Molecular Diagnostics for Melanoma: Methods and Protocols*, Methods in Molecular Biology, vol. 1102, DOI 10.1007/978-1-62703-727-3_1, © Springer Science+Business Media New York 2014

benefit in occasional patients, with a very low frequency of responses that were highly relevant for those patients with benefit since these tended to be very durable, many times lasting years. However, these immunotherapies were far from desirable since multiple active vaccination approaches had proven to have very low immunological potency, and nonspecific immune stimulating such as the cytokines interleukin-2 (IL-2) or interferon-alpha (IFN-α) had to be administered at the highest (barely tolerated) doses to result in a low frequency of clinical benefit.

The big clinical improvements provided by the recently widely available therapies for advanced melanoma are based on a refined understanding of oncogenic signaling pathways in cancer cells and how immune responses to cancer are regulated. Therapies based on inhibiting mutated BRAF signaling and blocking negative immune checkpoint regulatory proteins have provided the first clinical trials demonstrating improvements in overall survival in patients with metastatic melanoma.

2 Targeted Therapies Blocking Melanoma Driver Oncogenic Signaling

Insights into the genetic alterations in melanoma allowed understanding what gives this cancer the oncogenic signals to proliferate. Over 70 % of skin and mucosal melanomas have activating mutations in the receptor tyrosine kinase (RTK) KIT, or the oncogenic proteins NRAS or BRAF [1, 2]. These are generally mutually exclusive mutations that all result in constitutive oncogenic signaling through the mitogen-activated protein kinase (MAPK) pathway governing cell proliferation and avoidance of apoptosis [1, 3]. The great majority of uveal melanomas have a distinct set of driver oncogenic mutations in *GNAQ* and *GNA11* [4, 5]. Together with the near universal alterations in cell cycle control, they provide the key oncogenic events to transform normal melanocytes into cancer cells [3]. These mutations are not randomly distributed among melanomas. As noted for the distinct mutations in uveal melanoma, different melanoma subtypes likely with different pathogenic events have a different set of driver oncogenic mutations: *KIT* mutations are more common in mucosal, acral, and lentiginous melanomas, *NRAS* mutations are more common in cutaneous melanomas in older adults, and *BRAF* mutations are more common in melanomas arising from intermittently sun exposed skin in younger adults [1, 6, 7]. The biological significance of the affected proteins and signaling pathways, their mutual exclusivity in the great majority of cases and their nonrandom distribution in distinct clinicopathological subtypes of melanoma provide clues to their importance and potential for therapeutic targeting.

The greatest therapeutic advance has been achieved in patients with mutations in *BRAFV600*, which is present in approximately

50 % of patients with metastatic melanoma. Small molecule inhibitors that displace ATP in the mutated *BRAFV600* threonine-serine kinase have been developed and demonstrated to have unprecedently high response rates [8]. Clinical studies with the type I (which bind to the activation state of the kinase) RAF kinase inhibitors vemurafenib (formerly PLX4032) and dabrafenib (formerly GSK2118436) demonstrated objective tumor responses in excess of 50 % of patients by strict RECIST criteria, with up to 85 % of patients having some kind of tumor response and a very low frequency of innate resistance [9–13]. These two BRAF inhibitors have demonstrated improvement in progression free survival (PFS) against the old standard chemotherapy agent dacarbazine [10, 13], while vemurafenib has also demonstrated improvident in overall survival (OS) in a randomized clinical trial [10].

The high specificity of these agents for the mutated BRAF kinase allows a wide therapeutic window, with most toxicities being manageable with dose adjustments or interruptions. The most common grade 3 or 4 toxicity with these agents is the development of cutaneous squamous cell carcinomas (cuSCC), most of them of keratoacanthoma (KA) subtype. These toxicities are usually easily managed by simple surgical excision and do not preclude continued therapy. The pathobiology of their appearance has been elucidated through the phenomenon of paradoxical MAPK activation [14, 15], where cells with preexisting upstream mutations, most frequently in *HRAS* and *KRAS*, are transactivated to proliferate through MAPK signaling [16, 17]. Despite the initial tumor responses and early benefit in PFS and OS, the majority of patients demonstrate disease progression frequently within months. The mechanisms how *BRAFV600* mutant metastatic melanoma develops acquired resistance to BRAF inhibitors are different from the prevalent gatekeeper mutations with other ATP-competitive small molecule targeted inhibitor therapies for cancer. In fact, melanomas seem to develop a wide array of mechanisms to overcome BRAF inhibition. These mechanisms either reactivate the MAPK pathway through secondary *NRAS* mutations, *BRAF* amplification, BRAF truncation, or MEK mutations, or provide alternative survival signaling by activating RTKs and downstream signaling through the PI3K/AKT pathway [18–26].

Furthermore, inhibiting MAPK signaling immediately downstream of mutated *BRAF* can be achieved with MEK inhibitors, which preclinical studies had shown to have preferential activity in the setting of the *BRAFV600*^{0} mutations [27]. In patients who had not previously received BRAF inhibitor-based therapy, a randomized clinical trial demonstrated that the MEK inhibitor trametinib (GSK1120211) improved both PFS and OS over dacarbazine [28], providing another active agent for these patients. However, the antitumor activity is lower and the toxicities are higher with single agent MEK inhibitors compared to single agent BRAF inhibitors.

The rapid phase of development of targeted treatments for BRAF mutant metastatic melanoma has resulted in the testing of combined therapy with BRAF and MEK inhibitors. This combination has the theoretical ability to provide improved initial antitumor activity resultant from double inhibition of oncogenic signaling through the MAPK pathway [29], as well and providing longer duration of responses by preventing or treating acquired resistance [30]. At the same time, the combination of BRAF and MEK inhibitors has the potential to also decrease toxicities resultant from paradoxical MAPK activation, since the MEK inhibitor would block the BRAF inhibitor-induced MAPK activation in cells that are wild type for BRAF and have strong upstream signaling [16]. Early clinical testing of this combined therapy is highly encouraging [31], and formal testing of improvements in PFS and OS over single agent BRAF inhibitor therapy is ongoing.

3 Immune Modulation Overcoming Negative Regulatory Pathways

Therapies that attempt to activate a cytotoxic T lymphocyte (CTL) immune response against chronically expressed self-antigens, as are most tumor antigens, are negatively regulated by T cell-intrinsic negative costimulatory signaling known as immune checkpoints [32]. The recent advances in immunotherapy for melanoma have been based on the clinical application of antibodies blocking these immune checkpoints, in particular the cytotoxic T lymphocyte-associated antigen-4 (CTLA-4) and the programmed death receptor 1 (PD-1) [33]. These two negative immune regulatory receptors have very different biological roles, which may allow understanding their effects in the clinic [33, 34]. CTLA-4 is a negative costimulatory receptor that competes with CD28 for costimulatory signaling through CD80/CD86 upon T cell activation. The blockade of CTLA-4 releases negative regulation upon T cell activation in secondary lymphoid organs, and these T cells then need to circulate through the periphery and recognize cells expressing their cognate targets. Therefore, CTLA-4 blockade is relatively nonspecific for antitumor T cells and its clinical effects are likely to be delayed. On the contrary, PD-1 is expressed by chronically antigen-exposed T cells and it is engaged primarily in peripheral tissues upon recognition of the PD ligand 1 (PD-L1), which is an activation-induced ligand expressed in inflamed tissues and cancers. Therefore, PD-1 inhibits the final effector mechanism of CTLs that have already recognized antigen and have been negatively regulated by PD-L1 in the periphery. This predicts a more specific activation of T cells to cancer and chronic infections, while it should also provide more rapid antitumor activity.

These preclinical predictions correlate well with the clinical effects of CTLA-4 and PD-1/PD-L1 blocking antibodies. Two CTLA-4 blocking antibodies have been extensively tested in the clinic, ipilimumab (formerly MDX010) and tremelimumab (formerly CP-675,206) [35]. They both provided a low but reproducible level of antitumor activity in patients with metastatic melanoma, with the main feature of providing very long duration of tumor responses in roughly 10 % of treated patients, with responses lasting years [36–39]. Ipilimumab has been demonstrated to improve OS in two randomized clinical trials, one against a gp100 peptide vaccine and another in combination with dacarbazine against single agent dacarbazine [40, 41], leading to its regulatory approval in several countries. Tremelimumab was tested in a randomized clinical trial against dacarbazine or temozolomide but failed to demonstrate a statistically significant improvement in OS, with the major reason being a relatively high rate of use of ipilimumab in patients in the control chemotherapy arm [42]. These two agents are limited by their low frequency of tumor responses, their delayed tumor responses, and their frequency of 15–20 % of serious inflammatory and autoimmune toxicities, in particular colitis and endocrinopathies.

Early clinical testing of PD-1 and PD-L1 blocking antibodies suggests that they may have higher antitumor activity, more rapid tumor responses, and a lower frequency of toxicities. There are several PD-1 axis inhibitors in current clinical testing, with the most advanced programs using the anti-PD-1 nivolumab (formerly MDX1106) and the anti-PD-L1 MDX1105 [33]. Both of these agents have provided evidence of objective tumor responses in 20–30 % of patients with metastatic melanoma in phase 1 testing, with the majority being durable responses [43–45]. These encouraging results are being pursued in larger series and randomized clinical trials. Furthermore, the ability to detect PD-L1 in tumors may allow selecting patients whose immune response to melanoma is being blocked through the PD-1/PD-L1 interaction, with the potential for enriching for patients who are more likely to respond to these antibodies.

4 Conclusions

The rapid advancement of new therapies active in patients with metastatic melanoma has been achieved thanks to the clinical translation of preclinical scientific knowledge. These advances are in sharp contrast with the lack of significant progress when attempting to treat melanoma with nonspecific agents, in particular chemotherapy. The ability to understand mechanisms of response and resistance to BRAF inhibitor-based therapies and immune checkpoint blockade at a molecular level, and the rapid advancement of the knowledge brought through by the scientific community's renewed interest in melanoma, predicts that the pace of improvements in further developing effective therapies for this disease will continue in the near future.

References

1. Curtin JA, Fridlyand J, Kageshita T, Patel HN, Busam KJ, Kutzner H et al (2005) Distinct sets of genetic alterations in melanoma. N Engl J Med 353:2135–2147
2. Curtin JA, Busam K, Pinkel D, Bastian BC (2006) Somatic activation of KIT in distinct subtypes of melanoma. J Clin Oncol 24:4340–4346
3. Gray-Schopfer V, Wellbrock C, Marais R (2007) Melanoma biology and new targeted therapy. Nature 445:851–857
4. Van Raamsdonk CD, Bezrookove V, Green G, Bauer J, Gaugler L, O'Brien JM et al (2009) Frequent somatic mutations of GNAQ in uveal melanoma and blue naevi. Nature 457: 599–602
5. Van Raamsdonk CD, Griewank KG, Crosby MB, Garrido MC, Vemula S, Wiesner T et al (2010) Mutations in GNA11 in uveal melanoma. N Engl J Med 363:2191–2199
6. Viros A, Fridlyand J, Bauer J, Lasithiotakis K, Garbe C, Pinkel D et al (2008) Improving melanoma classification by integrating genetic and morphologic features. PLoS Med 5:e120
7. Long GV, Menzies AM, Nagrial AM, Haydu LE, Hamilton AL, Mann GJ et al (2011) Prognostic and clinicopathologic associations of oncogenic BRAF in metastatic melanoma. J Clin Oncol 29:1239–1246
8. Ribas A, Flaherty KT (2011) BRAF targeted therapy changes the treatment paradigm in melanoma. Nat Rev Clin Oncol 8:426–433
9. Flaherty KT, Puzanov I, Kim KB, Ribas A, McArthur GA, Sosman JA et al (2010) Inhibition of mutated, activated BRAF in metastatic melanoma. N Engl J Med 363: 809–819
10. Chapman PB, Hauschild A, Robert C, Haanen JB, Ascierto P, Larkin J et al (2011) Improved survival with vemurafenib in melanoma with BRAF V600E mutation. N Engl J Med 364:2507–2516
11. Sosman JA, Kim KB, Schuchter L, Gonzalez R, Pavlick AC, Weber JS et al (2012) Survival in BRAF V600-mutant advanced melanoma treated with vemurafenib. N Engl J Med 366:707–714
12. Falchook GS, Long GV, Kurzrock R, Kim KB, Arkenau TH, Brown MP et al (2012) Dabrafenib in patients with melanoma, untreated brain metastases, and other solid tumours: a phase 1 dose-escalation trial. Lancet 379:1893–1901
13. Hauschild A, Grob JJ, Demidov LV, Jouary T, Gutzmer R, Millward M et al (2012) Dabrafenib in BRAF-mutated metastatic melanoma: a multicentre, open-label, phase 3 randomised controlled trial. Lancet 380:358–365
14. Heidorn SJ, Milagre C, Whittaker S, Nourry A, Niculescu-Duvas I, Dhomen N et al (2010) Kinase-dead BRAF and oncogenic RAS cooperate to drive tumor progression through CRAF. Cell 140:209–221
15. Poulikakos PI, Zhang C, Bollag G, Shokat KM, Rosen N (2010) RAF inhibitors transactivate RAF dimers and ERK signalling in cells with wild-type BRAF. Nature 464:427–430
16. Su F, Viros A, Milagre C, Trunzer K, Bollag G, Spleiss O et al (2012) RAS mutations in cutaneous squamous-cell carcinomas in patients treated with BRAF inhibitors. N Engl J Med 366:207–215
17. Oberholzer PA, Kee D, Dziunycz P, Sucker A, Kamsukom N, Jones R et al (2012) RAS mutations are associated with the development of cutaneous squamous cell tumors in patients treated with RAF inhibitors. J Clin Oncol 30:316–321
18. Nazarian R, Shi H, Wang Q, Kong X, Koya RC, Lee H et al (2010) Melanomas acquire resistance to B-RAF(V600E) inhibition by RTK or N-RAS upregulation. Nature 468: 973–977
19. Poulikakos PI, Persaud Y, Janakiraman M, Kong X, Ng C, Moriceau G et al (2011) RAF inhibitor resistance is mediated by dimerization of aberrantly spliced BRAF(V600E). Nature 480:387–390
20. Shi H, Moriceau G, Kong X, Koya RC, Nazarian R, Pupo G et al (2012) Sensitivity of B-RAF/MEK1 double-mutant melanomas to B-RAF inhibitors. Cancer Discov 2(5): 414–424
21. Shi H, Moriceau G, Kong X, Lee MK, Lee H, Koya RC et al (2012) Melanoma whole-exome sequencing identifies (V600E)B-RAF amplification-mediated acquired B-RAF inhibitor resistance. Nat Commun 3:724

22. Straussman R, Morikawa T, Shee K, Barzily-Rokni M, Qian ZR, Du J et al (2012) Tumour micro-environment elicits innate resistance to RAF inhibitors through HGF secretion. Nature 487:500–504
23. Wilson TR, Fridlyand J, Yan Y, Penuel E, Burton L, Chan E et al (2012) Widespread potential for growth-factor-driven resistance to anticancer kinase inhibitors. Nature 487:505–509
24. Villanueva J, Vultur A, Lee JT, Somasundaram R, Fukunaga-Kalabis M, Cipolla AK et al (2010) Acquired resistance to BRAF inhibitors mediated by a RAF kinase switch in melanoma can be overcome by cotargeting MEK and IGF-1R/PI3K. Cancer Cell 18:683–695
25. Johannessen CM, Boehm JS, Kim SY, Thomas SR, Wardwell L, Johnson LA et al (2010) COT drives resistance to RAF inhibition through MAP kinase pathway reactivation. Nature 468:968–972
26. Wagle N, Emery C, Berger MF, Davis MJ, Sawyer A, Pochanard P et al (2011) Dissecting therapeutic resistance to RAF inhibition in melanoma by tumor genomic profiling. J Clin Oncol 29(22):3085–3096
27. Solit DB, Garraway LA, Pratilas CA, Sawai A, Getz G, Basso A et al (2006) BRAF mutation predicts sensitivity to MEK inhibition. Nature 439:358–362
28. Flaherty KT, Robert C, Hersey P, Nathan P, Garbe C, Milhem M et al (2012) Improved survival with MEK inhibition in BRAF-mutated melanoma. N Engl J Med 367:107–114
29. Smalley KS, Flaherty KT (2009) Integrating BRAF/MEK inhibitors into combination therapy for melanoma. Br J Cancer 100:431–435
30. Lo RS (2012) Combinatorial therapies to overcome B-RAF inhibitor resistance in melanomas. Pharmacogenomics 13:125–128
31. Flaherty KT, Infante JR, Daud A, Gonzalez R, Kefford RF, Sosman J et al (2012) Combined BRAF and MEK inhibition in melanoma with BRAF V600 mutations. N Engl J Med 367:1694–1703
32. Korman AJ, Peggs KS, Allison JP (2006) Checkpoint blockade in cancer immunotherapy. Adv Immunol 90:297–339
33. Pardoll DM (2012) The blockade of immune checkpoints in cancer immunotherapy. Nat Rev Cancer 12:252–264
34. Ribas A (2012) Tumor immunotherapy directed at PD-1. N Engl J Med 366(26): 2517–2519
35. Agarwala SS, Ribas A (2010) Current experience with CTLA4-blocking monoclonal antibodies for the treatment of solid tumors. J Immunother 33:557–569
36. Ribas A, Camacho LH, Lopez-Berestein G, Pavlov D, Bulanhagui CA, Millham R et al (2005) Antitumor activity in melanoma and anti-self responses in a phase I trial with the anti-cytotoxic T lymphocyte-associated antigen 4 monoclonal antibody CP-675,206. J Clin Oncol 23:8968–8977
37. Hodi FS, Mihm MC, Soiffer RJ, Haluska FG, Butler M, Seiden MV et al (2003) Biologic activity of cytotoxic T lymphocyte-associated antigen 4 antibody blockade in previously vaccinated metastatic melanoma and ovarian carcinoma patients. Proc Natl Acad Sci USA 100:4712–4717
38. O'Day SJ, Maio M, Chiarion-Sileni V, Gajewski TF, Pehamberger H, Bondarenko IN et al (2010) Efficacy and safety of ipilimumab monotherapy in patients with pretreated advanced melanoma: a multicenter single-arm phase II study. Ann Oncol 21:1712–1717
39. Camacho LH, Antonia S, Sosman J, Kirkwood JM, Gajewski TF, Redman B et al (2009) Phase I/II trial of tremelimumab in patients with metastatic melanoma. J Clin Oncol 27: 1075–1081
40. Hodi FS, O'Day SJ, McDermott DF, Weber RW, Sosman JA, Haanen JB et al (2010) Improved survival with ipilimumab in patients with metastatic melanoma. N Engl J Med 363:711–723
41. Robert C, Thomas L, Bondarenko I, O'Day S, M DJ, Garbe C et al (2011) Ipilimumab plus dacarbazine for previously untreated metastatic melanoma. N Engl J Med 364:2517–2526
42. Ribas A, Kefford R, Marshall MA, Punt CJA, Haanen JB, Marmol M et al (2013) A phase III randomized clinical trial comparing tremelimumab with standard-of-care chemotherapy in patients with advanced melanoma. J Clin Oncol 31(5):616–622
43. Brahmer JR, Drake CG, Wollner I, Powderly JD, Picus J, Sharfman WH et al (2010) Phase I study of single-agent anti-programmed death-1 (MDX-1106) in refractory solid tumors: safety, clinical activity, pharmacodynamics, and immunologic correlates. J Clin Oncol 28: 3167–3175
44. Brahmer JR, Tykodi SS, Chow LQ, Hwu WJ, Topalian SL, Hwu P et al (2012) Safety and activity of anti-PD-L1 antibody in patients with advanced cancer. N Engl J Med 366: 2455–2465
45. Topalian SL, Hodi FS, Brahmer JR, Gettinger SN, Smith DC, McDermott DF et al (2012) Safety, activity, and immune correlates of anti-PD-1 antibody in cancer. N Engl J Med 366:2443–2454

Chapter 2

Emerging Clinical Issues in Melanoma in the Molecularly Targeted Era

Ryan J. Sullivan and Michael B. Atkins

Abstract

The standard of care of patients with malignant melanoma is dramatically changing, hallmarked by the approval of three new agents for the treatment of malignant melanoma in 2011. In this changing therapeutic landscape, several clinical issues are emerging which will best be addressed through the application of advances in molecular analytics, diagnostics, and therapeutics. It is expected that dedicated and coordinated efforts in basic, translational, and clinical will be responsible for the next major breakthroughs in the care of patients with this dreaded disease. In this chapter, five critical, emerging clinical issues are presented with descriptions of approaches that might be expected to help solve these challenges to optimal patient care.

Key words BRAF, NRAS, Predictive biomarkers, Patient selection, Treatment sequencing

1 Introduction

With the FDA approval of pegylated interferon alpha, ipilimumab, and vemurafenib in 2011, the number of standard of care options for patients with high risk and metastatic melanoma functionally doubled. In fact, the number of agents approved in 2011 equaled the total number of agents approved for this disease over the previous 35 years (Fig. 1). Despite this progress, it is important to note that melanoma is the fifth and sixth leading cause of cancer in men and women, respectively, and is second in terms of potential life years lost [1]. It was estimated that over 76,000 Americans will be diagnosed with and over 9,000 will die of melanoma in 2013. The incidence of melanoma has increased steadily over the past 40 years and the mortality rates continue to increase most notably in patients over the age of 55. These numbers are sobering and highlight the need for continued progress in order build upon recent successes and continue to improve treatment outcomes for patients with high risk and advanced melanoma. Five clinical issues that merit further focus and attention by the melanoma research community are the following:

Magdalena Thurin and Francesco M. Marincola (eds.), *Molecular Diagnostics for Melanoma: Methods and Protocols*, Methods in Molecular Biology, vol. 1102, DOI 10.1007/978-1-62703-727-3_2, © Springer Science+Business Media New York 2014

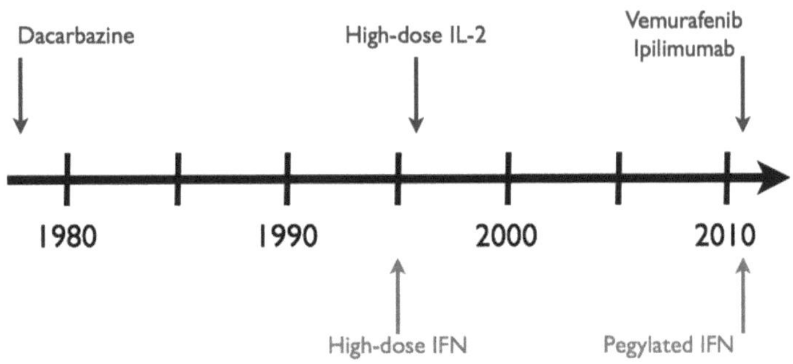

Fig. 1 Melanoma therapy FDA-approval timeline

1. Improving adjuvant therapy
2. Enhanced patient selection for immunotherapy
3. Identifying the ideal sequence of systemic therapy for advanced disease
4. Improving the efficacy of BRAF inhibitor-based therapy
5. Developing "targeted" therapies for hard-to-target subgroups

2 Improving Adjuvant Therapy

The standard of care for patients with intermediate to high-risk melanoma (Stage II and III) has been a topic of great debate in the oncology community for decades [2]. Currently, there are two FDA-approved therapies, high-dose interferon alpha 2b and pegylated interferon alpha 2b. Both agents are associated with an improvement in disease free survival; however, this translates only into a minor improvement in overall survival [3, 4]. While adjuvant therapy for breast cancer is typically associated with 50 % or greater reductions in disease-related mortality, interferon (either approved formulation) is associated with no better than a 10–15 % improvement in survival [3, 5–7].

While the benefit of adjuvant interferon is limited, it may be possible to identify which patients are most appropriate for therapy. For example, with the adoption of sentinel lymph node sampling, a number of patients with thin (T1) or intermediate thin (T2) melanoma are being upstaged to Stage IIIA disease and thus eligible for interferon therapy [8]. This subset of patients has a lower risk of disease-related mortality than patients with Stage IIB or IIC melanoma [9]. Given that this is a newly defined population of patients, there is no data from prospectively randomized clinical trials that defines the benefit from a course of interferon to these patients. However, patients with an ulcerated primary melanoma and a microscopic sentinel lymph node biopsy appear to have the most benefit from pegylated interferon [10]. If this finding, which is the basis of a large phase III EORTC study (NCT00636168), proves to be true, then this will be the first validated, predictive biomarker of benefit to adjuvant therapy.

Other potential predictors of benefit to adjuvant interferon have also been evaluated. In particular, development of autoimmunity, either clinically identified or serologically defined, has been shown to be associated with a very low chance of relapse and subsequent disease-related mortality in patients treated with a high-dose interferon regimen [11]. Interestingly, this finding was not seen is a comprehensive evaluation of patients treated with pegylated interferon [12]. Whether these discrepant results are related to differences in the treatment, the patients enrolled in these studies, or simply reflect the limited value of this biomarker is unknown. No matter the reason, it may be a moot point unless pretreatment testing can predict which patients will develop autoimmunity. To date this has been elusive.

While interferon remains the only standard therapy for stage III melanoma, a number of other therapies have been evaluated. Two recently completed and reported studies in specific clinical subgroups of patients with high-risk melanoma highlight that other potentially effective adjuvant treatment options might exist for these patients. In the first study, patients with very high-risk (stage IIIB and IIIC patients) melanoma were randomized to either high-dose interferon or IL-2- and cisplatin-based biochemotherapy [13]. While a difference in overall survival was not seen between the two groups, there was a near doubling of relapse-free survival in the group who received biochemotherapy. This finding will likely not change the standard of care, since biochemotherapy is difficult to administer and overall survival was not improved, however the fact that such dramatic improvements in Recurrence Free Survival (RFS) did not translate into improvements in overall survival (OS) will likely give pause to the interpretation of RFS as a surrogate endpoint for efficacy in future adjuvant studies. The second study was a phase II study in Chinese patients with high-risk mucosal melanoma who were randomized to receive chemotherapy, interferon, or observation [14]. Improvement in relapse-free and overall survival was seen in patients treated with chemotherapy compared with patients who received either interferon or observation. Additionally, interferon was superior to observation in this study. Whether a distinct subset of patients can be identified who benefited most from adjuvant chemotherapy remains to be seen. Particular emphasis should be placed on determining the role of KIT mutation/amplification common in mucosal melanoma in predicting benefit or lack of benefit from therapy. In addition, validation of these results in another study that includes a proportion of patients from Western populations is also warranted.

Recently, changes to the standard of care for patients with unresectable stage III and stage IV melanoma have occurred. Whether the benefits of ipilimumab and/or vemurafenib in the metastatic setting will be translated into an improved cure rate in the adjuvant setting remains to be seen [15–18]. There are now two phase III studies of ipilimumab in the adjuvant setting. The first is a randomized, placebo-controlled study comparing ipilimumab therapy with placebo (NCT00636168) and the second a randomized, open-label study of ipilimumab at two different dose levels compared with high-dose interferon (ECOG 1609; NCT01274338). Neither study is mature enough to comment on either the safety or efficacy of adjuvant ipilimumab in this setting. Lastly, with the success of BRAF inhibitors in advanced melanoma, studies of adjuvant BRAF-directed therapy are beginning enrollment (vemurafenib—NCT01667419; dabrafenib + trametinib—NCT01597908).

With the application of newer therapies effective in stage IV disease to the adjuvant setting, there will likely be an enhanced need to determine which patients are most likely to benefit from a particular therapy. Part of this selection process will likely involve better assessment of a particular patient's recurrence risk. Currently, both tissue-based (AJCC features such as depth of invasion, ulceration, mitoses) and blood-based (serum RNA testing) prognostic biomarkers have been described [9, 19–21]. Whether these or other assays may offer predictive value is unknown. It is of great importance that biomarker development is built into adjuvant studies.

3 Enhanced Patient Selection for Immunotherapy

Based on the descriptions of spontaneous regressions in patients with melanoma and complete regressions in patients with melanoma treated with various immune-modulators, immunotherapy has been a mainstay in the treatment of patients with metastatic melanoma [22]. High-dose bolus interleukin-2 (HD IL-2) was the first immunotherapy FDA-approved for the treatment of patients with metastatic melanoma based on data presented on 270 patients entered onto eight clinical trials [23]. Objective responses were seen in 43 of the 270 patients (RR 16 %). There were 17 (6 %) complete responses (CRs) and 26 (10 %) partial responses (PRs). Most importantly, the median duration of response for complete responders exceeded 59 months [24]. In a more contemporary series of 208 patients treated with HD IL-2 at two tertiary referral centers, the CR and PR rates (6 % and 13 % respectively) were comparable to the historical RR, and similar durability of responses were seen [25]. While HD IL-2 remains an important option for patients with advanced melanoma, its toxicity limits its application to a select group of patients treated in specialized centers [23]. The extreme toxicity of HD IL-2 is characterized by the induction of a septic shock-like clinical picture with concomitant severe but reversible and therefore manageable multiorgan dysfunction. Delivery of therapy requires hospital admission to a highly skilled nursing unit with intensive care capabilities. Clearly the toxicity and restricted benefit of HD IL-2 highlight the need to improve the selection of patients for this treatment. Identifying subpopulations of patients with advanced melanoma who are more or less likely to benefit from treatment is a critical next step to improve its therapeutic index.

Recent studies have shown that certain subgroups of patients may indeed have differential benefit from HD IL-2. For example, an analysis of gene expression profiles in pretreatment tumor samples from patients with advanced melanoma treated with HD IL-2 suggested some expression signatures might predict benefit [26]. Despite a small sample size and a population enriched for responders (13 of 28 patients; 46 %), a nearly 2.5-fold difference in response rate was seen between patients designated as having a prespecified immune/inflammatory gene profile subset compared with a melanocytic antigen/growth factor subset. In a separate analysis, elevated pretreatment serum vascular endothelial growth factor (VEGF) and fibronectin levels have been shown to independently predict for poor outcome in patients treated with high-dose IL-2 [27]. Most recently, tumor NRAS mutational status in patients with metastatic melanoma treated with HD IL-2 was shown to be an important predictor of benefit [25]. Specifically, patients with tumors harboring an NRAS mutation had a higher response rate (45 %) compared to those with BRAF mutations (22 %) or no mutation in either BRAF or NRAS (12 %). This observation requires independent validation and if indeed validated it will be important to explore the mechanisms underlying this relationship.

Interestingly, the experience with HD IL-2 appears to be mirrored by the emerging results with the anti-cytotoxic T-lymphoctye antigen 4 (CTLA-4) antibody ipilimumab. As was previously mentioned, ipilimumab was FDA-approved in 2011 for the treatment of patients with metastatic melanoma. By inhibiting CTLA-4, it leads to the activation of cytotoxic T lymphocytes and subsequent antitumor effects [28]. Ipilimumab is associated with a response rate similar to HD-IL2 (10–15 %) and also like HD IL-2 appears to lead to durable benefit in a subset of patients [29]. However, one important distinction is that in contrast to HD IL-2, the more favorable toxicity profile of ipilimumab allows it to be administered to a broader spectrum of patients and in an outpatient setting [30]. This enabled the conduct of two prospectively randomized phase III trials, which established that ipilimumab produced an improvement in overall survival compared to a vaccine and dacarbazine [17, 18].

Even with its improved safety profile, severe autoimmune toxicity is still seen in 10–30 % of patients treated with ipilimumab frequently limiting its use to melanoma referral centers [31]. As with HD IL-2, it is critical to determine which patients are most or least likely to receive benefit for ipilimumab. To date, it appears that seropositivity of antibodies against the cancer/testis antigen NY-ESO-1 at baseline is predictive of benefit to ipilimumab, though it should be noted that patients who developed detectable seropositivity on treatment (seroconverted) experienced similar increased benefit as those with initial seropositivity [32]. Thus, even if this assay proves to be predictive of benefit, it might not be selective enough to exclude patients from treatment with ipilimumab. Another potential pretreatment predictive biomarker is the presence of various single-nucleotide polymorphisms (SNPs) of immune-related genes. While one group originally described that SNPs of the CTLA4 gene predicted benefit to therapy, a second group found that neither these SNPs nor any others of immune-related genes were predictive [33, 34]. More work in this area is clearly indicated. Lastly, while BRAF mutational status is not predictive of benefit and examination of the potential predictive value of NRAS mutational status (as suggested for IL-2) or other tumor molecular changes has yet to be performed [35].

CTLA-4 serves as one of the major immune checkpoints in the T-cell activation process [28]. A second key checkpoint is the programmed death 1 (PD-1) receptor pathway [36]. PD-1 is a receptor found on T-lymphocytes which, when engaged with its ligand, PD-L1, inhibits T-cell activation [36]. PD-L1 is expressed on macrophages as well as on tumor cells; that latter expression has been shown to be induced by IFN gamma release by immune infiltrating, tumor-specific CD8 positive T cells and is therefore a marker of nascent tumor recognition and attack by the immune system [36]. As such, it appears that PDL1 expression is one of the major mechanisms utilized by tumors to evade destruction by the immune system. Recently, monoclonal antibodies to both PD-1 and PD-L1 have been developed and are currently being tested in the clinic [37, 38]. BMS-936559 is an anti-PD-L1 antibody that showed responses in patients harboring a variety of solid tumors including in 9 of 55 patients with metastatic melanoma [38]. Treatment with the anti-PD-1 antibody MDX-1106 (BMS-936558) has also led to tumor responses in patients with solid tumors including 26 of 94 (28 %) patients with advanced melanoma [37]. Additionally, both of these agents appear to be associated with relatively limited toxicity; though treatment-related deaths have been reported due to pneumonitis. In an effort to define a patient population benefiting for PD-1 blockade, a subset of patients treated on the phase I study of MDX-1106 had pretreatment tumor samples evaluated for PD-L1 expression [37]. Positive PD-L1 expression was defined as membranous expression by more than 5 % of tumor cells in the examined specimen. In this subset analysis of 42 patients, the response rate in patients with tumors exhibiting PD-L1 expression was 36 % (9/25) compared to 0 % (0/17) in those with tumors lacking PD-L1 expression [37]. While this finding needs prospective validation, it represents an example of linking drug development with testable, pretreatment biomarkers in an attempt to identify the patients most likely to benefit. The extent to which PD-L1 expression represents a surrogate for tumor immune recognition and infiltration and its ability to be a general predictor of immunotherapy responsiveness is also being further explored [39]. Further, how other pretreatment biomarkers discussed above (i.e. inflammatory gene expression analysis, BRAF/NRAS mutation, serum VEGF) relate to and/or complement PD-L1 expression to better predict response to immunotherapy is unknown, but certainly worth studying.

4 Identifying the Ideal Sequence of Systemic Therapy for Advanced Disease

There are now four FDA-approved therapies for patients with metastatic melanoma, with more expected in the coming years. While this can only be considered a good development, the availability of multiple treatment options does raise questions regarding how best to sequence therapy. Although current data on this question is limited; some prospective and retrospective data has been reported that can help providers make critical treatment decisions.

It appears that prior high-dose IL-2 does not impact either toxicity or potential efficacy of treatment with ipilimumab or vemurafenib. This data comes from subgroup analyses in both the phase III study of ipilimumab vs. GP100 vaccine and the BRIM2 study (phase II vemurafenib) [17, 40]. Specifically, in the ipilimumab study the overall survival advantage seen with ipilimumab compared to GP100 vaccine was similar whether patients had or had not received prior HD IL-2 [17]. In the BRIM2 study, the response rate was essentially identical amongst patients who had or had not received prior IL-2 [40]. While there is limited data regarding the effectiveness of HD IL-2 treatment following ipilimumab, it has been shown in a small, single-center series that IL-2 therapy after ipilimumab is associated with a higher rate of colitis and possibly a better response rate [41]. There is currently no data about HD IL-2 therapy given subsequent to BRAF-inhibitor treatment, though immunotherapy (mainly ipilimumab) following BRAF-inhibitor therapy has been the subject of a recent report [42]. In this multi-institutional, retrospective series 10 patients were treated with ipilimumab following progression on vemurafenib. None of the patients had a response to therapy, all had progressed by 6 months, and only three survived past 6 months.

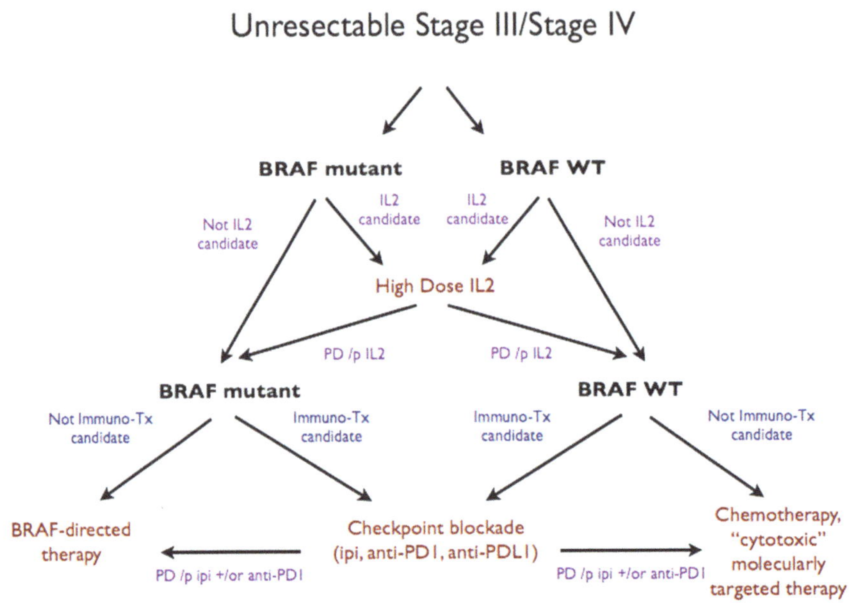

Fig. 2 2012 Treatment algorithm for unresectable or metastatic melanoma

In the coming years it will be absolutely essential to determine the optimal sequencing of existing therapies and additional therapies as they are approved. This will require studies that randomize patients to a sequence of therapies as opposed to one treatment at a time. The first sequence trial has been proposed in the US Intergroup mechanism and will randomize patients with BRAF mutant melanoma to either the sequence of ipilimumab followed by vemurafenib or vemurafenib followed by ipilimumab. Based on the currently available information, Fig. 2 shows one potential treatment algorithm.

Of note, as is described below; there is some rationale for combining various therapies (i.e. vemurafenib and ipilimumab; HD IL-2 and vemurafenib; HD IL-2 and ipilimumab). While the development of such combination regimens might make the sequencing questions moot, it will like raise issues of cost and toxicity that will heighten the need for predictive biomarkers.

5 Improving the Efficacy of BRAF Inhibitor-Based Therapy

Single-agent treatment with either of the selective BRAF inhibitors, vemurafenib and dabrafenib, and the MEK inhibitor trametinib has been shown to improve outcome in patients with advanced, BRAF-mutant melanoma compared with treatment with dacarbazine in randomized, phase III studies [15, 43, 44]. Unfortunately, these treatments while producing significant and rapid tumor regression in the majority of patients, appear to delay

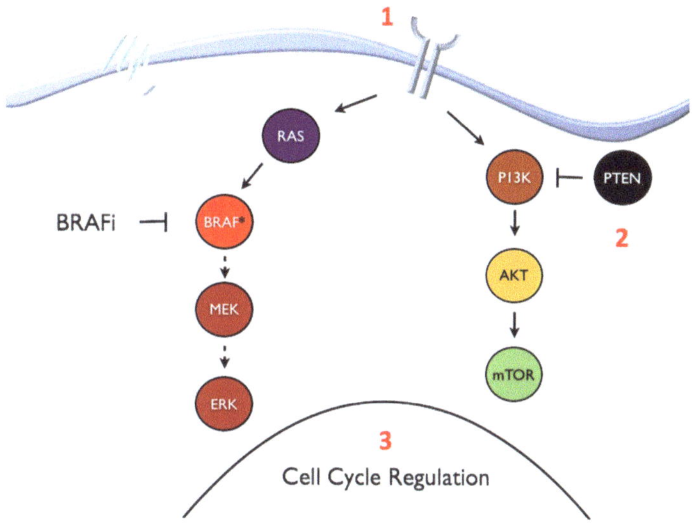

Fig. 3 Extrinsic mechanisms of BRAF-inhibitor resistance: (1) Hepatocyte growth factor upregulation leading to CMET activation; (2) PTEN loss; (3) Cell cycle dysregulation

rather than prevent death from melanoma. Tumor resistance to BRAF-directed therapy typically develops within a median of 5–8 months following treatment initiation, (range of 2 months to 2 years) [15, 40, 43–46]. BRAF-inhibitor resistance has been described as an increasingly complex process that includes both intrinsic and acquired mechanisms [47].

It is now clear that there are identifiable, pretreatment factors that predict poor outcomes in patients treated with BRAF-directed therapy. These include, as shown in Fig. 3, molecular changes within the tumor such as whether the tumor suppressor phosphate and tensin (PTEN) has been lost, whether certain cell cycle regulators are abnormally expressed (i.e. cyclin D amplification), and whether the tumor microenvironment secretes certain growth factors such as hepatocyte growth factor (HGF) [48–51]. It can be expected that clinical trials will test BRAF inhibitors in combination with inhibitors of each of these resistance associated pathways such as phosphotidylinositol-3-kinase (PI3K) inhibitors (PTEN loss), CDK4/6 inhibitors (cell cycle disruption), and HGF or CMET inhibitors (HGF expression).

In addition to intrinsic factors that predict worse outcome, various mechanisms of acquired resistance have been described (Fig. 4). In general, two major categories of mechanisms exist; those associated with reactivation of the MAPK pathway (ERK-dependent) and those that are not (ERK-independent) [52]. Upregulation of growth factor receptors such as the receptor tyrosine kinases–VEGF-receptor (VEGFR), platelet derived growth factor (PDGFR), and insulin-like growth factor 1 receptor (IGF-R1) can be associated

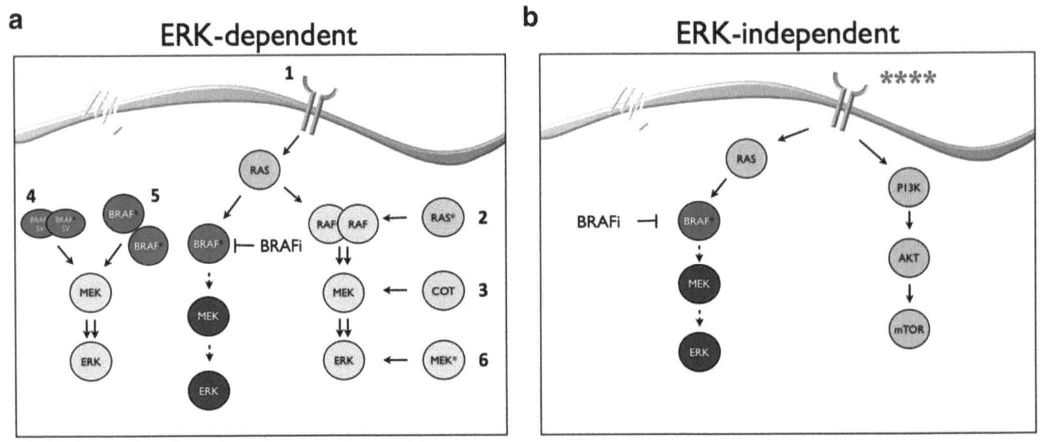

Fig. 4 Intrinsic mechanisms of resistance. ERK-dependent mechanisms (**a**) include (1) Receptor tyrosine kinase (RTK) hyperactivation/upregulation, (2) NRAS mutation, (3) Alternative MAPK activation (COT), (4) BRAFV600 splice variant, (5) BRAFV600 amplification, (6) MEK mutation. The ERK-independent mechanism (**b**) thus far is RTK hyperactivation/upregulation leading to PI3K pathway signaling

with either ERK reactivation or renewed growth independent of ERK-reactivation through upregulation of parallel signaling pathways, namely the PI3K pathway [53–55]. Other ERK-dependent methods of BRAF-inhibitor resistance include the development of concomitant upstream (NRAS) or downstream (MEK) mutations, increased expression of mutant BRAF, the emergence of mutant BRAF splice variants, and activation of alternative MAPKs (COT) [53, 54, 56–60]. It is important to note that each of these "intrinsic" mechanisms of resistance that emerge from genetic mutation, alteration, or amplification of MAPK pathway mediators actually represent subpopulations of cells which have a relative growth advantage in the presence of BRAF-directed therapy. While the sensitivity required to detect these aberrant cells at baseline is quite high, it is possible that the future application of next-generation sequencing techniques may help identify these subpopulations and help aid treatment selection.

Based on the finding that tumor ERK-reactivation occurs in a majority of patients treated with BRAF-inhibitors, the combination of a BRAF inhibitor (dabrafenib) plus a MEK inhibitor (trametinib) was studied in patients with BRAF mutant melanoma both prior to and following other BRAF-directed therapy [52]. Interestingly, this combination appears to be better tolerated than either single-agent alone (particularly with respect to rash, photosensitivity, and secondary squamous cell carcinomas) and has excellent clinical activity (RR 57 %) across multiple dose levels, and a median PFS of 10.8 months at the recommended phase II dose [61]. Of note, this combination also led to responses in patients who were previously treated and developed resistance to a BRAF-inhibitor (RR 18 %). Results from a randomized phase II study comparing the combination to single-agent dabrafenib are expected later this year. Also randomized phase III studies comparing the combination of dabrafenib and trametininb to either dabrafenib (NCT015979080) or vemurafenib (NCT01597908) have recently been launched in an effort to establish the utility of the combination relative to single agent therapy. Other BRAF-directed therapy plus molecularly targeted combinations aimed to impact acquired mechanisms of resistance are either opening soon (vemurafenib + bevacizumab—NCT01495988) or being planned.

Lastly, the combination of immunotherapy with BRAF-directed therapy is clearly appealing as it offers the opportunity to extend the benefit of BRAF-inhibition. Encouragingly, preclinical data has emerged that also appear to support potential synergy for this combination [62]. It has been recently shown that MAPK pathway inhibitors actually lead to an increase in melanocytic antigen expression, both in vitro and in patient tumors, and lead to an influx of CD-8+ T-Cells into tumors [63, 64]. Further, BRAF inhibitors are not immunosuppressive in any testable way, while MEK inhibitors appear to exert some immunosuppression [65]. Thus, a series of trials are now either open or being planned to combine various immunotherapies (ipilimumab, HD IL-2, anti-PD1/PD-L1 antibodies) with BRAF inhibitors (NCT01400451, NCT01603212, NCT01683188, NCT01656642).

6 Developing "Targeted" Therapies for Hard-to-Target Subgroups

With the preponderance of data and current research seemingly focused on immune checkpoint inhibitors and/or BRAF-directed therapy, it is easy to lose site of the fact that there are patients with other molecularly defined subgroups of melanoma who might benefit from targeted therapeutic approaches if specific and selective agents could be identified. While mutations in BRAF are seen in approximately 40–50 % of patients with melanoma, an additional 15–20 % of patients have NRAS mutations, and nearly 75 % of patients have aberrations in cell cycle regulatory proteins [66, 67]. Though there is no standard "targeted" therapy for patients with BRAF WT melanoma, promising data is emerging with a few agents in these previously hard-to-target subgroups.

Based on preclinical studies, MEK inhibitors have been predicted to have activity in patients with NRAS mutations [68]. Whether due to inadequate mutational analysis or ineffective agents, a number of early phase studies of MEK inhibitors were performed in patients with melanoma without substantial benefit [69, 70]. More recently, a trial of the MEK1/2 inhibitor MEK162 was performed in patients with NRAS mutations and showed modest activity (RR approximately 20 %) [71]. While this activity does not approach the effect of BRAF directed therapy in patients with

BRAF mutant melanoma, it is likely that MEK162 (and possibly other, similarly potent MEK1/2 inhibitors) will be used as the backbone of therapy for a number of combination trials.

KIT mutations or amplification is seen in a small minority of all patients with melanoma, in general, though up to 10–25 % in highly selected subgroups such as acral or mucosal disease [72, 73]. In all patients with melanoma, the KIT inhibitor imatininb has proven to be ineffective; however in patients with melanomas containing KIT mutations response rates approach 20 % [74–76]. Interestingly, all currently documented responses have occurred in patients with mutations of exons 11 or 13, suggesting that these are the patients who are most likely to benefit from this agent [74, 75]. Additionally, studies with dasatinib (NCT01092728) and nilotinib (NCT01028222) that are enriched or selected for patients with CKIT mutations are ongoing.

Lastly, a number of other mutations have recently been described in melanomas that may have therapeutic implications. These include the G-proteins GNAQ and GNA11 that are mutated in over 80 % of uveal melanoma, inactivating mutations of BRCA1 associated protein 1 (BAP1) seen in nearly 50 % of uveal melanoma (and >80 % of tumors that metastasize) and gain-of-function mutations in the GTPase RAC1 in 5 % of melanomas [77–81]. While there are no current therapies available for the treatment for these specific mutational subgroups, it is very likely that the ramifications of mutation are the upregulation of oncogenic proteins that could be inhibited with either small molecule inhibitors or novel therapeutic approaches.

7 Conclusions

We have identified five clinical issues deserving of considerable attention from the melanoma research community in the coming years; issues which have risen to the forefront following decades of fundamental research discoveries that are now being translated into clinical improvement for our patients. Through continued basic science, as well as translational and clinical research efforts, we expect the continued development of impactful therapeutic advances. An important component of this research will be the development of predictive biomarkers that will enable clinicians to better choose the optimal therapy for each patient with melanoma.

References

1. Siegel R, Naishadham D, Jemal A (2013) Cancer statistics, 2012. CA Cancer J Clin 63(1):11–30
2. Ascierto PA, Kirkwood JM (2008) Adjuvant therapy of melanoma with interferon: lessons of the past decade. J Transl Med 6:62
3. Kirkwood JM, Manola J, Ibrahim J, Sondak V, Ernstoff MS, Rao U (2004) A pooled analysis of eastern cooperative oncology group and intergroup trials of adjuvant high-dose interferon for melanoma. Clin Cancer Res 10:1670–1677

4. Eggermont AM, Suciu S, Santinami M et al (2008) Adjuvant therapy with pegylated interferon alfa-2b versus observation alone in resected stage III melanoma: final results of EORTC 18991, a randomised phase III trial. Lancet 372:117–126
5. Mocellin S, Pasquali S, Rossi CR, Nitti D (2010) Interferon alpha adjuvant therapy in patients with high-risk melanoma: a systematic review and meta-analysis. J Natl Cancer Inst 102:493–501
6. Berry DA, Cirrincione C, Henderson IC et al (2006) Estrogen-receptor status and outcomes of modern chemotherapy for patients with node-positive breast cancer. JAMA 295:1658–1667
7. Peto R, Davies C, Godwin J et al (2012) Comparisons between different polychemotherapy regimens for early breast cancer: meta-analyses of long-term outcome among 100,000 women in 123 randomised trials. Lancet 379:432–444
8. Balch CM, Buzaid AC, Soong SJ et al (2001) Final version of the American Joint Committee on Cancer staging system for cutaneous melanoma. J Clin Oncol 19:3635–3648
9. Balch CM, Gershenwald JE, Soong SJ et al (2009) Final version of 2009 AJCC melanoma staging and classification. J Clin Oncol 27:6199–6206
10. Eggermont AM, Suciu S, Testori A et al (2012) Ulceration and stage are predictive of interferon efficacy in melanoma: results of the phase III adjuvant trials EORTC 18952 and EORTC 18991. Eur J Cancer 48:218–225
11. Gogas H, Ioannovich J, Dafni U et al (2006) Prognostic significance of autoimmunity during treatment of melanoma with interferon. N Engl J Med 354:709–718
12. Bouwhuis MG, Suciu S, Testori A et al (2010) Phase III trial comparing adjuvant treatment with pegylated interferon Alfa-2b versus observation: prognostic significance of autoantibodies—EORTC 18991. J Clin Oncol 28:2460–2466
13. Flaherty LE, Moon J, Atkins MB et al (2012) Phase III trial of high-dose interferon alpha-2b versus cisplatin, vinblastine, DTIC plus IL-2 and interferon in patients with high-risk melanoma (SWOG S0008): an intergroup study of CALGB, COG, ECOG, and SWOG. J Clin Oncol 30
14. Lian B, Mao LL, Cui CL et al (2012) Phase II randomized study of high-dose interferon alfa-2b (HDI) versus chemotherapy as adjuvant therapy in patients with resected mucosal melanoma. J Clin Oncol 30
15. Chapman PB, Hauschild A, Robert C et al (2011) Improved survival with vemurafenib in melanoma with BRAF V600E mutation. N Engl J Med 364:2507–2516
16. Hauschild A, Grob JJ, Demidov LV et al (2012) Dabrafenib in BRAF-mutated metastatic melanoma: a multicentre, open-label, phase 3 randomised controlled trial. Lancet 380:358–365
17. Hodi FS, O'Day SJ, McDermott DF et al (2010) Improved survival with ipilimumab in patients with metastatic melanoma. N Engl J Med 363:711–723
18. Robert C, Thomas L, Bondarenko I et al (2011) Ipilimumab plus dacarbazine for previously untreated metastatic melanoma. N Engl J Med 364:2517–2526
19. Panka DJ, Sullivan RJ, Mier JW (2010) An inexpensive, specific and highly sensitive protocol to detect the BrafV600E mutation in melanoma tumor biopsies and blood. Melanoma Res 20:401–407
20. Kitago M, Koyanagi K, Nakamura T et al (2009) mRNA expression and BRAF mutation in circulating melanoma cells isolated from peripheral blood with high molecular weight melanoma-associated antigen-specific monoclonal antibody beads. Clin Chem 55:757–764
21. Hoshimoto S, Faries MB, Morton DL et al (2012) Assessment of prognostic circulating tumor cells in a phase III trial of adjuvant immunotherapy after complete resection of stage IV melanoma. Ann Surg 255:357–362
22. Sullivan RJ, Atkins MB (2010) Cytokine therapy in melanoma. J Cutan Pathol 37(Suppl 1):60–67
23. Atkins MB, Lotze MT, Dutcher JP et al (1999) High-dose recombinant interleukin 2 therapy for patients with metastatic melanoma: analysis of 270 patients treated between 1985 and 1993. J Clin Oncol 17:2105–2116
24. Atkins MB, Kunkel L, Sznol M, Rosenberg SA (2000) High-dose recombinant interleukin-2 therapy in patients with metastatic melanoma: long-term survival update. Cancer J Sci Am 6(Suppl 1):S11–S14
25. Joseph RW, Sullivan RJ, Harrell R et al (2012) Correlation of NRAS mutations with clinical response to high-dose IL-2 in patients with advanced melanoma. J Immunother 35:66–72
26. Sullivan RJ, Hoshida Y, Brunet J et al (2009) A single center experience with high-dose IL-2 treatment for patients with advanced melanoma and pilot investigation of a novel gene expression signature as a predictor of response. J Clin Oncol 27(suppl): abstr 9003
27. Sabatino M, Kim-Schulze S, Panelli MC et al (2009) Serum vascular endothelial growth factor and fibronectin predict clinical response to high-dose interleukin-2 therapy. J Clin Oncol 27:2645–2652
28. Wolchok JD, Saenger Y (2008) The mechanism of anti-CTLA-4 activity and the negative regulation of T-cell activation. Oncologist 13(suppl 4):2–9

29. Wolchok JD, Neyns B, Linette G et al (2010) Ipilimumab monotherapy in patients with pretreated advanced melanoma: a randomised, double-blind, multicentre, phase 2, dose-ranging study. Lancet Oncol 11:155–164
30. Wolchok JD, Weber JS, Hamid O et al (2010) Ipilimumab efficacy and safety in patients with advanced melanoma: a retrospective analysis of HLA subtype from four trials. Cancer Immun 10:9
31. Weber JS, Kahler KC, Hauschild A (2012) Management of immune-related adverse events and kinetics of response with ipilimumab. J Clin Oncol 30:2691–2697
32. Yuan J, Adamow M, Ginsberg BA et al (2011) Integrated NY-ESO-1 antibody and CD8+ T-cell responses correlate with clinical benefit in advanced melanoma patients treated with ipilimumab. Proc Natl Acad Sci USA 108: 16723–16728
33. Breunis WB, Tarazona-Santos E, Chen R, Kiley M, Rosenberg SA, Chanock SJ (2008) Influence of cytotoxic T lymphocyte-associated antigen 4 (CTLA4) common polymorphisms on outcome in treatment of melanoma patients with CTLA-4 blockade. J Immunother 31: 586–590
34. Hamid O, Schmidt H, Nissan A et al (2011) A prospective phase II trial exploring the association between tumor microenvironment biomarkers and clinical activity of ipilimumab in advanced melanoma. J Transl Med 9:204
35. Shahabi V, Whitney G, Hamid O et al (2012) Assessment of association between BRAF-V600E mutation status in melanomas and clinical response to ipilimumab. Cancer Immunol Immunother 61:733–737
36. Pardoll DM (2012) The blockade of immune checkpoints in cancer immunotherapy. Nat Rev Cancer 12:252–264
37. Topalian SL, Hodi FS, Brahmer JR et al (2012) Safety, activity, and immune correlates of anti-PD-1 antibody in cancer. N Engl J Med 366(26):2443–2454
38. Brahmer JR, Tykodi SS, Chow LQ et al (2012) Safety and activity of anti-PD-L1 antibody in patients with advanced cancer. N Engl J Med 366(26):2455–2465
39. Taube JM, Anders RA, Young GD et al (2012) Colocalization of inflammatory response with B7-h1 expression in human melanocytic lesions supports an adaptive resistance mechanism of immune escape. Sci Transl Med 4:127–137
40. Sosman JA, Kim KB, Schuchter L et al (2012) Survival in BRAF V600-mutant advanced melanoma treated with vemurafenib. N Engl J Med 366:707–714
41. Smith FO, Goff SL, Klapper JA et al (2007) Risk of bowel perforation in patients receiving interleukin-2 after therapy with anti-CTLA 4 monoclonal antibody. J Immunother 30:130
42. Ackerman A, McDermott DF, Lawrence DP et al (2012) Outcomes of patients with malignant melanoma treated with immunotherapy prior to or after vemurafenib. J Clin Oncol 30:8569
43. Flaherty KT, Robert C, Hersey P et al (2012) Improved survival with MEK inhibition in BRAF-mutated melanoma. N Engl J Med 367(2):107–114
44. Hauschild A, Agarwala SS, Trefzer U et al (2009) Results of a phase III, randomized, placebo-controlled study of sorafenib in combination with carboplatin and paclitaxel as second-line treatment in patients with unresectable stage III or stage IV melanoma. J Clin Oncol 27:2823–2830
45. Falchook GS, Long GV, Kurzrock R et al (2012) Dabrafenib in patients with melanoma, untreated brain metastases, and other solid tumours: a phase 1 dose-escalation trial. Lancet 379:1893–1901
46. Flaherty KT, Puzanov I, Kim KB et al (2010) Inhibition of mutated, activated BRAF in metastatic melanoma. N Engl J Med 363: 809–819
47. Sullivan RJ, Flaherty K (2013) MAP kinase signaling and inhibition in melanoma. Oncogene 32(19):2373–2379
48. Nathanson KL, Martin A, Letrero R, D'Andrea KP, O'Day S, Infante JR, Falchook GS, Millward M, Curtis CM, Ma B, Gagnon RC, Lebowitz PF, Long GV, Kefford RF (2011) Tumor genetic analyses of patients with metastatic melanoma treated with the BRAF inhibitor GSK2118436 (GSK436). In: ASCO, 2011, Chicago. J Clin Oncol (suppl): abstr 8501
49. Smalley KS, Lioni M, Dalla Palma M et al (2008) Increased cyclin D1 expression can mediate BRAF inhibitor resistance in BRAF V600E-mutated melanomas. Mol Cancer Ther 7:2876–2883
50. Straussman R, Morikawa T, Shee K et al (2012) Tumour micro-environment elicits innate resistance to RAF inhibitors through HGF secretion. Nature 487:500–504
51. Wilson TR, Fridlyand J, Yan Y et al (2012) Widespread potential for growth-factor-driven resistance to anticancer kinase inhibitors. Nature 487:505–509
52. Bollag G, Hirth P, Tsai J et al (2010) Clinical efficacy of a RAF inhibitor needs broad target blockade in BRAF-mutant melanoma. Nature 467:596–599
53. Johannessen CM, Boehm JS, Kim SY et al (2010) COT drives resistance to RAF inhibition through MAP kinase pathway reactivation. Nature 468:968–972

54. Nazarian R, Shi H, Wang Q et al (2010) Melanomas acquire resistance to B-RAF(V600E) inhibition by RTK or N-RAS upregulation. Nature 468:973–977
55. Villanueva J, Vultur A, Lee JT et al (2010) Acquired resistance to BRAF inhibitors mediated by a RAF kinase switch in melanoma can be overcome by cotargeting MEK and IGF-1R/PI3K. Cancer Cell 18:683–695
56. Wagle N, Emery C, Berger MF et al (2011) Dissecting therapeutic resistance to RAF inhibition in melanoma by tumor genomic profiling. J Clin Oncol 29:3085–3096
57. Poulikakos PI, Persaud Y, Janakiraman M et al (2011) RAF inhibitor resistance is mediated by dimerization of aberrantly spliced BRAF(V600E). Nature 480:387–390
58. Shi H, Moriceau G, Kong X et al (2012) Melanoma whole-exome sequencing identifies (V600E)B-RAF amplification-mediated acquired B-RAF inhibitor resistance. Nat Commun 3:724
59. Tap WD, Gong KW, Dering J et al (2010) Pharmacodynamic characterization of the efficacy signals due to selective BRAF inhibition with PLX4032 in malignant melanoma. Neoplasia 12:637–649
60. Emery CM, Vijayendran KG, Zipser MC et al (2009) MEK1 mutations confer resistance to MEK and B-RAF inhibition. Proc Natl Acad Sci USA 106:20411–20416
61. Weber JS, Flaherty KT, Infante JR, Falchook GS, Kefford R, Daud A, Hamid O, Gonzalez R, Kudchadkar RR, Lawrence DP, Burris HA, Long GV, Algazi AP, Lewis KD, Kim KB, Puzanov I, Sun P, Little SM, Patel K, Sosman JA (2012) Updated safety and efficacy results from a phase I/II study of the oral BRAF inhibitor dabrafenib (GSK2118436) combined with the oral MEK 1/2 inhibitor trametinib (GSK1120212) in patients with BRAFi-naive metastatic melanoma. In: ASCO, 2012, Chicago. J Clin Oncol (suppl): abstr 8510
62. Koya RC, Mok S, Otte N et al (2012) BRAF inhibitor vemurafenib improves the antitumor activity of adoptive cell immunotherapy. Cancer Res 72:3928–3937
63. Boni A, Cogdill AP, Dang P et al (2010) Selective BRAFV600E inhibition enhances T-cell recognition of melanoma without affecting lymphocyte function. Cancer Res 70: 5213–5219
64. Wilmott JS, Long GV, Howle JR et al (2012) Selective BRAF inhibitors induce marked T-cell infiltration into human metastatic melanoma. Clin Cancer Res 18:1386–1394
65. Comin-Anduix B, Chodon T, Sazegar H et al (2010) The oncogenic BRAF kinase inhibitor PLX4032/RG7204 does not affect the viability or function of human lymphocytes across a wide range of concentrations. Clin Cancer Res 16:6040–6048
66. Omholt K, Platz A, Kanter L, Ringborg U, Hansson J (2003) NRAS and BRAF mutations arise early during melanoma pathogenesis and are preserved throughout tumor progression. Clin Cancer Res 9:6483–6488
67. McArthur GA, Young RJ, Sheppard KE et al (2012) Clinical significance of genomic alterations of the CDK4-pathway and sensitivity to the CDK4 inhibitor PD 0332991 in melanoma. J Clin Oncol 30
68. Solit DB, Garraway LA, Pratilas CA et al (2006) BRAF mutation predicts sensitivity to MEK inhibition. Nature 439:358–362
69. Adjei AA, Cohen RB, Franklin W et al (2008) Phase I pharmacokinetic and pharmacodynamic study of the oral, small-molecule mitogen-activated protein kinase kinase 1/2 inhibitor AZD6244 (ARRY-142886) in patients with advanced cancers. J Clin Oncol 26:2139–2146
70. Banerji U, Camidge DR, Verheul HM et al (2010) The first-in-human study of the hydrogen sulfate (Hyd-sulfate) capsule of the MEK1/2 inhibitor AZD6244 (ARRY-142886): a phase I open-label multicenter trial in patients with advanced cancer. Clin Cancer Res 16:1613–1623
71. Ascierto PA, Berking C, Agawala SS et al (2012) Efficacy and safety of oral MEK162 in patients with locally advanced and unresectable or metastatic cutaneous melanoma harboring BRAFV600 or NRAS mutations. In: ASCO, 2012, Chicago. J Clin Oncol
72. Curtin JA, Fridlyand J, Kageshita T et al (2005) Distinct sets of genetic alterations in melanoma. N Engl J Med 353:2135–2147
73. Curtin JA, Busam K, Pinkel D, Bastian BC (2006) Somatic activation of KIT in distinct subtypes of melanoma. J Clin Oncol 24:4340–4346
74. Carvajal RD, Antonescu CR, Wolchok JD et al (2011) KIT as a therapeutic target in metastatic melanoma. JAMA 305:2327–2334
75. Guo J, Si L, Kong Y et al (2011) Phase II, open-label, single-arm trial of imatinib mesylate in patients with metastatic melanoma harboring c-Kit mutation or amplification. J Clin Oncol 29:2904–2909
76. Wyman K, Atkins MB, Prieto V et al (2006) Multicenter phase II trial of high-dose imatinib mesylate in metastatic melanoma: significant toxicity with no clinical efficacy. Cancer 106:2005–2011
77. Van Raamsdonk CD, Bezrookove V, Green G et al (2009) Frequent somatic mutations of GNAQ in uveal melanoma and blue naevi. Nature 457:599–602

78. Van Raamsdonk CD, Griewank KG, Crosby MB et al (2010) Mutations in GNA11 in uveal melanoma. N Engl J Med 363:2191–2199
79. Harbour JW, Onken MD, Roberson ED et al (2010) Frequent mutation of BAP1 in metastasizing uveal melanomas. Science 330:1410–1413
80. Hodis E, Watson IR, Kryukov GV et al (2012) A landscape of driver mutations in melanoma. Cell 150:251–263
81. Krauthammer M, Kong Y, Ha BH et al (2012) Exome sequencing identifies recurrent somatic RAC1 mutations in melanoma. Nat Genet 44:1006–1014

Chapter 3

Integrating Molecular Biomarkers into Current Clinical Management in Melanoma

Ragini Kudchadkar, Geoffrey Gibney, and Vernon K. Sondak

Abstract

Personalized melanoma medicine has progressed from histopathologic features to serum markers to molecular profiles. Since the identification of activating *BRAF* mutations and subsequent development of drugs targeting the mutant BRAF protein, oncologists now need to incorporate prognostic and predictive biomarkers into treatment decisions for their melanoma patients. Examples include subgrouping patients by genotype profiles for targeted therapy and the development of serologic, immunohistochemical, and genotype profiles for the selection of patients for immunotherapies. In this chapter, we provide an overview of the current status of *BRAF* mutation testing, as well as promising serologic and molecular profiles that will impact patient care. As further research helps clarify the roles of these factors, the clinical outcomes of melanoma patients promise to be greatly improved.

Key words Melanoma, Biomarkers, Targeted therapy

1 Introduction

Since the introduction of pathologic prognostic factors by Clark in 1969 [1] and Breslow in 1970 [2], clinicians have used histopathologic criteria as "biomarkers" to estimate prognosis and formulate decisions regarding surgical and adjuvant therapy for patients with cutaneous melanoma. Limitations of pathologic assessment were readily evident, and clinicians and researchers have long sought additional, more reliable biomarkers to help explain why some patients with very favorable primary melanomas rapidly relapsed and died, while others with multiple high-risk features survived for decades without evidence of recurrence. Meanwhile, progress in the treatment of metastatic melanoma lagged far behind, and when responses to treatment did occur they were seemingly random and unpredictable events. The new millennium saw melanoma research enter into a new "molecular era," characterized by fundamental improvements in our understanding of the biology of melanoma

Magdalena Thurin and Francesco M. Marincola (eds.), *Molecular Diagnostics for Melanoma: Methods and Protocols*, Methods in Molecular Biology, vol. 1102, DOI 10.1007/978-1-62703-727-3_3, © Springer Science+Business Media New York 2014

development and progression as well as the biology of the host immune response to tumors in general and melanoma in particular. Over the past decade, these advances in biology have translated directly into improved treatments and biomarkers that enable the appropriate selection of patients for those treatments, and offer the promise of many more improvements to come. In this chapter, we will briefly review currently used biomarkers and preview those most likely to have an impact in the foreseeable future, all with an eye toward how these biomarkers are best integrated into modern clinical management of patients with melanoma across the entire spectrum of disease stage.

2 Primary Tumor Biomarkers

The science of biomarker development in melanoma began with studies of primary cutaneous tumors and involved correlating histopathologic findings with outcome as measured by the development of regional lymph node and/or distant metastasis as well as death from melanoma. Clark's level of invasion relative to the layers of the epidermis and dermis [1] and Breslow's measured depth of invasion beneath the granular layer of the epidermis [2] were supplemented by the presence of tumor ulceration [3] and quickly became established tools for the management of clinically localized melanoma. Soon thereafter, however, came the realization of the limitations of these basic histopathologic features in fully defining prognosis.

3 Predicting Recurrence/Nodal Metastasis

The development of sentinel lymph node biopsy for surgical staging of clinically normal regional lymph nodes [4] improved the ability to discriminate which patients with melanomas of a given thickness or level would develop distant recurrence and die from their disease [5]. At the same time, it increased the impetus for more reliable indicators of which patients were at sufficient risk of nodal metastasis to merit consideration for the procedure, and for predictors of patients who would develop distant metastasis despite a negative sentinel lymph node.

3.1 Ulceration and Mitosis

Although primary tumor ulceration remains one of the most reliable prognostic features in cutaneous melanoma, the biology underlying its development and the reasons for its impact on prognosis remain poorly understood. Ulceration is also very infrequently encountered until a primary melanoma has progressed to at least 1.5–2.0 mm in thickness, so ulceration has proven to be of little help in discriminating which thinner melanomas would be most likely to metastasize to the regional nodes and beyond. Primary tumor mitotic count was proposed as an alternative, and was shown to have advantages over ulceration as a prognostic factor [6]. Like so many biomarkers to follow, difficulties with technique, reproducibility, and assigning consistent and optimum values for low, moderate, and high risk initially hampered the incorporation of mitotic count into clinical practice. Over time, however, the impact of mitotic count on the likelihood of sentinel node metastasis was recognized [7], and eventually mitotic rate became incorporated into the AJCC/IUCC staging system for melanoma [8]. Concerns regarding interobserver variability in the identification and counting of mitotic figures remain, and have spurred the development of more reliable markers of mitosis. Antibodies to phosphohistone 3, a protein that is phosphorylated during mitosis, have shown potential to improve the identification of mitoses through immunohistochemistry [9, 10], and may enhance the prognostic value of mitotic counts [11].

3.2 Tumor Infiltrating T Cells (TIL)

The presence of tumor infiltrating lymphocytes (TIL) in primary cutaneous melanoma tumors was first described by Clark et al. in 1969 [1]. Since then, multiple studies have demonstrated that increased lymphocyte infiltration is associated with a better overall prognosis [12, 13]. Incorporation of TIL as a factor in clinical management has been relatively limited, although new approaches (outlined below) may lead to the eventual incorporation of TIL as a predictive factor for immunotherapy of advanced disease. Many other biomarkers are in development for predicting nodal and distant metastasis. This represents a fertile area of research with the potential to directly impact surgical and adjuvant therapy decisions in melanoma patients.

4 FISH/CGH in Diagnostically Challenging Lesions

Biomarkers can be helpful in the work up of diagnostically challenging pigmented lesions, because pigmented lesions are not always easily classified as malignant melanoma or completely benign. Terminology such as Spitzoid tumor of uncertain malignant potential (STUMP), melanocytic tumor of uncertain malignant potential (MELTUMP), superficial atypical melanocytic proliferation of uncertain significance (SAMPUS), atypical Spitz tumor (AST), and atypical melanocytic proliferation (AMP) have been used to refer to lesions that have histologic features of both benign melanocytic proliferations and malignant melanoma [14]. Therefore, markers are needed to help distinguish a benign lesion from a potentially malignant one, especially when traditional immunohistochemical methods do not suffice.

Molecular analytic techniques to evaluate the multiple chromosomal aberrations present in melanoma are frequently used. Fluorescence in situ hybridization (FISH) is a commercially available test and can be performed on formalin-fixed tissue [15, 16]. However, this method can have false positive results, particularly in regards to tetraploidy. Comparative genomic hybridization is another method to evaluate for genetic abnormalities in a specimen [17]. However, until recently, this test has only been available on a research basis and the predictive value for ambiguous lesions is uncertain [18]. The characteristic chromosomal abnormality of benign Spitz nevi is a gain in the short arm of chromosome 11 [19]; when this abnormality is present it can support that diagnosis in an otherwise atypical but not clearly malignant lesion.

While genetic evaluations can be helpful in selected ambiguous lesions, however, neither FISH nor CGH abnormalities alone are sufficient to call a lesion malignant. These tests must be used in the context of all traditional histopathologic parameters and are just one piece of the puzzle. Neither FISH nor CGH are recommended for routine use on pigmented lesions, and all results should be interpreted in context with all other findings by a pathologist with expertise in atypical melanocytic proliferations.

5 Identifying Primary Site in Melanoma of Unknown Primary Origin

Occasionally, patients will be diagnosed with metastatic melanoma involving a lymph node or visceral organ where no primary source of melanoma has been identified. This has been termed melanoma of unknown primary origin, and documented to occur in 2–9 % of patients [20]. Some cases originally thought to represent unknown primary metastatic melanoma may actually represent primary clear cell sarcomas at visceral sites [21]. Histopathologic features and immunohistochemical markers, such as S-100, HMB-45, and Melan-A, may not be definitive in these instances. The presence of the characteristic *EWS/ATF1* gene rearrangement secondary to a t(12;22)(q13;q12) translocation, demonstrable either by FISH or RT-PCR, supports the diagnosis of clear cell sarcoma [22]. Conversely, the presence of a *BRAF* or *NRAS* mutation supports the diagnosis of melanoma. Recent data indicate that unknown primary melanoma tumors have mutation profiles more similar to that of cutaneous melanomas as opposed to those arising from acral, mucosal, or uveal origin [23]. These data support the theory that the great majority of unknown primary melanomas arise from a cutaneous site.

6 Biomarkers for Targeted Therapy of Metastatic Disease

6.1 *BRAF*

The recognition that mutations in the *BRAF* gene were frequent in cutaneous melanomas [24], particularly those arising in association with intermittent rather than chronic sun damage [25], led in just a few years to clinical trials of selective BRAF inhibitors such as vemurafenib and dabrafenib. Randomized phase III trials have demonstrated a survival benefit for treatment with vemurafenib or dabrafenib compared to dacarbazine chemotherapy [26, 27], and the benefits of trametinib appear to be of a similar nature [28]. The availability of these drugs led to the need for a well-validated, reproducible *BRAF* mutation test. Testing for this mutation has changed the way clinicians manage metastatic disease, as most treatment algorithms have this as the first branching point for decision making. This assessment will only be valid if the *BRAF* mutation test is accurate, and not all tests are created equal. With multiple methods of determining the *BRAF* mutation status of the tumor, clinicians are left with determining on their own which test is best for their patient. Sanger sequencing, the proprietary cobas 4800 BRAF V600 Mutation Test®, and pyrosequencing are the most common methods used in the United States today. We will review the pros and cons of each method.

When analyzing a melanoma DNA sequence for a *BRAF* mutation, the focus is primarily on detecting a single amino acid substitution occurring at valine 600 (*BRAF* V600). The most common mutation in the 600 codon, V600E, is the result of a valine-to-glutamic acid conversion [29]. A number of less common variants exist, including V600K, V600D, and V600R. The alternative variants are present in approximately 10–20 % of *BRAF* mutant melanomas and tend to be more frequent in the elderly patients with melanoma [29, 30]. Therefore, the ideal test will recognize all these potential alterations.

Traditional direct sequencing (Sanger) has been widely used in many clinical laboratories for the testing of multiple different mutations, including *BRAF* mutations. This form of genetic sequencing is often considered the first generation of the sequencing technologies. This method identifies linear sequences of nucleotides by electrophoretic separation of randomly terminated extension products [31]. This method is readily available and accurate but has limited sensitivity for detecting mutations that are present in low percentages of a specimen. Compared to other available tests, sequencing is costly and relatively slow. For example, it has been estimated that it would take almost 60 years to sequence an entire human genome using Sanger-based sequencing [32]. Currently, it takes approximately 3 days to determine the *BRAF* mutational status of a melanoma specimen with this approach, and that specimen must harbor at least 20 % of the DNA with the mutant sequence. Therefore, this is not the ideal method to test specimens with only a small amount of tumor DNA present, such as may be obtained from a fine-needle aspiration biopsy.

During the clinical development of vemurafenib, a companion diagnostic test was also developed and ultimately approved by the FDA. This test is referred to as the cobas 4800 BRAF V600 Mutation Test®, and uses paraffin-embedded tissue samples and real-time polymerase chain reaction (RT-PCR) amplification of target DNA with a complementary primer pair and two oligonuleotide probes labeled with different fluorescent dyes: one probe to detect wild-type *BRAF* sequence and the other to detect the V600E mutation sequence. As compared to Sanger method, studies have shown that the cobas test has a lower assay failure rate and is more sensitive in the detection of V600E mutations [33, 34]. The detection rate of alternative V600 mutations is lower, however, with only 70 % of V600K mutations detected. Clinicians must take this fact into account, especially when testing tumors from elderly patients whose tumors are more likely to harbor these alternative mutations [29, 30]. Use of the cobas assay is mandated for participation in many clinical trials involving vemurafenib, particularly those sponsored by the drug's manufacturer.

The *BRAF* mutation test currently used by many academic centers uses pyrosequencing technology, targeting mutations in *BRAF* exon 15. Paraffin embedded tissue is sectioned and de-paraffinized. The tumor area in the section is outlined by a pathologist and the tumor area is micro-dissected and used for DNA extraction. The sequences to be analyzed are amplified using PCR and then sequenced using pyrosequencing. This test can detect a mutation with very low levels of mutated DNA in the tumor specimen. If there are 5 % or more mutant tumor cells in the specimen, the mutation will routinely be detected. This test covers over 95 % of known *BRAF* mutations with a specificity of 100 % during validation against the V600E results from a reference lab [35]. Overall, pyrosequencing is an accurate, sensitive method of detection of V600E, which also has increased sensitivity over cobas in detecting alternative V600 mutations.

At present, the choice of which test to use is often determined by availability more than any other factor. Many academic institutions are using pyrosequencing, in part because the need to know which specific mutation in V600 is present may be of significance for new drug development and clinical trials. However, given the widespread availability of the cobas 4800 BRAF V600 Mutation Test® that was approved along with vemurafenib, much of the oncologic community relies on this form of *BRAF* testing. Because this test is highly specific for detecting the V600E mutation, one can be confident with initiating BRAF inhibitor therapy based on a positive result for a mutation. However, clinicians must keep in mind that this test may not detect alternative mutations in the V600 codon with a high degree of sensitivity or specificity. Getting results quickly can also be very important when deciding which test to use; both cobas and pyrosequencing can have results to the provider in about 5 days, much shorter than traditional Sanger sequencing. Combined with the increased sensitivity of the other methods, this has led to decreased use of Sanger sequencing for the detection of *BRAF* mutations in melanoma patients.

In 2013, dabrafenib and trametinib were FDA approved as first-line therapies for *BRAF* mutant melanoma. This now adds to the choices available for *BRAF* targeted approaches. It is important to note that the phase III trials of dabrafenib (BREAK-3) and trametinib (METRIC) in metastatic melanoma utilized a different *BRAF* test than the cobas assay used for vemurafenib [26–28]. It is an allele-specific PCR assay developed by GSK collaborators (bioMeieux S.A.). This assay is now called the THxID™*BRAF* kit for use on the ABI 7500 Fast DX RT-PCR instrument and was approved by the FDA in May 2013 as a companion diagnostic for these *BRAF* targeted therapeutics. The THxID™*BRAF* assay specifically identifies *BRAF* V600E and V600K mutations, whereas the cobas assay was designed to identify the *BRAF* V600E mutation and is now known to incidentally detect other V600 mutations. With regards to the latter, the cobas test is reported as positive or negative result, which does not specifically tell if the mutation happens to be one of the less common non-V600E *BRAF* mutations. This begs the question of which diagnostic test to use for *BRAF* targeted therapies. Will clinicians need to use different tests for different drugs even if the target of the drug is the same? The logical answer is no at this time; however, the sensitivity and specificity of each test, as well as the cost and time to obtain a result, will need to be considered. From a practical standpoint, *BRAF* results from a CLIA-certified laboratory should be sufficient for treatment decisions. As routine genomic testing is expanded beyond *BRAF* in melanoma, tissue availability may also dictate the type of *BRAF* testing utilized, as single gene pyrosequencing will generally require less tumor DNA than more sophisticated platforms such as Sequonom®, SnapShot®, and Illumina®.

After deciding which test to use, the clinician also needs to decide which pathologic specimen to test. Most clinicians test the most recent pathology, which is often the biopsy specimen that confirmed the stage IV melanoma diagnosis. However, it is not infrequent that there is not enough tissue in the biopsy to test. Therefore one must decide whether to rebiopsy a metastasis or test previously obtained pathology specimens, such as the primary tumor or lymph node metastasis.

Similar rates of *BRAF* mutations are present in primary and metastatic melanomas, suggesting that *BRAF* mutations occur early and remain relatively consistently present though disease progression [36]. Colombino et al. also evaluated the prevalence and distribution of *BRAF* mutations in melanoma progression [37].

Two-hundred-ninety-one melanoma specimens were evaluated from 132 patients. Paired samples from primary melanomas and synchronous or asynchronous metastases from the same patients were evaluated. The concordance rate reported between mutation status of primary and metastatic lesions in 46 patients with paired samples was very high: 93 % of lymph node metastases, 96 % of visceral lesions, 80 % of brain metastases and 75 % of skin recurrences had identical mutation status as the primary tumor. When there was a discrepancy, it was primarily from the primary site being wild-type and the metastasis harboring a *BRAF* mutation, though isolated exceptions were noted.

This distribution of mutations can help a clinician determine the best specimen to test. Overall, given the high rate of concordance of metastatic lesions to primary, it is reasonable to test whatever tissue specimen is easiest to access. Therefore, re-biopsy for testing is not recommended routinely unless no other specimen is available. The concordance rate, however, is clearly not 100 %. There are clinical scenarios where clinicians must consider the possibility that a tumor with a negative *BRAF* mutation test might still harbor a treatment-sensitive mutation. In particular, given the relatively high prevalence of a *BRAF* V600E mutation in melanomas in young adults with a superficial spreading or nodular melanoma [30], if the initial testing in these cases comes back negative, retesting may be a reasonable way to proceed. Conversely, elderly patients whose initial testing was done with the cobas method may benefit from retesting using pyrosequencing or Sanger sequencing in view of the higher incidence of non-V600E mutations in melanomas in older patients.

Other methods of *BRAF* mutation testing are under development, including protein-based and serologic assays, which clinicians will likely encounter in the future. Several studies have now demonstrated that a monoclonal antibody directed against V600E BRAF protein (VE1) can identify the mutant protein in melanoma, epithelial ovarian tumors, and papillary thyroid carcinomas [38–40]. While immunohistochemical detection of BRAF mutations would simplify diagnostic testing, the reliability of the VE1 antibody compared to standard techniques, such as PCR-based assays and pyrosequencing, has not yet been definitively determined. Even if it is as accurate for detecting V600E mutations, there would still be a need for further testing of other *BRAF* mutations that are sensitive to BRAF inhibitor therapy.

Also promising is the ability to detect mutant BRAF in serologic assays by techniques involving circulating melanoma cells and free DNA. Using a technique called BEAMing technology, baseline *BRAF* V600E and V600K mutations were assayed in plasma samples from 91 patients on the phase II study of dabrafenib (BREAK-2) [41]. There was an overall agreement of 83 % and 96 % between plasma and tumor *BRAF* V600E and V600K results, respectively. Also, higher circulating free DNA levels of *BRAF*

V600E fraction were associated with greater tumor burden, lower overall response rate, and shorter progression-free survival. Another method, capable of detecting as little as one *BRAF* V600E mutant melanoma cell in 400,000 peripheral blood lymphocytes using a proprietary assay of DNA amplification and restriction endonuclease cleavage, has been developed [42]. Interestingly, serologic *BRAF* V600E levels correlated to BRAF inhibitor response and predicted therapeutic failure at least 4 weeks in advance of clinical or radiographic progression. Although these strategies for *BRAF* mutations are not ready for routine clinical use, these may become important techniques available to clinicians in the future for identify melanoma patients with *BRAF* mutations and for monitoring treatment responses.

Finally, even in patients who are not candidates for BRAF inhibitor therapy, knowledge of the *BRAF* mutation status may provide important prognostic information. At present, several studies of the prognostic significance of *BRAF* mutation have been published [29, 43–45]. This topic is addressed further in a later chapter.

6.2 Alternative Mutations: NRAS, CKIT, GNQA/GNA11

Alternative mutations that are found in melanoma, such as *NRAS*, *CKIT*, and *GNQA/GNA11*, are not routinely tested for as there are no approved agents in melanoma that directly target these genetic alterations. However, trials of agents that block these pathways are available and therefore testing is becoming increasing more important in making therapeutic decisions for patients. Mutations in these genes are almost always mutually exclusive, meaning that a tumor does not harbor both an *NRAS* and a *BRAF* mutation or both an *NRAS* and *CKIT* mutation [25].

NRAS mutations are present in approximately 20 % of tumors from melanoma patients and mostly occur within exon 1 (codon 12) and exon 2 (codon 61) [46]. *NRAS* mutation status has been associated with older age and mucosal melanomas as well as thicker tumors with high mitotic rates [47, 48]. Given the lack of approved direct therapeutic options for subjects harboring the *NRAS* mutation, routine testing in patients with metastatic melanoma is not recommended. However, patients whose tumors are *BRAF* wild-type can consider *NRAS* testing on a clinical trial.

6.3 CKIT Mutations

CKIT amplifications and mutations are seen in an even smaller portion of cases, about 2–3 % of all melanomas but perhaps as many as 10–30 % of acral-letiginous and mucosal melanomas [49]. Chronic-sun damaged cutaneous melanoma may also have a higher incidence of *CKIT* aberrations. Imatinib is a multi-tyrosine kinase inhibitor, approved for chronic myelogenous leukemia, which has now been studied as a CKIT inhibitor in metastatic melanoma patients whose disease harbors *CKIT* amplifications and/or mutations [50, 51]. While *CKIT* amplification does increase pathway signaling, activating mutations in exon 11 and 13 of the

CKIT gene better predict for clinical response to imatinib. In three phase II trials of imatinib in metastatic melanoma with *CKIT* aberrations, a response rate of 35–54 % was seen in patients with exon 11 or 13 *CKIT* mutant melanoma whereas limited benefit was observed in patients with *CKIT* amplifications or other mutations [52–55]. Very low responses rates are seen in unselected melanoma populations given CKIT inhibitors [56]. Therefore, *CKIT* testing should entail sequencing of exon 11 and 13. Given the limited options for this population of patients, off-label treatment with these agents is often considered. For this reason, it is reasonable to test mucosal and acral-letiginous melanomas for *CKIT* mutations, particularly in the absence of an activating *BRAF* mutation. As *CKIT* profiling is not routinely available at most institutions and sendout testing may take up to 4–6 weeks, we would not recommend withholding other therapeutic options while awaiting results. Also, we would not recommend routine testing for *CKIT* mutations in cutaneous (non-chronic sun damaged) or uveal melanoma.

6.4 GNAQ and GNA11 Mutations

GNAQ and *GNA11* mutations are found primarily in uveal melanomas, with almost 80 % of uveal melanomas harboring one of these mutations [57, 58]. Uveal melanomas have not been found to harbor the *BRAF* mutation commonly seen in cutaneous primaries. However, *BRAF* mutations have been identified in 27–58% of conjunctival melanomas [59]. While direct targeting of GNAQ or GNA11 has not been possible, activating mutations in these G-proteins are known to signal through the MAPK pathway [60]. There is now interest in developing MEK inhibitors as targeted therapy for *GNAQ* and *GNA11* mutant melanoma. Indeed, a randomized phase II trial of the MEK inhibitor selumetinib, compared to temozolomide, demonstrated clinical benefit in uveal melanoma patients [61]. However, there is no FDA-approved agent specifically for *GNAQ/GNA11* mutant melanoma, which largely relegates this genotyping to clinical trial purposes at the present time.

Other important genetic alterations have been identified in uveal melanoma. These include germline mutations in the BRCA1-Associated Protein (*BAP-1*) gene, which predispose individuals to more aggressive uveal melanomas [62–64]. Familial BAP-1 syndromes have recently been characterized as well. Though currently this is an area of research interest only, one can perceive testing individuals with uveal melanoma for prognostic purposes in the near future. There is also new data risk stratifying patients with resected uveal melanoma based on a 15-gene expression profile (GEP) [65]. This divides patients into two subgroups: class 1 (low metastatic risk) and class 2 (high metastatic risk). The GEP class modeling demonstrated clear prognostic significance, independent of other factors such as TMN staging and chromosome 3 loss [65]. This test is now available for clinical use under the name Decision DX-UM by Castle Biosciences.

7 Biomarkers for Immunotherapy

Melanoma has been long regarded as an immunogenic malignancy based on tumor infiltration of lymphocytes, spontaneous regression of tumors, and the identification of T cell reactivity against a variety of melanoma antigens [66]. Over the years, multiple immune-based therapeutic strategies have been investigated with clinical and immunologic responses seen in patients treated with interleukin-2 (IL-2) [67], ipilimumab [68], and more recently, anti-programmed cell death-1 (anti-PD1) therapy [69]. While some patients will achieve durable remission with immunotherapy, a majority of melanoma patients do not experience regression in their disease. A biomarker that can predict response to immunotherapy is a much needed tool for medical oncologists to help guide treatment decisions for their patients.

While there are no approved immunotherapy biomarker tests to aid in patient care for melanoma, studies have shown that several serologic and tumor profiles are associated with patient outcomes. Tumor-infiltrating lymphocytes (TIL) are a biomarker of outcome in primary melanoma (see above). To date, no data have shown a clear association between TIL in metastatic melanomas and therapeutic response or long-term outcome. TIL have been used experimentally, however, for adoptive cell therapy, in which tumors are harvested for ex vivo TIL expansion then reinfused with subsequent IL-2 after non-myeloablative lymphodepleting chemotherapy [70, 71]. Recently, organized collections of TIL with architecture recapitulating the structure of lymph nodes ("ectopic" lymph nodes) have been recognized in tumors [72], and a chemokine gene expression signature predicted the presence of these structures in metastatic melanoma deposits and may potentially represent a selection marker for tumors more likely to respond to immunotherapy [73].

Retrospective studies of patients treated with IL-2 have demonstrated associations between clinical outcomes and both serum interleukin-6 level and tumor *NRAS* status. Pretreatment interleukin-6 levels were elevated in 43 % of metastatic melanoma patients prior to IL-2 based therapy, which was associated with shorter overall survival compared to patients with normal interleukin-6 levels (median 4.5 months vs. 10.8 months, $P < 0.0002$) [74]. In another study of 208 patients treated with high-dose IL-2, the response rate for patients with *NRAS* mutant melanoma was 47 % as compared to 23 % and 12 % seen in patients with *BRAF* mutant and wild-type melanoma, respectively [75]. Progression-free and overall survival also favored patients with *NRAS* mutant melanoma. It remains unclear if interleukin-6 or *NRAS* genotype will be associated with responses to ipilimumab or anti-PD1 therapy. Of note, a retrospective analysis of *BRAF* V600E status on 80 patients treated with ipilimumab on the CA184004 phase II trial showed no difference in disease control rates between patients with *BRAF* V600E mutant and *BRAF* wild-type tumors [76]. Both interleukin-6 and *NRAS* mutational status will need to be analyzed prospectively in immunotherapy trials to confirm their roles as biomarkers.

One of the more recent promising immunotherapy strategies in melanoma is targeting PD1 on regulatory T cells and PD-ligand-1 (PD-L1). PD1 is a co-inhibitor receptor on regulatory T cells that interacts with PDL1, which is expressed by various immune and malignant cells, including 14–40 % of metastatic melanoma tumors [77]. Preclinical models have shown that PD1/PD-L1 interaction leads to immune evasion by the tumor cells, which can be reversed by blocking either PD1 or PD-L1 [78, 79]. The phase I data for anti-PD1 and anti-PD-L1 monoclonal antibodies has shown impressive immunologic responses and objective tumor responses in melanoma patients ranging from 17 % to 38 % [69, 80–82]. Investigators are now exploring whether assaying PD-L1 by immunohistochemistry will serve as a predictive biomarker for this class of therapy. Interestingly, data from the anti-PD1 study of nivolumab has shown that 16 out of 25 patients with positive tumor PD-L1 expression experienced an objective response while none of the 17 patients with negative tumor PD-L1 expression responded to therapy [69]. Other studies have also shown higher response rates with patients whose tumors express PD-L1 by immunohistochemistry [82]. However, patients with no PD-L1 expression on their melanoma have also demonstrated objective responses to anti-PD1 therapy. As many melanoma patients are now enrolling on anti-PD1 and anti-PD-L1 clinical trials, it will be important to continue assessing PD-L1, as well as other biomarkers, which may help with patient decisions in the future.

8 Adjuvant Interferon

While the past few years have seen major advances in the management of advanced metastatic melanoma, there is also reason to be optimistic about the future of adjuvant therapy for this disease. Improved biomarkers of prognosis, including genomic or other biomarkers to identify and quantitate metastatic potential and/or the presence of residual tumor cells after surgery, would allow avoidance of treatment toxicity for patients who were cured by surgery alone and focus attention on the patients who stand to gain most from adjuvant therapy. Biomarkers could also help identify those patients most likely to respond (or be resistant) to therapy, allowing those least likely to respond to "standard" treatment to be entered directly into clinical trials [83]. One relevant example is the identification of single nucleotide polymorphisms in the interleukin-28 gene that may predict interferon sensitivity or resistance in viral hepatitis [84]. Finally, immunologic therapies that can eliminate cells bearing specific antigens may find an increasingly important role in adjuvant therapy, leading to increased reliance on biomarkers to identify appropriate candidates [85]. Two forms of interferon-alfa have been approved for the adjuvant therapy of node-positive melanoma, high-dose native interferon-alfa for 1 year [86] and pegylated interferon-alfa for 5 years [87]. It has been proposed that primary tumor ulceration may be a powerful biomarker for sensitivity to interferon [88], particularly in patients with sentinel node metastases [89]. This provocative observation merits further validation in prospective clinical trials.

9 Conclusions

In this exciting era of a personalized approach to the management of melanoma patients, oncologists will need to be knowledgeable of the evolving role of melanoma-specific biomarkers. Already, metastatic melanoma patients are categorized into two genetically defined groups: *BRAF* mutant and *BRAF* wild-type. Moreover, the groundwork is being laid for a broader landscape of biomarkers that may ultimately establish a more complex patient classification based on understanding tumor genotype and signaling pathway aberrations combined with host immune response factors. This will not be simple: the roles of evolving tumor biology during disease progression and treatment will have to be taken into account. Furthermore, intratumoral heterogeneity exists in melanoma, and may need to be incorporated into treatment decisions in ways that are as yet unknown. But by tackling these challenges, we have every reason to expect that we can greatly enrich the quality and the length of the lives of our melanoma patients.

References

1. Clark WH Jr, From L, Bernadino EA et al (1969) The histogenesis and biologic behavior of primary human malignant melanomas of the skin. Cancer Res 29:705–727
2. Breslow A (1970) Thickness, cross-sectional area and depth of invasion in the prognosis of cutaneous melanoma. Ann Surg 172:902–908
3. Balch CM, Murad TM, Soong S-J et al (1978) A multifactorial analysis of melanoma: prognostic histopathological features comparing Clark's and Breslow's staging methods. Ann Surg 188:732–742
4. Morton DL, Wen DR, Wong JH et al (1992) Technical details of intraoperative lymphatic mapping for early stage melanoma. Arch Surg 127:392–399
5. Morton DL, Thompson JF, Cochran AJ et al (2006) Sentinel-node biopsy or nodal observation in melanoma. N Engl J Med 355: 1307–1317
6. Azzola MF, Shaw HM, Thompson JF et al (2003) Tumor mitotic rate is a more powerful prognostic indicator than ulceration in patients with primary cutaneous melanoma: an analysis of 3661 patients from a single center. Cancer 97:1488–1498
7. Sondak VK, Taylor JM, Sabel MS et al (2004) Mitotic rate and younger age are predictors of sentinel lymph node positivity: lessons learned from the generation of a probabilistic model. Ann Surg Oncol 11:247–258
8. Thompson JF, Soong S-J, Balch CM et al (2011) Prognostic significance of mitotic rate in localized primary cutaneous melanoma: an analysis of patients in the multi-institutional American Joint Committee on Cancer melanoma staging database. J Clin Oncol 29: 2137–2141
9. Casper DJ, Ross KI, Messina JL et al (2010) Use of anti-phosphohistone H3 immunohisto-

chemistry to determine mitotic rate in thin melanoma. Am J Dermatopathol 32:650–654
10. Schimming TT, Grabellus F, Roner M et al (2012) pHH3 immunostaining improves interobserver agreement of mitotic index in thin melanomas. Am J Dermatopathol 34: 266–269
11. Ladstein RG, Bachmann IM, Straume O et al (2012) Prognostic importance of the mitotic marker phosphohistone H3 in cutaneous nodular melanoma. J Invest Dermatol 132: 1247–1252
12. Clemente CG, Mihm MC Jr, Bufalino R et al (1996) Prognostic value of tumor infiltrating lymphocytes in the vertical growth phase of primary cutaneous melanoma. Cancer 77: 1303–1310
13. Tuthill RJ, Unger JM, Liu PY et al (2002) Risk assessment in localized primary cutaneous melanoma: a Southwest Oncology Group study evaluating nine factors and a test of the Clark logistic regression prediction model. Am J Clin Pathol 118:504–511
14. Zedek DC, McCalmont TH (2011) Spitz nevi, atypical spitzoid neoplasms, and spitzoid melanoma. Clin Lab Med 31:311–320
15. Zembowicz A, Yang SE, Kafanas A et al (2012) Correlation between histologic assessment and fluorescence in situ hybridization using MelanoSITE in evaluation of histologically ambiguous melanocytic lesions. Arch Pathol Lab Med 136:1571–1579
16. Zimmermann AK, Hirschmann A, Pfeiffer D et al (2010) FISH analysis for diagnostic evaluation of challenging melanocytic lesions. Histol Histopathol 25:1139–1147
17. Moore SR, Persons DL, Sosman JA et al (2008) Detection of copy number alterations in metastatic melanoma by a DNA fluorescence in situ hybridization probe panel and array comparative genomic hybridization: a Southwest Oncology Group study (S9431). Clin Cancer Res 14:2927–2935
18. Scolyer RA, Murali R, McCarthy SW et al (2010) Histologically ambiguous ("borderline") primary cutaneous melanocytic tumors: approaches to patient management including the roles of molecular testing and sentinel lymph node biopsy. Arch Pathol Lab Med 134:1770–1777
19. Ali L, Helm T, Cheney R et al (2010) Correlating array comparative genomic hybridization findings with histology and outcome in spitzoid melanocytic neoplasms. Int J Clin Exp Pathol 3:593–599
20. de Waal AC, Aben KK, van Rossum MM et al (2012) Melanoma of unknown primary origin: a population-based study in the Netherlands. Eur J Cancer 49:676–683
21. Lyle PL, Amato CM, Fitzpatrick JE et al (2008) Gastrointestinal melanoma or clear cell sarcoma? Molecular evaluation of 7 cases previously diagnosed as malignant melanoma. Am J Surg Pathol 32:858–866
22. Yang L, Chen Y, Cui T et al (2012) Identification of biomarkers to distinguish clear cell sarcoma from malignant melanoma. Hum Pathol 43:1463–1470
23. Dutton-Regester K, Kakavand H, Aoude L et al (2013) Melanomas of unknown primary have a mutational profile consistent with cutaneous sun exposed melanoma. Pigment Cell Melanoma Res 26:852–860
24. Davies H, Bignell GR, Cox C et al (2002) Mutations of the BRAF gene in human cancer. Nature 417:949–954
25. Curtin JA, Fridlyand J, Kageshita T et al (2005) Distinct sets of genetic alterations in melanoma. N Engl J Med 353:2135–2147
26. Chapman PB, Hauschild A, Robert C et al (2011) Improved survival with vemurafenib in melanoma with BRAF V600E mutation. N Engl J Med 364:2507–2516
27. Hauschild A, Grob JJ, Demidov LV et al (2012) Dabrafenib in BRAF-mutated metastatic melanoma: a multicentre, open-label, phase 3 randomised controlled trial. Lancet 380:358–365
28. Flaherty KT, Robert C, Heresy P et al (2012) Improved survival with MEK inhibition in BRAF-mutated melanoma. N Engl J Med 372:107–114
29. Long GV, Menzies AM, Nagrial AM et al (2011) Prognostic and clinicopathologic associations of oncogenic BRAF in metastatic melanoma. J Clin Oncol 29:1239–1246
30. Menzies AM, Haydu LE, Visintin L et al (2012) Distinguishing clinicopathologic features of patients with V600E and V600K BRAF-mutant metastatic melanoma. Clin Cancer Res 18:3242–3249
31. Sanger F, Nicklen S, Coulson AR (1977) DNA sequencing with chain-terminating inhibitors. Proc Natl Acad Sci U S A 74:5463–5467
32. Hert DG, Fredlake CP, Barron AE (2008) Advantages and limitations of next-generation sequencing technologies: a comparison of electrophoresis and non-electrophoresis methods. Electorphoresis 29:4618–4626
33. Anderson S, Bloom KJ, Vallera DU et al (2012) Multisite analytic performance studies of a real-time polymerase chain reaction assay for the detection of BRAF V600E mutations in formalin-fixed, paraffin-embedded tissue specimens of malignant melanoma. Arch Pathol Lab Med 136:1385–1391
34. Halait H, Demartin K, Shah S et al (2012) Analytical performance of a real-time PCR-based assay for V600 mutations in the BRAF gene, used as the companion diagnostic test for the novel BRAF inhibitor vemurafenib in metastatic melanoma. Diagn Mol Pathol 21:1–8

35. Spittle C, Ward MR, Nathanson KL et al (2007) Application of a BRAF pyrosequencing assay for mutation detection and copy number analysis in malignant melanoma. J Mol Diagn 9:464–471
36. Casula M, Colombino M, Satta MP et al (2004) BRAF gene is somatically mutated but does not make a major contribution to malignant melanoma susceptibility: the Italian Melanoma Intergroup Study. J Clin Oncol 22:282–292
37. Colombino M, Capone M, Lissia A et al (2012) BRAF/NRAS mutation frequencies among primary tumors and metastases in patients with melanoma. J Clin Oncol 30:2522–2529
38. Long GV, Wilmott JS, Capper D et al (2013) Immunohistochemistry is highly sensitive and specific for the detection of V600E BRAF mutation in melanoma. Am J Surg Pathol 37:61–65
39. Capper D, Preusser M, Habel A et al (2011) Assessment of BRAF V600E mutation status by immunohistochemistry with a mutation-specific monoclonal antibody. Acta Neuropathol 122: 11–19
40. Koperek O, Kornauth C, Capper D et al (2012) Immunohistochemical detection of the BRAF V600E-mutated protein in papillary thyroid carcinoma. Am J Surg Pathol 36:844–850
41. Long GV, Trefzer U, Davies MA et al (2012) Dabrafenib in patients with Val600Glu or Val600Lys BRAF-mutant melanoma metastatic to the brain (BREAK-MB): a multicentre, open-label, phase 2 trial. Lancet Oncol 13:1087–1095
42. Panka DJ, Sullivan RJ, Mier JW (2010) An inexpensive, specific and highly sensitive protocol to detect the BrafV600E mutation in melanoma tumor biopsies and blood. Melanoma Res 20:401–407
43. Bucheit AD, Suklawer E, Jakob JA et al (2013) Clinical characteristics and outcomes with specific BRAF and NRAS mutations in patients with metastatic melanoma. Cancer 119:3821–3829
44. Moreau S, Saiag P, Aegerter P et al (2012) Prognostic value of BRAF V600 mutations in melanoma patients after resection of metastatic lymph nodes. Ann Surg Oncol 19:4314–4321
45. Ardekani GS, Jafarnejad SM, Tan L et al (2012) The prognostic value of *BRAF* mutation in colorectal cancer and melanoma: a systematic review and meta-analysis. PLoS One 7:e47054
46. Lee JH, Choi JW, Kim YS (2011) Frequencies of BRAF and NRAS mutations are different in histological types and sites of origin of cutaneous melanoma: a meta-analysis. Br J Dermatol 164:776–784
47. Jakob JA, Bassett RL Jr, Ng CS et al (2012) NRAS mutation status is an independent prognostic factor in metastatic melanoma. Cancer 118:4014–4023
48. Kelleher FC, McArthur GA (2012) Targeting NRAS in melanoma. Cancer J 18:132–136
49. Davies MA, Samuels Y (2010) Analysis of the genome to personalize therapy for melanoma. Oncogene 29:5545–5555
50. Hodi FS, Friedlander P, Corless CL et al (2008) Major response to imatinib mesylate in KIT-mutated melanoma. J Clin Oncol 26:2046–2051
51. Lyle M, Long G (2013) Diagnosis and treatment of KIT-mutant metastatic melanoma. J Clin Oncol 31:3176–3181
52. Carvajal RD (2013) Another option in our KIT of effective therapies for advanced melanoma. J Clin Oncol 26:3173–3175
53. Guo J, Si L, Kong Y et al (2011) Phase II, open-label, single-arm trial of imatinib mesylate in patients with metastatic melanoma harboring c-Kit mutation or amplification. J Clin Oncol 29:2904–2909
54. Carjaval RD, Antonescu CR, Wolchok JD et al (2011) KIT as a therapeutic target in metastatic melanoma. JAMA 305:2327–2334
55. Hodi FS, Corless CL, Giobbie-Hurder A et al (2013) Imatinib for melanomas harboring mutationally activated or amplified KIT arising on mucosal, acral, and chronically sun-damage skin. J Clin Oncol 26:3182–3190
56. Handolias D, Hamilton AL, Salemi R et al (2010) Clinical responses observed with imatinib or sorafenib in melanoma patients expressing mutations in KIT. Br J Cancer 102: 1219–1223
57. Van Raamsdonk CD, Bezrookove V, Green G et al (2009) Frequent somatic mutations of GNAQ in uveal melanoma and blue naevi. Nature 457:599–602
58. Van Raamsdonk CD, Griewank KG, Crosby MB et al (2010) Mutations in GNA11 in uveal melanoma. N Engl J Med 363:2191–2199
59. Weber JL, Smalley KS, Sondak VK et al (2013) Conjunctival melanomas harbor BRAF and NRAS mutations—Letter. Clin Cancer Res, epub ahead of print.
60. Patel M, Smyth E, Chapman PB et al (2011) Therapeutic implications of emerging molecular biology of uveal melanoma. Clin Cancer Res 17:2087–2100
61. Carvajal RD, Sosman JA, Quevedo F et al (2013) Phase II study of selumetinib (sel) versus temozolomide (TMZ) in Gnaq/Gna11(Gq/11) mutant (mut) uveal melanoma (UM). J Clin Oncol; Abs 9003
62. Abdel-Rahman MH, Pilarski R, Cebulla CM et al (2011) Germline BAP1 mutation predisposes to uveal melanoma, lung adenocarcinoma, meningioma, and other cancers. J Med Genet 48:856–859
63. Wiesner T, Obenauf AC, Murali R et al (2011) Germline mutations in BPA1 predispose to melanocytic tumors. Nat Genet 43:1018–1021

64. Njauw CJ, Kim I, Piris A et al (2012) Germline BAP1 inactivation is preferentially associated with metastatic ocular melanoma and cutaneous-ocular melanoma families. PLoS ONE 7:e35295
65. Oken MD, Worley LA, Char DH et al (2012) Collaborative Ocular Oncology Group Report No. 1: Prospective validation of a multi-gene prognostic assay in uveal melanoma. Ophthalmology 119:1596–1603
66. Weber J (2011) Immunotherapy for melanoma. Curr Opin Oncol 23:163–169
67. Keilholz U, Conradt C, Legha SS et al (1998) Results of interleukin-2-based treatment in advanced melanoma: a case record-based analysis of 631 patients. J Clin Oncol 16:2921–2929
68. Hodi FS, O'Day SJ, McDermott DF et al (2010) Improved survival with ipilimumab in patients with metastatic melanoma. N Engl J Med 363:711–723
69. Topalian SL, Hodi FS, Brahmer JR et al (2012) Safety, activity, and immune correlates of anti-PD-1 antibody in cancer. N Engl J Med 366:2443–2454
70. Rosenberg SA, Yang JC, Sherry RM et al (2011) Durable complete responses in heavily pretreated patients with metastatic melanoma using T-cell transfer immunotherapy. Clin Cancer Res 17:4550–4557
71. Pilon-Thomas S, Kuhn L, Ellwanger S et al (2012) Efficacy of adoptive cell transfer of tumor-infiltrating lymphocytes after lymphopenia induction for metastatic melanoma. J Immunother 35:615–620
72. Coppola D, Nebozhyn M, Khalil F et al (2011) Unique ectopic lymph node-like structures present in human primary colorectal carcinoma are identified by immune gene array profiling. Am J Pathol 179:37–45
73. Messina JL, Fenstermacher DA, Eschrich S et al (2012) 12-chemokine gene signature identifies lymph node-like structures in melanoma:potential for patient selection for immunotherapy? Sci Rep 2:765
74. Hoejberg L, Bastholt L, Johansen JS et al (2012) Serum interleukin-6 as a prognostic biomarker in patients with metastatic melanoma. Melanoma Res 22:287–293
75. Joseph RW, Sullivan RJ, Harrell R et al (2012) Correlation of NRAS mutations with clinical response to high-dose IL-2 in patients with advanced melanoma. J Immunother 35:66–72
76. Shahabi V, Whitney G, Hamid O et al (2012) Assessment of association between BRAF-V600E mutation status in melanomas and clinical response to ipilimumab. Cancer Immunol Immunother 61:733–777
77. Gadiot J, Hooijkaas AI, Kaiser AD et al (2012) Overall survival and PD-L1 expression in metastasized malignant melanoma. Cancer 117:2192–2201
78. Dong H, Strome SE, Salomao DR et al (2002) Tumor-associated B7-H1 promotes T-cell apoptosis: a potential mechanism of immune evasion. Nat Med 8:793–800
79. Iwai Y, Ishida M, Tanaka Y et al (2002) Involvement of PD-L1 on tumor cells in the escape from host immune system and tumor immunotherapy by PD-L1 blockade. Proc Natl Acad Sci USA 99:12293–12297
80. Brahmer JR, Tykodi SS, Chow LQ et al (2012) Safety and activity of anti-PD-L1 antibody in patients with advanced cancer. N Engl J Med 366:2455–2465
81. Hamid O, Robert C, Daud A et al (2013) Safety and tumor responses with lambrolizumab (anti-PD-1) in melanoma. N Engl J Med 369:134–144
82. Weber JS, Kudchadkar RR, Gibney GT et al (2013) Safety, efficacy, and biomarkers of nivolumab With vaccine in ipilimumab-refractory or -naive melanoma. J Clin Oncol, epub ahead of print.
83. Kirkwood JM, Tarhini AA (2009) Biomarkers of therapeutic response in melanoma and renal cell carcinoma: potential inroads to improved immunotherapy. J Clin Oncol 27:2583–2585
84. Pearlman BL (2011) The IL-28 genotype: how it will affect the care of patients with hepatitis C virus infection. Curr Gastroenterol Rep 13:78–86
85. Peled N, Oton AB, Hirsch FR et al (2009) MAGE A3 antigen-specific cancer immunotherapeutic. Immunotherapy 1:19–25
86. Kirkwood JM, Sondak VK, Hersey P et al (2009) Adjuvant systemic therapy for high-risk melanoma patients. In: Balch CM, Houghton AN, Sober AJ, Soong S-J, Atkins MB, Thompson JF (eds) Cutaneous melanoma, 5th edn. Quality Medical Publishing, St Louis, MO, pp 669–692
87. Eggermont AM, Suciu S, Santinami M et al (2008) Adjuvant therapy with pegylated interferon alfa-2b versus observation alone in resected stage III melanoma: final results of EORTC 18991, a randomized phase III trial. Lancet 372:117–126
88. Eggermont AM, Suciu S, Testori A et al (2012) Ulceration and stage are predictive of interferon efficacy in melanoma: results of the phase III adjuvant trials EORTC 18952 and EORTC 18991. Eur J Cancer 48:218–225
89. Eggermont AM, Suciu S, Testori A et al (2012) Long-term results of the randomized phase III trial EORTC 18991 of adjuvant therapy with pegylated interferon alfa-2b versus observation in resected stage III melanoma. J Clin Oncol 30:3810–3818

Part II

Biomarkers for Prediction of Response and Resistance to Treatment

Chapter 4

Advances in Adjuvant Therapy: Potential for Prognostic and Predictive Biomarkers

Diwakar Davar, Ahmad A. Tarhini, Helen Gogas, and John M. Kirkwood

Abstract

Melanoma is the third most common skin cancer but accounts for the majority of skin cancer-related mortality. The rapidly rising incidence and younger age at diagnosis has made melanoma a leading cause of lost productive years of life and has increased the urgency of finding improved adjuvant therapy for melanoma. Interferon-α was approved for the adjuvant treatment of resected high-risk melanoma following studies that demonstrated improvements in relapse-free survival and overall survival that were commenced nearly 30 years ago. The clinical benefits associated with this agent have been consistently observed across multiple studies and meta-analyses in terms of relapse rate, and to a smaller and less-consistent degree, mortality. However, significant toxicity and lack of prognostic and/or predictive biomarkers that would allow greater risk–benefit ratio have limited the more widespread adoption of this modality.

Recent success with targeted agents directed against components of the MAP-kinase pathway and checkpoint inhibitors have transformed the treatment landscape in metastatic disease. Current research efforts are centered around discovering predictive/prognostic biomarkers and exploring the options for more effective regimens, either singly or in combination.

Key words Melanoma, Adjuvant, Interferon, IFN-α, CTLA-4, Ipilimumab, BRAF, Vemurafenib, Debrafenib, MEK, Trametinib

1 Introduction

In 2012 alone, invasive melanoma accounted for approximately 76,180 new cases and 9,250 deaths in the USA alone according to US Surveillance, Epidemiology, and End Results (SEER) registry estimates [1]. The increasing incidence of this disease, tripling the rate observed in the Caucasian population over the last two decades, adds national and international importance to this most lethal of all cancers of the skin, the largest organ of the human body.

When discovered early, definitive surgical resection is often curative for melanoma. However, patients with advanced disease (>stage IIB) are at increased risk of recurrence and death. Adjuvant interferon-α (IFN-α), originally licensed by the US Food and Drug

Magdalena Thurin and Francesco M. Marincola (eds.), *Molecular Diagnostics for Melanoma: Methods and Protocols*, Methods in Molecular Biology, vol. 1102, DOI 10.1007/978-1-62703-727-3_4, © Springer Science+Business Media New York 2014

Administration (US FDA) on the basis of a low but reproducible reduction in risk of relapse, has been the mainstay of adjuvant therapy in high-risk disease for the preceding two decades.

Following early experiments that suggested broad anti-tumor effects in various laboratory models through a variety of potential mechanisms, multiple international and US Intergroup trials were conducted that tested various doses and schedules to derive maximal therapeutic benefit. High-dose interferon (HDI) comprising an induction phase (20 MU/m^2 daily for 5 days per week for 4 weeks) followed by a subcutaneous maintenance phase (10 MU/m^2 for 48 weeks) has reliably and reproducibly demonstrated improvement in relapse-free survival (RFS) and, to a lesser extent, overall survival (OS) in patients with high-risk cutaneous melanoma [2]. European trials studying the pegylated form of interferon (peg IFN-α) have shown improvement in RFS although, unlike the experience with HDI, no impact upon overall survival (OS) has been observed.

The advances of the past decade have elucidated some of the molecular underpinnings and elements of host immunological response to melanoma and have resulted in transformational new therapies targeting the MAP kinase signaling pathway (RAS/RAF/MEK/ERK) and immune checkpoints (CTLA-4, PD-1). The BRAF inhibitor vemurafenib and the CTLA-4 blocking antibody ipilimumab have independently demonstrated survival benefits in phase III trials leading to regulatory approval for these new treatment options in the setting of advanced disease. However, their potential role in the adjuvant and neo-adjuvant arenas remains a topic of ongoing investigation.

This chapter will focus on the indications for adjuvant therapy, current management of high-risk resected melanoma, ongoing adjuvant and neo-adjuvant trials and the development of prognostic and predictive biomarkers in this arena.

1.1 Indications for Adjuvant Therapy

Adjuvant therapy is indicated in patients whose risk of recurrence following definitive surgery remains high, and is pursued with the intent of treating micro-metastatic disease and thereby reducing the risk of local and distant relapse. As not all patients have the same risk, and among those at risk, not all may benefit from adjuvant systemic therapy, the decision to pursue adjuvant therapy requires assessment of an individual patient's risk for recurrence and fractional likelihood of reducing risks of recurrence or mortality, weighed against the risks and the costs of treatment.

A number of independent prognostic factors have been identified based on analysis of data obtained from patients compiled in the American Joint Committee on Cancer (AJCC) Melanoma Staging Database and these form the basis of the revised 2009 AJCC staging manual for melanoma [3]. These include:

- *Primary tumor thickness*—single greatest predictor of recurrence and survival which are directly commensurate to thickness measured in millimeters.
- *Ulceration*—adversely affects survival at every T sub-stage such that ulceration in any given T level is associated with a similar risk of death and relapse as the next higher non-ulcerated T level (i.e. T2b–T3a).
- *Mitotic rate*—defined as the number of mitoses per square millimeter in the primary tumor with the threshold of significance being $1/mm^2$. High mitotic rate connotes a more aggressive phenotype and being the second most powerful predictor of survival after tumor thickness is strongly associated with adverse outcomes. In sub-mm lesions (T1), mitotic rate separates T1a (non-ulcerated T1 melanomas with a mitotic rate of less than $1/mm^2$) from T1b lesions (ulcerated T1 melanomas with a mitotic rate of greater than $1/mm^2$).
- *Lymph node burden*—risk of lymph node involvement increases with tumor thickness by approximately 2–5 % for Breslow's depth ≤1.00 mm and reaches 34 % for T4 lesions [3]. Survival decreases commensurate with increasing lymph node tumor burden—5 year survival rates for stage IIIA, IIIB, and IIIC disease ranging from 78 % to 59 % and 40 % respectively. The importance of accurate assessment of lymph node involvement was underscored by two changes in AJCC 7th edition staging system: (a) use of immunohistochemistry to define nodal disease rather than hematoxylin and eosin (H&E) staining alone, and (b) inclusion of micro-metastases (0.1–1.0 mm) in addition to macro-metastases (>1.0 mm) in defining lymph node involvement. However, patients with sub-micrometastases (<0.1 mm) tend to perform similarly as patients with sentinel lymph node (SLN) negative disease [4].
- *Systemic burden of disease—number* of metastatic sites and *sites* of distant metastases are important prognostic factors. Patients with distant skin, subcutaneous, and lymph node metastases (M1a) disease, pulmonary metastases (M1b), and extrapulmonary visceral metastases (M1c) have 1-year survival rates of 62 %, 53 % and 33 % respectively. Patients with elevated *serum lactate dehydrogenase (LDH) enzyme level* perform as poorly as patients with non-lung visceral metastases suggesting that elevated LDH levels are a marker of a more aggressive phenotype.

Although the majority of patients present with early stage disease (stage I) in which surgery alone is largely curative, a significant number present with intermediate-risk (stage IIA) and high-risk (stages IIB–IIIC) disease in which the risk of recurrence ranges from 30 % to 80 %. Adjuvant therapy with HDI or enrollment in a clinical trial is currently indicated for patients who present with high-risk disease whose risk of recurrence exceeds 30 %.

1.2 Current Management of High-Risk Resected Melanoma

The past several years have seen evaluation both in randomized and in nonrandomized trials of multiple agents without clear advances. These trials have evaluated agents including nonspecific immune stimulants (BCG, levamisole), cytokines (IFN-α, IL-2), single-agent and combination chemotherapeutics [dacarbazine; cisplatin, vinblastine, and dacarbazine (CVD); lomustine (CCNU)], and hormonal agents like megestrol acetate.

Early trials suggested similar antitumor response rates for immunomodulators and single-agent chemotherapy in metastatic disease (~13–24 %)—but the long-term durable responses observed in a third of patients responding to immunotherapies such as IFN-α sparked the broader clinical investigation of this agent in the adjuvant setting for high-risk resected melanoma. Of the agents tested, IFN-α emerged as the most promising on the basis of three US Eastern Cooperative Oncology Group (ECOG) studies—E1684, E1690, and E1694, as well as trials of the North Central Cancer Treatment Group, the World Health Organization (WHO), and Austrian, French as well as more recent Italian (IMI), Hellenic, German (ADO or DeCOG), and other European trials of the European Organization for Treatment of Cancer (EORTC).

The mechanism of action for IFNα in melanoma is now understood to be primarily immunomodulatory rather than directly cytotoxic, anti-angiogenic, or anti-proliferative. The mechanisms of immunosuppression exerted by melanoma lie beyond this review of adjuvant therapy, but our understanding of how melanoma subverts the host anti-tumor immune responses through multiple mechanisms currently being dissected include the modulation of major histocompatibility antigens, antigen processing, and the expression of inhibitory ligands (PD-L1) that suppress the cytotoxic T-cell response; induction of tolerance through production of immunosuppressive factors ranging from cytokines such as IL-10 and VEGF; JAK/Src-mediated upregulation of STAT3 signaling that appears to be constitutive in melanoma, and apparent from the atypical nevic precursors of melanoma have been particularly important to the analysis of immune function restoration achieved by the type I IFNs, and IFN-α2b in particular [5–8].

IFN-α directly mobilizes effector T-cells: a neo-adjuvant study of patients with IIIB/C melanoma treated with HDI reported that IFN-α administration resulted in an influx of CD8+ cytotoxic T-cells and CD11c+/83+/86+ DCs in a fashion that correlated with clinical responses [9]. Gajewski and colleagues have reported that type 1 IFNs are critical to the priming of anti-tumor CD8+ T-cells via CD8α+ DCs—where in vivo expression of IFN-α or IFN-β in a murine model by retroviral transduction led to total rejection of melanoma [10]. Critchley-Thorne et al. and Simmons et al. have shown that T cell signaling defects found in association with advanced melanoma are restored by incubation of peripheral blood lymphocytes with high, but not low concentrations of IFN-α [11, 12]. These laboratory translational investigations and others that are currently in progress are likely to define mechanisms of immunosuppression induced by the tumor that are assailable with new therapeutic agents that interrupt mutationally activated pathways of signaling that are the basis of tumor progression [Ferrone S, Zarour H, Davar D, Kirkwood JM unpublished data].

E1684 tested the HDI regimen (IFN-α2b I.V. 20 MU/m^2 daily for 5 days for 4 weeks as induction followed by S.C. 10 MU/m^2 thrice weekly for 48 weeks as maintenance) versus placebo in patients with deep primary tumors (T4N0M0) and/or regional lymph node metastases (TxN1-3M0) in a randomized phase III trial [13]. When first reported in 1996 at a median follow-up of 6.9 years, investigators noted statistically significant improvements in both RFS and OS. However, updated survival statistics at 12.6 years revealed an attenuation of the benefits of HDI in E1684—particularly in relation to the impact upon overall survival that has been interpreted as the result of competing causes of death in an elderly patient cohort [14]. Long term studies of the basis of mortality in these and subsequent phase III trial populations have never been undertaken, but are an important agenda for the field.

The toxicity of HDI as pursued in E1684 with Grade III (67 %) and IV (9 %) toxicity prompted consideration of alternative regimens—and ECOG led intergroup US studies E1690 and E1694 compared E1684's HDI regimen to a lower dose regimen (E1690) and to a ganglioside vaccine comprised of GM2/KLH/QS-21 (E1694) respectively [15, 16]. The former trial included an observation arm while the latter did not, given the emergence of a survival benefit in E1684 in the interim. Although both studies reported improvements in RFS, only E1694 reported an OS benefit. Both clinical trials accrued high-risk patients defined as deep primary melanomas of T4 or greater, or node positive disease. E1690 was conducted at a time in which lymph node sampling/removal had not yet become the standard of care and hence regional lymphadenectomy was not uniformly performed in E1690 patients. This led to the situation where patients assigned to the observation arm who experienced lymph node relapse had the opportunity to cross over to receive HDI as this had been approved by regulatory agencies in mid-1995, and where second line HDI treatment given to the majority of patients who had failed with resectable regional lymph node relapse could be demonstrated to be associated with RFS benefit as noted on retrospective analysis, and may have eroded the chance to document OS benefit. The aggregate results of these three phase III studies was reviewed following the initial regulatory approval of HDI on the basis of E1684, and has led to sustained approval of this single therapy across the world for the adjuvant therapy of high-risk disease as defined by the E1684.

The goals of adjuvant therapy have always been considered first in relation to improved survival of melanoma, although trials apart from those of HDI noted above have introduced consideration of relapse-free (RFS), distant metastasis, or disease-free survival (DMFS, particularly in EORTC) beyond the unequivocal goal of overall survival (OS) as addressed in 1684, 1690, and 1694. The morbidity associated with the year-long regimen prompted investigators in Europe and elsewhere to consider lower-dose regimens that might be able to be delivered for longer periods of therapy, if needed, to achieve goals superior to those achieved by the E1684 HDI regimen. A broad variety of regimens were subsequently assessed including intermediate-dose regimens tested in EORTC 18952 (stage IIB/III), EORTC 18991 (T3/4N0M0), and the Nordic IFN trial (stage IIB-IIIB); low-dose regimens (3 MU S.C. thrice weekly) were tested in the WHO Melanoma Program Trials 16 (stage III), UKCCCR AIM-High trial (stage IIB/III), the Scottish trial (stage IIB/III) and the 2010 German DeCOG study (T3anyN); and very-low-dose regimen (1 MU S.C. every other day) tested in EORTC 18871 (stage IIB/III). Although variably associated with improvements in RFS, none of the alternative dosage trials reported any OS benefit. A 2008 DeCOG study has reported an OS benefit for low-dose regimen that has not been observed in multiple other low-dose IFNα trials—though it should be noted that this trial was powered to assess the LDI/dacarbazine combination rather than LDI regimen per se. The results of the high-dose, intermediate-dose, and low-dose trials are summarized in Table 1 [17–30].

Survival analysis in E1684 suggested that the bulk of the RFS benefit appeared to occur early underscoring the importance of the induction phase of the regimen. ECOG E1697 was intended to prospectively evaluate this observation in patients with intermediate-risk and high-risk melanoma defined as T3 or greater primary tumors or microscopic node positive disease (N1a-2a). Patients were randomized to standard HDI induction only versus observation [31]. After 1,150 of a planned 1,420 patients were enrolled and treated, study investigators reported that neither RFS nor OS were impacted (5-year survival rate 0.82 for IFN and 0.85 for observation) leading to early closure for futility. The Hellenic Cooperative Oncology Group conducted a noninferiority randomized phase III trial of the induction portion of a modified HDI versus the full year of a modified-dosage HDI in 353 eligible patients [32]. At a median follow-up of 5 years, the RFS difference was less than the prespecified noninferiority boundary of 15 % and authors concluded that the 1-month regimen was not inferior in terms of RFS. However, the reduced dose employed in this modified HDI regimen has not previously been tested against observation or any other control, and this together with the small size confound interpretation of these results.

Table 1
Phase III studies of adjuvant IFN-α in high-risk resected melanoma

Study reference	Number of patients eligible for analysis	TNM stage	Therapy and IFN sub-species	Dose and schedule –treatment arm	Median follow-up at time of reporting (years)	DFS/RFS	OS	% Node positive	Biomarkers evaluated
High dose									
NCCTG 83-7052 [17]	262	II–III (T2-4N0M0/ TanyN+M0)	IFNα-2a versus observation	I.M. 20 MU/m² thrice weekly for 4 months	6.1	NS	NS	61	None reported
ECOG E1684 [13]	287	II–III (T4N0M0/ TanyN+M0)	IFNα-2b versus observation	I.V. 20 MU/m² 5 days a week for 4 weeks → then → SC 10 MU/m² 3 days a week for 48 weeks	12.6	HR: 1.38 (HDI vs. obs) (S)	HR: 1.22 (HDI vs. obs) (S at 6.9 years but NS at 12.6 years)	89	None
ECOG E1690 [15]	642	II–III (T4N0M0/ TanyN+M0)	IFNα-2b–high dose versus low dose versus observation	High Dose: *Induction*—I.V. 20 MU/m² 5 days a week for 4 weeks *Maintenance*—S.C. 10 MU/m² 3 days a week for 48 weeks Low dose: S.C. 3 MU/m² 2 days a week for 2 years	4.3	HR: 1.28 (HDI vs. obs) (S) 1.19 (LDI vs. obs) (NS) RFS: 44 % (HDI) versus 40 % (LDI) versus 35 % (obs)	HR: 1.0 (HDI vs. obs) (NS) 1.04 (LDI vs. obs) (NS) OS: 52 % (HDI) versus 53 % (LDI) versus 55 % (obs)	74	Peripheral blood HLA-A phenotype and blood immune profile studied in subset of patients (corollary E2690) [54]
ECOG E1694 [16]	774	II–III (T4N0M0/ TanyN+M0)	IFNα-2b versus GMK vaccine	*Induction*—I.V. 20 MU/m² 5 days a week for 4 weeks *Maintenance*—S.C. 10 MU/m² 3 days a week for 48 weeks	2.1	HR: 1.49 (HDI vs. GMK) (S) RFS: 25 % (HDI) versus 39 % (GMK)	HR: 1.38 (HDI vs. GMK) (S) OS: 78 % (HDI) versus 73 % (GMK)	77	Serum protein S100 at baseline ≥0.15 μg/L [HR = 1.39 for poorer OS (S); correlation with poorer RFS (NS)] [55]

(continued)

Table 1
(continued)

Study reference	Number of patients eligible for analysis	TNM stage	Therapy and IFN sub-species	Dose and schedule –treatment arm	Median follow-up at time of reporting (years)	DFS/RFS	OS	% Node positive	Biomarkers evaluated
ECOG E2696 [18]	107	II–IV	GMK vaccination with concurrent HDI (Arm A) versus GMK vaccination with HDI beginning D28 (Arm B) versus GMK vaccination alone (Arm C)	HDI: *Induction*—I.V. 20 MU/m^2 5 days a week for 4 weeks *Maintenance*—S.C. 10 MU/m^2 3 days a week for 48 weeks GMK vaccination: GM2-KLH/QS-21 on D1, 8, 15, 22 then weeks 12, 24,36	2.4	HR: 1.75 (C vs. A) (S) 1.96 (C vs. B) (S) RFS: Not reached (A) versus 30.72 months (B) versus 14.8 months (C)	HR: not reported OS: Not reached (A, B, or C)	Not Available	Serum protein S100 at baseline ≥0.08 μg/L (HR = 1.96 for poorer RFS; S) [56] Serum protein S100 at 1 year ≥0.08 μg/L (HR = 5.7 for poorer OS; S) [56] ANA, anti-TPO, anti-TG, AMA, ACL (NS) [56]
Italian Melanoma Intergroup [19]	330	III (TanyN1-3M0)	Intensified IFNα-2b (IHDI) every other month versus IFNα-2b for 1 year	IHDI: I.V. 20 MU/m^2 5 days a week for 4 weeks every other month for 4 cycles Standard HDI: *Induction*—I.V. 20 MU/m^2 5 days a week for 4 weeks *Maintenance*—S.C. 10 MU/m^2 3 days a week for 48 weeks	5.0	Median RFS: 47.9 months (IHDI) versus 35.6 months (HDI) (NS) 5 year RFS: 45.8 % (IHDI) versus 44.3 % (HDI)	Median OS: 88.7 months 5 year OS: 60.1 % (IHDI) versus 82.6 % (HDI) (NS)	100	N/A

Intermediate dose									
EORTC 18952 [20]	1,388	II–III (T4N0M0 or TanyN+M0)	IFNα-2b for 1 year versus 2 year versus observation	*Induction*—I.V. 10 MU 5 days a week for 4 weeks	4.7	DMFI HR: 0.93 (13 months vs. obs) (NS)	DMFS HR: 0.95 (13 months vs. obs) (NS)	74	Serum protein S100 ≥0.2 μg/L (HR = 5.57 for poorer DMFS; S) [57]
				Maintenance—S.C. 10 MU 3 days a week for 1 year *OR* S.C. 5 MU 3 days a week for 2 years					ANA, anti-TG, ACL development (HR = 0.41 for improved RFS; S before adjusting for guarantee-time bias) [58]
						0.83 (25 months vs. obs) (S)	0.85 (25 months vs. obs) (NS)		ANA, anti-TG, ACL development (HR = 0.81 for improved RFS; NS after adjusting for guarantee-time bias) [58]
									Higher ferritin and lower CRP ratios (not prognostic) [59]
EORTC 18991 [21, 33, 34]	1,256	III (TanyN+M0)	PEG IFNα-2b for 5 year versus observation	*Induction*—S.C. 6 μg/kg/week for 8 weeks *Maintenance*—S.C. 3 μg/kg/week for 5 years	7.6	34.8 months (IFN) versus 25.6 months (obs); S	Not reported	100	ANA, anti-TG, ACL development (HR = 0.56 for improved RFS; S before adjusting for guarantee-time bias) [59]
									ANA, anti-TG, ACL development (HR = 1.19 for improved RFS; NS after adjusting for guarantee-time bias) [60]

(continued)

Table 1 (continued)

Study reference	Number of patients eligible for analysis	TNM stage	Therapy and IFN sub-species	Dose and schedule –treatment arm	Median follow-up at time of reporting (years)	DFS/RFS	OS	% Node positive	Biomarkers evaluated
Nordic IFN [22]	855	IIB-IIIB (T4N0M0 or TanyN1-2M0)	IFNα-2b for 1 year versus 2 years versus observation	Observation (A) versus S.C. 10 MU 5 days a week for 4 weeks then S.C. 10 MU 3 days a week for 1 year (B) versus S.C. 10 MU 5 days a week for 4 weeks then S.C. 10 MU 3 days a week for 2 years (C)	6.0	23.2 months (A) versus 37.8 months (B) versus 28.6 months (C) IFN versus obs & IFN 1 year versus obs (S); IFN 2 year versus obs (NS)	56.1 months (A) versus 72.1 months (B) versus 64.3 months (C) (NS)	81	ANA, anti-TG, ACL development (HR = 0.51 for improved RFS; S before adjusting for guarantee-time bias) [58] ANA, anti-TG, ACL development (HR = 0.85 for improved RFS; NS after adjusting for guarantee-time bias) [58]
Low dose									
Austrian Melanoma Cooperative Group (AMCG) [23]	311	II (T2-4N0M0)	IFNα-2a versus observation	S.C. 3 MU 7 days a week for 3 weeks → then → S.C. 3MU 3 days a week for 1 year	3.4	RFS/DMFS not reported Rate of relapse: (24.0 % LDI vs. 36.3 % obs)	Not available	0	N/A
French Melanoma Cooperative Group (FCGM) [24]	499	II (T2-4N0M0)	IFNα-2a versus observation	S.C. 3MU 3 days a week for 18 months	>3	HR: 0.74 (LDI vs. obs) (S)	HR: 0.70 (LDI vs. obs) (S)	0	N/A

WHO Melanoma Program Trial 16 [25]	444	III (TanyN+M0)	IFNα-2a versus observation	S.C. 3MU 3 days a week for 36 months	7.3	NS	NS	100	N/A
Scottish Melanoma Cooperative Group [26]	96	II–III (T3-4N0M0/ TanyN+M0)	IFNα-2a versus observation	S.C. 3 MU 3 days a week for 6 months	>6	NS	NS	Not available	N/A
EORTC 18871/DKG 80-1 [27]	728	II–III (T3-4N0M0/ TanyN+M0)	IFNα-2b versus IFN-γ versus ISCADOR M® versus observation	IFN-α2b: S.C. 1MU every other day for 12 months IFN-γ: S.C. 0.2 mg every other day for 12 months	8.2	NS	NS	58	N/A
UKCCCR/ AIM HIGH [28]	674	II–III (T3-4N0M0/ TanyN+M0)	IFNα-2a versus observation	S.C. 3 MU 3 days a week for 24 months	3.1	NS	NS	Not available	N/A
DeCOG [29]	840	III (T3anyN+M0)	IFNα-2a	S.C. 3 MU 3 days a week for 18 months (A) versus 5 years (B)	4.3	5 years DMFS 81.9 % (A) versus 79.7 % (B) (NS)	5 years OS 85.9 % (A) versus 84.9 % (B) (NS)	Not available	N/A
DeCOG [30]	444	III (TanyN+M0)	IFNα-2a	S.C. 3MU 3 days a week for 24 months (A) versus S.C. 3MU 3 days a week for 24 months + DTIC 850 mg/m² every 4–8 weeks for 24 months (B) versus observation (C)	3.9	HR: 0.69 (A) versus 1.01 (B) versus 1.0 (C)	HR: 0.62 (A) versus 0.96 (B) versus 1.0 (C)	100 %	N/A

NS not significant, *S* significant, *HR* hazard ratio, *DFS* disease-free survival, *DMFS* distant metastases-free survival, *OS* overall survival, *ANA* anti-nuclear antibody, ***anti-TPO*** anti-thyroid peroxidase antibody, ***anti-TG*** anti-thyroglobulin antibody, *AMA* anti-mitochondrial antibody, *ACL* anti-cardiolipin autoantibodies

The Italian Melanoma Group evaluated the same hypothesis using an intensified regimen—4 cycles of induction dosing for a month with HDI administered every other month (intensified HDI, IHDI) compared to the standard E1684 full-year regimen—in a randomized phase III study [19]. Although RFS and OS were improved in the IHDI arm compared to the standard HDI arm, the differences were not statistically significant. However, given that the overall toxicity profiles were relatively similar in both groups, an argument can be made for this shorter (and more feasible) regimen.

The pegylated form of IFN-α allows once-weekly administration without sacrificing potency. Several EORTC trials assessed various pegylated IFN-α schedules to determine if similar benefits could be obtained. EORTC 18991 was an adjuvant study in which 1,256 patients with resected AJCC stage III melanoma were randomized in a nonblinded fashion to either pegylated IFN-α for 5 years versus observation. The choice of an extended duration of therapy (5 years) was designed to assess whether the benefit of IFN eroded after cessation of therapy—as suggested by earlier European trials of low-dose IFN [20, 23]. Study investigators presented initial results in 2007—noting a significant improvement in RFS (HR = 0.82, $p = 0.011$) with no improvement in either of the original primary endpoints of the study, DMFS or OS at 3.8 years median follow-up [33]. Patients with microscopic node-positive disease appeared to benefit predominantly in comparison to the other groups with no evidence of any benefit in the macroscopic nodal disease (N2) subset. Although the study results were published early, the study was criticized due to the lack of maturity of the results, given their lesser magnitude compared to E1684 (which was first reported at 6.9 years median follow-up). Nonetheless, the results served as the basis for a successful application for FDA approval of pegylated IFN-α (Sylatron™, Merck Corporation) for adjuvant therapy of stage III melanoma with either microscopic or macroscopic nodal involvement following definitive surgical resection including complete lymphadenectomy.

Recently, the mature results of this trial were published [34]. At mature follow-up, the overall RFS benefit has diminished from the prior HR of 0.82 to a current HR of 0.87 (95 % CI, 0.76–1.00) and the prior significance has diminished to a marginal ($p = 0.055$) without significant benefits in the originally specified endpoints of DMFS/OS. Subgroup analysis suggests that patients with microscopic nodal disease and ulcerated primaries derive relatively greater RFS benefit while patients with N2 disease lack benefit in any parameter. In light of these results, practitioners should consider several factors when deciding between HDI and pegylated IFN-α: first, the overall hazard of benefit in PFS terms is greater with conventional high-dose IFN—HR 0.69 at 6.9 years and 0.72 at 12.6 years (E1684) versus HR 0.82 at 3.8 years and 0.87 at more mature 7.6 years with pegylated IFN-α as tested in EORTC 18991. Second, the collective US intergroup experience over time demonstrates RFS and OS in patients with macroscopic as well as microscopic nodal disease while pegylated IFN-α has no benefit in this sub-group of patients whose risk of recurrence/death is the highest in all of the trials of various dosages and formulations of IFN over the years. The quest for biomarkers that would allow the more selective application of IFN in general for adjuvant therapy of melanoma is thus even more compelling for pegylated IFN-α; for the present and apart from biomarkers that may allow the improvement of therapeutic index for IFNs, pegylated IFN-α may be considered for patients with N1 disease who are either unwilling or unable to tolerate the HDI regimen.

The benefit of adjuvant IFN-α has been comprehensively evaluated in several meta-analyses [35, 36], a systematic review [37] and a pooled data analysis [38]. The 2003 meta-analysis by Wheatley and colleagues pooled data from 12 randomized controlled trials (RCT) that compared varying doses of IFN-α to observation and demonstrated RFS (significant) and OS (nonsignificant) benefits with a trend towards improved outcomes in patients receiving higher doses of IFN-α. The second meta-analysis by Wheatley and colleagues in 2007 utilized individual patient level data from 13 RCTs that included vaccine and observation comparators and concluded that IFN-α significantly improved RFS and OS as did a more recent 2010 meta-analysis of 14 RCTs. The accumulated evidence reliably indicates that adjuvant HDI reduces RFS by 30 % with a lesser impact on OS.

1.3 Ongoing Adjuvant Trials

The current agenda of cooperative group trials for adjuvant therapy involve the introduction of new targeted molecular signaling inhibitor therapies (BRAF, MEK), and inhibitors of immune checkpoints (anti-CTLA-4, anti-PD1, and anti-PDL1) and next-generation immunotherapeutic options that are summarized in Table 2. Building upon the earlier observations of Ives et al., in the meta-analysis which demonstrated a potential selective advantage of patients with ulcerated primary melanomas receiving adjuvant IFN, and trials that have shown this in the EORTC including 18952 and 18991 the proposed EORTC 18081 is designed to prospectively test the benefit of 2 years of pegylated IFN-α versus observation in patients with node-negative melanoma and ulcerated primaries greater than 1 mm (T2-4bN0M0, $n = 1{,}200$).

MAGE-A3 is a tumor-associated protein expressed in >60 % of metastatic melanoma that elicits humoral and cell-mediated immune responses in the autologous host. Previously, a phase II trial of MAGE-A3 vaccine (GSK Biologicals, Rixensart, Belgium) showed objective responses in 5/72 treated patients and long lasting

Table 2
Ongoing adjuvant studies in high-risk resected melanoma

Study reference	Estimated enrollment	Study design	Primary endpoint	Secondary endpoint(s)	Dose and schedule—treatment arm	Start date	Estimated completion	Biomarker evaluation
EORTC 18081 (NCT01502696)	1,200	Phase III, randomized, open-label study in T2b-4bN0M0 melanoma	RFS	OS, DMFS, quality of life	Pegylated IFN-α2b 3 μg/kg weekly injections for 2 years	April 2012	April 2020	Unknown
COMBI-AD (NCT01682083)	850	Phase III, randomized, double-blinded study in high-risk (IIIA-C) resected BRAF V600E/K mutant melanoma	RFS	OS, DMFS, FFR, safety, toxicity	Dabrafenib 150 mg B.I.D. AND Trametinib 2 mg once daily versus placebos for 12 months	November 2012	July 2015	Unknown
Adjuvant dabrafenib (NCT01682213)	23	Open label phase II study in high-risk (IIIC) resected BRAF V600E/K mutant melanoma	RFS	OS, safety, toxicity	Dabrafenib 150 mg B.I.D. per cycle (28 days) for 4 cycles	September 2012	September 2014	Unknown

Adjuvant vemurafenib (NCT01667419)	725	Phase III, randomized, double-blinded study in high-risk (IIC or IIIA-C) resected BRAF V600E mutant melanoma	DFS	OS, DMFS, quality of life, pharmacokinetics, safety, toxicity	Vemurafenib 960 mg B.I.D. versus placebo for 12 months	September 2012	June 2016	Unknown
E1609 (NCT01274338)	1,500	Phase III, randomized, open-label study in high-risk (IIIB-C or resected IVA) resected melanoma	RFS, OS	Toxicity, global quality of life	Ipilimumab in 2 dose levels vs. HDI Ipilimumab: *Induction*—3/10 mg/kg q3weeks for 4 doses *Maintenance*—3/10 mg/kg q6weeks until week 48 then q12weeks afterwards HDI: *Induction*—I.V. 20 MU/m^2 5 days a week for 4 weeks *Maintenance*—S.C. 10 MU/m^2 3 days a week for 48 weeks	May 2011	May 2018	Ipilimumab—MDSC, Treg, IL-17 HDI—S100B

(continued)

Table 2
(continued)

Study reference	Estimated enrollment	Study design	Primary endpoint	Secondary endpoint(s)	Dose and schedule—treatment arm	Start date	Estimated completion	Biomarker evaluation
EORTC 18071 (NCT00636168)	950	Phase III, randomized, open-label study in T2b-4bNxM0 melanoma following resection	RFS	OS, DMFS, quality of life, quality-of-life-adjusted survival	Ipilimumab versus placebo Ipilimumab: *Induction*—10 mg/kg q3weeks for 4 doses *Maintenance*—10 mg/kg q6weeks until week 48 then q12weeks afterwards	June 2008	September 2014	Unknown
MAGE-A3 vaccine (NCT00796445)	1,349	Phase III, randomized, open-label study in T2b-4bN0M0 melanoma	DFS	OS, DMFS, anti-MAGE-A3 and anti-protein D seropositivity status, quality of life	MAGE-A3 vaccine with 2 adjuvants including QS-21 (Stimulon™, Agenus), and a proprietary Toll-like receptor 9 agonist (VaxImmune™, Coley Pharmaceuticals)	December 2008	October 2016	Expression of MAGE-A3 Antigen-Specific Cancer Immuno-therapeutic (ASCI) gene signature

OS overall survival, *RFS* relapse-free survival, *DFS* disease-free survival, *DMFS* distant metastasis-free survival, *FFR* freedom from relapse, *DLT* dose-limiting toxicities

stable disease in 11/72 patients [39]. A phase III trial of the vaccine combined with two potent new immunopotentiators including a toll-like receptor 9 agonist designed to induce potent antibody and CD8+ T-cell responses completed accrual in 2011 and results of this trial are awaited in 2013.

Ipilimumab (Yervoy™, Medarex Inc/Bristol-Myers Squibb) is a fully humanized immunoglobulin G1κ monoclonal antibody that competitively inhibits CTLA-4. CTLA-4 and PD-1 are T-cell surface receptors that down modulate T-cell responses following binding of cognate ligands present on antigen presenting cells—B7-1/2 and PD-L1, respectively. By blocking negative regulators known as immune checkpoints, CTLA-4 (and PD-1) inhibitors appear to enhance T-cell activation and proliferation in early nodal phases of the immune response to melanoma, and later tissue-based immune responses to melanoma. Ipilimumab has demonstrated improved survival in two large RCTs involving different dosages (10 mg/kg and 3 mg/kg), directed at different settings (untreated first line versus relapsed prior treated patients) and compared against different controls (dacarbazine versus gp 100 peptide vaccine) [40, 41]. EORTC 18071 is prospectively comparing ipilimumab at 10 mg/kg to placebo in stage III melanoma following resection in 950 patients. Accrual has completed and results are expected in 2013. ECOG's companion study (E1609) is an open-label RCT that seeks to compare ipilimumab at 2 dose levels (3 mg/kg and 10 mg/kg) to HDI in highest-risk melanoma (stage IIIB-C and resected stage IV).

The mitogen-activated protein (MAP) kinase pathway comprises several (RAS/RAF/MEK/ERK) serine/threonine-specific protein kinases that direct cellular responses to a diverse array of stimuli including growth signals. Activating mutations in BRAF are present in approximately 40–60 % of cutaneous melanomas most of which are V600E mutations and result in unregulated cellular proliferation. MEK lies directly downstream of RAF and is an attractive target as MEK inhibition would effectively target BRAF- and RAS-mutant melanoma.

When compared against dacarbazine in previously untreated patients with metastatic melanoma, the BRAF V600E inhibitor vemurafenib (Zelboraf™, Roche/Plexxikon) demonstrated improved overall survival and decreased risk of tumor progression with an overall response rate (ORR) of 48 %. Dabrafenib (GSK2118436, Glaxo-SmithKline) is another BRAF inhibitor with activity in V600E and V600K mutants that appears similar in efficacy, and different in its profile of toxicities that are in general, well tolerated for both agents. In a phase III trial that compared dabrafenib to dacarbazine in previously untreated patients with advanced V600E mutant melanoma, dabrafenib demonstrated significant improvement in PFS over dacarbazine with a confirmed response rate of 53 % [42]. Trametinib (GSK1120212, Glaxo-SmithKline) is a MEK inhibitor that has also demonstrated improved

PFS and OS in V600E/K mutant melanoma when tested against dacarbazine or paclitaxel [43].

Success in the metastatic setting has prompted the development of investigations of these agents in the adjuvant setting. Currently there are three proposed or initiated studies evaluating RAF/MEK inhibitors either singly or in combination for adjuvant treatment of melanoma. COMBI-AD (NCT01682083) and NCT01667419 are randomized, double-blind phase III studies enrolling high-risk stage III patients to placebo versus combined RAF/MEK inhibition with dabrafenib and trametinib (COMBI-AD) or RAF inhibition alone with vemurafenib (NCT01667419). Primary endpoints are RFS (COMBI-AD) and disease-free survival (NCT01667419) with the proposed duration of treatment in both studies being 12 months. Investigators from Memorial Sloan-Kettering Cancer Center are performing a phase II adjuvant study of 4 cycles of monthly dabrafenib in resected stage IIIC patients with RFS as a primary endpoint (NCT01682213). These trials are slated to open in 2013 with estimated completion between 2014 and 2016.

RAF/MEK inhibition is associated with the acquisition of resistance at a median PFS of 4.8–5.3 months. The treatment of patients who have progressed on RAF/MEK inhibitors has been problematic—and an important consideration for adjuvant therapy has to be the longer term (years in the future) impact of the drug to be tested. The rationale and mechanism of action for the agents under evaluation are important to consider for adjuvant therapy, given the lack of durability of direct antitumor effects with BRAF inhibitors alone, and BRAF-MEK inhibitor combinations to date. There is emerging evidence of immunological effects with BRAF inhibitors alone and these lend support to the notion that BRAF inhibitors might add to the impact of immunotherapy in the adjuvant setting [44, 45]. We have proposed the sequenced combination of BRAF inihibitors prior to IFNα, for which the clinical experience with BRAF inhibitors provides partial support, and additional evidence preclinical evidence is also promising (Ferrone, Zarour, Davar & Kirkwood unpublished). The consideration of BRAF inhibitors and MEK inhibitors together has been advanced in view of the reduced toxicity and potential to prolong the interval to progression with the combination. However, the impact of MEK inhibitors upon the immune response needs to be evaluated, as the potential inhibition of immune responses in the adjuvant setting may be a larger issue. The use of tyrosine kinase inhibitors (TKIs) in EGFR-mutant lung cancer suggests that *timing* of recurrence is associated with resistance mediated by EGFR kinase domain mutation (T790M) observed *on treatment*, but not *after treatment*. Thus, it may be that recurrence after finite intervals of BRAF inhibitor therapy may still allow successful retreatment with BRAF inhibitors at later intervals [46].

1.4 Prognostic and Predictive Biomarkers

The identification of predictive and prognostic biomarkers of therapy for melanoma is the highest priority for translational research in melanoma both in the advanced and in the adjuvant settings of disease, to allow the individualization of therapy to optimize efficacy and minimize toxicity and cost. While the effort to individualize therapy will ultimately refine the population to be treated, this narrowing of the therapeutic window will be more than compensated by the improvement in the therapeutic index.

One potential avenue for tailoring adjuvant IFN therapy lies in the pathologic variable of primary tumor ulceration already discussed. The aggregate data from EORTC 18952 and 18991 in 2,644 patients report that ulceration is strongly correlated with benefit from intermediate dosage or pegylated IFN-α [20, 33]. The more limited Sunbelt melanoma trial also identified ulceration as a predictive factor, but neither the Sunbelt trial nor the EORTC trials have adopted rigorous pathology review for subjects enrolled into these trials, so they rely upon institutional pathology reporting that has not been verified [47, 48]. Unfortunately, the US Intergroup trials conducted to date and the E1684 pivotal study have not identified ulceration as a predictive factor and these studies have uniformly required central pathology review. The possibility that a gene signature will predict the benefit of immunotherapy has already been noted, and the MAGE A3 DERMA vaccine trial for Stage IIIB melanoma is accompanied by a prospective formal gene signature analysis that may further refine the application of this vaccine, and enhance the potential therapeutic index of this vaccine [49]. Gene signatures of the tumor may guide future therapies apart from vaccines such as MAGE A3, and current questions in regard to the pathological variable of tumor ulceration may ultimately be understood in terms of the genetic profile of the tumor.

The development of autoimmunity has been advanced as a surrogate of IFN response following on observations of autoimmune thyroid and cutaneous depigmentary response with IL-2 [50]. The prospective clinical and serological analysis in the Hellenic Oncology Group trial 13A/98 provided rigorous evidence that the development of autoimmunity was associated with statistically significant improvements in RFS and OS in patients with melanoma treated with adjuvant IFN [51]. Analyses of US Intergroup trials E2696 and E1694 have shown a correlation between improved survival and HDI-induced autoimmunity, but did not have the advantage of assessing clinical features of autoimmunity [52]. US Intergroup trial E1697 evaluated 1 month induction only course of adjuvant IFN-α2b versus observation in patients with intermediate-risk resected melanoma. Following interim analysis that suggested futility, the trial was closed early. However biomarker analysis in 268 patients suggested that month IL2Rα, IL-12p40, and IFN levels at 1 month in the treatment group significantly predicted 1 year RFS (Kirkwood et al., presented at

ASCO 2013). Other analyses using different methodologies in relation to intermediate-dosage IFN regimens and focusing only on the serological development of autoimmunity have confirmed this correlation, but lacked prospective clinical evaluations [53]. These analyses are delineated in the "Biomarkers Evaluated" section of Table 1.

Other candidate biomarkers include methylthioadenosine phosphorylase (MTAP) protein expression, YKL-40 (a mammalian chitinase-like protein) levels, S100B, melanoma-inhibiting activity (MIA), and tumor-associated antigen 90 immune complex (TA90IC)—reviewed in detail elsewhere [54–60]. While these candidate biomarkers have, to varying degrees, been linked with outcomes on retrospective analyses they have not been evaluated as markers for IFN adjuvant therapy for melanoma.

2 Conclusions

Multiple prior US and European intergroup studies (E1684, E1690, E1694, EORTC 18952, and EORTC 18991) have demonstrated in aggregate that adjuvant therapy with IFN-α reliably consistently improves RFS and to a lesser magnitude, OS in patients with deep primary melanomas, and in those with nodal disease—without differential effects in resected nodal disease of macroscopic and microscopic extent. The pivotal study and subsequent evaluations of HDI have revealed benefit across the operable high-risk disease spectrum, and no differential benefit according to disease bulk, or the presence of primary tumor ulceration. The benefits of high-dose recombinant IFN upon OS appears to be real, but less in magnitude than upon RFS, and diminish with long-term follow-up past 10 years. Trials of pegylated IFN-α show improvement in RFS without any evidence of an impact upon OS, and the magnitude of the benefit upon RFS is less than that of HDI, and restricted to patient populations with microscopic nodal disease, where the benefit, like that of other lower-dose regimes, has been linked with primary tumor ulceration. Although certain clinical features have been advanced that may allow the improvement in the therapeutic index of IFN (such as ulceration of the primary and laboratory indices of immune reactivity) (such as the development of autoimmunity, MTAP expression, and serum levels of YKL-40, S100B, MIA, and TA90IC), predictive biomarkers used to predict therapeutic benefit to IFN adjuvant therapy, or any of the newer candidate immunomodulators are still lacking. These are the compelling need of the field, as we develop new immune checkpoint inhibitors, signaling pathway inhibitors, and combinations for adjuvant therapy. E1609, the current US Intergroup trial, will evaluate candidate blood biomarkers of immunotherapeutic benefit with anti-CTLA4 blocking antibody ipilimumab, as well as IFNα and EORTC 18081 will evaluate the role of Peg-IFNα in patients with ulcerated primaries (T2b-4b) to shed light on this issue in the future.

The past several years have witnessed an exponential increase in our understanding of the molecular events underpinning melanoma tumorigenesis and the subtleties of the host-tumor immune interactions, culminating in regulatory approval of the BRAF inhibitor vemurafenib and the CTLA-4 inhibitor ipilimumab in advanced melanoma.

These agents have transformed the therapeutic landscape in advanced melanoma—where molecular profiling of BRAF and NRAS is now routine in patients with metastatic disease. The role of these genetic mutations in guiding adjuvant therapy is likely in the future, but for the large population without identified BRAF or NRAS mutations, immunotherapeutic options with either IL-2 or ipilimumab are considerations in metastatic disease, and IFN-α has an established role in the adjuvant setting. Despite the impressive and frequent remission of advanced metastatic BRAFV600E melanoma with vemurafenib (ORR 48.4 %), and the recently identified immunological effects of this agent, the relatively short duration of response secondary to the rapid acquisition of resistance at a median PFS of 5.3 months is an issue for adjuvant application of this agent as a single intervention. Ipilimumab has demonstrated durable responses in a significant but small proportion of patients in two phase III trials involving different dosages against different comparators in the treatment-naïve and previously untreated populations. The low ORR of 10.9–15.2 % may be improved in the adjuvant setting for this agent, as has been observed with IFNα, where a response rate of 16 % in advanced disease translates to a hazard ratio of 0.67 or relapse reduction of 33 %. This is the basis for current efforts to evaluate ipilimumab in randomized trials for high-risk resected melanoma compared against HDI in ECOG 1609 (ipilimumab at 10 mg/kg and 3 mg/kg vs. HDI) and against placebo in EORTC 18071 (ipilimumab 10 mg/kg vs. placebo). Vemurafenib and the dabrafenib/tremetinib combination are each being considered for evaluation randomized trials in similar high-risk groups.

Our understanding of the mechanism of action for IFN, and now for ipilimumab, has arisen from neoadjuvant studies conducted over the years and argues for the prospective application of this approach to accelerate the development of combinations of immunotherapy and molecularly-targeted therapy in the neoadjuvant setting. This approach provides us the needed access to essential biomarker information, and a rapid read-out of correlations between the antitumor effects at the level of tumor tissue that is otherwise lost in the adjuvant postoperative treatment setting. The effort to optimize our new agents and combinations as well as sequences of these agents will be best served by the pursuit of neoadjuvant studies in parallel with the definitive clinical evaluation of these approaches. Clinical trials currently underway may answer these questions and for now, patients with high-risk melanoma who are unable to participate in clinical trials are reasonably offered high-dose IFN-α following surgery.

Funding

This work was supported by Award Number P50 CA121973 from the National Cancer Institute. The content is solely the responsibility of the authors and does not necessarily represent the official views of the National Cancer Institute or the National Institutes of Health.

References

1. Howlader N, Noone AM, Krapcho M, Neyman N, Aminou R, Altekruse SF, Kosary CL, Ruhl J, Tatalovich Z, Cho H, Mariotto A, Eisner MP, Lewis DR, Chen HS, Feuer EJ, Cronin KA (eds) SEER cancer statistics review, 1975–2009 (Vintage 2009 populations), National Cancer Institute. Bethesda, MD, http://seer.cancer.gov/csr/1975_2009_pops09/, based on November 2011 SEER data submission, posted to the SEER web site, 2012
2. Tarhini AA, Kirkwood JM (2012) How much of a good thing? What duration for interferon Alfa-2b adjuvant therapy? J Clin Oncol 30(31):3773–3776
3. Balch CM, Gershenwald JE, Soong SJ et al (2009) Final version of 2009 AJCC melanoma staging and classification. J Clin Oncol 27(36):6199–6206
4. van Akkooi AC, Nowecki ZI, Voit C et al (2008) Sentinel node tumor burden according to the Rotterdam criteria is the most important prognostic factor for survival in melanoma patients: a multicenter study in 388 patients with positive sentinel nodes. Ann Surg 248(6): 949–955
5. Stewart TJ, Abrams SI (2008) How tumors escape mass destruction. Oncogene 27:5894–5903
6. Sato T, McCue P, Masuoka K et al (1996) Interleukin 10 production by human melanoma. Clin Cancer Res 2:1383–1390
7. Enk AH, Jonuleit H, Saloga J, Knop J (1997) Dendritic cells as mediators of tumor-induced tolerance in metastatic melanoma. Int J Cancer 73:309–316
8. Kirkwood JM, Farkas DL, Chakraborty A et al (1999) Systemic interferon-alpha (IFN-alpha) treatment leads to Stat3 inactivation in melanoma precursor lesions. Mol Med 5(1):11–20
9. Moschos SJ, Edington HD, Land SR et al (2006) Neoadjuvant treatment of regional stage IIIB melanoma with high-dose interferon alfa-2b induces objective tumor regression in association with modulation of tumor infiltrating host cellular immune responses. J Clin Oncol 24(19):3164–3171
10. Gajewski TF, Fuertes M, Spaapen R et al (2011) Molecular profiling to identify relevant immune resistance mechanisms in the tumor microenvironment. Curr Opin Immunol 23(2):286–292
11. Critchley-Thorne RJ, Yan N, Nacu S et al (2007) Down-regulation of the interferon signaling pathway in T lymphocytes from patients with metastatic melanoma. PLoS Med 4(5): e176
12. Simons DL, Lee G, Kirkwood JM, Lee PP (2011) Interferon signaling patterns in peripheral blood lymphocytes may predict clinical outcome after high-dose interferon therapy in melanoma patients. J Transl Med 9:52
13. Kirkwood JM, Strawderman MH, Ernstoff MS et al (1996) Interferon alfa-2b adjuvant therapy of high-risk resected cutaneous melanoma: the Eastern Cooperative Oncology Group Trial EST 1684. J Clin Oncol 14:7–17
14. Kirkwood JM, Manola J, Ibrahim J et al (2004) A pooled analysis of eastern cooperative oncology group and intergroup trials of adjuvant

high-dose interferon for melanoma. Clin Cancer Res 10(5):1670–1677
15. Kirkwood JM, Ibrahim JG, Sondak VK et al (2000) High- and low-dose interferon alfa-2b in high-risk melanoma: first analysis of intergroup trial E1690/S9111/C9190. J Clin Oncol 18(12):2444–2458
16. Kirkwood JM, Ibrahim JG, Sosman JA et al (2001) High-dose interferon alfa-2b significantly prolongs relapse-free and overall survival compared with the GM2-KLH/QS-21 vaccine in patients with resected stage IIB-III melanoma: results of intergroup trial E1694/S9512/C509801. J Clin Oncol 19(9): 2370–2380
17. Creagan ET, Dalton RJ, Ahmann DL et al (1995) Randomized, surgical adjuvant clinical trial of recombinant interferon alfa-2a in selected patients with malignant melanoma. J Clin Oncol 13(11):2776–2783
18. Kirkwood JM, Ibrahim J, Lawson DH et al (2001) High-dose interferon alfa-2b does not diminish antibody response to GM2 vaccination in patients with resected melanoma: results of the Multicenter Eastern Cooperative Oncology Group Phase II Trial E2696. J Clin Oncol 19(5):1430–1436
19. Chiarion-Sileni V, Guida M, Romanini A et al for Italian Melanoma Intergroup (IMI) (2011) Intensified high-dose intravenous interferon alpha 2b (IFNa2b) for adjuvant treatment of stage III melanoma: a randomized phase III Italian Melanoma Intergroup (IMI) trial [ISRCTN75125874]. J Clin Oncol 29(suppl):abstr 8506
20. Eggermont AM, Suciu S, MacKie R et al (2005) Post-surgery adjuvant therapy with intermediate doses of interferon alfa 2b versus observation in patients with stage IIb/III melanoma (EORTC 18952): randomised controlled trial. Lancet 366(9492):1189–1196
21. Bouwhuis MG, Suciu S, Testori A et al (2010) Phase III trial comparing adjuvant treatment with pegylated interferon Alfa-2b versus observation: prognostic significance of autoantibodies—EORTC 18991. J Clin Oncol 28(14): 2460–2466
22. Hansson J, Aamdal S, Bastholt L et al (2011) Two different durations of adjuvant therapy with intermediate-dose interferon alfa-2b in patients with high-risk melanoma (Nordic IFN trial): a randomised phase 3 trial. Lancet Oncol 12(2):144–152
23. Pehamberger H, Soyer HP, Steiner A et al (1998) Adjuvant interferon alfa-2a treatment in resected primary stage II cutaneous melanoma. Austrian Malignant Melanoma Cooperative Group. J Clin Oncol 16(4):1425–1429
24. Grob JJ, Dreno B, de la Salmonière P et al (1998) Randomised trial of interferon alpha-2a as adjuvant therapy in resected primary melanoma thicker than 1.5 mm without clinically detectable node metastases. French Cooperative Group on Melanoma. Lancet 351(9120): 1905–1910
25. Cascinelli N, Belli F, MacKie RM et al (2001) Effect of long-term adjuvant therapy with interferon alpha-2a in patients with regional node metastases from cutaneous melanoma: a randomised trial. Lancet 358(9285):866–869
26. Cameron DA, Cornbleet MC, Mackie RM et al (2001) Adjuvant interferon alpha 2b in high risk melanoma—the Scottish study. Br J Cancer 84(9):1146–1149
27. Kleeberg UR, Suciu S, Bröcker EB, for EORTC Melanoma Group in cooperation with the German Cancer Society (DKG) et al (2004) Final results of the EORTC 18871/DKG 80-1 randomised phase III trial. rIFN-alpha2b versus rIFN-gamma versus ISCADOR M versus observation after surgery in melanoma patients with either high-risk primary (thickness >3 mm) or regional lymph node metastasis. Eur J Cancer 40(3):390–402
28. Hancock BW, Wheatley K, Harris S et al (2004) Adjuvant interferon in high-risk melanoma: the AIM HIGH Study—United Kingdom Coordinating Committee on Cancer Research randomized study of adjuvant low-dose extended-duration interferon alfa-2a in high-risk resected malignant melanoma. J Clin Oncol 22(1):53–61
29. Hauschild A, Weichenthal M, Rass K et al (2010) Efficacy of low-dose interferon {alpha}2a 18 versus 60 months of treatment in patients with primary melanoma of >= 1.5 mm tumor thickness: results of a randomized phase III DeCOG trial. J Clin Oncol 28(5): 841–846
30. Garbe C, Radny P, Linse R et al (2008) Adjuvant low-dose interferon {alpha}2a with or without dacarbazine compared with surgery alone: a prospective-randomized phase III DeCOG trial in melanoma patients with regional lymph node metastasis. Ann Oncol 19(6):1195–1201
31. Agarwala SS, Lee SJ, Flaherty LE et al (2011) Randomized phase III trial of high-dose interferon alfa-2b (HDI) for 4 weeks induction only in patients with intermediate- and high-risk melanoma (Intergroup trial E1697). J Clin Oncol 29(suppl): abstr 8505
32. Pectasides D, Dafni U, Bafaloukos D et al (2009) Randomized phase III study of 1 month versus 1 year of adjuvant high-dose interferon alfa-2b in patients with resected high-risk melanoma. J Clin Oncol 27(6): 939–944
33. Eggermont AM, Suciu S, Santinami M et al (2008) Adjuvant therapy with pegylated

interferon alfa-2b versus observation alone in resected stage III melanoma: final results of EORTC 18991, a randomised phase III trial. Lancet 372(9633):117–126
34. Eggermont AM, Suciu S, Testori A et al (2012) Long-term results of the randomized phase III trial EORTC 18991 of adjuvant therapy with pegylated interferon alfa-2b versus observation in resected stage III melanoma. J Clin Oncol 30(31):3810–3818
35. Wheatley K, Ives N, Hancock B et al (2003) Does adjuvant interferon-alpha for high-risk melanoma provide a worthwhile benefit? A meta-analysis of the randomised trials. Cancer Treat Rev 29:241–252
36. Mocellin S, Pasquali S, Rossi CR et al (2010) Interferon alpha adjuvant therapy in patients with high-risk melanoma: a systematic review and metaanalysis. J Natl Cancer Inst 102:493–501
37. Lens MB, Dawes M (2002) Interferon alfa therapy for malignant melanoma: a systematic review of randomized controlled trials. J Clin Oncol 20:1818–1825
38. Wheatley K, Hancock B, Gore M et al (2007) Interferon-{alpha} as adjuvant therapy for melanoma: an individual patient data meta-analysis of randomised trials. J Clin Oncol 25(18 suppl):abstract 8526
39. Kruit W, Suciu S, Dreno B et al (2011) Active immunization toward the MAGE-A3 antigen in patients with metastatic melanoma: four-year follow-up results from a randomized phase II study (EORTC16032-18031). J Clin Oncol 29(suppl): abstr 8535
40. Hodi FS, O'Day SJ, McDermott DF et al (2010) Improved survival with ipilimumab in patients with metastatic melanoma. N Engl J Med 363(8):711–723
41. Robert C, Thomas L, Bondarenko I et al (2011) Ipilimumab plus dacarbazine for previously untreated metastatic melanoma. N Engl J Med 364(26):2517–2526
42. Hauschild A, Grob JJ, Demidov LV et al (2012) Dabrafenib in BRAF-mutated metastatic melanoma: a multicentre, open-label, phase 3 randomised controlled trial. Lancet 380(9839):358–342.
43. Flaherty KT, Robert C, Hersey P et al (2012) Improved survival with MEK inhibition in BRAF-mutated melanoma. N Engl J Med 367(2):107–114
44. Boni A, Cogdill AP, Dang P et al (2010) Selective BRAFV600E inhibition enhances T-cell recognition of melanoma without affecting lymphocyte function. Cancer Res 70(13):5213–5219
45. Wilmott JS, Long GV, Howle JR et al (2012) Selective BRAF inhibitors induce marked T-cell infiltration into human metastatic melanoma. Clin Cancer Res 18(5):1386–1394
46. Oxnard GR, Janjigian YY, Arcila ME et al (2011) Maintained sensitivity to EGFR tyrosine kinase inhibitors in EGFR-mutant lung cancer recurring after adjuvant erlotinib or gefitinib. Clin Cancer Res 17(19): 6322–6328
47. McMasters KM, Ross MI, Reintgen DS et al (2008) Final results of the Sunbelt Melanoma Trial. J Clin Oncol 26(suppl): abstr 9003
48. Eggermont AM, Spatz A, Lazar V, Robert C (2012) Is ulceration in cutaneous melanoma just a prognostic and predictive factor or is ulcerated melanoma a distinct biologic entity? Curr Opin Oncol 24(2):137–140
49. Trefzer U, Jouary T, Robert C et al (2010) FC13 DERMA Phase III trial of MAGE-A3 immunotherapy as adjuvant treatment in stage III melanoma: MAGE-A3 gene expression frequency and baseline demographics. Melanoma Res 20:e34–e35
50. Atkins MB, Mier JW, Parkinson DR et al (1988) Hypothyroidism after treatment with interleukin-2 and lymphokine-activated killer cells. N Engl J Med 318(24):1557–1563
51. Gogas H, Ioannovich J, Dafni U et al (2006) Prognostic significance of autoimmunity during treatment of melanoma with interferon. N Engl J Med 354(7):709–718
52. Tarhini AA, Stuckert J, Lee S, Sander C, Kirkwood JM (2009) Prognostic significance of serum S100B protein in high-risk surgically resected melanoma patients participating in Intergroup Trial ECOG 1694. J Clin Oncol 27(1):38–44
53. Bouwhuis MG, Ten Hagen TL, Suciu S, Eggermont AM (2011) Autoimmunity and treatment outcome in melanoma. Curr Opin Oncol 23(2):170–176
54. Davar D, Tarhini AA, Kirkwood JM (2012) Adjuvant therapy for melanoma. Cancer J 18(2):192–202
55. Tarhini AA, Stuckert J, Lee S, Sander C, Kirkwood JM (2009) Prognostic significance of serum S100B protein in high-risk surgically resected melanoma patients participating in Intergroup Trial ECOG 1694. J Clin Oncol 27(1):38–44
56. Stuckert JJ, Tarhini AA, Lee S et al (2007) Interferon alfa-induced autoimmunity and serum S100 levels as predictive and prognostic biomarkers in high-risk melanoma in the ECOG-intergroup phase II trial E2696. J Clin Oncol 2007 ASCO Annual Meeting Proceedings Part I, vol 25, no. 18S (June 20 Supplement): 8506
57. Bouwhuis MG, Suciu S, Kruit W et al (2011) Prognostic value of serial blood S100B

determinations in stage IIB-III melanoma patients: a corollary study to EORTC trial 18952. Eur J Cancer 47(3):361–368

58. Bouwhuis MG, Suciu S, Collette S et al (2009) Autoimmune antibodies and recurrence-free interval in melanoma patients treated with adjuvant interferon. J Natl Cancer Inst 101(12):869–877
59. Bouwhuis MG, Collette S, Suciu S et al (2011) Changes of ferritin and CRP levels in melanoma patients treated with adjuvant interferon-α (EORTC 18952) and prognostic value on treatment outcome. Melanoma Res 21(4):344–351
60. Bouwhuis MG, Suciu S, Testori A et al (2010) Phase III trial comparing adjuvant treatment with pegylated interferon Alfa-2b versus observation: prognostic significance of autoantibodies—EORTC 18991. J Clin Oncol 28(14): 2460–2466

Chapter 5

Immunologic Monitoring of Cancer Vaccine Trials Using the ELISPOT Assay

Lisa H. Butterfield and Mary Jo Buffo

Abstract

Cancer vaccines are designed to activate an immune response to tumor-specific or tumor-associated antigens expressed by the tumor. Cancer vaccines take many forms, including synthetic peptides, tumor cells and lysates, cell lines, and autologous antigen presenting cells like dendritic cells. The target antigens may be known, or "defined" in the vaccine, or unknown. In melanoma, more so than in other cancers, a large number of immunogenic "shared" antigens (tumor-specific or tumor-associated) have been identified. This allows for vaccination of groups of patients with the same vaccine, and also allows for testing for melanoma tumor immunity even when the vaccine does not include defined antigens. For the cancer vaccine field, the goal of a prognostic or predictive biomarker has yet to be achieved. However, the primary immunologic goal of any cancer vaccine is the induction (or amplification) of an immune response against the tumor, therefore the primary goal of immunologic monitoring in this setting, is testing for that response. In this chapter, we present standardized methodology from a central immunologic monitoring laboratory for melanoma cancer vaccine immune response assessment by the Enzyme-Linked Immunosorbant Spot (ELISPOT) assay. This assay allows for enumeration of antigen-specific cells in a plate format. We present the Interferon (IFN)-γ-producing lymphocyte assay, but the platform is easily adjusted to several cell types and several secreted molecules.

Key words Cancer vaccine, Immunologic monitoring, Dendritic cells, ELISPOT, T cells

1 Introduction

The goals of immunologic monitoring in cancer vaccine trials are, first, to determine the effects of vaccination and, second, to identify predictive and/or prognostic biomarkers of response [1, 2]. Recommendations on important parameters of immune biomarker assessments were recently published [3].

1.1 Development of the ELISPOT Assay

The enzyme-linked immunospot assay (ELISPOT) assay was originally developed in the early 1980s [4] and was quickly modified to detect antibody and quantify antigen-specific T cells via secretion of effector molecules such as cytokine, granzyme B, or perforin at the single-cell level [5–7]. Computerized, standardized counting

Magdalena Thurin and Francesco M. Marincola (eds.), *Molecular Diagnostics for Melanoma: Methods and Protocols*, Methods in Molecular Biology, vol. 1102, DOI 10.1007/978-1-62703-727-3_5, © Springer Science+Business Media New York 2014

methods were also developed early [8, 9] and response definitions have been addressed from a statistical standpoint [10]. Comparisons between the ELISPOT and other assays have been conducted [11–13] and many critical technical parameters have been identified [14, 15]. Several groups have led efforts at careful standardization of this assay [16–18], but the most wide-reaching effort has been the iterative proficiency panel program of the Cancer Immunotherapy Consortium [19]. These panels have identified additional important assay parameters and led to greater standardization and reproducibility in the field. They have addressed many procedural steps such as cells handling, serum source and serum-free medium that may be superior, to reduce variability [20], as well as spot data analysis [19]. In vitro stimulation before analysis has been tested [21], and testing for secretion of other cytokines, like IL-5, has been published [22]. If harmonization of immune assays can be achieved they can become a reliable and widely acceptable tool for monitoring of immune responses in clinical trials immunotherapy efforts.

1.2 Clinical Trial Results Using the ELISPOT

The ELISPOT assay has great potential as a diagnostic tool and it is currently the best-suited assay for evaluation of T cell responses on the clinical trial scale. There have been a number of recent trials utilizing the ELISPOT assay which have demonstrated a correlation between immune response and clinical outcome. In smaller trials, there are many examples demonstrating successful vaccination, as well as clinical correlations [23–26], however a recent large, multicenter cooperative group vaccine trial, in which the ELISPOT assays were performed in a central laboratory under standardized conditions, also showed a statistically significant correlation between immune response and clinical outcome, when response was measured functionally, by ELISPOT [27] but not when phenotypically measured by Major Histocompatibility (MHC) tetramer [28].

1.3 Outline of Major Steps in the ELISPOT Assay

The assay is based on the principle of an ELISA. Cells or peptides are applicable for stimulation of responder cells, and they are all plated directly on a filter-bottom microtiter plate coated with an antibody against the effector molecule of interest. Following a stimulation period, the effector molecule, such as IFN-γ, granzyme B, or IL-5, is visualized by a secondary antibody conjugated with an enzyme or biotin and then the corresponding substrate or avidin is added (respectively). The ELISPOT assay described in this protocol involves the need for the coating step and several incubation steps: precoating plates with capture monoclonal antibody (mAb), biotin conjugated detection antibody, enzyme conjugated avidin, and substrate for color development.

Day 1—Coating plates 1–3 days prior to the detection of interferon (IFN)-γ using ELISPOT assay. Nitrocellulose-backed plates are coated with capture antibody (Ab), i.e., anti-human INFγ mAb 1-D1K with the final coating concentration of 10 μg/mL.

Day 2—Blocking, peptide preparation, CD8 separation, CD4 separation, and cell preparation.

(a) Thawing and adjusting peripheral blood mononuclear cells (PBMC).

(b) Blocking of the ELISPOT plate.

(c) Plating INFγ secreting cells.

Day 3—IFN-γ development (18–24 h post incubation).

(a) Addition of mAB 7-B6-Biotin Detection Antibody at 2 μg/mL.

(b) Addition of Avidin-Peroxidase Complex.

(c) Color development with Peroxidase substrate AEC.

(d) Reading the ELISPOT plate.

2 Materials

2.1 Equipment

1. Centrifuge—standard benchtop model.
2. Incubator—humidified, 5 % CO_2, 37 °C.
3. Laminar flow hood.
4. Microscope, bright field.
5. CTL-ImmunoSpot® Reader/Analyzer (Cellular Technology Ltd., Model S5 UV Analyzer).
6. Hemacytometer.
7. MiniMACS Separation Magnet (Miltenyi Biotec).

2.2 Materials

1. MultiScreen HA 96-well sterile nitrocellulose filter containing plates (Millipore).
2. Eppendorf (or similar) repeating pipettor.
3. Sterile combitips (2.5 and 5.0 mL).
4. Variable pipettors (P10, P20, P100, P200, P1000).
5. Multichannel pipette capable of accurately dispensing 50–200 μL.
6. Sterile pipette tips.
7. Conical tubes, polypropylene, sterile (15, 50 mL).
8. Sterile serological disposable pipettes (1, 2, 5, 10 mL).
9. Sterile polypropylene round-bottom tubes (14 and 5 mL).
10. Filter units 50 mL, 0.22 μm for sterilizing solutions (Nalgene).
11. Filter units 500 mL, 0.22 μm for sterilizing solutions (Nalgene).
12. Squeeze bottle with tip cut to large bore.

13. Blue absorbent protective pads for drying plates.
14. Syringe filter for sterilizing reagents, 0.2 μm pore, 25 mm diameter.
15. Syringes (10 and 20 mL).
16. Needle 18 g 1½ inch.
17. Sterile reagent reservoirs.
18. MACS® Separation Columns for CD4⁺ or/and CD8⁺ T cells selection, MS + columns (Miltenyi Biotec,).
19. MACS® Pre-Separation Filters (Miltenyi Biotec).

2.3 Reagents

1. Sterile H_2O (Baxter).
2. RPMI-1640 medium.
3. AIM V serum-free assay medium (Gibco).
4. Fetal Bovine Serum (FBS).
5. Bovine Serum Albumin (BSA).
6. L-Glutamine-200 mM (L-Glut).
7. Penicillin-Streptomycin (Pen-Strep).
8. Tween-20.
9. EDTA.
10. 100 % pure Ethyl Alcohol, 200 proof, absolute, anhydrous ACS/USP grade.
11. Stemsol Dimethyl Sulfoxide sterile (DMSO) 99 %, (Protide Pharmaceuticals, Inc.).
12. Phosphate buffered saline (PBS) sterile, 10 mM (1×) and 10× (pH 7.4).
13. Wash Buffer (sterile 1× PBS, 0.05 % Tween-20).
14. Blocking Solution (RPMI, 10 % FBS, 1 % L-glut, 1 % Pen-Strept).
15. IFN-γ Coating Antibody mAb 1-D1K 1 mg/mL (Mabtech, Sweden).
16. IFNγ Biotinylated Detection Antibody mAb 7-B6-1-Biotin 1 mg/mL (Mabtech, Sweden).
17. Avidin Biotinylated Horseradish Peroxidase Complex (Vectastain Elite ABC Kit) (Vector Laboratories).
18. AEC Peroxidase Substrate kit (3-amino-9-ethylcarbazole) (Vector Laboratories).
19. Detection Antibody Diluent (1× PBS, 0.5 % BSA).
20. Vectastain ABC Diluent (1× PBS, 0.1 % Tween-20).
21. Phorbol 12-Myristate 13-Acetate (PMA), for stimulation of PBMC, Stock solution (1 mg/mL) (Sigma).
22. Ionomycin (ION) for stimulation of PBMC, Stock (10 mM) 1 mg Ionomycin (Sigma).

23. 2× PMA/ION Working Solution (2 ng/mL PMA, 2 μM Ionomycin).
24. Orthoclone OKT3 antibody specific for human CD3 complex, Stock solution (1 mg/mL) (eBioscience). Working Solution (5 μg/mL).
25. Peptides for T cell stimulation, stock solutions (1 mg/mL).
26. Normal control PBMC, cryopreserved.
27. MACS Buffer for cell separation (1× PBS, 0.5 % BSA, 2 mM EDTA).

3 Methods

3.1 Day 1: Coating Plates 1–3 Days Prior to the IFN-γ ELISPOT Assay (See Note 1)

Perform under the laminar flow in sterile conditions.

1. Coat the plates with IFN-γ-specific mAB 1-D1K with the final coating concentration of 10 μg/mL (Mabtech, stock 1 mg/mL) (*see* **Note 2**). Check the current concentration of the capture Ab for its current lot. For example, for one plate add the following in a 50 mL sterile conical tube:

   (a) 6 mL 1× PBS.

   (b) 60 μL mAB 1-D1K Ab stock.

   Mix thoroughly on a vortex and pour into a sterile reservoir.
2. With a multichannel pipette or an Eppendorf repeating pipettor, add 50 μL of the 10 μg/mL solution of mAB 1-D1K to each well of the 96 well plate for all plates to be completed. Swirl or tap the plate gently to ensure the entire surface of the well bottom is covered.
3. Cover the plates and incubate overnight at 4 °C in a sealed zip lock bag, with a "humidity pad," to avoid evaporation. Make sure that the plates are stored flat.

3.2 Day 2: Blocking, Peptide Preparation, CD8 Separation, CD4 Separation, and Cell Preparation

Work under the laminar flow in sterile conditions.

3.2.1 Preparation of Reagents

1. Warm AIM V assay medium in 37 °C waterbath.
2. Thaw DNAse thaw medium in 37 °C waterbath.
3. Remove Blocking Solution from the refrigerator and allow it to warm to room temperature.
4. Prepare working solution of PMA/ION according to reagent preparation. Place at 4 °C until use. Prepare working solution of OKT3 Ab immediately prior to the addition of plated cells.

5. Degas MACS Buffer if CD8 and/or CD4 separations are to be performed (*see* **Note 3**). Pour MACS buffer into a vacuum filter unit (0.22 μm), then replace lid on filter unit and tape around the lid to form a seal. Attach the vacuum hose to the filter unit. Turn on vacuum and let stand for 20 min to degas. Return MACS buffer to 4 °C after degassing.

3.2.2 Thawing and Adjusting PBMC

1. Thaw patient PBMC and frozen normal control according to the Procedure for Thawing Cells, using DNAse containing wash solutions (*see* **Note 4**).
2. Resuspend the patient cells and the frozen normal control in 5 mL of AIM V media.
3. Count the cells manually using Hemacytometer Trypan Blue Dye Exclusion Test for cell count and viability and report on worksheet.
4. Once the total number of cells has been determined, continue with CD8 and/or CD4 separations (separate procedure) (*see* **Note 3**) or adjust PBMC concentrations for direct ELISPOT. Separation of $CD8^+$ or $CD4^+$ is not always necessary. Whole PBMC can be plated in ELISPOT.
5. Adjust the concentration of responder cells according to the specific protocol requirements.
6. Adjust the concentration of cells to 1×10^6 cells/mL in AIM V or 5×10^5 cells/mL in AIM V buffer.
7. Keep cells at 4 °C until it is time to plate the assay. Let cells rest at least 2 h from thaw time.

3.2.3 Blocking of the ELISPOT Plate

1. After coating with anti INFγ antibody is completed discard all liquid within the plates by dumping into a sterile waste container.
2. Wash ELISPOT plate with sterile 1× PBS; using a multichannel pipette, add 180–200 μL of sterile 1× PBS to each well and let stand for 3 min.
3. Discard the PBS in the plates by sterilely dumping the liquid into the waste container. Do not allow the nitrocellulose membrane to dry.
4. Repeat the wash step four more times for a total of five washes.
5. On sterile gauze, turn plates upside-down and gently tap out any excess liquid still remaining in the plates. Do not allow the nitrocellulose membrane to dry.
6. Using a multichannel pipette, add 180 μL of Blocking Solution to each well for blocking.
7. Cover all plates with the plate lid and incubate at 37 °C, 5 % CO_2 for a minimum of 1 h. Use ELISPOT plates on the same day that they are washed and blocked.

	Sample 1			Sample 2			Sample 3			NC		
	1	2	3	4	5	6	7	8	9	10	11	12
A	Responders 1 x 10^5	→	→	Responders 1 x 10^5	→	→	Responders 1 x 10^5	→	→	NC 1 x 10^5	→	→
B	OKT3 + Resp 1 x 10^5	→	→	OKT3 + Resp 1 x 10^5	→	→	OKT3 + Resp 1 x 10^5	→	→	OKT3 + NC 1 x 10^5	→	→
C	APC only + Resp 1 x 10^5	→	→	APC only + Resp 1 x 10^5	→	→	APC only + Resp 1 x 10^5	→	→	APC only	→	→
D	Stimulus 1 + Resp 1 x 10^5	→	→	Stimulus 1 + Resp 1 x 10^5	→	→	Stimulus 1 + Resp 1 x 10^5	→	→	Media Only	→	→
E	Stimulus 2 + Resp 1 x 10^5	→	→	Stimulus 2 + Resp 1 x 10^5	→	→	Stimulus 2 + Resp 1 x 10^5	→	→	PMA/Ion + NC 2 x 10^4	→	→
F	Stimulus 3 + Resp 1 x 10^5	→	→	Stimulus 3 + Resp 1 x 10^5	→	→	Stimulus 3 + Resp 1 x 10^5	→	→	NC 2 x 10^4	→	→
G	Stimulus 4 + Resp 1 x 10^5	→	→	Stimulus 4 + Resp 1 x 10^5	→	→	Stimulus 4 + Resp 1 x 10^5	→	→			
H	Stimulus 5 + Resp 1 x 10^5	→	→	Stimulus 5 + Resp 1 x 10^5	→	→	Stimulus 5 + Resp 1 x 10^5	→	→			

Fig. 1 A sample 96-well plate design for an ELISPOT assay, with each condition plated in triplicate. The antigen being tested (for example, MART-1/Melan-A, gp100, tyrosinase, MAGE-A3, NY-ESO-1, all commonly tested, immunogenic shared antigens) can be used as peptides added to PBMC, peptides pulsed onto APC like T2 cells or autologous dendritic cells (DC), or as antigens in protein or recombinant vector form pulsed with autologous APC. *NC* normal control PBMC, *OKT3* anti CD3 antibody, *APC* antigen presenting cell(s), *Resp* responders (PBMC or purified $CD4^+$ or $CD8^+$ T cells), *Stimulus* the antigen being tested (for example, MART-1/Melan-A, gp100, tyrosinase, MAGE-A3, NY-ESO-1)

3.2.4 Plating Cells

1. Under sterile conditions, remove blocking solution from the plate by flicking out the contents into a sterile waste container.
2. Using a 2.5 mL Eppendorf combitip with a pipette tip on the end or a P100 pipette, pipet 100 μL of (responder) cells (not more than 1×10^5 cells/well) to each well, making sure that the pipette tip DOES NOT touch or tear the nitrocellulose membrane. Avoid any splashing.
3. Plate controls: Using a 2.5 mL Eppendorf combitip with a pipette tip on the end or a P100 pipette, pipet 100 μL of each adjusted normal control (NC) suspension into their corresponding wells. Add 100 μL of OKT3 Ab, 100 μL of PMA/Ionomycin [for polyclonal stimulation of T cells through either the T cell receptor (OKT3) or directly intracellularly through protein kinase C (PMA/ionomycin)] and 100 μL of AIM V media to the appropriate wells (*see* Fig. 1).
4. Using a 2.5 mL Eppendorf combitip with a pipette tip on the end or a P100 pipette, pipet the appropriate number of Antigen Presenting Cells (APCs) to the appropriate wells for PBMC/purified T cell stimulation (*see* Fig. 1; **Notes 5** and **6**).
5. Cover all plates and incubate at 37 °C, 5 % CO_2 for 18–24 h to enable IFN-γ release and capture on the nitrocellulose filter, preferably 18 h (*see* **Note** 7).

3.2.5 Day 3: IFN-γ Development (18–24 h Post Incubation)

Part I: Addition of mAB 7-B6-Biotin Detection Antibody

1. Dispose of liquid in the plates by flicking contents into a sink lined with paper towel.
2. Using a wash bottle with tip cut to large bore, fill each well with wash solution (1× PBS, 0.05 % Tween-20).
3. Let the wash solution sit in the wells for 3 min for each plate.
4. Dispose of wash in the plates by dumping the liquid into the sink.
5. Repeat washing the plates in the same manner for a total of six washes.
6. After the last wash, tap plates upside-down on a blue absorbent pad before going on to the next step. Do not allow the nitrocellulose membrane to dry.
7. Make working solution of mAB 7-B6-1-Biotin conjugate (Mabtech, stock 1 mg/mL).
8. For example, for one plate add the following in a 50 mL sterile conical for 2 μg/mL concentration of Ab:
   (a) 6 mL Detection Ab Diluent, sterile (1× PBS, 0.5 % BSA).
   (b) 12 μL of 1 mg/mL mAB 7-B6-1 Stock Solution.
9. Mix thoroughly and pass through a sterile 0.2 μm syringe filter using a 10 or 20 mL syringe and put into a reagent reservoir.
10. Using a multichannel pipet, add 50 μL of the diluted antibody to each well.
11. Cover plates and incubate at 37 °C, 5 % CO_2 for 2 h.

Part II: Addition of Avidin-Peroxidase Complex

1. 5–10 min before the end of the 2 h incubation, prepare the Vectastain Elite Avidin-Peroxidase Complex (ABC Reagent). Add to a 50 mL sterile conical, per plate, the following:
   (a) 10 mL sterile Vectastain ABC diluent (0.1 % Tween 20, 1× PBS).
   (b) One drop reagent A.
   (c) One drop reagent B.
2. Vortex Avidin-Peroxidase Complex thoroughly and let it stand at room temperature for 30 min.
3. Dispose of liquid in the plates by flicking contents into a sink lined with paper towel.
4. Using a wash bottle with tip cut to large bore, fill each well with wash solution.
5. Let the wash solution sit in the wells for 3 min for each plate.
6. Dispose of wash in the plates by dumping the liquid into the sink.
7. Repeat washing the plates in the same manner for a total of six washes.

8. After the last wash, tap plates upside-down on a blue absorbent pad before going on to the next step. Remove the excess wash buffer, but do not let the nitrocellulose membrane dry.
9. Add 100 μL of the ABC Reagent to each well using a multi-channel pipette.
10. Cover plates and incubate at room temperature for 1 h in the dark.

Part III: Color Development with AEC Substrate

1. Dispose of liquid in the plates by flicking contents into a sink lined with paper towel.
2. Using a wash bottle with tip cut to large bore, fill each well with wash solution.
3. Let the wash solution sit in the wells for 3 min for each plate.
4. Dispose of wash in the plates by dumping the liquid into the sink.
5. Repeat washing the plates in the same manner for a total of three washes.
6. Gently tap the plates approximately ten times upside-down on a blue absorbent pad to expel any excess liquid in the plates.
7. Continue to wash three more times using 1× PBS instead of wash solution.
8. During the final PBS wash, prepare the AEC substrate solution in a 50 mL conical:
   (a) 10 mL sterile water.
   (b) Four drops buffer solution, *mix thoroughly by inverting conical.*
   (c) Six drops AEC stock solution, *mix thoroughly by inverting conical.*
   (d) Four drops H_2O_2, mix the solution thoroughly.
9. After the last wash, tap plates upside-down on a blue absorbent pad before going on to the next step. Remove the excess wash buffer, but do not let the nitrocellulose membrane dry.
10. Add 100 μL of AEC substrate solution to each well. Incubate in the dark for 3½–5 min (*see* **Note 8**). All plates should incubate with the AEC substrate the same amount of time.
11. Stop reaction by placing plates under running tap water. Rinse thoroughly for a minimum of 5 min.
12. Immediately remove the under tray from the plate by gently peeling the tray from the plate. Gently blot the bottom of the wells on a paper towel, and air dry the plate in the dark overnight. The plate must dry completely before reading spots.

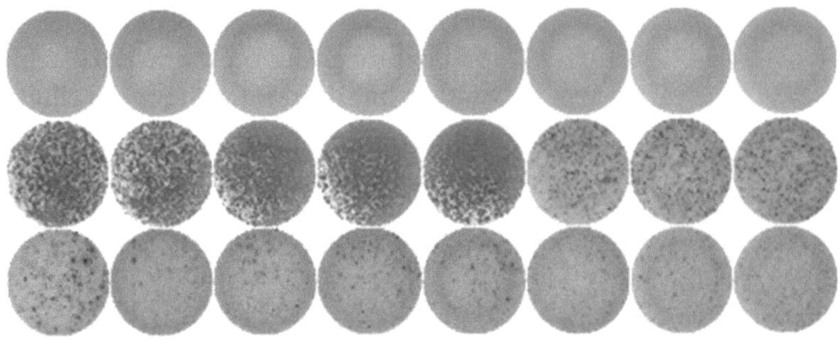

Fig. 2 Example of an IFNγ ELISPOT plate developed with AEC, showing positive and negative control wells

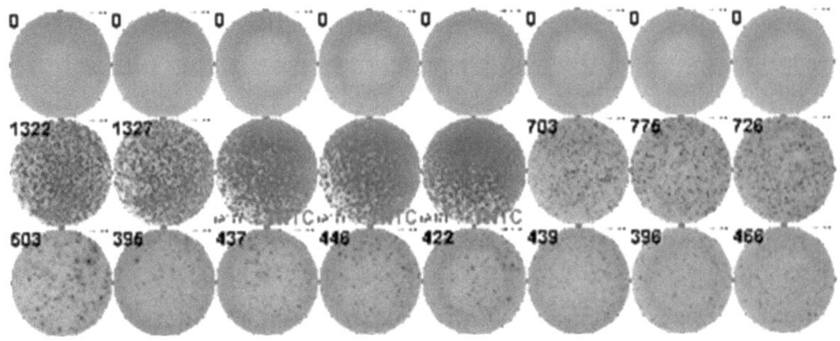

Fig. 3 Example of the IFNγ ELISPOT plate in Fig. 2, with spot counts and quality control (QC) generated with the CTL Technologies ELISPOT plate reader. "TNTC" indicates that the spots were "too numerous to count" accurately

Reading the ELISPOT Plate

Read the ELISPOT plate according to the CTL Analyzer and Immunospot Program. Figure 2 shows an example of an IFN-γ ELISPOT assay result. Figure 3 shows the same wells of the same ELISPOT plate after analysis by the CTL Technologies ELISPOT plate reader, showing well counts (*see* **Note 9**).

4 Notes

1. Plan the assay and prepare an assay template so that each condition is run in triplicate (*see* Fig. 1). Peptides/antigens are to be organized in a manner so that they will be run in order of priority. The priority and specific peptides are protocol specific. This is a critical step that assures a maximum number of test samples per plate and organizes samples ahead of time to make plating the assay easier.
2. Label the plate with your initials, coating antibody, date, and a plate number if coating more than one plate. Plates can be coated up to 3 days prior to assay. ELISPOT plates can be coated on Friday afternoon for Monday assays.

3. Separation of CD4 and CD8 T cells using magnetic-activated cell sorting (MACS) system from Miltenyi. The $CD8^+$ and $CD4^+$ T cell isolation kits are designed for negative selection by depleting non-$CD8^+$ and $CD4^+$ cells using cocktail of biotin-labelled antibodies and anti-biotin superparamagnetic microbeads that are retained in magnetic field on MACS® Separation Columns. CD8 and CD4 positive cells that pass through these columns can be used for functional characterization using ELISPOT assay.
4. Cells that die during freeze–thawing release DNA strands that cause cell clumping and aggregation. Therefore, the use of DNAse-containing wash solutions is recommended while thawing PBMC.
5. If Antigen Presenting Cells (APC) are to be utilized in the ELISPOT assay, pulsing cells (often HLA-$A2^+$ T2 cells) with peptides requires a 2–4 h incubation in serum-free medium, while complex (full length protein) antigens may require overnight incubation with APC (such as immature dendritic cells). Therefore, allow enough time at the beginning of assay setup to perform this process. Pulsing step varies according to the APC type.
6. When a specific antigen is tested (for example, MART-1/Melan-A, gp100, tyrosinase, MAGE-A3, NY-ESO-1, all commonly tested, immunogenic shared antigens) peptides can be added directly to PBMC, peptides can be pulsed onto APC like T2 cells or autologous dendritic cells (DC), or added as antigens in protein or recombinant vector form first pulsed with autologous APC for several hours.
7. During the 18–24 h incubation period (Subheading 3.2.4, step 5), DO NOT open and close the incubator repeatedly as this will interfere with spot clarity.
8. Do not exceed 5 min because of background staining.
9. A reference plate is scanned once per day prior to any ELISPOT plates for all protocols. This ensures that the instrument is operating properly.

References

1. Butterfield LH, Disis ML, Khleif SN et al (2010) Immuno-oncology biomarkers 2010 and beyond: perspectives from the iSBTc/SITC biomarker task force. J Transl Med 8:130
2. Fox BA, Schendel DJ, Butterfield LH et al (2011) Defining the critical hurdles in cancer immunotherapy. J Transl Med 9:214
3. Butterfield LH, Palucka AK, Britten CM et al (2011) Recommendations from the iSBTc-SITC/FDA/NCI workshop on immunotherapy biomarkers. Clin Cancer Res 17:3064–3076
4. Czerkinsky CC, Nilsson LA, Nygren H et al (1983) A solid-phase enzyme-linked immunospot (ELISPOT) assay for enumeration of specific antibody-secreting cells. J Immunol Methods 65:109–121
5. Asai T, Storkus WJ, Whiteside TL (2000) Evaluation of the modified ELISPOT assay for gamma interferon production in cancer patients receiving antitumor vaccines. Clin Vaccine Immunol 7:145–154
6. Cox JH, Ferrari G, Janetzki S (2006) Measurement of cytokine release at the single cell level using the ELISPOT assay. Methods 38:274–282
7. Snyder JE, Bowers WJ, Livingstone AM et al (2003) Measuring the frequency of mouse and

human cytotoxic T cells by the Lysispot assay: independent regulation of cytokine secretion and short-term killing. Nat Med 9:231–235
8. Cui Y, Chang L-J (1997) Computer-assisted, quantitative cytokine enzyme-linked immunospot analysis of human immune effector cell function. Biotechniques 22:1146–1149
9. Herr W, Linn B, Leister N et al (1997) The use of computer-assisted video image analysis for the quantification of CD8+ T lymphocytes producing tumor necrosis factor α spots in response to peptide antigens. J Immunol Methods 203:141–152
10. Moodie Z, Price L, Gouttefangeas C et al (2010) Response definition criteria for ELISPOT assays revisited. Cancer Immunol Immunother 59:1489–1501
11. Whiteside TL, Zhao Y, Tsukishiro T et al (2003) Enzyme-linked immunospot, cytokine flow cytometry, and tetramers in the detection of T-cell responses to a dendritic cell-based multipeptide vaccine in patients with melanoma. Clin Cancer Res 9:641–649
12. Maecker HT, Hassler J, Payne JK et al (2008) Precision and linearity targets for validation of an IFN-γ ELISPOT, cytokine flow cytometry, and tetramer assay using CMV peptides. BMC Immunol 9:9
13. Speiser DE, Pittet MJ, Guillaume P et al (2004) Ex vivo analysis of human antigen-specific CD8+ T-cell responses: quality assessment of fluorescent HLA-A2 multimer and interferon-γ ELISPOT assays for patient immune monitoring. J Immunother 27:298–308
14. Maecker HT, Moon J, Bhatia S et al (2005) Impact of cryopreservation on tetramer, cytokine flow cytometry, and ELISPOT. BMC Immunol 6:17
15. Bull M, Lee D, Stucky J et al (2007) Defining blood processing parameters for optimal detection of cryopreserved antigen-specific responses for HIV vaccine trials. J Immunol Methods 322:57–69
16. Xu Y, Theobald V, Sung C et al (2008) Validation of a HLA-A2 tetramer flow cytometric method, IFNgamma real time RT-PCR, and IFNgamma ELISPOT for detection of immunologic responses to gp100 and MelanA/MART-1 in melanoma patients. J Transl Med 6:61
17. Dubey S, Clair J, Fu T-M et al (2007) Detection of HIV vaccine-induced cell-mediated immunity in HIV-seronegative clinical trial participants using an optimized and validated enzyme-linked immunospot assay. J Acquir Immune Defic Syndr 45:20–27
18. Zhang W, Caspell R, Karulin AY et al (2009) ELISPOT assays provide reproducible results among different laboratories for T-cell immune monitoring-even in hands of ELISPOT-inexperienced investigators. J Immunotoxicol 6:227–234
19. Janetzki S, Panageas KS, Ben-Porat L et al (2007) Results and harmonization guidelines from two large-scale international Elispot proficiency panels conducted by the Cancer Vaccine Consortium (CVC/SVI). Cancer Immunol Immunother 57:303–315
20. Janetzki S, Price L, Britten CM et al (2010) Performance of serum-supplemented and serum-free media in IFNγ Elispot assays for human T cells. Cancer Immunol Immunother 59:609–618
21. Meidenbauer N, Harris DT, Spitler LE et al (2000) Generation of PSA-reactive effector cells after vaccination with a PSA-based vaccine in patients with prostate cancer. Prostate 43:88–100
22. Bennouna J, Hildesheim A, Chikamatsu K et al (2002) Measurements of helper type T-cell responses in humans using ELISPOT assays for IL-5. J Immunol Methods 261:145–156
23. Butterfield LH, Ribas A, Dissette VB et al (2003) Determinant spreading associated with clinical response in dendritic cell-based immunotherapy for malignant melanoma. Clin Cancer Res 9:998–1008
24. Welters MJ, Kenter GG, de Vos van Steenwijk PJ et al (2010) Success or failure of vaccination for HPV16-positive vulvar lesions correlates with kinetics and phenotype of induced T-cell responses. Proc Natl Acad Sci U S A 107: 11895–11899
25. Slingluff CL, Petroni GR, Yamshchikov GV et al (2004) Immunologic and clinical outcomes of vaccination with a multiepitope melanoma peptide vaccine plus low-dose interleukin-2 administered either concurrently or on a delayed schedule. J Clin Oncol 22:4474–4485
26. Linette GP, Zhang D, Hodi S et al (2005) Immunization using autologous dendritic cells pulsed with the melanoma-associated antigen gp100-derived G280-9V peptide elicits CD8+ immunity. Clin Cancer Res 11:7692–7699
27. Kirkwood JM, Lee S, Moschos SJ et al (2009) Immunogenicity and antitumor effects of vaccination with peptide vaccine +/- granulocyte-monocyte colony-stimulating factor and/or IFN-alpha2b in advanced metastatic melanoma: eastern cooperative oncology group phase II Trial E1696. Clin Cancer Res 15:1443–1451
28. Schaefer C, Butterfield LH, Lee S et al (2012) Function but not phenotype of melanoma peptide-specific CD8+ T cells correlate with survival in a multi-epitope peptide vaccine trial (ECOG 1696). Int J Cancer 131:874–884. doi:10.1002/ijc.26481

Chapter 6

Markers for Anti-cytotoxic T-lymphocyte Antigen 4 (CTLA-4) Therapy in Melanoma

Michael A. Postow, Jianda Yuan, Shigehisa Kitano, Alexander M. Lesokhin, and Jedd D. Wolchok

Abstract

Therapeutic strategies that block Cytotoxic T lymphocyte antigen-4 (CTLA-4) enhance antitumor immunity and prolong the lives of patients with metastatic melanoma. However, only a subset of patients benefit, and responses are often delayed due to heterogeneous response kinetics. Ongoing monitoring of the immunologic effects of therapy and correlating these immunologic changes with patient outcomes continue to be important goals to better identify possible mechanisms of clinical activity of these agents. This chapter introduces the major areas of investigation in monitoring patients treated with CTLA-4 blockade and provides specific details of our experience performing selected assays.

Key words Ipilimumab, Tremelimumab, CTLA-4, Immunologic response biomarkers, Absolute lymphocyte count, Inducible costimulator, Myeloid-derived suppressor cells, NY-ESO-1 antigen

1 Introduction

Cytotoxic T lymphocyte antigen-4 (CTLA-4) is an inhibitory molecule that is expressed on the cell surface of activated T cells and is essential for the maintenance of immunologic homeostasis. Therapeutic strategies that block CTLA-4 have been shown to increase immunologic responses and augment antitumor immunity. Two antibodies that block CTLA-4, ipilimumab (Yervoy™, Bristol-Myers Squibb, Princeton, NJ) and tremelimumab (MedImmune, Gaithersburg, MD), have been evaluated in phase III clinical trials where an overall survival (OS) benefit for patients with metastatic melanoma treated with ipilimumab has been demonstrated [1, 2].

Despite this improvement in OS, only a subset of patients benefit from CTLA-4 blockade. Some patients experience mechanism-based toxicity, referred to as immune-related adverse events (irAEs) or adverse events of special interest (AEOSI) [3].

Magdalena Thurin and Francesco M. Marincola (eds.), *Molecular Diagnostics for Melanoma: Methods and Protocols*, Methods in Molecular Biology, vol. 1102, DOI 10.1007/978-1-62703-727-3_6, © Springer Science+Business Media New York 2014

We and others have been interested in assessing the immunologic status of patients undergoing therapy with CTLA-4 blockade to understand presumed mechanisms of antitumor immunity and/or AEOSI induced by these agents.

In this chapter, we first introduce the major efforts investigating quantifiable immunologic parameters associated with benefit and toxicity from CTLA-4 blockade. We then share detailed methods of the standard operating procedures we use to perform these immunologic assays. We conclude by sharing specific aspects of our experience as it pertains to the methods described. Though ipilimumab and tremelimumab have both been evaluated as CTLA-4 blocking therapies, we have chosen to focus the majority of this chapter on selected markers relevant to ipilimumab, the current commercially approved CTLA-4 blocking antibody and the agent with which we have had the most extensive experience.

1.1 Absolute Lymphocyte Count

The absolute lymphocyte count (ALC) is a readily accessible value in nearly all clinical laboratories as it constitutes part of the complete blood count (CBC) routinely performed by automated analyzers. Several retrospective analyses have shown that the ALC correlates positively with improved clinical outcomes following ipilimumab therapy. In the largest analysis, 379 patients from three phase II trials were analyzed [4]. Patients who achieved clinical benefit from ipilimumab (stable disease ≥24 weeks, partial response, and/or complete response) had a greater mean increase in ALC after starting therapy than patients who had progressive disease ($p = 0.0013$). Similar results were found prospectively in 64 patients [4].

The ALC has also been shown to correlate with overall survival. In a separate study, 51 patients treated with ipilimumab at 10 mg/kg whose ALC was ≥1,000/μL prior to the third dose of ipilimumab had improved survival compared to patients whose ALC <1,000/μL [5]. This finding was similar for 137 patients treated with ipilimumab at 3 mg/kg, even when adjusting for M-stage, lactate dehydrogenase (LDH), and number of prior therapies [6]. Since the ALC reflects a heterogeneous lymphocyte population including T cells, B cells, and to a lesser degree, natural killer (NK) cells, the specific cell population predominantly responsible for the association with clinical benefit and overall survival in these analyses remains the subject of ongoing evaluation.

1.2 Analyses of Specific T Cell Populations

Flow cytometry analyses of lymphocyte subpopulations in the peripheral blood and tumor have revealed suggestions of the most relevant lymphocyte subsets that correlate with benefit from ipilimumab. One study of 35 patients showed that patients who achieved clinical benefit from ipilimumab had a greater absolute increase in the number of CD8+ T cells compared to patients who did not benefit ($p = 0.0294$). The absolute increase in CD4+ T cells did not differ significantly between patients who achieved clinical benefit and those who did not ($p = 0.2237$) [7].

The type and degree of tumor infiltrating lymphocytes (TIL) have also been investigated. Earlier investigations into ipilimumab biomarkers revealed that the ratio of CD8+ T cells to Forkhead Box P3 (FoxP3)+T regulatory cells was associated with therapy-induced tumor necrosis [8]. These results are consistent with a dedicated biomarker study of ipilimumab, where an increase in TIL during therapy was associated with a higher likelihood of clinical benefit ($p = 0.005$) [9].

Cell surface marker expression on T cells has also been examined to further characterize T cell responses during CTLA-4 therapy. Increased levels of the human leukocyte antigen (HLA)-DR and CD45RO on CD4+ and CD8+ T cells in peripheral blood after ipilimumab treatment have been reported in several studies [10–13]. There was no correlation, however, between the elevation of HLA-DR or CD45RO and clinical response to ipilimumab. An independent study of 12 patients treated with tremelimumab suggested similar effects, although there was some correlation with clinical benefit in this small cohort [14].

Inducible costimulator (ICOS) is expressed on the cell surface after T cell activation and plays a role in T cell expansion and survival [15]. Ipilimumab was administered as neoadjuvant therapy in a study of six patients with bladder cancer undergoing cystoprostatectomy. After ipilimumab treatment, the frequency of CD4+ T cells that expressed ICOS increased in both the peripheral blood and bladder tumor tissue [16]. In a retrospective analysis of 14 patients with melanoma, a sustained increase over 12 weeks of CD4+ICOS^{hi} T cells in the peripheral blood correlated with improved survival [17]. These results are consistent with those from another study in which ipilimumab was shown to result in a pharmacodynamic increase in ICOS^{hi}, proliferating (Ki67+), CD4+ and CD8+ T cells [18]. In this study, decreased levels of Ki67+CD8+ T cells were significantly associated with the development of irAEs.

1.3 Tumor Antigen-Specific Immunity

In addition to efforts monitoring T cell subpopulations during treatment with CTLA-4 blockade, characterization of antigen-specific antibody and T cell responses has similarly led to associations between immunologic changes and benefit from CTLA-4 therapy. Serological studies have evaluated antibody responses against a number of tumor-associated antigens, including, but not limited to MAGE, Melan-A, MART-1, gp-100, and tyrosinase. Humoral responses against the cancer-testis antigen, NY-ESO-1, however, have been the most thoroughly described.

NY-ESO-1 is a well-characterized cancer-testis antigen expressed in 30–40 % of melanomas [19]. In a study of 144 melanoma patients treated with ipilimumab (most of whom received ipilimumab at 10 mg/kg), the 22 who had a detectable antibody titer by enzyme-linked immunosorbent assay (ELISA) against NY-ESO-1 prior to ipilimumab were more likely to experience clinical benefit than those with no detectable NY-ESO-1 antibody titer (12/22; 55 % vs. 36/118; 31 %, respectively, $p=0.0481$) [20]. It is possible that antibody responses to NY-ESO-1 serve as a surrogate for broader mechanisms of antitumor immunity, rather than direct mediators.

Antigen-specific T cells have also been evaluated as a potential biomarker for CTLA-4 blockade. In a case report of a patient who experienced a complete remission to ipilimumab, a high percentage of melan-A-specific CD8+ T cells was seen in histologic analysis of regressing tumor tissue and in peripheral blood [21]. Though not all patients were treated with anti-CTLA-4 therapy, in another study, the prognostic value of functional T cells responding to the tumor-associated antigens NY-ESO-1 and Melan-A was evaluated. Of the 84 patients with metastatic melanoma, those who had increased functional T cells to NY-ESO-1 and Melan-A had improved survival by Cox regression analysis [22]. In the study of 144 ipilimumab treated patients with melanoma, NY-ESO-1-seropositive patients with associated CD8+ T cells experienced more frequent clinical benefit (10 of 13; 77 %) than those with undetectable CD8+ T-cell response (one of seven; 14 %; $p=0.02$; relative risk = 5.4, two-tailed Fisher test), as well as a significant survival advantage ($p=0.01$; hazard ratio = 0.2, time-dependent Cox model) [20]. Despite these findings, the presence of these cells supports, but does not confirm their mechanistic role in tumor control as they may be a surrogate for other mechanisms of antitumor immunity. Whether this finding is relevant in a population of patients who all receive anti-CTLA-4 therapy remains unknown.

1.4 Myeloid-Derived Suppressor Cells

Myeloid-derived suppressor cells (MDSC) are a heterogeneous population of immunosuppressive monocytic cells. Though MDSC have been described differently, in patients with melanoma, they are typically classified as CD14+/HLA-DR$^{low/-}$ cells, based upon this cell population's ability to suppress lymphocyte function [23]. MDSC have been shown to be increased in patients with melanoma, and the quantity of MDSC has been shown to correlate with melanoma disease activity [24, 25].

We have been investigating MDSC as a biomarker for melanoma patients undergoing treatment with ipilimumab. In a pilot study of 26 patients with metastatic melanoma undergoing treatment with ipilimumab at 10 mg/kg, we evaluated the quantity and functional capabilities of MDSC in the peripheral blood.

Prior to ipilimumab treatment, a lower MDSC quantity was associated with improved overall survival (HR 1.07, $p=0.002$), even when adjusting for pretreatment ALC and lactate dehydrogenase (LDH) [26]. Efforts are ongoing to evaluate this finding in a larger cohort of patients and determine whether this finding is specific for ipilimumab treatment.

2 Materials

2.1 Peripheral Blood Collection, Cell Separation, and Cryopreservation

1. Cell Preparation Tubes (CPT) containing sodium heparin (BD Vacutainer, Franklin Lakes NJ).
2. RPMI 1640 media supplemented with L-glutamine (2 mM final, GIBCO/BRL), 25 % Human Serum Albumin(HSA) (Alpine Biologics).
3. Pooled Human Serum (PHS), heat inactivated at 56 °C for 30 min (Gemini Bio-Products, Woodland CA).
4. Dimethylsulfoxide (DMSO) (Sigma-Aldrich).
5. Autologous plasma.
6. Guava easyCyte flow cytometer to measure cell viability and count the cells (Millipore).

2.2 Monitoring of Activated T Cell Subpopulations by Flow Phenotype Staining

1. Fluorochrome labeled antibodies: CD278 (ICOS)-PE-Cy7, CD3-Pacific Blue, CD8-PE-Cy5, CD25-PE, and FOXP3-APC (eBioscience); and CD4-ECD (Beckman Coulter Inc.).
2. Fixation/Permeabilization solution (1×) for use prior to intracellular FOXP3 staining (eBioscience).
3. Permeabilization buffer (1×) for use following Fixation buffer, washing and cell suspension prior to FOXP3 staining (eBioscience).
4. Antibody Isotype controls for the appropriate fluorochrome-conjugated mouse IgG_{1a} or IgG_{2a} from same companies (eBioscience, Beckman Coulter and BD Bioscience).
5. Fluorescence-activated cell sorting (FACS) buffer: 1 % fetal calf serum (FCS) in 1× PBS EDTA (10 mM phosphate buffered saline, pH 7.4, 1 mM EDTA).
6. CYAN ADP High-Performance Flow Cytometer with multiple laser excitation sources with Summit software (Dako Cytomation California Inc., Carpinteria, CA).
7. FlowJo software for data analysis (version 9.2) (TreeStar, Inc.).

2.3 Monitoring of Antigen-Specific Humoral Immune Responses by Enzyme-Linked Immunosorbent Assay (ELISA) Using NY-ESO-1 Antigen as an Example

1. Full-length NY-ESO-1 protein and control proteins including dihydrofolate reductase (DHFR) are supplied in 8 M urea or PBS and diluted to a final concentration of 1 μg/mL (Ludwig Institute for Cancer Research, New York branch). Protein dilutions are prepared in PBS.
2. The second antibody: goat anti-human IgG-AP (Alkaline Phosphatase)-conjugate (Southern Biotech, Inc. Birmingham).
3. AttoPhos AP Fluorescent Substrate (Promega).
4. AttoPhos buffer to reconstitute the AttoPhos Substrate (Promega).
5. Ready to use AttoPhos working solution: weigh 36 mg Attophos substrate, add to 60 mL Attophos buffer, store at 4 °C up to 1 month.
6. Blocking buffer (5 % nonfat dry (NF) milk in PBS): 500 mL PBS, 150 μg sodium azide and 25 g NF-milk fortified with Vitamins A&D.
7. Wash-buffers: 1× PBS; 1× PBS and 0.1 % Tween-20 (Tw20).
8. Stop solution: 2 N NaOH (in distilled water).
9. A pool of healthy donor sera.
10. ELISA plates (FluoroNunc Maxisorp ELISA plates, Thermo Scientific, Rochester, NY).
11. Microplate Washer ELx405 series (Biotek).
12. Biostack, automated microplate stacking device (Biotek).
13. Microplate ELISA reader (Synergy L, Biotek).

2.4 Monitoring of Antigen-Specific Cellular Responses by Tetramer and Intracellular Cytokine Staining

1. Fluorochrome-labeled antibodies: CD3 PE-Cy7, CD45RA ECD, CD4 ECD (Beckman Coulter); CCR7 FITC (R&D system); CD28 PerCPCy5.5 and CD3 Pacific Blue (BD Biosciences); and CD8 APC-AF750, CD27 APC, IL-2 APC, MIP1-beta PE, TNF-alpha PE-Cy7, and IFN-gamma FITC (BD Pharmingen).
2. Fluorochrome labeled tetramers: PE-NY-ESO-$1_{94\text{-}102}$ (MPFATPMEA) loaded HLA/B*3501, and PE-NY-ESO-$1_{157\text{-}165}$ (SLLMWITQC) loaded HLA/A0201 tetramer (Tetramer Core, Ludwig Institute of Cancer Research, Lausanne Branch, Switzerland). MHC class I negative tetramer control (Beckman Coulter). Concentration of each tetramer was determined by the staining on thawed frozen tetramer positive T cells.
3. NY-ESO-1 overlapping peptides (20-mer overlapped by ten amino acids) (JPT Peptide Technologies GmbH, Berlin, Germany). Peptides were resuspended in DMSO/PBS at the final concentration of 10 % (vol/vol) and stored at −20 °C. Peptides were thawed the day of the assay and diluted to the required concentration. They were never frozen nor thawed more than once.

4. DAPI (4′ 6-diamino-2-phenylindole, Dihydrochloride) nucleic acid stain (Invitrogen).
5. Interleukin (IL)-2 (10 IU/mL, Chiron, Emeryville).
6. IL-15 (10 ng/mL, R&D Systems).
7. Brefeldin A and monensin to block cytokine secretion (BD Bioscience).
8. PE-Cy5-CD107a antibody for detection of degranulating lymphocytes (5 μL/mL BD Pharmingen).
9. Mark I Irradiator (JL Shepard and Associated, San Fernando CA).

2.5 Myeloid-Derived Suppressor Cell Flow Phenotype Staining

1. Lineage-specific antibody (CD3/CD16/CD19/CD20/CD56) cocktail-FITC conjugate (special-ordered BD Pharmingen).
2. The following fluorochrome labeled other antibodies: CD14-PerCP Cy5.5, CD11b-APC Cy7, and CD33-PE-Cy7 (BD Pharmingen); and HLA-DR-ECD (Beckman Coulter).
3. Isotype controls: the appropriate fluorochrome-conjugated mouse IgG_1, IgG_k, IgG_{2a}, or IgG_{2bk} from same companies (BD Pharmingen and Beckman Coulter).

3 Methods

3.1 Blood Collection, Cell Separation, and Cryopreservation

1. Collect whole blood from healthy donors or patients in Vacutainer® Cell Preparation Tubes (CPT™).
2. Spin CPT tubes at 1,000 × *g* average (~2,500 rpm Beckman GH-3.8 rotor), slow acceleration, no brake, at room temperature for 25 min.
3. Collect the plasma to be used in other experiments. Harvest the interface and pool cells from interfaces in several 15 mL centrifuge tubes. Top off with RPMI media.
4. Spin at 600–650 × *g* (1,500 rpm Beckman GH-3.8 rotor) in cold centrifuge (4 °C) for 10 min.
5. Aspirate supernatant and resuspend pellet in RPMI media before each wash (approximately 45 mL).
6. Spin at 200–235 × *g* (1,100 rpm Beckman GH-3.8 rotor) in cold centrifuge (4 °C) for 10 min.
7. Aspirate supernatant and resuspend pellet in RPMI media before each wash (approximately 45 mL).
8. Repeat **steps 6** and 7 twice.
9. Count cells either using Trypan Blue at appropriate dilution to count ~100 cells or Guava cell analyzer.
10. For cryopreservation resuspend peripheral blood mononuclear cells (PBMC) in autologous plasma or human serum albumin with 10 % DMSO, keep frozen at −80 °C for 2–3 days and then store in liquid nitrogen.

3.2 Monitoring of Activated T Cell Subpopulations by Flow Phenotype Staining

1. Wash 0.5 million PBMCs with 2 mL FACS buffer.
2. Resuspend the cells in 50 μL FACS buffer and stain with 1 μL ICOS-PE-Cy7 antibody and the following antibodies: 3 μL CD3-Pacific Blue, 1 μL CD4-ECD, 1 μL CD8-PE-Cy5 and 2 μL CD25-PE. Incubate at 4 °C for 30 min.
3. Rewash the cells with FACS buffer, fix and permeabilize the cells with 250 μL 1× fixation/permeabilization solution at 4 °C for 30 min before washing with 2 mL 1× permeabilization buffer.
4. Add 5 μL FOXP3-APC antibody at 4 °C for 60 min before a final washing with 1× permeabilization buffer.
5. Resuspend the cells in 400 μL FACS buffer and perform flow cytometry analysis and acquire data on a CYAN flow cytometer with Summit software.
6. Perform data analysis by using FlowJo software.
7. Use isotype controls for the appropriate fluorochrome-conjugated mouse IgG_{1a} or IgG_{2a} for setting up the gate (*see* **Note 1**).

3.3 Monitoring of Antigen-Specific Humoral Immune Responses by ELISA

1. Prepping of ELISA plates: Add 1 μg/mL of desired antigen (e.g., NY-ESO-1) in PBS (30 μL/well). Incubate overnight at 4 °C or at room temperature for 2 h.
2. Shake off contents of plates, wash three times with 1× PBS and blot dry with paper towels.
3. Block with 5 % NF milk in PBS (30 μL/well) and incubate at 4 °C overnight or at room temperature for 2 h.
4. Shake off contents and wash as in **step 2**.
5. Prepare human serum dilution in blocking buffer in 96-well dilution trays. Usual serum dilutions are fourfold: 1:100, 1:400, 1:1,600, etc.
6. Shake off last wash, blot dry with paper towel and add serum dilutions (30 μL/well) incubate at 4 °C overnight.
7. Shake off contents and wash 3× with 1× PBS and 0.1 % Tw20, and 3× with 1× PBS using Microplate Washer and Biostack.
8. Shake off last wash, blot dry with paper towel and add second antibody (goat anti-human IgG-AP) at appropriate dilution 1:4,000 in blocking buffer (30 μL/well) and incubate at room temperature for 1 h.
9. Shake off contents and wash as in **step 7**.
10. Shake off last wash, blot dry, and add 30 μL AttoPhos working solution containing AP substrate and incubate in dark for 30 min.
11. Stop color development by adding 15 μL stop solution (2 N NaOH).

12. Fluorescence signal (Excitation at 450/50 nm and Emission at 580/50 nm with gain of 25) is measured using ELISA plate reader with Biostack (Optics position top 510 nm, lightsource Tungsten, detection method fluorescence, read type endpoint) (*see* **Note 2**).

3.4 Monitoring of Tumor Antigen-Specific Cellular Responses by Tetramer and Intracellular Cytokine Staining

3.4.1 In Vitro Stimulation with T Cell-Specific Peptides

1. Resuspended thawed PBMCs in 10 % pooled human serum (PHS) in RPMI 1640 medium and plate at 2.5×10^6 cells per well.
2. Pulse $2.5 \times 10e^6$ autologous PBMCs with 20-mer NY-ESO-1 overlapping peptides (10 μg/mL) at room temperature for 1 h, then irradiate with 30 Gy and culture with the responder cells at 1:1 ratio.
3. The culture medium contains IL-2 (10 IU/mL) and IL-15 (10 ng/mL). Change media every 2–3 days during the in vitro stimulation.
4. After 10 days of in vitro culture, harvest the cells and analyze by flow cytometry for tetramer staining and intracellular cytokine staining.

3.4.2 Tetramer Staining

1. Incubate $5 \times 10e^5$ cells with 0.5 μL of corresponding tetramer in 50 μL FACS buffer, 0.05 mM EDTA, 0.01 % sodium azide at 37 °C for 15 min, followed by the surface antigen-specific antibodies at room temperature for another 15 min.
2. Wash the cells with FACS buffer once and resuspend in 300 μL FACS buffer for flow cytometric acquisition.
3. Cells are considered positive for tetramer staining when they form a clear population with mean fluorescence intensity that is ≥1 log above the MHC Class I negative tetramer control (*see* **Note 3**).
4. Collect events (≥10^5) after live gating on lymphocytes by forward and side scatter. Use DAPI stain to gate out dead cells for tetramer staining (*see* Fig. 1 for example data showing an increase in NY-ESO-1 T cells during ipilimumab therapy).

3.4.3 Intracellular Cytokine Staining

1. For intracellular cytokine and staining detection of multiple parameters including expression of IFN-γ, IL-2, TNF-α, MIP-1β, and CD107a, harvest $2 \times 10e^6$ cultured T cells at Day 10 and resuspend in 1 mL 10 % PHS RPMI medium (*see* **Note 4**).
2. Restimulate the cells with the addition of corresponding peptides at 37 °C for the first 2 h and then in the presence of 5 μg/mL each of Brefeldin A and monensin for 4 h.
3. Add PE-Cy5-CD107a specific antibody (5 μL/mL or concentration 2.5 μg/mL) prior to stimulation. Harvest and wash the cells with 2 mL FACS buffer once.

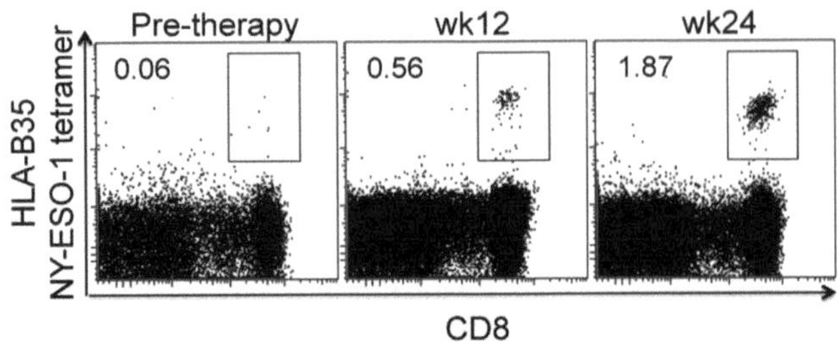

Fig. 1 Ipilimumab induced the expansion of NY-ESO-1$_{94\text{-}102}$ (MPFATPMEA) HLA/B*3501 tetramer + CD8+ T cells. PBMCs from both pre-therapy and post-therapy (week 12 and week 24) in a melanoma patient treated with 10 mg/kg of ipilimumab were cultured with NY-ESO-1 overlapping peptide for 10 days as described in Subheading 3.4. NY-ESO-1$_{94\text{-}102}$ (MPFATPMEA) HLA/B*3501 staining was performed on harvested T cells. A greater number of NY-ESO-1$_{94\text{-}102}$ (MPFATPMEA) HLA/B*3501 tetramer + CD8+ T cells were detected at week 12 and week 24 after ipilimumab treatment

4. Resuspend a total of $10e^6$ cells in FACS buffer and stain with the panel of antibodies for appropriate phenotypic cell surface markers and functional cytokine antibodies following fixation/permeabilization as described at Subheading 3.2.
5. Cells are analyzed by flow cytometry on a CYAN flow cytometer with Summit software to acquire the data. Perform further analysis on FlowJo software.

3.5 Myeloid-Derived Suppressor Cell Phenotype Staining

1. Wash thawed $5 \times 10e^5$ PBMCs from melanoma patients before and after treatment with 2 mL FACS buffer (*see* **Note 5**).
2. Add the following fluorochrome-conjugated antibodies: Lineage-specific antibodies (CD3/CD16/CD19/CD20/CD56) cocktail-FITC, and CD14-PerCP Cy5.5, CD11b-APC Cy7, CD33-PE-Cy7, and HLA-DR-ECD, and incubate at 4 °C for 20 min.
3. Include the appropriate fluorochrome-conjugated mouse IgG_1, IgG_k, IgG_{2a}, or IgG_{2bk} as isotype controls.
4. Detect the stained cells by using a CYAN flow cytometer. Use FlowJo software for all analysis (*see* **Note 5** and Fig. 2 for example gating strategy).

4 Notes

1. We optimize our phenotype flow staining for CD4 + ICOS^{hi} T cells by performing each analysis in duplicate or triplicate and staining each PBMC sample for isotype control as well. In our experience, the frequency of CD4 + ICOS^{hi} T cells is much higher in the tumor than in the peripheral blood. Therefore, we apply the gate of 0.5 % in the isotype control

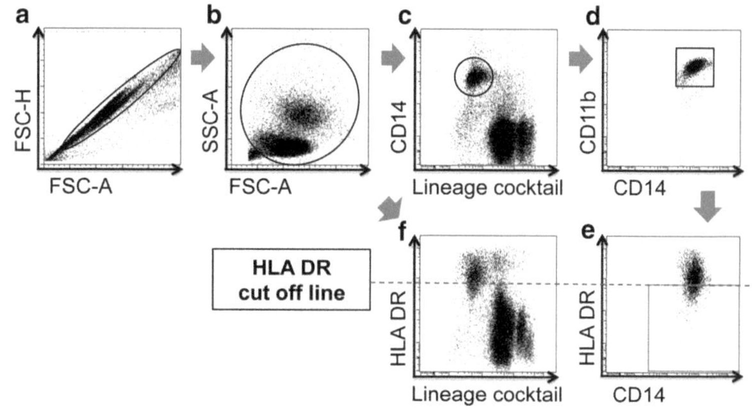

Fig. 2 MDSC gating strategy. MDSC are characterized as a CD14+CD11b+ population that is HLA-DR$^{low/-}$. After gating on single cells with forward scatter (FSC)-A and FSC-H selection (**a**), the myeloid population is gated based on side scatter (SSC) (**b**). Then, using our lineage cocktail (Subheading 3.5), we select CD14 positive cells that are lineage negative (**c**). The majority of these CD14 positive cells are CD11b positive (**d**). Finally, the selection of HLA-DR$^{low/-}$ cells in this population (**e**) is based upon the HLA-DR expression level on lymphocyte populations (lineage positive cells, **f**)

tube to select the real sample. We define a persistent increase in CD4+ICOS^{hi} expression as a ≥2-fold increase in % CD4+ICOS^{hi} expression at week 7 or 12 over baseline that is sustained at week 12.

2. We perform the analysis of serum samples by ELISA in a blinded fashion to the knowledge of clinical results. We test sera in 4× serial dilutions, starting from 1/100, for IgG reactivity against full-length NY-ESO-1. Using the control protein, DHFR, is essential to assess antibody specificity. Positive control sera with known reactivity on each plate are used to validate the assays. We usually do not detect antibody reactivity to DHFR in sera from patients with ipilimumab, assuring ourselves of its capabilities as a negative control. We also perform an extrapolation of antibody titers based on a pool of healthy donor sera with no reactivity to NY-ESO-1. We consider reciprocal titers positive if greater than 100.

3. We assess tumor antigen-specific T cell response by either tetramer or intracellular cytokine staining. To determine tetramer positive T-cell responses, we calculate the standard deviation of the pre-therapy replicate values taken at baseline. A tetramer T-cell response at any post-therapy time point is considered positive if it has a value ≥3 standard deviations than the mean value at baseline and has an absolute value of >0.1 %.

4. For intracellular cytokine staining, CD107a-specific antibody should be added to the culture prior to the stimulation.

We then determine each cytokine response by subtracting the background cytokine production in an unstimulated sample. Specificity of tumor antigen-specific T cell responses is considered significant if >3-fold over control (unpulsed target cells). Patients are considered to have an increase in T cell response if the frequency of T cells detected in at least one post-therapy sample exceeded that found in the baseline sample by three-fold, and the response has an absolute value of at least 0.1 %. The data analysis program Simplified Presentation of Incredibly Complex Evaluations (SPICE software, version 5.2.2) has been kindly provided by M. Roederer, NIH, Bethesda, MD. We use this software to analyze and generate graphical representations of T cell responses detected by polychromatic flow cytometry.

5. For MDSC analysis, we have found that peripheral blood samples should ideally be processed within 5–6 h from the patient's blood draw. In our experience, expression levels by mean fluorescence intensity (MFI) of HLA-DR molecules on CD14 + CD11b+ cells increase with greater time in the blood collection tube. Consequently, the sensitivity of flow cytometry in detecting MDSC elevation is lost if the samples are processed after an overnight interval. The definition of MDSC (HLA-DR$^{low/-}$ on CD14 + CD11b+ population) depends on the gating strategy. We draw the cut-off line between HLA-DR high and low—based on HLA-DR expression level on lymphocyte populations (lineage positive cells) within each sample, which are HLA-DR high and stable over time.

Acknowledgements

We would like to thank Erika Ritter and Teresa Rasalan for their critical review of the book chapter.

References

1. Hodi FS, O'Day SJ, McDermott DF et al (2010) Improved survival with ipilimumab in patients with metastatic melanoma. N Engl J Med 363:711–723
2. Robert C, Thomas L, Bondarenko I et al (2011) Ipilimumab plus dacarbazine for previously untreated metastatic melanoma. N Engl J Med 364:2517–2526
3. Topalian SL, Hodi FS, Brahmer JR et al (2012) Safety, activity, and immune correlates of anti-PD-1 antibody in cancer. N Engl J Med 366:2443–2454
4. Berman D, Wolchok J, Weber J et al (2009) Association of peripheral blood absolute lymphocyte count (ALC) and clinical activity in patients (pts) with advanced melanoma treated with ipilimumab. J Clin Oncol 27(suppl): 15s.3020 (abstr)
5. Ku GY, Yuan J, Page DB et al (2010) Single-institution experience with ipilimumab in advanced melanoma patients in the compassionate use setting: lymphocyte count after 2 doses correlates with survival. Cancer 116: 1767–1775
6. Postow M, Yuan J, Panageas K et al (2012) Evaluation of the absolute lymphocyte count as a biomarker for melanoma patients treated with the commercially available dose of ipilimumab (3mg/kg). J Clin Oncol 30(suppl):8575, abstr

7. Yang A, Kendle RF, Ginsberg BA et al (2010) CTLA-4 blockade with ipilimumab increases peripheral CD8+ T cells: correlation with clinical outcomes. J Clin Oncol 28(suppl):15s.2555, abstr
8. Hodi FS, Butler M, Oble DA et al (2008) Immunologic and clinical effects of antibody blockade of cytotoxic T lymphocyte-associated antigen 4 in previously vaccinated cancer patients. Proc Natl Acad Sci USA 105: 3005–3010
9. Hamid O, Schmidt H, Nissan A et al (2011) A prospective phase II trial exploring the association between tumor microenvironment biomarkers and clinical activity of ipilimumab in advanced melanoma. J Transl Med 9:204
10. Phan GQ, Yang JC, Sherry RM et al (2003) Cancer regression and autoimmunity induced by cytotoxic T lymphocyte-associated antigen 4 blockade in patients with metastatic melanoma. Proc Natl Acad Sci USA 100: 8372–8377
11. Attia P, Phan GQ, Maker AV et al (2005) Autoimmunity correlates with tumor regression in patients with metastatic melanoma treated with anti-cytotoxic T-lymphocyte antigen-4. J Clin Oncol 23:6043–6053
12. Maker AV, Phan GQ, Attia P et al (2005) Tumor regression and autoimmunity in patients treated with cytotoxic T lymphocyte-associated antigen 4 blockade and interleukin 2: a phase I/II study. Ann Surg Oncol 12:1005–1016
13. Maker AV, Yang JC, Sherry RM et al (2006) Intrapatient dose escalation of anti-CTLA-4 antibody in patients with metastatic melanoma. J Immunother 29:455–463
14. Comin-Anduix B, Lee Y, Jalil J et al (2008) Detailed analysis of immunologic effects of the cytotoxic T lymphocyte-associated antigen 4-blocking monoclonal antibody tremelimumab in peripheral blood of patients with melanoma. J Transl Med 6:22
15. Burmeister Y, Lischke T, Dahler AC et al (2008) ICOS controls the pool size of effector-memory and regulatory T cells. J Immunol 180:774–782
16. Liakou CI, Kamat A, Tang DN et al (2008) CTLA-4 blockade increases IFNgamma-producing CD4+ICOShi cells to shift the ratio of effector to regulatory T cells in cancer patients. Proc Natl Acad Sci USA 105: 14987–14992
17. Carthon BC, Wolchok JD, Yuan J et al (2010) Preoperative CTLA-4 blockade: tolerability and immune monitoring in the setting of a presurgical clinical trial. Clin Cancer Res 16(10):2861–2871
18. Wang W, Yu D, Sarnaik AA et al (2012) Biomarkers on melanoma patient T Cells associated with ipilimumab treatment. J Transl Med 10:146
19. Jungbluth AA, Chen YT, Stockert E et al (2001) Immunohistochemical analysis of NY-ESO-1 antigen expression in normal and malignant human tissues. Int J Cancer 92:856–860
20. Yuan J, Adamow M, Ginsberg BA et al (2011) Integrated NY-ESO-1 antibody and CD8+ T-cell responses correlate with clinical benefit in advanced melanoma patients treated with ipilimumab. Proc Natl Acad Sci U S A 108:16723–16728
21. Klein O, Ebert LM, Nicholaou T et al (2009) Melan-A-specific cytotoxic T cells are associated with tumor regression and autoimmunity following treatment with anti-CTLA-4. Clin Cancer Res 15:2507–2513
22. Weide B, Zelba H, Derhovanessian E et al (2012) Functional T cells targeting NY-ESO-1 or Melan-A are predictive for survival of patients with distant melanoma metastasis. J Clin Oncol 30:1835–1841
23. Filipazzi P, Valenti R, Huber V et al (2007) Identification of a new subset of myeloid suppressor cells in peripheral blood of melanoma patients with modulation by a granulocyte-macrophage colony-stimulation factor-based antitumor vaccine. J Clin Oncol 25: 2546–2553
24. Poschke I, Mougiakakos D, Hansson J et al (2010) Immature immunosuppressive CD14+HLA-DR-/low cells in melanoma patients are Stat3hi and overexpress CD80, CD83, and DC-sign. Cancer Res 70: 4335–4345
25. Postow MA, Callahan MK, Barker CA et al (2012) Immunologic correlates of the abscopal effect in a patient with melanoma. N Engl J Med 366:925–931
26. Kitano S, Postow M, Cortez C et al (2012) Myeloid-derived suppressor cell quantity prior to treatment with ipilimumab at 10mg/kg to predict for overall survival in patients with metastatic melanoma. J Clin Oncol 30(suppl):2518, abstr

Chapter 7

Marker Utility for Combination Therapy

Ester Simeone, Antonio M. Grimaldi, and Paolo A. Ascierto

Abstract

Melanoma is a heterogeneous disease for which monotherapies are likely to fail in the majority of patients due to genomic variations between individuals. Novel treatments, such as vemurafenib and ipilimumab, offer clinical promise in metastatic melanoma and the increased potential for combined therapeutic strategies, necessary given the differences in response between patients. Together with these new approaches, the development of clinically relevant biomarkers that predict treatment outcomes are required to ensure these new therapies are targeted at those patients most likely to benefit. Here we review the utility of some potential biomarkers of treatment response in patients with metastatic melanoma.

Key words Metastatic melanoma, BRAF inhibitors, Vemurafenib, Immune therapy, Anti-PD1, Ipilimumab, Combination therapy, Biomarkers, Molecular profiling

1 Introduction

Melanoma is a heterogeneous disease for which monotherapies are likely to fail in the majority of patients due to genomic variations between individuals. However, in metastatic melanoma there are now two important broad classes of drug therapies that offer significant clinical promise. These are the small molecules that specifically target particular mutated genes, such as the BRAF inhibitors (vemurafenib and dabrafenib), MEK inhibitors (NRAS mutated population), and c-Kit inhibitors, and the monoclonal antibodies (mAbs) directed against specific T-cell receptors, such as anti-CTLA4 (ipilimumab) and anti-PD1 [1–8].

Vemurafenib and ipilimumab are approved for the treatment of metastatic melanoma, with both having shown a positive effect on progression-free survival (PFS) and overall survival (OS) in phase III clinical trials [1, 6]. However, despite their promise, both drugs have therapeutic limitations. Although vemurafenib can result in a dramatic, rapid clinical response (within 15 days), this is not maintained over the longer-term in most patients, with

Magdalena Thurin and Francesco M. Marincola (eds.), *Molecular Diagnostics for Melanoma: Methods and Protocols*, Methods in Molecular Biology, vol. 1102, DOI 10.1007/978-1-62703-727-3_7,

a median time to relapse of 7–8 months. Moreover, 10–20 % of patients do not have an initial response to vemurafenib therapy. This intrinsic and/or acquired resistance to vemurafenib (and the other BRAF inhibitor, dabrafenib) is currently being investigated in preclinical studies. Conversely, ipilimumab does not have a major beneficial impact on clinical response rates, but can prolong survival and has the potential to change the tumour into a chronic disease (in approximately 20 % of patients), even when the tumour load is still present [6]. This finding has resulted in the classic Response Evaluation Criteria in Solid Tumors (RECIST) criteria being modified with the new immune-related response criteria (irRC) to reflect the additional response patterns observed with ipilimumab and other immune therapy in metastatic melanoma [9].

Given the variations in response to different treatments between patients, the future of melanoma treatment is likely to focus on the use of combined therapeutic approaches involving targeted therapy, immunotherapy, chemotherapy, surgery, and vaccination etc. [10]. For example, the first combination study of dabrafenib plus tramatenib has already shown encouraging results [11]. In addition, the promising results already seen with other novel compounds, such as the MEK inhibitors [3, 4] and anti-PD1 [8], will increase the opportunities for various other combination therapy strategies. Together with the increasing use of combination therapy, the development of biomarkers that can help predict treatment outcomes is required to ensure that these costly new treatments are targeted at those patients most likely to benefit.

2 Tumor Gene Profiling for Predicting Outcome and Response to Treatment

Genetic alterations, somatic or inherited, play a fundamental role in the pathogenesis of melanoma. Thus, identifying genetic variants and their roles in critical pathways and the development of aggressive phenotypes is important in identifying new targets for melanoma therapy. Genetic variations in susceptibility to melanoma and pathogenesis lead to different molecular subsets of melanomas, which in turn may indicate the need for different therapeutic approaches.

Immunohistochemical and mutational analyses have shown that inactivation and impairment of the p16CDKN2A gene are present at steadily increasing rates as lesions move from primary melanoma to melanoma metastases, correlating with disease progression and cell proliferation. The relative risk of carrying a CDKN2A mutation for patients with melanoma significantly increases with the presence of familial occurrence of melanoma (likelihood of CDKN2A germline mutations increasing according to the number of affected family members), multiple primary melanomas, and early age of onset [12].

Recently, a synergistic relationship between germline MC1R variants and somatic BRAF mutations has been suggested, whereby MC1R variant genotypes seem to confer a significantly increased risk of developing BRAF-mutant melanoma in skin not damaged by sunlight. It has been hypothesized that intermittent sun exposure may indirectly induce BRAF mutations through the impairment of MC1R and an increased production of free radicals [12]. Since this correlation has not been confirmed in Australia, it could be speculated that differences in patients' geographical origins and/or the genetic backgrounds of patient populations may play an important role in determining such geographical discrepancies [12]. This consideration could be important for future personalized treatment. Additional information about melanoma susceptibility could be obtained from genome-wide association studies that aim to identify common genetic variants contributing to melanoma risk [12].

Focusing mainly on BRAF, evidence has suggested poor correlation between pathogenetic mutations in the primary tumor and in metastasis in individuals. This could be explained by the presence of polyclonality in the primary tumor, similar to the recent finding for melanocytic nevi and in line with the recent stem cells progression model. However, in a recent study in which 291 tumor tissues from 132 patients with melanoma were screened, we observed a good intra-patient correlation between primary and metastatic lesions [13]. Thus, different molecular mechanisms generate different subsets of melanoma patients with distinct disease aggressiveness, clinical behavior, and response to therapy. As such, the characterization of molecular mechanisms that can help better categorize different subsets of patients might influence the optimal management approach and help inform better therapeutic decision-making.

One possible approach in the identification of biomarkers is cDNA microarray analysis, which has enabled the identification of putative melanoma biomarkers by virtue of their differential expression in distinct phases of melanoma progression [14]. Application of cDNA microarray analysis has, for example, led to the development of multimarker diagnostic and prognostic assays that are nearing clinical application. More recently, this approach has led to the discovery that Pleckstrin homology domain-interacting protein (PHIP), involved in the IGF pathway, represents a positive prognostic factor for PHIP-overexpressing melanomas [14].

Studies based on gene expression profiling in identical lesions before and after different types of immune therapy demonstrated a unique molecular signature in the tumor microenvironment when rejection occurred. Among these signature genes, interferon regulatory factor-1 (IRF-1) upregulation has been the key immune modulator associated with responsiveness, not only in melanoma but also in the response of genital warts to imiquimod, and carcinoid tumors and chronic myeloid leukemia to interferon-α [14]. High-dose IL-2-induced melanoma regression is associated with upregulation of NKGC5, T-cell receptor alpha chain, and HLA I-related transcripts. The best self-controlled study is the analysis of patients with mixed treatment responses. With identical genetic make-up and immune pressure, the differences between the phenotypes of separate and distinct lesions emphasize the importance of tumor microenvironment. This study revealed that antigen presentation machinery in responsive metastases was significantly enhanced compared with progressive lesions [14].

With regard to prediction of immune responsiveness and survival, Wang [14] identified 100 genes with significant differential expression by tumor-infiltrating lymphocytes (TILs) from 13 complete responders and 40 nonresponders. However, when the tumors that were the source of the TILs were studied, no clear predictors of their phenotype could be identified, suggesting that response or progression could result from intrinsic genetics of the patient rather than the specific genetics of the tumor.

In conclusion, clinical outcomes of patients treated by immune therapy are determined by multiple factors that may be redundant, synergistic or contrasting. To fully understand each component's contribution to the outcome, a systems biology approach needs to be applied.

3 Markers of Intrinsic Resistance to BRAF Inhibitors

Although the presence of an activating BRAF mutation is generally predictive of a response to BRAF inhibitors, a significant proportion of BRAF V600E mutated melanoma cell lines show signs of intrinsic drug resistance [15–17]. Similar findings were observed in the different clinical trials of vemurafenib, where between 10 and 20 % of patients with BRAF V600E mutated melanomas did not meet the RECIST criteria threshold for a response [1, 18, 19]. Melanomas are known to have complex mutational profiles and harbor concurrent alterations in many genes including CDK2, CDK4, MITF, and AKT3. How these genes and possibly others impact upon the biological behavior of melanoma cells and modulate the response to BRAF inhibitors is not yet understood but may explain the lack of therapeutic response in some BRAF V600E mutated melanoma patients. In melanoma cells, constitutive BRAF/MEK/ERK signaling drives cell cycle entry and uncontrolled growth by increasing cyclin D1 expression. It is now well established that inhibition of BRAF in BRAF V600E mutant melanoma cell lines leads to both inhibition of cyclin D1 expression and cell cycle arrest. A recent array comparative genomic (aCGH) analysis of a large panel of melanoma cell lines and tumor specimens showed 17 % had a BRAF V600E mutation in conjunction with amplification of cyclin D1 [20]. In Western blot experiments, the amplified cell lines had increased cyclin D1 protein expression and showed intrinsic resistance to SB590885, a BRAF-inhibitor [20].

There is already good evidence from breast cancer that the expression and mutational status of the tumor suppressor PTEN is an important predictor of intrinsic resistance to targeted therapy agents such as trastuzumab and gefitinib [21]. In these instances, tumors that are PTEN negative, or those with high basal PI3K/AKT signaling showed a marked impairment of therapy-induced apoptosis and were associated with significantly worse therapeutic response [21]. Different studies in melanoma support these assumption and identified loss of PTEN, observed in >10 % of melanoma specimens, as being predictive for an attenuated apoptotic response following treatment with vemurafenib [15]. In the context of PTEN loss, BRAF inhibition led to an increase in AKT signaling that suppressed the pro-apoptotic protein BAD [22]. However, it was shown that BRAF inhibitor resistance could be overcome by treating the BRAF V600E/PTEN null melanoma cell lines with the combination of a BRAF inhibitor and a PI3K inhibitor. This dual BRAF/PI3K inhibition restored the nuclear accumulation of FOXO3a, upregulated BIM expression, and significantly enhanced the level of apoptosis [15]. FOXO3a is a member of the Forkhead family of transcription factors that regulates cell survival and growth through the activation or suppression of a diverse array of oncogenesis-related genes such as BIM, Fas-Ligand, cyclin D1, and GADD45 [23]. There is good evidence that inactivation of FOXO3a is a prerequisite for the transformation of many cell types, and cytoplasmic FOXO3a accumulation is known to be a negative prognostic factor for breast cancer [23]. Moreover, there is some suggestion that increased insulin like growth factor (IGF)-1 signaling may be involved in the mechanisms underlying the BRAF inhibitor-induced increase of AKT signaling [15].

4 NRAS Mutation as Predictive Factor

The presence of a BRAF or NRAS mutation is associated with a higher risk of central nervous system (CNS) involvement at initial stage IV melanoma diagnosis and the presence of an NRAS mutation has been reported by Jacob et al. to correlate with poorer survival from time of melanoma diagnosis [24]. However, different survival analyses of NRAS-mutation patients have reported discordant results. While a prospective study of 249 Australian melanoma patients reported shorter melanoma-specific survival after the initial melanoma diagnosis for NRAS patients compared with wild type (WT) patients [25], another prospective study identified no significant difference in overall survival from initial melanoma diagnosis among NRAS-mutant melanoma patients [26]. Moreover, a retrospective study of 109 patients, including 82 with metastatic disease, demonstrated that the NRAS-mutated tumor genotype was associated with increased overall survival (compared with the BRAF-mutated and WT tumor genotypes) [27].

The data from Jacob et al. support the view that patients who have melanoma with an NRAS mutation represent a distinct cohort with a highly aggressive disease and shorter survival with stage IV disease [24]. However, the role of NRAS mutations for selecting and/or prioritizing anti-cancer treatment, including cytotoxic chemotherapy and targeted agents, is unknown at this time. Clinical data for RAS-mutated melanomas treated with BRAF inhibitors is lacking. However, preclinical data have demonstrated a paradoxical stimulation of the MAPK signaling pathway and thus enhanced tumor growth in melanoma cells harboring mutant RAS [28, 29]. Moreover, a Q61K mutation was found in a tumor from a patient with acquired resistance to vemurafenib [30].

Promising data on MEK162 in an ongoing phase II trial of patients with BRAF and NRAS mutated advanced melanoma were recently reported [4]. MEK162, a small molecule selective inhibitor of the kinases MEK1 and MEK2, showed clinical activity and good tolerability in this patient population. Response rate was 21 %, disease control rate was 68 %, and median PFS was 3.65 months (95 % CI 2.53–5.39 months) for patients with NRAS mutations [4]. This is the first targeted therapy to show activity in patients with NRAS-mutated melanoma, a cohort that accounts for around 18 % of all mutations of metastatic melanoma.

5 Tumor-Specific Circulating Cell-Free DNA (cfDNA) BRAF-Mutated to Predict Clinical Outcome in Patients Treated with the BRAF Inhibitors

Tumor-specific circulating cell-free DNA (cfDNA) levels in blood increase with tumor burden and decrease following treatment. cfDNA can harbor gene aberrations, such as BRAF mutations, consistent with the tumor. Thus, cfDNA could be a useful biomarker of prognostic value and therapeutic response. BREAK-2 was an open-label, single-arm, phase II study that evaluated efficacy, safety, and tolerability of the BRAF inhibitor, dabrafenib, in BRAF V600E/K mutation positive metastatic melanoma patients [31]. The exploratory objectives of the BREAK-2 trial were to evaluate whether tumor and cfDNA BRAF mutations are correlated, whether cfDNA levels correlate with baseline tumor burden, and if clinical outcome could be predicted by cfDNA mutations. In this study, BRAF mutation status was established using an allele-specific polymerase chain reaction (PCR) assay in tumor samples, while cfDNA BRAF mutation status was evaluated using BEAM technology. Baseline plasma samples were available for 91 of 92 patients. The overall agreement between tumor and cfDNA BRAF V600E and V600K mutation status was 83 %, and 96 %, respectively. Higher cfDNA V600E mutated fraction was associated with higher baseline tumor burden (Odds ratio [OR] = 0.73; $p < 0.0001$; $n = 60$); lower overall response rate (ORR) (OR = 0.83; 95 % CI = 0.72–0.96; $p = 0.0134$; $n = 46$) and shorter PFS (HR = 1.09; $p = 0.0006$; $n = 46$). Median PFS was 27.4 weeks in the overall V600E patient population ($n = 76$) and 20.0 weeks in the cfDNA V600E patient population ($n = 46$). Otherwise, the response endpoints were comparable between the two populations. There was no correlation between V600K mutated fraction ($n = 14$) and any efficacy endpoints [32].

Therefore cfDNA appears useful for detecting BRAF mutations in patients treated with dabrafenib and increasing V600E mutated fraction was associated with reduced ORR and shorter PFS, suggesting higher amounts of mutated cfDNA in V600E mutation positive patients predicts poorer clinical outcome. This approach could be useful in identifying patients who can benefit or not from treatment with the BRAF inhibitors and possible combination therapies.

6 BRAF Inhibitors and Ipilimumab: Possible Immunological Effect of Vemurafenib

Two important drugs are now available for the treatment of two specific groups of melanoma: patients: vemurafenib for patients with a genetic alteration (i.e. V600 BRAF, NRAS, cKit), and ipilimumab for those without mutation. For both these agents, approaches to help improve their efficacy are required. While the results of an ongoing clinical trial of these drugs used in combination are awaited [33], one possible strategy is to use these two agents in a sequential manner i.e. vemurafenib (or other BRAF inhibitor) to reduce the tumour and then ipilimumab to maintain the response, or ipilimumab first and then vemurafenib to reduce the tumour load. Both these strategies have a scientific rationale [34].

Ribas et al. showed in an in vitro model, in which peripheral blood mononuclear cell and metastatic melanoma cells were exposed to increasing concentrations of PLX4032, that the viability and function of T-lymphocytes were maintained [33]. These preliminary results may support the feasibility of combining a BRAF inhibitor with immunotherapy, even though they must be confirmed in clinical studies. Another important observation comes from Boni et al., who showed that PLX4720 (a PLX4032 analogue) may increase melanoma antigen expression on melanoma cell lines and so facilitate the recognition of melanoma cells by melanoma-specific lymphocytes [34].

Other evidence for combining chemotherapy with immunotherapy is provided by preclinical and clinical studies, which have highlighted the crucial importance of timing in combination treatment. In many cases, the best way to improve efficacy was shown to be sequential use, with chemotherapy being followed by immunotherapy [35]. We have previously investigated both possible sequential regimens: BRAF inhibitors (vemurafenib or dabrafenib) followed by ipilimumab and ipilimumab followed by BRAF inhibitors [36]. Our experience was a retrospective, single-institution analysis of patients treated with vemurafenib 960 mg or dabrafenib 150 mg twice-daily and ipilimumab 3 mg/kg every 3 weeks for four doses. Eligible patients tested positive for the BRAFV600 mutation and had sequentially received treatment with vemurafenib or dabrafenib followed by ipilimumab, or vice versa. 34 BRAF-mutation positive patients were eligible, comprising 6 patients who received ipilimumab followed by a BRAF inhibitor, and 28 patients treated with a BRAF inhibitor who subsequently received ipilimumab. Of these 28 patients, 12 (43 %) had rapid disease progression resulting in death and were unable to complete ipilimumab treatment as per protocol. Median overall survival for patients with rapid disease progression was 5.7 months (95 % CI: 5.0–6.3), compared with 18.6 months (95 % CI: 3.2–41.3; $p<0.0001$) for those patients who were able to complete ipilimumab treatment. Baseline factors associated with rapid progression were elevated lactate dehydrogenase, a performance status of 1 and the presence of brain metastases. Patients were more likely to have rapid disease progression if they had at least two of these risk factors at baseline (Fig. 1). Our analysis suggests it may be possible to identify those patients at high risk of rapid disease progression upon relapse with a BRAF inhibitor who might not have time to subsequently complete ipilimumab treatment. We hypothesize that these BRAF-mutation positive patients may benefit from being treated with ipilimumab before a BRAF inhibitor.

7 Chemotherapy and BRAF Inhibitors

Another interesting area of investigation is the role of chemotherapy in combination and/or in sequence with a BRAF inhibitor. Yang et al. [35] showed that among chemotherapies, temozolomide may

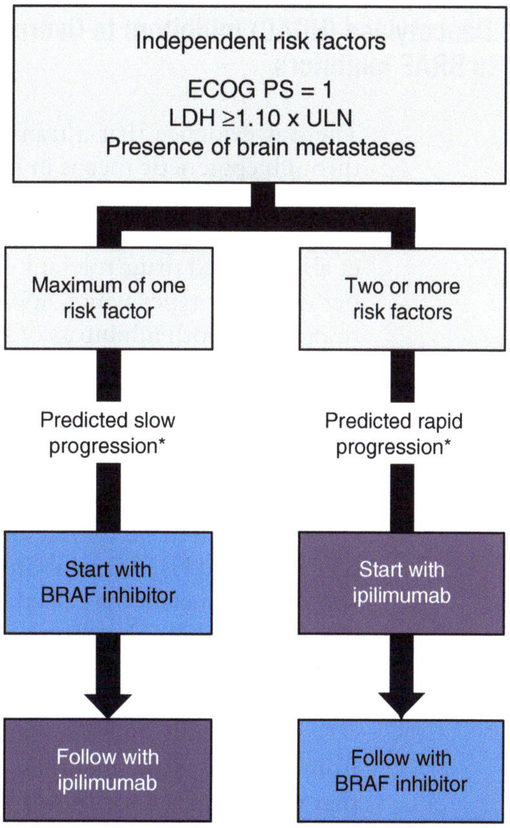

Fig. 1 Suggested algorithm for the sequential use of ipilimumab and BRAF inhibitors in patients with metastatic, BRAFV600 mutation-positive melanoma [34]

have a synergistic effect with BRAF inhibitors. In a preclinical model, the efficacy of chemotherapy against melanoma depended on the regulation of expression of NF-kB-mediated anti-apoptotic genes. The constitutive activation of NF-kB on melanoma cells contributes to intrinsic resistance to systemic chemotherapy and/or biotherapy. The role of V600E mutation on NF-kB is that of activation and this mediates the expression of many anti-apoptotic, pro-proliferative, and pro-metastatic genes [35]. Furthermore, temozolomide may inhibit NF-kB, but not ERK and it has been shown to confer anti-tumour activity in melanoma in vivo [35]. This preclinical study may provide the basis of evidence for potential synergistic effect of a B-RAF inhibitor and temozolomide in metastatic melanoma treatment. The NF-kB status could be a possible marker for the association of temozolamide with BRAF inhibitors. However, further studies are necessary.

8 Histone Deacetylase (HDAC) Inhibitors to Overcome Resistance to BRAF Inhibitors

There is evidence that a transient drug-tolerant state can emerge through epigenetic means in individual cells, through activation of IGFR-1 signaling and an altered chromatin state mediated through the histone demethylase RBP2/KDM5A/Jarid1A [37]. Sharma et al. identified drug-tolerant cells in cultures derived from a number of tumor types which appeared to be important in the escape response to both inhibitors of RTK signaling and cytotoxic chemotherapy drugs [37]. Interestingly, the drug-tolerant population also emerged in cultures established from single cells, demonstrating the reversible, switchable nature of this phenotype. From a therapeutic standpoint, tolerance could be abrogated by the inhibition of IGFR-1 signaling or through use of histone deacetylase (HDAC) inhibitors. Of relevance to melanoma and BRAF inhibitor resistance, HDAC inhibition was found to induce at least some apoptosis in melanoma cells that were resistant to the BRAF inhibitor AZ628 [37]. The characterization of the preexisting subpopulation of cells that escape BRAF inhibitor therapy is central to managing resistance.

New insights into the nature of drug-tolerant cells have come from a recent study identifying a minor subset of melanoma cells that were required for tumor maintenance and expressed high levels of the H3K4 histone demethylase Jarid1B [38]. These cells tended to be present at low levels within the melanoma population, proliferated very slowly, and underwent a marked expansion when treated with either BRAF inhibitors or cytotoxic chemotherapeutic drugs [38].

Further study will be required to determine whether simultaneous treatment with inhibitors of BRAF and HDAC is sufficient to prevent the onset of resistance, and whether the expansion of Jarid1B-expressing melanoma cells is a critical step in the emergence of drug resistance.

9 Ipilimumab and Possible Predictive Markers

Ipilimumab, a mAb directed against cytotoxic T-lymphocyte-associated antigen-4 (CTLA-4) was the first agent approved for the treatment of unresectable or metastatic melanoma that showed an overall survival benefit in a randomized phase III trial [6]. However, to date, no clinical parameter has consistently been found to be a surrogate or predictive marker for response and the identification of a biomarker to identify patients who might benefit from ipilimumab treatment remains an important goal. It has been suggested that the absolute lymphocyte count (ALC) > 1,000/μL after two

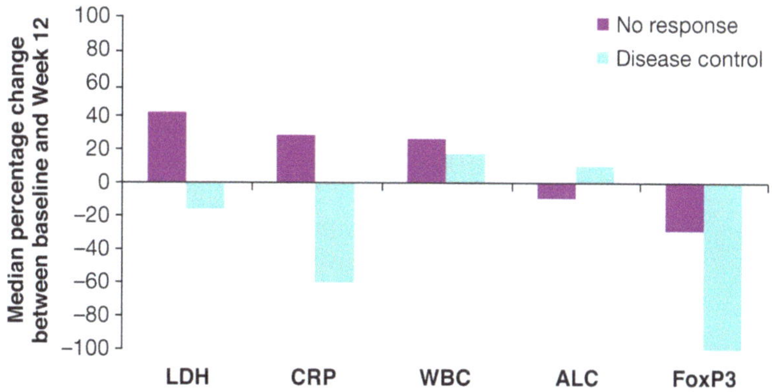

Fig. 2 Percentage change in immunological markers among patients with and without disease control

ipilimumab treatments (week 7) could be a possible marker and seems to correlate with clinical benefit and OS [39]. Another important biomarker could be the expression of the inducible costimulator (ICOS) molecule [40], which was shown to correlate with clinical outcome in a small cohort of melanoma patients treated with ipilimumab and to be necessary for optimal anti-tumor responses mediated by anti-CTLA-4 [40]. Biomarkers in the tumor microenvironment have also been demonstrated to be associated with clinical activity in patients treated with ipilimumab [41]. In fact, it was shown that clinical activity was related to high expression of FOXP3 and IDO at baseline and an increase from baseline in TILs (at week 4) in tumor biopsies.

We have investigated potential immunological markers in patients with metastatic melanoma treated with ipilimumab 3 mg/kg, including lactate dehydrogenase (LDH), c-reactive protein (CRP), flow cytometry circulating Treg cell analysis, ALC and white blood cell (WBC) count evaluated in blood at baseline and at weeks 4, 7, 10, and 12 after first tumour assessment [42]. Among the 95 patients evaluated, 36 had a complete response, partial response or stable disease according to irRC at week 24 (disease control rate of 38 %). We also demonstrated that tumour response was independent of BRAF and NRAS mutational status [42]. We found significant associations between some of these potential markers and the tumour response to ipilimumab. In responders, decreased levels of LDH, CRP, and circulating Treg cells and increased ALC levels were observed (Fig. 2). Compared with patients who had no change in the level of these markers, these changes between baseline and week 12 were significantly associated with survival (LDH and CRP, $p<0.0001$; ALC: $p=0.01$; FoxP3, $p=0.008$). Estimated median overall survival was 7.8 months (95 % CI: 5.0–10.6). Further clinical or translational studies are required to verify these data and identify robust markers of clinical benefit.

Patients with melanoma have a predominant and early involvement of immunological dysfunctions affecting myeloid cells. In particular, CD14+HLA-DRneg/low, representing *bona fide* myeloid derived suppressor cells (MDSC) in this tumor histology [40], accumulate in the peripheral blood of melanoma patients from the very start of the disease (stage IIB and C) and can be detected as infiltrating components of primary lesions, suggesting a potential involvement of these cells in melanoma progression. CD14+HLA-DRneg/low spontaneously release a large array of immunosuppressive and pro-tumorigenic cytokines and chemokines, and inhibit proliferation and function of activated T cells mostly through TGFb secretion. Since patients with lower frequency of CD14+HLA-DRneg/low and lower TGFb serum levels mount better immune responses to anti-tumor vaccine [40], CD14+HLA-DRneg/low down-modulation could be an opportunity to enhance immunotherapy. As such, studies are undergoing to identify potential pharmacological tools interfering with MDSC differentiation and function both in vitro and in vivo, in melanoma patients.

10 Other Promising Immunotherapies and Possible Combinations: Immune Score and Gene Signature to Predict Outcome and Response

The promising efficacy observed in response to anti-CTLA-4 therapy has set the stage for the development of more T-cell immunomodulatory approaches for cancer treatment. There are several antibodies in various stages of preclinical/clinical development that offer exciting possibilities for use in combination with anti-CTLA-4 mAbs. These include antibodies against CD137 (a costimulatory molecule that is rapidly induced on CD4+ and CD8+ T cells after activation and enhances T-cell activation/proliferation on cross-linking), programmed death-1 receptor (PD-1), a receptor that binds to the negative T-cell costimulatory molecule, programmed death ligand-1 (PD-L1), promoting T-cell apoptosis and dampening the immune response, and anti-CD40 and anti-OX-40 (CD134), which have an immunostimolatory effect on the immune system.

As mentioned above, PD-1 is a surface molecule that delivers inhibitory signals important to maintain T-cell functional silence against their cognate antigens. It has two known ligands: B7-H1/PD-L1 (hereafter B7-H1), the predominant mediator of PD-1 dependent immunosuppression, and B7-DC/PD-L2. PD-L1 is expressed on hematopoietic cells and can be upregulated on activation. PD-L1 is also found in tissues such as pancreatic islets, heart, endothelium, small intestine, and placenta. Tumor cells that express PD-L1 use this pathway as a mechanism to evade recognition/destruction by the immune system. PD-L2 expression is restricted only to macrophages and dendritic cells and is also upregulated on activation. In murine tumor models, B7-H1 expression confers immune resistance, and interrupting PD-1:B7-H1 interactions has an antitumor effect. B7-H1 is highly upregulated in many murine and human tumors (either in tumor cells or nontransformed cells in the tumor microenvironment, such as antigen-presenting cells), and its expression is associated with poor outcome for patients with certain epithelial cancers [43]. PD-L1 expression on melanoma cells might be a good marker for poor prognosis and for response to treatment with anti-PD1/PDL1 [43]. As a result, human anti-PD1 and anti PD-L1 mAbs are in clinical development. Phase I trials with anti-PD1 have been very encouraging, particularly those involving repeated doses in which durable objective responses have been observed with a reasonable safety profile [43]. As a new type of drug in cancer therapy, the development of immunostimulatory mAbs may require reshaping of drug response evaluation criteria and the rationale for combining these promising therapies with each other and with other more conventional strategies.

Other promising immunotherapies in the treatment of melanoma are vaccine [44], oncolitic immunotherapy (e.g. OncoVEXGM-CSF) [44], Darleukine (a fusion protein, consisting of the human vascular targeting antibody L19 and human interleukin-2) [45], and Treg depletors (as in the experience based on the use of denileukin diftitox) [46]. However, as already discussed, the next challenge will be to optimize the treatment of individual patients using these active agents sequentially or in combination with each other or with traditional anticancer modalities such as chemotherapy, radiation, or surgery [10].

The adaptive immune response influences the behavior of human tumors. In fact, characterization of the tumor-infiltrating immune cells in large cohorts of human colorectal cancers by gene expression profiling and in situ immunohistochemical staining to evaluate the expression levels of genes related to inflammation, TH1 adaptive immunity, and immunosuppression, suggested that TH1 adaptive immunity has a beneficial effect on clinical outcome [12]. Tissue microarrays to investigate the in situ adaptive immune response in the center of the tumor (CT) and the invasive margin (IM) of 415 CRCs showed that tumors from patients without recurrence had higher immune cell densities (CD3,CD8, GZMB, and CD45RO) within each tumor region (CT and IM), than did those from patients whose tumors had recurred. For all the markers of the combined analysis of CT plus IM regions, it was demonstrated that coordinated adaptive immune reaction more than tumor invasion predicts clinical outcome. Collectively, the immunological data (type, density, and location of immune cells within the tumor samples) were found to be a better predictor of patient survival than the histopathology [12].

This has resulted in the concept of "immune contexture," the combination of immune variables associating the nature, density, functional orientation, and distribution of immune cells within the tumor of a natural in situ immune reaction [47, 48]. In order to understand the mechanisms underlying immune responses in colorectal cancer, data integration, and biomolecular network reconstruction have been applied. The presence of specific chemokines (CX3CL1, CXCL10, CXCL9) correlate with high densities of T-cell subpopulations within specific tumor regions and their high expression is associated with prolonged disease-free survival [47, 49]. The prognostic significance of an immune score ("immunoscore") based on the evaluation of CD45RO-CT/IM and CD8-CT/IM was compared with that of the tumor extension criteria using the American Joint Committee on Cancer/International Union Against Cancer-TNM (AJCC/UICC-TNM) staging system. Assessment of CD8+ cytotoxic T lymphocytes in combined tumor regions provided an indicator of tumor recurrence beyond that predicted by AJCC/UICC-TNM staging [49, 50]. Similarly there is a correlation between the extent of immune cell density, tumor stage, and relapse in melanoma. In addition, for most of the malignancies a correlation between lymphocytic infiltration and survival benefit for patients with cancers was demonstrated [49, 50]. These findings, though a revision of the current indicators of clinical outcome, may help to better identify the high-risk patients who would benefit from adjuvant therapy.

Antigen-specific cancer immunotherapeutic approaches have been developed in the last decade [50]. These are aimed at educating the immune system to eradicate cancer cells by targeting specific antigens present on the tumors cells. MAGE-A3 antigen, one of these specific tumor antigens, is expressed by up to 76 % of metastatic melanomas [51]. In a phase I dose-escalation study, patients with metastatic MAGE-A3 positive melanoma were immunized with recombinant MAGE-A3 protein associated with the immunostimulant AS02B to evaluate the safety profile and the clinical response following immunization. All dosage levels were well tolerated and no dose-toxicity relationship was observed [51]. Clinical activity was mainly observed in early metastatic disease and no differences in immunogenicity were reported between different doses of protein tested (30, 100, 300 mg) [51]. In a subsequent phase II study in patients with MAGE-A3 positive cutaneous melanoma to evaluate MAGE-A3 recombinant protein combined with different immunostimulants (AS) AS15 or AS02B (NCT00086866), both MAGE-A3 ASCI formulations were well tolerated with rec-MAGE-A3 plus AS15 seeming to be more active than rec-MAGE-A3 plus AS02B. The patients receiving rec-MAGE-A3 plus AS15 also developed a more frequent and robust immune response. The main outcome of this study was the selection of the AS15 as adjuvant system for further development [51]. These results represent a second positive signal of clinical activity for MAGE-A3, since clinical activity was also reported in a double-blind, placebo-controlled phase II study of patients with non-small-cell lung cancer (NSCLC) (NCT00290355) [52]. Phase III trials have now been initiated in melanoma (DERMA trial: resected MAGE-A3 plus pIIIB/pIIIC melanoma randomized to rec-MAGE-A3 plus AS15 or placebo—NCT00796445) and NSCLC (MAGRIT trial: resected MAGE-A3+ NSCLC pIB/II/IIIA randomized to rec-MAGE-A3 plus AS15 or placebo with or without prior chemotherapy—NCT00480025).

Moreover, gene profiling of melanoma tumors taken before MAGE-A3 immunization has led to the identification of a gene signature that may predict the clinical outcomes of MAGE-A3 treatment. Most of the genes identified in the gene signature were immune-related, suggesting that the presence of a specific tumor-environment prior to MAGE-A3 treatment influences its efficacy. The predictive value of the melanoma signature was also tested in NSCLC and showed that patients with the gene signature are more likely, but not certain, to benefit from MAGE-A3 immunization [51, 52]. The gene signature is currently under validation.

Ultimately, future study about the immunoscore and gene signature will be useful to help identify subgroups of patients who can benefit from different type of immunotherapy and could mean the start of an era of personalized immunotherapy.

11 Ipilimumab Plus Anti-PD1

A phase I study of ipilimumab in combination with anti-PD-1 is currently ongoing. However, several preclinical studies have shown possible markers of activity. Mangsbo et al. [53] explored single or combined antibody blockade of CTLA-4 and PD-1 alone or combined with the toll-like receptor agonists CpG or bacillus Calmette-Guérin for treatment of murine experimental bladder cancer. In therapeutic studies, tumors were rejected by anti-CTLA-4 while anti-PD-1 suppressed tumor growth. The combination had no additive effect compared with anti-CTLA-4 alone. However, elevated levels of circulating CD107a expressing CD8 T cells were found in the anti-CTLA-4 plus anti-PD-1 group [53]. In addition, levels of antinuclear antibodies correlated inversely with tumor size. When either CpG or bacillus Calmette-Guérin were combined with anti-CTLA-4, anti-PD-1, or anti-PD-L1, CpG in combination with anti-CTLA-4 or anti-PD-1 increased the survival of mice, with anti-PD-1 plus CpG being superior to either agent alone. CpG plus anti-CTLA-4 or anti-PD-1 increased the numbers of circulating tumor-specific

CD107a expressing CD8 T cells as well as activated (CD25FoxP3-) CD4 splenocytes [43]. Further, the numbers of Tregs in the tumor area of treated animals were decreased after anti-CTLA-4 or anti-PD-1 plus CpG therapy. Thus, the combination of CpG with CTLA-4 or PD-1 blockade improved long-term survival and led to increased levels of tumor-reactive T cells and reduced numbers of Tregs at the tumor site [53].

Clearly, all markers potentially useful for treatment with ipilimumab or anti-PD1 as single agents may also be useful for the combined therapy approach.

12 Does Chemotherapy Have a Role in Combination with Ipilimumab?

It has been suggested that chemotherapy-induced spreading of tumor antigens might amplify the anti-tumour activity of ipilimumab. This hypothesis has been investigated in a large, international, multicentre phase III trial (NCT00324155) that compared dacarbazine plus ipilimumab 10 mg/kg with dacarbazine plus placebo. Patients ($n = 502$) were treated in the front-line metastatic setting every 3 weeks for four doses followed by maintenance therapy. Although the ORR was not notably different between the two groups, the cohort receiving ipilimumab plus dacarbazine had a statistically significant improvement in the primary endpoint of OS compared to placebo plus dacarbazine (11.2 months vs 9.1 months). This is the first study that demonstrated the efficacy of a possible combination in metastatic melanoma patients [7]. However, it is unclear if this result may be due to ipilimumab alone instead of the combination dacarbazine plus ipilimumab. The Italian Network for Tumor Biotherapy (NIBIT) designed a study to investigate the clinical and immunologic efficacy of the combination of ipilimumab and fotemustine in metastatic melanoma patients with or without brain metastases [54]. The NIBIT-M1 is a phase II, open-label, single-arm study that enrolled unresectable stage III or IV cutaneous melanoma patients in seven NIBIT centers. Eligible patients had ECOG performance status of 0 or 1, had received one prior systemic treatment and presented with asymptomatic brain metastases. Ipilimumab was administered intravenously (IV) at 10 mg/kg every 3 weeks for four doses for the first 12 weeks and then once weekly from week 12 to 24; IV fotemustine was administered at 100 mg/m^2 weekly for 3 weeks, and every 3 weeks from week 9. The primary objective was to assess the immune-response disease control rate (irDCR: complete/partial response or stable disease) using the irRC [9]. A total of 86 patients were enrolled, of whom 20 had brain metastases. The irDCR was 46.5 % (95 % CI, 35.7–57.6 %), and the 1-year OS rate was 52.6 % (95 % CI, 41.8–63.4). The median OS was 13.3 months (95 % CI, 8.9–19.9).

Such preliminary results are suggestive of the efficacy and safety of the combination fotemustine plus ipilimumab in patients with melanoma. Of course, these results should be confirmed in a prospective study.

Ongoing trials are also exploring other combinations with temozolomide, paclitaxel, and carboplatin. Future studies will evaluate the best chemotherapeutic drug to combine with ipilimumab. Of particular interest for melanoma is the ability of Nab-paclitaxel or ABI-007 (and not paclitaxel) to bind SPARC (secreted protein acidic and rich in cysteine), a protein highly expressed on malignant melanocytes. SPARC, or osteonectin, belongs to the family of matricellular proteins that modulate cell-matrix interactions and cellular functions. SPARC promotes epithelial/mesenchymal-like changes and cell migration. This is a potentially important pathway in delivering ABI-007 to the tumor at high concentrations and may explain superior clinical activity seen with single agent ABI-007 therapy in patients with previously treated stage IV melanoma compared with prior studies of paclitaxel [55].

13 Conclusions

New treatments now offer significant clinical potential in patients with metastatic melanoma. Both vemurafenib and ipilimumab have shown a positive effect on survival in phase III clinical trials and other compounds have also shown promising results. These novel therapies offer the potential for various combined therapeutic strategies, some of which are currently being investigated. With the development of these new approaches, comes the need for clinically predictive biomarkers that can help ensure that expensive new drugs are targeted at those patients who are most likely to benefit. Various biomarkers that appear to be associated with better response or intrinsic resistance to BRAF inhibition or ipilimumab have been identified. However, more research is required to confirm the clinical utility of these markers.

References

1. Chapman PB, Hauschild A, Robert C et al (2011) Improved survival with vemurafenib in melanoma with BRAF V600E mutation. N Engl J Med 364:2507–2516
2. Hauschild A, Grob JJ (2012) Demidov LV, et al Dabrafenib in BRAF-mutated metastatic melanoma: a multicentre, open-label, phase 3 randomised controlled trial. Lancet 380:358–365
3. Flaherty KT, Robert C, Hersey P et al (2012) Improved survival with MEK inhibition in BRAF-mutated melanoma. N Engl J Med 367:107–114
4. Ascierto PA, Schadendorf D, Berking C et al (2013) MEK162 for patients with advanced melanoma harbouring NRAS or Val600 BRAF mutations: a non-randomised, open-label phase 2 study. Lancet Oncol 14:249–256

5. Carvajal RD, Antonescu CR, Wolchok JD et al (2011) KIT as a therapeutic target in metastatic melanoma. JAMA 305:2327–2334
6. Hodi FS, O'Day SJ, McDermott DF et al (2010) Improved survival with ipilimumab in patients with metastatic melanoma. N Engl J Med 363:711–723
7. Robert C, Thomas L, Bondarenko I et al (2011) Ipilimumab plus dacarbazine for previously untreated metastatic melanoma. N Engl J Med 364:2517–2526
8. Topalian SL, Hodi FS, Brahmer JR et al (2012) Safety, activity, and immune correlates of anti-PD-1 antibody in cancer. N Engl J Med 366:2443–2454
9. Wolchok JD, Hoos A, O'Day S et al (2009) Guidelines for the evaluation of immune therapy activity in solid tumors: immune-related response criteria. Clin Cancer Res 15:7412–7420
10. Ascierto PA, Streicher HZ, Sznol M (2010) Melanoma: a model for testing new agents in combination therapies. J Transl Med 8:38
11. Flaherty KT, Infante JR, Daud A et al (2012) Combined BRAF and MEK inhibition in melanoma with BRAF V600 mutations. N Engl J Med 367:1694–1703
12. Ascierto PA, De Maio E, Bertuzzi S et al (2011) Future perspectives in melanoma research. Meeting report from the "Melanoma Research: a bridge Naples-USA. Naples, December 6th-7th, 2010". J Transl Med 9:32
13. Colombino M, Capone M, Lissia A et al (2012) BRAF/NRAS mutation frequencies among primary tumors and metastases in patients with melanoma. J Clin Oncol 30:2522–2529
14. Wang E, Zhao Y, Monaco A et al (2012) A multifactorial genetic model for prognostic assessment of high risk melanoma patients receiving adjuvant interferon. PLoS One 7:e40805
15. Paraiso KH, Xiang Y, Rebecca VW et al (2011) PTEN loss confers BRAF inhibitor resistance to melanoma cells through the suppression of BIM expression. Cancer Res 71:2750–2760
16. Tap WD, Gong KW, Dering J et al (2010) Pharmacodynamic characterization of the efficacy signals due to selective BRAF inhibition with PLX4032 in malignant melanoma. Neoplasia 12:637–649
17. Sondergaard JN, Nazarian R, Wang Q et al (2010) Differential sensitivity of melanoma cell lines with BRAFV600E mutation to the specific Raf inhibitor PLX4032. J Transl Med 8:39
18. Flaherty KT, Puzanov I, Kim KB et al (2010) Inhibition of mutated, activated BRAF in metastatic melanoma. N Engl J Med 363: 809–819
19. Sosman JA, Kim KB, Schuchter L et al (2012) Survival in BRAF V600-mutant advanced melanoma treated with vemurafenib. N Engl J Med 366:707–714
20. Smalley KS, Lioni M, Palma MD et al (2008) Increased cyclin D1 expression can mediate BRAF inhibitor resistance in BRAF V600Emutated melanomas. Mol Cancer Ther 7:2876–2883
21. Keniry M, Parsons R (2008) The role of PTEN signaling perturbations in cancer and in targeted therapy. Oncogene 27:5477–5485
22. Boisvert-Adamo K, Aplin AE (2008) Mutant B-RAF mediates resistance to anoikis via Bad and Bim. Oncogene 27:3301–3312
23. Yang JY, Hung MC (2009) A new fork for clinical application: targeting forkhead transcription factors in cancer. Clin Cancer Res 15:752–757
24. Jakob JA, Bassett RL Jr, Ng CS et al (2012) NRAS mutation status is an independent prognostic factor in metastatic melanoma. Cancer 118:4014–4023
25. Devitt B, Liu W, Salemi R et al (2011) Clinical outcome and pathological features associated with NRAS mutation in cutaneous melanoma. Pigment Cell Melanoma Res 24:666–672
26. Ellerhorst JA, Greene VR, Ekmekcioglu S et al (2011) Clinical correlates of NRAS and BRAF mutations in primary human melanoma. Clin Cancer Res 17:229–235
27. Ugurel S, Thirumaran RK, Bloethner S et al (2007) B-RAF and N-RAS mutations are preserved during short time in vitro propagation and differentially impact prognosis [serial online]. PLoS One 2:e236
28. Hatzivassiliou G, Song K, Yen I et al (2010) RAF inhibitors prime wild-type RAF to activate the MAPK pathway and enhance growth. Nature 464:431–435
29. Poulikakos PI, Zhang C, Bollag G et al (2010) RAF inhibitors transactivate RAF dimers and ERK signalling in cells with wild-type BRAF. Nature 464:427–430
30. Nazarian R, Shi H, Wang Q et al (2010) Melanomas acquire resistance to B-RAF(V600E) inhibition by RTK or N-RAS upregulation. Nature 468:973–977
31. Ascierto PA, Minor D, Ribas A et al (2013) Phase II Trial (BREAK-2) of the BRAF Inhibitor Dabrafenib (GSK2118436) in Patients With Metastatic Melanoma. J Clin Oncol 31:3205–3211
32. Long GV, Ascierto PA, Grob JJ et al (2012) Tumor-specific circulating cell-free DNA (cfDNA) BRAF mutations (muts) to predict clinical outcome in patients (pts) treated with the BRAF inhibitor dabrafenib (GSK2118436). J Clin Oncol 30(Suppl):8518, abstract
33. Koya RC, Mok S, Otte N et al (2012) BRAF inhibitor vemurafenib improves the antitumor activity of adoptive cell immunotherapy. Cancer Res 72:3928–3937
34. Boni A, Cogdill AP, Dang P et al (2010) Selective BRAFV600E inhibition enhances

T-cell recognition of melanoma without affecting lymphocyte function. Cancer Res 70:5213–5219
35. Yang J, Amiri KI, Burke JR et al (2006) BMS-345541 targets inhibitor of kappaB kinase and induces apoptosis in melanoma: involvement of nuclear factor kappaB and mitochondria pathways. Clin Cancer Res 12:950–960
36. Ascierto PA, Simeone E, Giannarelli D et al (2012) Sequencing of BRAF inhibitors and ipilimumab in patients with metastatic melanoma: a possible algorithm for clinical use. J Transl Med 10:107
37. Sharma SV, Lee DY, Li B, Quinlan MP et al (2010) A chromatin-mediated reversible drug-tolerant state in cancer cell subpopulations. Cell 141:69–80
38. Roesch A, Fukunaga-Kalabis M, Schmidt EC et al (2010) A temporarily distinct subpopulation of slow-cycling melanoma cells is required for continuous tumor growth. Cell 141:583–594
39. Callahan MK, Wolchok JD, Allison JP (2010) Anti-CTLA-4 antibody therapy: immune monitoring during clinical development of a novel immunotherapy. Semin Oncol 37:473–484
40. Fu T, He Q, Sharma P (2011) The ICOS/ICOSL pathway is required for optimal antitumor responses mediated by anti-CTLA-4 therapy. Cancer Res 71:5445–5454
41. Hamid O, Schmidt H, Nissan A et al (2011) A prospective phase II trial exploring the association between tumor microenvironment biomarkers and clinical activity of ipilimumab in advanced melanoma. J Transl Med 9:204
42. Simeone E, Gentilcore G, Romano A et al (2012) Immunological and biological changes during ipilimumab (Ipi) treatment and their correlation with clinical response and survival. J Clin Oncol 30(Suppl):8573, abstract
43. Simeone E, Ascierto PA (2012) Immunomodulating antibodies in the treatment of metastatic melanoma: the experience with anti-CTLA-4, anti-CD137, and anti-PD1. J Immunotoxicol 9:241–247
44. Hu JC, Coffin RS, Davis CJ et al (2006) A phase I study of OncoVEXGM-CSF, a second-generation oncolytic herpes simplex virus expressing granulocyte macrophage colony-stimulating factor. Clin Cancer Res 12: 6737–6747
45. Eigentler TK, Weide B, de Braud F et al (2011) A dose-escalation and signal-generating study of the immunocytokine L19-IL2 in combination with dacarbazine for the therapy of patients with metastatic melanoma. Clin Cancer Res 17:7732–7742
46. Telang S, Rasku MA, Clem AL et al (2011) Phase II trial of the regulatory T cell-depleting agent, denileukin diftitox, in patients with unresectable stage IV melanoma. BMC Cancer 11:515
47. Oshita C, Takikawa M, Kume A et al (2012) Dendritic cell-based vaccination in metastatic melanoma patients: phase II clinical trial. Oncol Rep 28:1131–1138. doi:10.3892/or.2012.1956
48. Fox BA, Schendel DJ, Butterfield LH et al (2011) Defining the critical hurdles in cancer immunotherapy. J Transl Med 9:214
49. Galon J, Pagès F, Marincola FM et al (2012) The immune score as a new possible approach for the classification of cancer. J Transl Med 10:1
50. Allen T, Gundrajakuppam L (2012) A role of immunotherapy in metastatic malignant melanoma. Cent Nerv Syst Agents Med Chem 12:182–188
51. Peled N, Oton AB, Hirsch FR, Bunn P (2009) MAGE A3 antigen-specific cancer immunotherapeutic. Immunotherapy 1:19–25
52. Tyagi P, Mirakhur B (2009) MAGRIT: the largest-ever phase III lung cancer trial aims to establish a novel tumor-specific approach to therapy. Clin Lung Cancer 10:371–374
53. Mangsbo SM, Sandin LC, Anger K et al (2010) Enhanced tumor eradication by combining CTLA-4 or PD-1 blockade with CpG therapy. J Immunother 33:225–235
54. Di Giacomo AM, Ascierto PA, Pilla L et al (2012) Ipilimumab and fotemustine in patients with advanced melanoma (NIBIT-M1): an open-label, single-arm phase 2 trial. Lancet Oncol 13:879–886
55. Hersh EM, O'Day SJ, Ribas A et al (2010) A phase 2 clinical trial of nab-paclitaxel in previously treated and chemotherapy-naive patients with metastatic melanoma. Cancer 116: 155–163

Chapter 8

Assaying for BRAF V600E in Tissue and Blood in Melanoma

David J. Panka, James W. Mier, and Ryan J. Sullivan

Abstract

The Braf^{V600E} mutation has been detected in patients with metastatic melanoma, colon, thyroid, and other cancers. Studies suggested that tumors with this mutation are especially sensitive to BRAF inhibitors-hence the need to reliably determine the BRAF status of tumor specimens. The present technologies used to screen for this mutation fail to address the problems associated with infiltrating stromal and immune cells bearing wild-type BRAF alleles and thus may fail to detect the presence of mutant BRAF^{V600E} tumors. We have developed a rapid, inexpensive method of BRAF analysis that reduces the contamination of wild-type BRAF sequences from tumor biopsies. The protocol involves a series of PCR amplifications and restriction digestions that take advantage of unique features of both wild-type and mutant BRAF RNA at codon 600. Using this protocol, mutant BRAF can be detected in RNA from mixed populations with as few as 0.1 % BRAF^{V600E} mutant containing cells.

Key words BRAF^{V600E}, Biomarker, Target, Melanoma test, TspR1restriction digestion, Vemurafenib, Dabrafenib, Trametanib

1 Introduction

1.1 Why Assay for BRAF V600E in Melanoma?

Metastatic melanoma is currently the fifth and sixth most common cancer in American men and women, respectively, and remains one of the few cancers with a rising incidence [1, 2]. Over 9,000 people are expected to die in the United States in 2012 from this disease. Recent treatment advances have been made which has led to the FDA approval of both zelboraf, a BRAF inhibitor, and ipilimumab, an immunotherapy, for the treatment of patients with advanced melanoma [3–5]. Unfortunately, resistance to either drug rapidly occurs and eventually the overwhelming majority of these patients will die of their disease. Efforts are needed to develop biomarkers which would allow for better treatment selection for melanoma patients and for following patients while they are being treated. With BRAF targeted therapy now established as a standard therapy for metastatic melanoma, the development of highly-sensitive, blood-based assays have the potential to greatly improve the care of patients with BRAF activating mutations.

Magdalena Thurin and Francesco M. Marincola (eds.), *Molecular Diagnostics for Melanoma: Methods and Protocols*, Methods in Molecular Biology, vol. 1102, DOI 10.1007/978-1-62703-727-3_8, © Springer Science+Business Media New York 2014

Fifty percent of patients with cutaneous melanoma have a tumor that harbors an oncogenic BRAF (V600E) mutation [6]. In practice, current BRAF mutational methods are only capable of testing archival tissue and have limited sensitivity. Very often a patient who previously was diagnosed with an early stage melanoma who recurs would have a fine needle aspiration performed to confirm the diagnosis, and performing BRAF mutational analysis can be challenging due to the small amount of tissue that is obtained during such procedures. Analyzing blood for the BRAF mutation would prove to be a more efficient and possibly more reliable method of determining a patient's BRAF status.

Tumor resistance to BRAF-directed therapy typically develops within 6–8 months following initial tumor regression [3, 7–9]. Importantly, each described resistance mechanism involves the retention of the initiating BRAF mutation [10–15]. As the mechanisms of resistance are just now being studied, assays which would identify developing resistance at an earlier time-point than standard clinical or radiographic assessments will have the ability to assist clinicians and researchers in determining the next treatment option for patients whose disease is progressing on BRAF-directed therapy. This is particularly important due to the fact that a number of patients treated with BRAF inhibitors progress quite quickly following initial disease regression [7, 8]. It is thought that more advanced notice of disease progression when disease growth is more modest would allow for a more timely shift in treatment. In addition, earlier detection of disease progression would also predictably allow investigators to analyze tumors or circulating tumor cells (CTCs) in these patients with a goal of determining the specific mechanism of resistance for an individual patient. This would have the added value of predicting which therapy would be most appropriate for any individual patient.

Over the next 12 months, it is expected that multiple trials will open to test the effectiveness of BRAF-directed therapy in patients with resected, high-risk disease. In patients with resected disease, the current standard of care for adjuvant therapy is interferon alpha, which has reproducibly been shown to improve disease-free survival but not overall survival [16]. Further, while the development of serologic or clinical evidence of autoimmunity has been associated with a marked improvement in overall survival in patients treated with adjuvant interferon, there has never been a reliable pretreatment biomarker that predicts which patients are more likely to benefit from this therapy [17]. It is critical that trials with adjuvant BRAF inhibitors have access to biomarkers predictive of benefit. One such biomarker would be a detectable BRAF mutation in tissue, as it is clear that patients with advanced melanoma only benefit from BRAF-directed therapy if they have a tumor with a detectable BRAF mutation, however assessment of BRAF mutations in primary melanoma samples may be complicated by substantial tumor heterogeneity [18, 19]. This may lead to both false negatives and false positives, as it may not be clear which of the heterogeneous clones will ultimately establish metastasis. While it is uncertain whether detectable or high levels of circulating BRAF will be prognostic of a poor outcome or predictive of benefit to adjuvant BRAF-directed therapy, it is critical to evaluate both the predictive and prognostic qualities of blood-based BRAF assays in patients enrolled in adjuvant trials of BRAF inhibitors, as it is more likely that circulating cells are the subpopulations of primary melanomas are more reflective of the cells that will recur.

Finally, the recommended optimal follow-up of patients who are currently rendered disease free with surgery for their melanoma is unknown. Namely, the current National Comprehensive Cancer Network (NCCN) guidelines do not recommend any blood analysis for such patients and only concede that considerations be made towards routine imaging in patients with higher risk disease [20]. The development and validation of a blood-based prognostic biomarker would offer the potential to improve these guidelines and potential help direct radiographic imaging. As an example, it is conceivable that the positive predictive value of cross-sectional imaging would be much higher in the context of a rising biomarker, much the way it is in patients with concerning symptoms, then when imaging is performed at randomly selected intervals.

1.2 Outline of the Protocol

The protocol described here [21] was designed to efficiently and accurately determine the V600E BRAF status of any tumor biopsy without the need for expensive instrumentation and reagents. The wild-type (WT) BRAF has a Valine at position 600 encoded by a GTG codon. The V600E mutant has a Glutamic acid at that position encoded by a GAG codon. As outlined in Fig. 1a, the protocol involves a series of PCR amplifications and restriction digestions that discriminate between wild-type and mutant BRAF at codon 600. An initial RT-PCR is followed by digestion with TspR1 endonuclease, which preferentially digests the wild-type (TACAGTGAA) sequence but not the V600E mutated (TACAGAGAA) PCR product. In addition, none of the other less frequently reported V600 mutations (V600D, V600M, V600G, V600A, V600R, V600K, V600G) are substrates for TspR1. A second nested PCR using the digested material follows. This PCR product is subjected to sequencing using either of the nested oligonucleotides (other V600 mutations can be identified here). The PCR product is also subjected to a third PCR (product 140 bp) using a unique nested forward oligonucleotide which creates an Xba 1 restriction site in the amplified product only with the mutant sequence (*see* Fig. 1b).

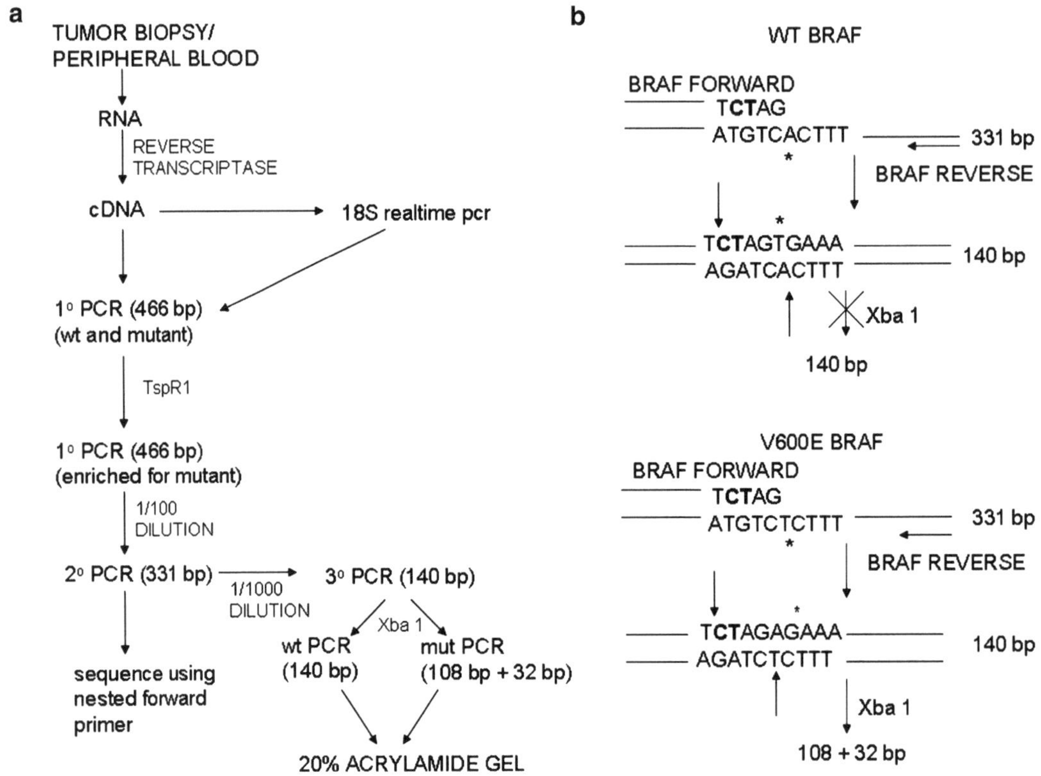

Fig. 1 (**a**) Schematic outline of the protocol determining the BRAF 600 codon status, as described in Subheading 1.2. (**b**) The final PCR uses a unique forward primer with mismatches at positions -3 and -4 (*bold letters*). This creates an Xba 1 restriction site if the mutant Adenine (A) and not the wild-type (WT) Thymidine (T) is present in the secondary PCR template. Digestion with Xba 1 produces products of 108 and 32 bp. *Arrows* indicate the potential Xba 1 cleavage site. Reproduced from [21] with permission from Lippincott Williams and Wilkins

1.3 Validation of the Protocol

The protocol [21] was initially used to examine two cell lines: A375, a melanoma line with a $BRAF^{V600E}$ mutation and 786-0, a kidney cancer cell line with a WT BRAF. As shown in Fig. 2, the PCR product digested with Xba 1 from the A375 has the predicted 108 and 32 bp fragments indicative of $BRAF^{V600E}$ status while the PCR product (140 bp) from the 786-0 shows no evidence of digested fragments characteristic of WT BRAF. The sequence around the mutation site confirms the results from the Xba 1 digest, namely that the BRAF sequence from the A375 has the predicted mutated GAG codon at position 600, while the BRAF from 786-0 has the predicted WT GTG codon.

1.4 The Sensitivity of the Protocol and the Need for the TspR1 Digestion

The TspR1 digestion was added after the initial PCR as a consequence of excessive contamination by wild-type BRAF in tumor biopsy samples from surrounding and infiltrating normal cells. To illustrate the need for the TspR1 digestion, 1 μg of total RNA from 786-0 and A375 cells was mixed in varying ratios in the presence

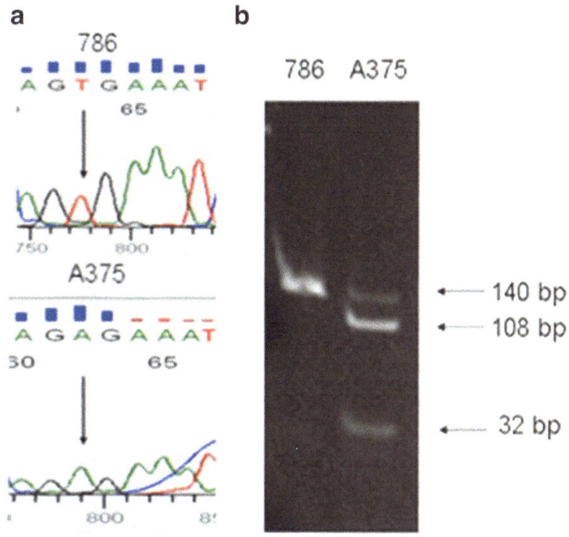

Fig. 2 The sequence in BRAF codon 600 and the accompanying Xba 1 digestion of WT and mutant BRAF cell lines (786-0) and (A375), respectively. The *arrows* in the sequence indicate the mutation site. The undigested (140 bp) and Xba 1-digested (108 and 32 bp) fragments are indicated. Reproduced from [21] with permission from Lippincott Williams and Wilkins

and absence of TspR1. As shown in Fig. 3, in the presence of TspR1 the digested PCR fragment, evidence of mutant BRAF could be detected from as little as a 1:1,000 (mutant:wild-type) dilution. On the other hand, without the addition of TspR1, in order to detect mutant BRAF nearly equal quantities of mutant and wild type were required, a restriction that may not be possible without refined microdissection of tissue biopsies.

1.5 An Analysis of Melanoma Tumor Biopsies

We next applied this method to melanoma tumor biopsies. In tissue, we utilized the protocol to detect the mutations at a two log-fold greater sensitivity (1:999) than standard assays. To date greater than 70 biopsies have been examined from paraffin-embedded archived and fresh frozen tissue. Fig. 4 shows representative findings with the corroborative sequencing information. Variations are observed indicative of the degree of normal tissue in the biopsy sample. Of particular note, pure wild-type BRAF tissue never shows any evidence of Xba 1-digested PCR fragments as seen with samples D and F and also show no evidence of an Adenine (A) at the mutation site. On the other hand there are varying degrees of $Braf^{V600E}$ positivity. Samples such as C and E have strong mutant signals, sample B has equivalent mutant and wild type signals, as evidenced by the overlapping A and T curves at the mutation site and finally sample A has a weak mutant signal as determined by both the Xba 1 digest and the sequence information (note: even though the sequencing software registers T at codon 600 in

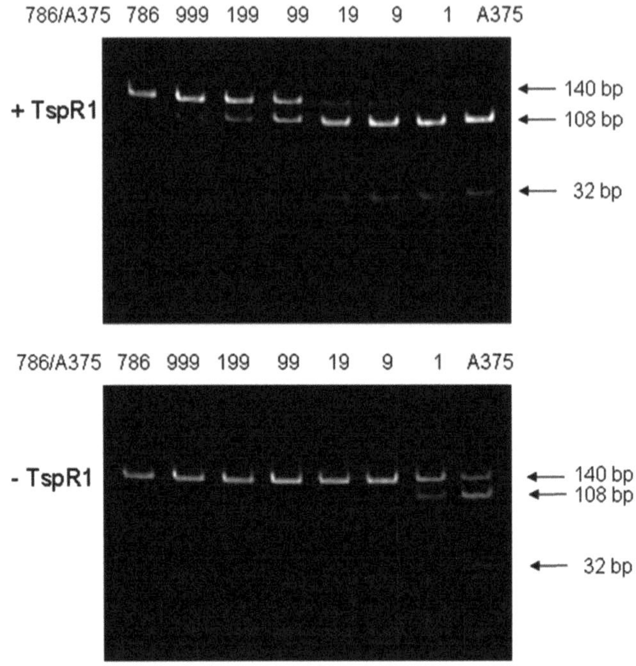

Fig. 3 Accessing the sensitivity of the method in the presence and absence of TspR1 restriction enzyme. Varying ratios of WT (786-0) to mutant (A375) BRAF containing RNA were subjected to the digestion withTspR1 (*top*) or processed without the endonuclease treatment (*bottom*). The undigested (140 bp) and digested fragments (108 and 32 bp) are indicated following Xba I treatment. Reproduced from [21] with permission from Lippincott Williams and Wilkins

samples A and B, there is clearly evidence of an A signal at this position in both samples). Importantly, in all cases where there is evidence of Xba 1-digested material the sequence always shows some evidence of an adenine at the mutation site.

1.6 Detection of the BRAF^{V600E} Mutation in the Presence of Peripheral Blood Lymphocytes

In order to detect CTCs from a metastatic melanoma patient with a known BRAF^{V600E} mutation, the protocol was modified by increasing the number of cycles in the second PCR to 45. In order to determine the sensitivity of the assay in blood, varying numbers of several melanoma cell lines and short-term cultures were mixed with 400,000 PBLs from a normal donor. Fig. 5a shows that the assay can detect variations in expression levels of V600E BRAF in a dose dependent manner. For some lines as many as 1,000 cells were necessary in order to detect an Xba 1-digested band whereas in other lines V600E BRAF Xba 1-digested products can be detected with as few as 1 (A375) to 5 (WM1862) cells in 400,000 PBLs. As shown in the A375 and SK MEL 5 titrations, normal PBLs without added tumor cells show no evidence of Xba 1-digested bands. This level of detection is theoretically high enough to detect the mutation in CTCs which are reportedly found in patients with melanoma at a range of from 1 to 100 per

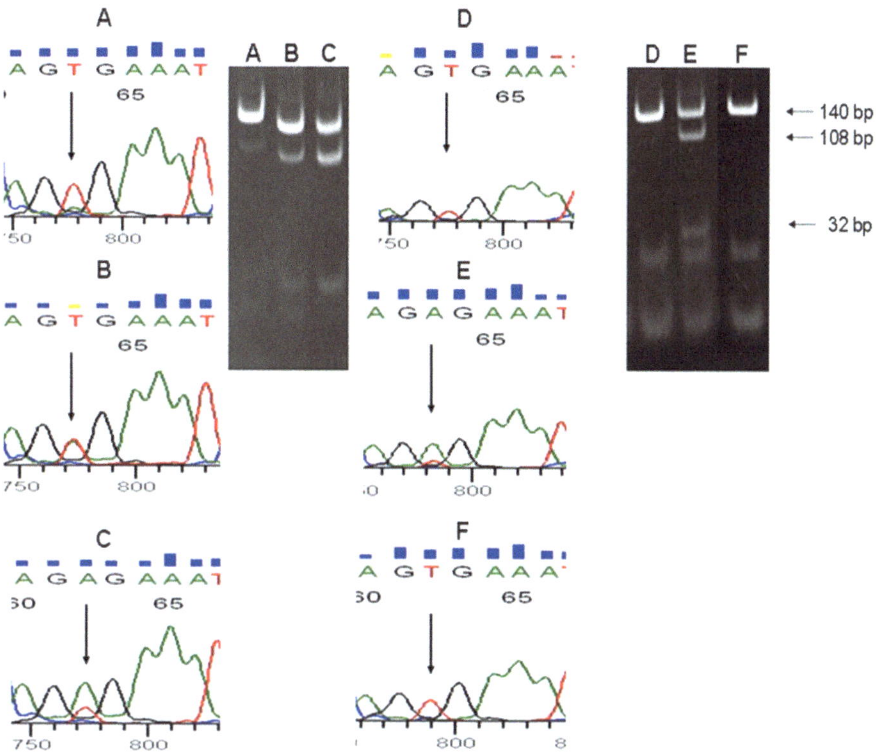

Fig. 4 Testing the protocol on melanoma biopsies. The sequence analysis of BRAF codon 600 and the accompanying gel electrophoresis profiles of Xba 1 digestion for six melanoma tumor biopsies (**a–f**). The *arrows* in the sequence indicate the mutation site. The undigested (140 bp) and Xba 1-digested fragments (108 and 32) are shown. The intensity of the 108 bp band correlates with the relative peak height of adenine (*green*) to thymidine (*red*) at BRAF codon 600. Reproduced from [21] with permission from Lippincott Williams and Wilkins

million peripheral blood lymphocytes [22]. The assay was next applied to the blood of a patient with metastatic melanoma with a known BRAF^{V600E} mutation. As shown in Fig. 5b, Xba 1-digested PCR fragments were easily detected with either 1 or 10 μg of starting RNA from the patient's PBLs but undetected with either 1 or 10 μg of RNA from a normal donor.

We have since applied this blood-based assay to detect the mutation in the blood of patients with known tissue BRAF^{V600E} mutation prior to their enrollment on the clinical trials of vemurafenib (zelboraf) or dabrafenib/trametanib [23]. The mean quantitation of the 108 bp fragment relative to the pretreatment levels for both treatment groups was determined. Importantly, each patient had a decrease in the amount of BRAF^{V600E} mutant RNA with either treatment during clinical improvement, either on imaging or via improvement of tumor-related symptoms. The mean BRAF^{V600E} mutant RNA level eventually increased in both trials in the setting of disease progression. Importantly, it appears that the BRAF level increases, on average, 6–8 weeks in advance of documented radiographic disease progression by RECIST ($p < .026$) [23].

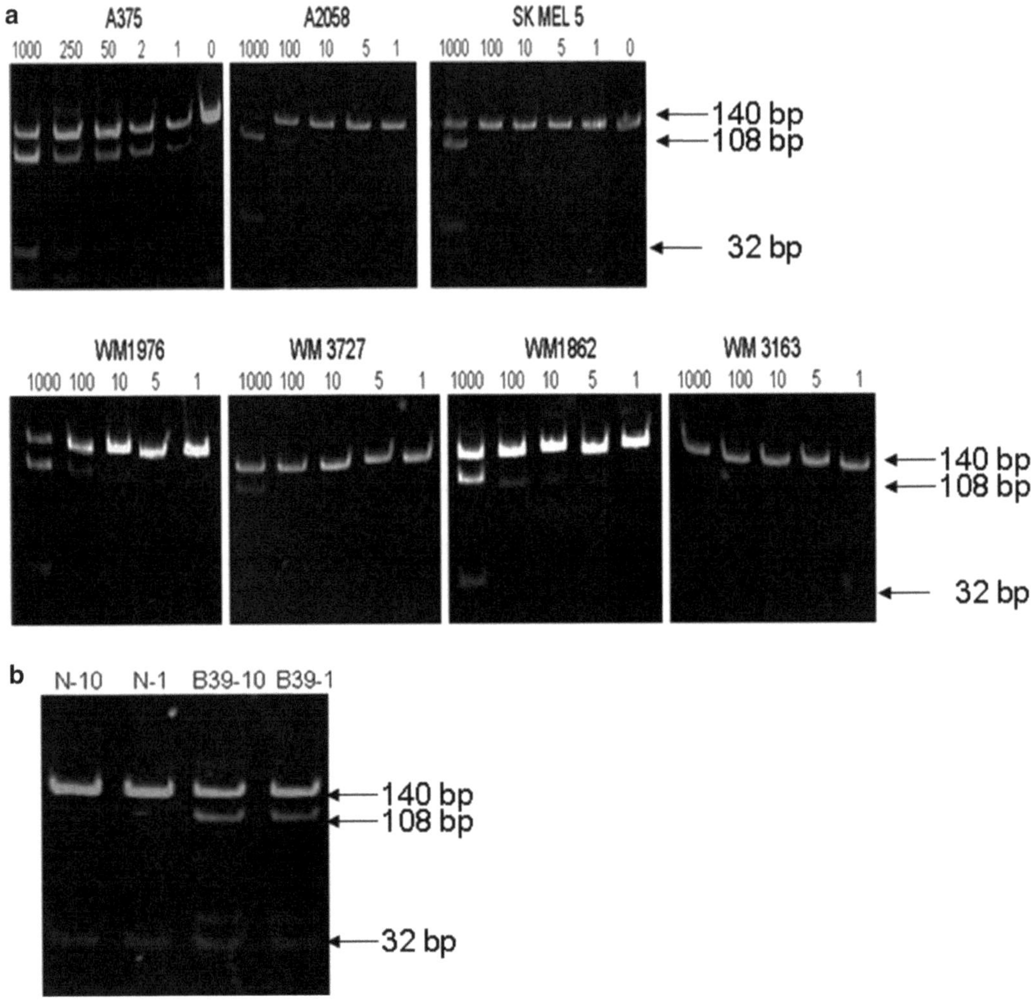

Fig. 5 Testing the protocol in the presence of peripheral blood lymphocytes. (**a**) Xba 1 digestion of the BRAF PCR products from samples containing varying ratios of BRAF mutant A375, A2058, SK MEL 5, WM 1976, WM 3727, WM 1862, and WM 3163 melanoma cells in 400,000 PBLs. Data are presented as the number of melanoma cells in 400,000 PBLs. (**b**) Xba 1 digestion of the BRAF PCR product from PBLs from a normal donor (N) and a patient with a known V600E mutation (B39). One or 10 μg of RNA was used in the assay. Reproduced from [21] with permission from Lippincott Williams and Wilkins

1.7 Comparison to Other Methods

We have presented an inexpensive, specific and highly sensitive method to detect the $BRAF^{V600E}$ mutation. Alternative methods make use of real-time PCR [24, 25], mass spectrometry [26, 27], allelic-specific PCR [28–31], PCR using locked oligonucleotides to suppress wild type sequences [31–33] or direct sequencing [34, 35] of RNA or DNA to preferentially distinguish the mutant V600E from wild type BRAF. Methods that incorporate real-time PCR tend to be expensive due to the use of fluorescent probes and the need for expensive real-time PCR instrumentation or access to core facilities. These methods cost in the range of US$50–80/sample. However once the PCR conditions are optimized with respect to annealing temperature, real-time PCR has the advantage of specificity albeit to the detriment of sensitivity. The protocol presented here can generate BRAF status for any sample for under US$10. In addition, none of these other methods offer the sensitivity and specificity of this protocol. Methods involving real-time PCR reported sensitivity in which as little as 10 % of the total tissue is composed of V600E positive cells. Even the Sequenom method which relies on mass spectrometry to distinguish between mutant and wild type differences requires at least 20 % mutant sequences. The methods which have reported to be nearly as sensitive and specific as well as inexpensive and simple as the method reported here are allelic-specific PCR [28–31] and locked oligonucleotides in conjunction with PCR. They report the ability to detect 1–2 % BRAF mutant sequence in a pool of wild-type sequence. This is still several orders of magnitude less sensitive than our protocol. As was shown in Fig. 3, mutant product can be detected in the presence of a 1000-fold excess of wild-type RNA. Since many tumor biopsies contain a large amount of normal skin tissue, it is likely that these other methods have missed the presence of mutant BRAF and thus underestimate the frequency of the $BRAF^{V600E}$ mutation in patients with metastatic melanoma. Our protocol reduces the background from wild-type BRAF with the use of TspR1, a restriction enzyme that preferentially digests only the wild-type sequence from the first PCR product. Although quite effective at digesting the wild-type PCR fragment the digestion is not complete, leaving enough wild-type products for the rest of the assay to allow for detection of pure wild-type tumors. In fact this enzyme has previously been used to access BRAF mutations [34, 36]. In those reports the presence of undigested PCR product was claimed to be indicative of BRAF V600E mutant transcripts. Those findings need to be questioned in light of our observation about the incomplete digestion by TspR1. What may be interpreted as mutant PCR fragment may in fact be undigested wild-type fragments.

The power of the protocol is in its superior sensitivity and therefore can be used for the detection of CTCs from patients with metastatic melanoma and possibly other cancers where the $BRAF^{V600E}$ mutation has been documented such in colon [37–39], thyroid [28, 34, 40–42] and other cancers [43–45]. In fact, with a simple modification of the cycle number in the second PCR, one melanoma cell was detected in a mixture with 400,000 PBLs. Potentially using this protocol, disease progression, disease regression, and disease recurrence can be documented. In addition this protocol can be used to detect microscopic disease in sentinel lymph nodes which would otherwise be undetected by standard immunohistochemistry.

Finally, many protocols use DNA as a template for analysis due to concerns about RNA degradation in paraffin-embedded tumor biopsies. As a consequence of the extreme PCR amplification of the cDNA that arose from the RNA in the tissue, this protocol is able to tolerate some RNA degradation and still detect a BRAF PCR signal. In fact using this protocol, we have yet to observe a tissue sample where the final BRAF PCR product was not amplified. This concern is not an issue with fresh blood or tissue samples where RNA isolation is performed immediately. As a consequence using RNA as a template, this protocol allows for a greater degree of sensitivity than DNA-based assays, especially those melanoma cells that have high expression levels of V600E BRAF RNA.

One of the limitations of the current assay is that the insertion of the Xba1 one site during the tertiary PCR step only allows for assaying the $BRAF^{V600E}$ mutation specifically. While this is the commonest oncogenic $BRAF^{V600}$ mutation, other mutations such as V600D and V600K make up 2–20 % of $BRAF^{V600}$ mutations [6].

While we acknowledge that significantly more work is required to fully explore the clinical utility of this assay, we are encouraged by our compelling, initial findings. It is our opinion that this type of testing will ultimately be shown to have clinical utility and become a useful tool in caring for patients with BRAF-mutant malignancies.

2 Materials

2.1 Cell lines, Tissue, and Peripheral Blood Acquisition

1. Melanoma cell lines A375, A2058, and SK MEL 5 and kidney cancer cell line 786-0 (ATCC, Manassas, VA).
2. Melanoma short-term cultures WM1976, 1862, 3163, and 3727 (Meenhard Herlyn, Wistar Institute, Philadelphia, PA).
3. Tumor samples and peripheral blood lymphocytes were from patients with advanced melanoma as part of an IRB approved tissue banking protocol (DFHCC 02-017 or 11-181).

2.2 Isolation of Peripheral Blood Lymphocytes

1. Histopaque 1077 (Sigma)-for creating Ficoll gradients for cell separation.
2. 10× Phosphate buffered saline (PBS, pH 7.4).
3. Fetal bovine serum (FBS)-for making freezing media.
4. Dimethyl sulfoxide (DMSO)-for making freezing media.
5. Freezing media: 5 % DMSO, 95 % fetal bovine serum.
6. Polypropylene centrifuge tubes (50 cc).
7. Nunc freezing vials (1.5 ml).

2.3 Isolation of Total RNA

1. Trizol reagent (Life Technologies).
2. Chloroform.
3. Propanol.
4. Sterile water (RNase and DNase free).
5. Spectrophotometer for quantitating RNA.
6. Autoclaved Eppendorf tubes (1.5 ml).

2.4 Synthesis of cDNA

1. Autoclaved Eppendorf tubes (0.6 ml; USA Scientific) (*see* **Note 1**).
2. First strand synthesis buffer (5×, Invitrogen): 250 mM Tris–HCI (pH 8.3), 375 mM KC1, 15 mM MgCl2.
3. 0.1 M Dithiothreitol (DTT, Invitrogen).
4. Moloney Murine Leukemia Virus (M-MLV) Reverse Transcriptase (RT) (200 units/μl; Invitrogen).
5. rRNAsin RNase inhibitor (40 U/μl; Promega).
6. 10 mM dNTPs.
7. Oligo (dT)15 primer (500 μg/ml; Promega).

2.5 Real-Time PCR for 18S RNA

1. Master Mix (2×, proprietary mix; ABI product).
2. 18S RNA oligonucleotide set (proprietary mix; ABI part # 4308329) (*see* **Note 2**).
3. 96-well plates with caps (SABiosciences).
4. Real-time PCR thermal cycler (Applied Biosystems 7000 Sequence Detection System).

2.6 PCRs and Restriction Digestions

1. PCR Master mix (2×, 50U/ml of Taq DNA polymerase supplied in a proprietary reaction buffer, pH 8.5, 400 μM dATP, 400 μM dGTP, 400 μM dCTP, 400 μM dTTP, 3 mM MgCl2, Promega).
2. Oligonucleotides (custom synthesized from Life Technologies):

BRAF F1 (200 μM)	5′(CCATATCATTGAGACCAAATTTGAGATG)3′
BRAF R1 (200 μM)	5′(GGCACTCTGCCATTAATCTCTTCATGG)3′
BRAF F2 (200 μM)	5′(ACGCCAAGTCAATCATCCACAGAG)3′
BRAF R2 (200 μM)	5′(CCGTACCTTACTGAGATCTGGAGACAGG)3′
BRAF F3 (200 μM)	5′(TCACAGTAAAAATAGGTGATTTTGGTCTAGCTCTAG)3′
BRAF R3 (200 μM)	5′(GCTGTATGGATTTTTATCTTGCATTC)3′

3. Nucleospin Extract II Column (Clontech).
4. TspR1 restriction enzyme (10 U/μl, New England Biolabs).

5. XbaI restriction enzyme (20 U/μl, New England Biolabs).
6. Buffer 4 for restriction endonuclease digestion (10×, 200 mM Tris–acetate, 500 mM Potassium acetate, 100 mM Magnesium acetate, 10 mM DTT, pH 7.9, at 25 °C, New England Biolabs).
7. Bovine serum albumin (BSA, 10 mg/ml; New England Biolabs).
8. Autoclaved Eppendorf tubes (0.6 ml, USA Scientific) (*see* **Note 1**).
9. MJ Thermal Cycler (PTC-100).

2.7 Polyacrylamide Gel Electrophoresis and Desitometry

1. 20 % polyacrylamide/Tris–Borate–EDTA (TBE) gels (Life Technologies).
2. TBE buffer (5×) (Life Technologies).
3. Gel loading buffer (6×) with 0.1 % Bromphenol blue.
4. SYBR Safe DNA gel stain-for staining gel (*see* **Note 3**).
5. XCell SureLock™ mini cell electrophoresis system (Life Technologies).

3 Methods

3.1 Summary of the Protocol

This method is extremely sensitive. Therefore, care must be taken not to cross contaminate samples. Always use plugged tips and change tips between samples.

The protocol is based on standard methods for RNA isolation by the Trizol method and reverse transcription to cDNA using M-MLV reverse transcriptase and oligo $(dt)_{15}$ [46] and it can be used for cell lines, paraffin-embedded tissue, or Ficoll-purified peripheral blood lymphocytes (PBLs). The cDNA is subjected to real-time PCR for 18S RNA in order to normalize the quantity, as well as quality of the input RNA prior to the next step. The normalized cDNA is PCR amplified to produce a product of 466 bp including the mutation site at codon 600. After cleanup using a nucleospin extract column, the PCR product is digested with TspR1 rstriction enzyme. Only wild-type BRAF and not V600E mutant BRAF PCR product was digested by this enzyme The TspR1 digestion is not complete resulting in some PCR product containing wild-type sequence at position 600. A 1/20 dilution of the TspR1-digested material was then PCR amplified a second time using nested oligonucleotides producing a product of 331 bp which was enriched in PCR products containing the position 600 mutation. The conditions of the PCR were the same as the first PCR except instead of 40 cycles, the amplification was 35 cycles for tissue and cell lines and 45 cycles for PBLs. After a second cleanup using a nucleospin extract column, the DNA was subjected to sequencing using the nested forward primer. The forward primer has been designed with two mismatches at –4 and –3 from the 3′ end (*see* Fig. 1b). The resulting product (140 bp) from mutant but not wild-type transcripts contains an Xba1 restriction site. Digestion with Xba1 yielded products of 108 and 32 bp that indicate V600E BRAF.

3.2 Isolation of Peripheral Blood Lymphocytes

Peripheral blood lymphocytes were isolated by Ficoll density centrifugation [47] in a laminar flow hood (BL2).

1. Wearing gloves pour contents of green top heparinized blood collection tube into a 50 cc centrifuge tube.
2. Add 10 ml of PBS to green top tubes and pool with the blood in the 50 cc centrifuge tube.
3. Add 10 ml Histopaque to a new 50 cc centrifuge tube.
4. Carefully layer the blood on top of the Histopaque (*see* **Note 4**).
5. Centrifuge at 600 × *g* at room temperature for 12 min.
6. At the interface of the layers will be the PBLs (should be a white layer of cells). At the bottom of the tube will be the red cells. Remove some of the plasma above the interface with a 10 ml pipette (can be saved, but not needed for this protocol). Remove the cells at the interface with the same pipette, trying not to remove anything below the interface. Transfer to a new centrifuge tube.
7. Add enough PBS to fill the 50 cc tube.
8. Centrifuge at 400 × *g* at room temperature for 5 min.
9. Aspirate the liquid above the cellular pellet.
10. Add 2 ml freezing media to the pellet. Gently pipette up and down and aliquot into two Nunc freezing vials.
11. Store at –80 short term or in liquid nitrogen long term.

3.3 Isolation of RNA by the Trizol Method [48]

1. Add 1 ml Trizol to tissue sections or pelleted cells in a 1.5 ml eppendorf tube (*see* **Note 5**).
2. Vortex 30 s. Incubate at room temperature for 5 min.
3. Add 110 μl chloroform and vortex briefly to mix. Incubate at room temperature for 5 min.
4. Centrifuge at 15,700 × *g* at room temperature for 5 min.
5. The RNA is in the clear top layer. Carefully remove the top layers (~550 μl) and transfer to a new 1.5 ml Eppendorf tube.
6. Add 500 μl propanol to the tube and vortex briefly. Incubate at room temperature for 5 min.
7. Centrifuge at 15,700 × *g* at room temperature for 5 min.
8. Carefully aspirate the liquid above the RNA pellet.

9. Add 1 ml 70 % ethanol and centrifuge at 4 °C for 1 min.
10. Carefully aspirate the liquid above the RNA pellet.
11. Allow pellet to air dry on a paper towel.
12. Solubilize pellet with 50 μl sterile water.
13. Quantitate with a 1/20 dilution of the RNA using a spectrophotometer at 260 nm (*see* **Note 6**).

3.4 cDNA Synthesis by Reverse Transcription (See Note 7)

1. Mix the following in a single eppendorf tube:

1st strand buffer	4 μl
0.1 M DTT	2 μl
200 μM Oligo$(dT)_{15}$	0.5 μl
dNTPs (10 mM)	0.3 μl

2. If making a master mix aliquot 6.8 μl into each individual 0.6 ml eppendorf tube.
3. Add 3 μg RNA in 11.2 μl sterile water to respective tubes.
4. Program thermal cycler for 65 °C for 5 min, then 37 °C for 60 min and finally 95 °C for 5 min. Add 1 μλ RNasin and 1 μl RTase to each tube when thermal cycler reaches 37° (*see* **Note 8**).

3.5 Real-Time PCR for 18S RNA (See Note 2)

1. Mix the following in a single tube.

2× ABI Master Mix	25 μl
dH_20	20.5 μl
18S primer set and probe	2.5 μl

2. If making a master mix aliquot 48 μl into each well of a 96 well real-time PCR plate. Make enough of the master mix to account for each sample being run in duplicate.
3. Add 2 μl of the cDNA from Subheading 3.4 to two wells. Cap the wells.
4. Centrifuge the plate briefly (*see* **Note 9**).
5. Program the real-time instrument for 95 °C for 2 min followed by 40 cycles of 95 °C for 15 s, then 60 °C for 60 s.
6. Based on the results in this step, adjust the cDNA so that equivalent amounts are used in the next step (*see* **Note 10**).

3.6 PCR #1

1. Mix the following in a single Eppendorf tube:

2× PCR master mix	10 μl
BRAF F1	1 μl
BRAF R1	1 μl

2. When preparing a master mix aliquot 12 μl into each individual 0.6 ml Eppendorf tube.
3. Add equivalent cDNA totaling 8 μl based on the results in **step 6** of Subheading 3.5.
4. Program the thermal cycler to 94 °C for 2 min, followed by 40 cycles of 94 °C for 1 min, 60 °C for 2 min and 72 °C for 2 min, with a final incubation of 72 °C for 7 min.
5. Cleanup with a nucleospin extract column. Volume after cleanup: 30 μl.

3.7 Digestion with TspR1 to Reduce Wild-Type BRAF (See Note 11)

1. Mix the following in a single Eppendorf tube:

10× Buffer 4	3 μl
100× BSA	0.3 μl
water	22.2 μl
TspR1	3 μl

2. If making a master mix aliquot 28.5 μl into each individual 0.6 ml eppendorf tube.
3. Add 1.5 μl from **step 5** of Subheading 3.6 to each respective tube.
4. Using a thermal cycler, incubate at 65° for 16 h.
5. Add 570 μl water to each sample. Vortex for 10 s.

3.8 PCR #2 (See Note 12)

1. Mix the following in a single eppendorf tube:

2× PCR master mix	10 μl
BRAF F2	1 μl
BRAF R2	1 μl
Water	7 μl

2. When preparing a master mix aliquot 19 μl into each individual 0.6 ml eppendorf tube.
3. Add 1 μl from **step 5** of Subheading 3.7 to each respective tube.

4. Program the thermal cycler to 94 °C for min, followed by 35–45 cycles of 94 °C for 1 min, 60 °C for 2 min and 72 °C for 2 min, with a final incubation of 72 °C for 7 min.
5. Cleanup with a nucleospin extract column. Volume after cleanup: 30 μl (*see* **Note 13**).
6. Submit 10 μl for sequencing with 2 μl BRAF F2 (2 μM). Also dilute the product (**step 5** of Subheading 3.8) 1/1,000 with water.

3.9 PCR#3

1. Mix the following in a single Eppendorf tube:

2× PCR master mix	10 μl
BRAF F3	0.5 μl
BRAF R3	0.5 μl
Water	7 μl

2. When preparing a master mix aliquot 18 μl into each individual 0.6 ml Eppendorf tube.
3. Add 1 μl from the 1/1,000 dilution from **step 6** of Subheading 3.8 to each respective tube.
4. Program the thermal cycler to 94 °C for 2 min, followed by 30 cycles of 94 °C for 1 min, 54 °C for 2 min and 72 °C for 2 min, with a final incubation of 72 °C for 7 min.
5. Cleanup with nucleospin extract II column. Volume after cleanup: 30 μl.

3.10 Digestion with Xba1 and Polyacrylamide Gel Electrophoresis

1. Mix the following in a single Eppendorf tube:

10× Buffer 4	2 μl
100× BSA	0.2 μl
H_20	5.8 μl
Xba1	2 μl

2. If making a master mix aliquot 10 μl into each individual 0.6 ml eppendorf tube.
3. Add 10 μl from **step 5** of Subheading 3.9 to each respective tube.
4. Incubate at 37 °C for 2 h.
5. Add 4 μl 6× gel loading buffer with 0.1 % Bromphenol blue to each sample.

6. Load 12.5 μl onto a 20 % Polyacrylamide Gel in TBE buffer using an XCell Surelock gel system (any polyacrylamide system will do). Run at 135 V until the Bromphenol blue is about 1 cm from the bottom.
7. Separate plates and incubate gel in water with SYBR Safe DNA gel stain for 2 min with shaking.
8. Image and quantitate 108 bp fragment from the gel using BIORAD Gel Doc system and Image J software. 108 and 32 bp fragments are associated with the V600E BRAF; 140 bp undigested fragment is associated with wild-type BRAF.

4 Notes

1. We prefer the 0.6 ml locking centrifuge tubes from USA Scientific. It is important that the tubes do not open during any steps in the protocol.
2. We prefer using the 18S RNA oligonucleotide and probe set but any housekeeping gene can be used. This step is for normalizing the input RNA. Normalizing the input RNA by real-time PCR for 18S RNA is a critical step as dependence simply on 260 nm absorbance measurements can lead to assaying RNA of poor quality.
3. SYBR safe DNA gel stain is a safe alternative to ethidium bromide.
4. Hold the tube with the Histopaque as horizontal as possible as you slowly layer the blood, trying not to mix the layers. Alternately you can try to underlay the Histopaque below the blood but this can be messy.
5. One ml of Trizol is adequate for up to 10 million cells or an average 0.6 μm paraffin section.
6. One OD at 260 nm equals 40 μg/ml.
7. For this and the remaining steps we typically make master mixes of common reagents. For examples, if there are 9 RNA samples, a 10× mix will be made.
8. Combine the RNasin and reverse transcriptase as a mix, then add 2 μl to each tube.
9. Centrifuging prior to real-time PCR is important to prevent any air bubbles resting on the bottom of the wells.
10. To determine the amount of cDNA for each sample to use in the next step, the cycle numbers from the 18S RNA RT-PCR are compared. The difference in input cDNA is calculated by 2^n, where n represents the difference in cycle number for a particular fluorescence intensity. We generally set the sample

within a group with the greatest number of cycles (i.e., least amount of cDNA) to 1 and calculate the other samples relative to this one.

11. The TspR1 digestion was added to the protocol in order to reduce the amount of contaminating wild-type BRAF from surrounding and infiltrating normal tissue in the biopsy sample.
12. The number of cycles for the second PCR should be determined empirically based on the relative expression of $BRAF^{V600E}$ RNA in the various tissue subsets that are being assayed.
13. Nucleospin column is not necessary if one chooses not to sequence the second PCR product. Digested108 and 32 bp fragments are associated with the V600E BRAF, whereas140 bp undigested fragment is associated with WT BRAF.

References

1. Siegel R, Naishadham D, Jemal A (2012) Cancer statistics. CA Cancer J Clin 62:10–29
2. National Cancer Institute. Surveillance Epidemiology and End Results. http://seer.cancer.gov
3. Chapman PB, Hauschild A, Robert C et al (2011) Improved survival with vemurafenib in melanoma with BRAF V600E mutation. N Engl J Med 364:2507–2516
4. Hodi FS, O'Day SJ, McDermott DF et al (2010) Improved survival with ipilimumab in patients with metastatic melanoma. N Engl J Med 363:711–723
5. Robert C, Thomas L, Bondarenko I et al (2011) Ipilimumab plus dacarbazine for previously untreated metastatic melanoma. N Engl J Med 364:2517–2526
6. Davies H, Bignell GR, Cox C et al (2002) Mutations of the BRAF gene in human cancer. Nature 417:949–954
7. Flaherty KT, Puzanov I, Kim KB et al (2010) Inhibition of mutated, activated BRAF in metastatic melanoma. N Engl J Med 363:809–819
8. Sosman JA, Kim KB, Schuchter L et al (2012) Survival in BRAF V600-mutant advanced melanoma treated with vemurafenib. N Engl J Med 366:707–714
9. Kefford R, Arkenau H, Brown MP, Millward M, et al (2010) Phase I/II study of GSK2118436, a selective inhibitor of oncogenic mutant BRAF kinase, in patients with metastatic melanoma and other solid tumors. J Clin Oncol 28(15s):abstr 8503
10. Johannessen CM, Boehm JS, Kim SY et al (2010) COT drives resistance to RAF inhibition through MAP kinase pathway reactivation. Nature 468:968–972
11. Nazarian R, Shi H, Wang Q et al (2010) Melanomas acquire resistance to B-RAF(V600E) inhibition by RTK or N-RAS upregulation. Nature 468:973–977
12. Montagut C, Sharma SV, Shioda T et al (2008) Elevated CRAF as a potential mechanism of acquired resistance to BRAF inhibition in melanoma. Cancer Res 68:4853–4861
13. Poulikakos PI, Persaud Y, Janakiraman M et al (2011) RAF inhibitor resistance is mediated by dimerization of aberrantly spliced BRAF (V600E). Nature 480:387–390
14. Shi H, Moriceau G, Kong X et al (2012) Melanoma whole-exome sequencing identifies (V600E)B-RAF amplification-mediated acquired B-RAF inhibitor resistance. Nat Commun 3:724
15. Villanueva J, Vultur A, Lee JT et al (2010) Acquired resistance to BRAF inhibitors mediated by a RAF kinase switch in melanoma can be overcome by cotargeting MEK and IGF-1R/PI3K. Cancer Cell 18:683–695
16. Kirkwood JM, Manola J, Ibrahim J et al (2004) A pooled analysis of Eastern Cooperative Oncology Group and Intergroup trials of adjuvant high-dose interferon for melanoma. Clin Cancer Res 10:1670–1677
17. Gogas J, Ioannovich J, Dafni U et al (2006) Prognostic significance of autoimmunity during treatment of melanoma with interferon. N Engl J Med 354:709–718
18. Lin J, Goto Y, Murata H et al (2011) Polyclonality of BRAF mutations in primary melanoma and the selection of mutant alleles during progression. Br J Cancer 104:464–468
19. Yancovitz M, Litterman A, Yoon J et al (2012) Intra- and inter-tumor heterogeneity of BRAFV600E mutations in primary and

metastatic melanoma. PLoS One 7(1):e29336 (1–8)
20. NCCN Clinical Practice Guidelines in Oncology (NCCN Guidelines®): Melanoma version 3 2012. (2012) http://www.nccn.org/professionals/physicians_gls/pdf/melanoma.pdf
21. Panka DJ, Sullivan RJ, Mier JW (2010) An inexpensive, specific and highly sensitive protocol to detect the BrafV600E mutation in melanoma tumor biopsies and blood. Melanoma Res 20:401–407
22. Mocellin S, Hoon D, Ambrosi A et al (2006) The prognostic value of circulating tumor cells in patients with melanoma: a systemic review and meta-analysis. Clin Cancer Res 12:4605–4613
23. Sullivan RJ, Lawrence DP, Flaherty KT et al (2012) Predicting early relapse in patients with $BRAF^{V600E}$ melanoma with a highly sensitive blood BRAF assay. J Clin Oncol 30(suppl; abstr 8516)
24. Kitago M, Koyanagi K, Nakamura T et al (2009) mRNA expression and BRAF mutation in circulating melanoma cells isolated from peripheral blood with high molecular weight melanoma-associated antigen-specific monoclonal antibody beads. Clin Chem 55:757–764
25. Langland R, Sharp T, Tsai J et al (2006) Development of a companion diagnostic test for inhibitors of V600E BRAF. First AACR international conference on molecular diagnostics in cancer therapeutic development, 12–15 Sept 2006, abstr A13
26. McCullough RM, Cantor CR, Ding C (2005) High-throughput alternative splicing quantification by primer extension and matrix-assisted laser desorption/ionization time-of-flight mass spectrometry. Nucleic Acids Res 33:e99
27. Elvidge GP, Price TS, Glenny L et al (2005) Development and evaluation of real competitive PCR for high-throughput quantitative applications. Anal Biochem 339:231–241
28. Kwak JY, Kim EK, Kim JK et al (2010) Dual priming oligonucleotide-based multiplex PCR analysis for detection of BRAF(V600E) mutation in FNAB samples of thyroid nodules in BRAF(V600E) mutation-prevalent area. Head Neck 32:490–498
29. Miller CJ, Cheung M, Sharma A et al (2004) Method of mutation analysis may contribute to discrepancies in reports of (V599E)BRAF mutation frequencies in melanocytic neoplasms. J Invest Dermatol 123:990–992
30. Board RE, Ellison G, Orr MC et al (2009) Detection of BRAF mutations in the tumour and serum of patients enrolled in the AZD6244 (ARRY-142886) advanced melanoma phase II study. Br J Cancer 101:1724–1730
31. Morlan J, Baker J, Sinicropi D (2009) Mutation detection by real-time PCR: a simple, robust and highly selective method. PLoS One 4:e4584
32. Oldenburg RP, Liu MS, Kolodney MS (2008) Selective amplification of rare mutations using locked nucleic acid oligonucleotides that competitively inhibit primer binding to wild-type DNA. J Invest Dermatol 128:398–402
33. Dominguez PL, Kolodney MS (2005) Wild-type blocking polymerase chain reaction for detection of single nucleotide minority mutations from clinical specimens. Oncogene 24:6830–6834
34. Zatelli MC, Trasforini G, Leoni S et al (2009) BRAF V600E mutation analysis increases diagnostic accuracy for papillary thyroid carcinoma in fine-needle aspiration biopsies. Eur J Endocrinol 161:467–473
35. Domingo E, Laiho P, Ollikainen M et al (2004) BRAF screening as a low-cost effective strategy for simplifying HNPCC genetic testing. J Med Genet 41:664–668
36. Sidransky D, Cohen Y, Xing M (2008) BRAF mutation T1796A in thyroid cancers. US Patent 7,378,233, 27 May 2008
37. Oikonomou E, Makrodouli E, Evagelidou M et al (2009) BRAF(V600E) efficient transformation and induction of microsatellite instability versus KRAS(G12V) induction of senescence markers in human colon cancer cells. Neoplasia 11:1116–1131
38. French AJ, Sargent DJ, Burgart LJ et al (2008) Prognostic significance of defective mismatch repair and BRAF V600E in patients with colon cancer. Clin Cancer Res 14:3408–3415
39. Vandrovcova J, Lagerstedt-Robinsson K, Påhlman L et al (2006) Somatic BRAF-V600E mutations in familial colorectal cancer. Cancer Epidemiol Biomarkers Prev 15:2270–2273
40. Cradic KW, Milosevic D, Rosenberg AM et al (2009) Mutant BRAF(T1799A) can be detected in the blood of papillary thyroid carcinoma patients and correlates with disease status. J Clin Endocrinol Metab 94:5001–5009
41. Orru G, Coghe F, Faa G et al (2010) Rapid multiplex real-time PCR by molecular beacons for different BRAF allele detection in papillary thyroid carcinoma. Diagn Mol Pathol 19:1–8
42. Wojciechowska K, Lewinski A (2006) BRAF mutations in papillary thyroid carcinoma. Endocr Regul 40:129–138
43. Schiffman JD, Hodgson JG, VandenBerg SR et al (2010) Oncogenic BRAF mutation with CDKN2A inactivation is characteristic of a subset of pediatric malignant astrocytomas. Cancer Res 70:512–519
44. Jeong JH, Wang Z, Guimaraes AS et al (2008) BRAF activation initiates but does not maintain invasive prostate adenocarcinoma. PLoS One 3:e3949

45. Litterman AJ, Pollens D, Warycha, MA et al (2008) Tumor heterogeneity: evidence from BRAF V600E mutation detection. J Clin Oncol 26(May 20 suppl;abstr 20022)
46. Ju ST, Panka DJ, Cui H et al (1995) Fas(CD95)/FasL interactions required for programmed cell death after T-cell activation. Nature 373:444–448
47. Wilson BJ, Kocvara H (1975) A simple rapid method for layering blood on Ficoll-Isopaque gradients. J Immunol Methods 9:67–68
48. Chomczynski P, Sacchi N (1987) Single-step method of RNA isolation by acid guanidinium thiocyanate-phenol-chloroform extraction. Anal Biochem 162:156–159

Chapter 9

Selecting Patients for KIT Inhibition in Melanoma

Richard D. Carvajal, Omid Hamid, and Cristina R. Antonescu

Abstract

For many years, melanoma has been regarded as a single disease in terms of therapeutic considerations. The more recent identification of multiple molecular mechanisms underlying the development, progression, and prognosis of melanoma has led to a new paradigm for the management of this disease, has created new therapeutic opportunities, and has led to improved clinical outcomes. Such advances, however, are dependent upon methods that can reproducibly identify key molecular alterations within an individual tumor, define clinically relevant genetic subgroups of disease, and permit improved patient selection for targeted therapies.

Melanomas harboring genetic alterations of *KIT* have been demonstrated to constitute one such molecular subgroup of disease. In this chapter, we will discuss the biology of KIT in melanoma, review the rationale for and clinical data regarding KIT inhibition in melanomas harboring activating alterations of *KIT*, propose guidelines for the selection of patients for KIT inhibitor therapy, and, finally, present laboratory methods for *KIT* assessment in melanoma.

Key words Melanoma, KIT, Imatinib, Mucosal, Acral

1 Introduction

For many years, melanoma has been regarded as a single disease in terms of therapeutic considerations. Indeed, before 2011, U.S. Food and Drug Administration approved treatment options for advanced unresectable melanoma were limited to decarbazine (DTIC) [1] and interleukin-2 [2] irrespective of clinical, histological, or molecular features. However, the identification of multiple molecular mechanisms underlying the development, progression, and prognosis of melanoma has led to a new paradigm for the management of this disease, has created new therapeutic opportunities, and has led to improved clinical outcomes.

A major impetus towards the molecular classification of melanoma was the finding by the Wellcome Trust Sanger Institute in 2002 of oncogenic *BRAF* somatic mutations in 66 % of melanomas [3, 4]. This discovery led to the clinical evaluation of a number of inhibitors of the MAPK pathway in the *BRAF* mutant

Magdalena Thurin and Francesco M. Marincola (eds.), *Molecular Diagnostics for Melanoma: Methods and Protocols*, Methods in Molecular Biology, vol. 1102, DOI 10.1007/978-1-62703-727-3_9,

melanoma patient population, with unprecedented tumor responses observed and meaningful improvements in overall survival achieved. Vemurafenib, a small molecular inhibitor of mutant BRAF, was granted FDA approval in August 2011 based upon the results of the BRIM3 trial which demonstrated a relative reduction of 63 % in the risk of death and of 74 % in the risk of either death or disease progression, as compared with dacarbazine ($p<0.001$ for both comparisons) [4]. While the response rate was 5 % for those randomized to dacarbazine, the response rate was 48 % for vemurafenib. Subsequently, both dabrafenib (GSK2118436) [5], another selective BRAF inhibitor, as well as trametinib [6], a selective MEK inhibitor, were shown to improve outcomes when compared with dacarbazine in two additional randomized phase III trials (BREAK-3 and METRIC, respectively).

The dramatic efficacy observed with these agents in patients with melanoma harboring activating mutations in *BRAF* highlighted the critical need to consider the molecular heterogeneity of melanoma as we develop novel therapies for this disease. Bastian and colleagues demonstrated that four clinical subgroups of disease, including melanoma arising from nonchronically sun-damaged skin (non-CSD), melanoma arising from chronically sun-damaged skin (CSD), melanoma arising from mucosal surfaces, and melanoma arising from acral surfaces, are characterized by unique combinations of genome-wide aberrations in DNA copy number and oncogenic alterations [7].

The more common melanomas arising from non-CSD skin are associated with frequent activating mutations in *BRAF* and a relative increase in the frequency of *NRAS* mutations. Several groups have identified melanomas arising from the uveal tract of the eye to harbor distinct molecular alterations, with functionally activating mutations in *GNAQ* [8, 9] or *GNA11* [10] observed in approximately 80 % of uveal melanomas and loss of BAP1 in 84 % of metastatic tumor samples [11]. Although mutations in *BRAF* have been previously thought to be rare in uveal melanoma [12–14], such mutations can be identified when using techniques more sensitive than direct sequencing [15]; however, the relative scarcity of the *BRAF* mutation excludes a primary driving role for this mutation in uveal melanoma [15]. Melanomas arising from CSD, mucosal, or acral surfaces less commonly harbor oncogenic *BRAF* and *NRAS* mutations, but more commonly harbor alterations in the type III transmembrane receptor tyrosine kinase KIT [16, 17]. These mutually exclusive molecular alterations identify unique subsets of melanoma with distinct biological and therapeutic implications. By adopting a molecular classification system of melanoma, the heterogeneity of this disease is emphasized and the need for distinct therapeutic strategies for each subset is highlighted.

In this chapter, we will discuss the biology of KIT in melanoma, review the rationale for and clinical data regarding KIT inhibition in melanomas harboring activating alterations of *KIT*, propose guidelines for the selection of patients for KIT inhibitor therapy, and, finally, present laboratory methods for *KIT* assessment in melanoma.

1.1 Structure of KIT and KIT Signaling in Melanoma

KIT was first identified in 1987 and encodes a type III transmembrane receptor tyrosine kinase which is made up of five distinct domains including a glycosylated extracellular ligand binding domain containing five immunoglobulin-like repeats (encoded by exons 1–9), a hydrophobic transmembrane domain (encoded by exon 10), and an intracellular portion consisting of an inhibitory juxtamembrane domain (encoded by exon 11) and two intracellular tyrosine kinase domains (encoded by exons 12–21; Fig. 1) [18–20]. The juxtamembrane domain plays an auto-inhibitory role, preventing KIT activation in absence of ligand.

Stem cell factor (SCF; also known as KIT ligand, steel factor, or mast cell growth factor), the ligand for KIT, is also a glycosylated transmembrane protein. A proteolytic cleavage site within SCF can be introduced via alternative splicing and results in a soluble form of SCF [21]. Both the soluble and membrane-bound variants of SCF can bind to the extracellular domain of KIT, resulting in receptor dimerization and autophosphorylation of the

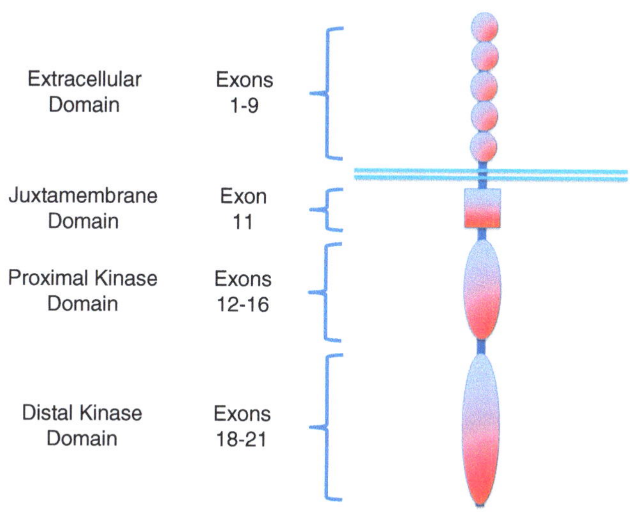

Fig. 1 Structure of the KIT protein. The N-terminal extracellular domain consists of five immunoglobulin-like regions (*circles*) that serve as the binding site for the KIT ligand, stem cell factor. Intracellularly, the juxtamembrane domain is responsible for preventing activation of the tyrosine kinase domains, unless ligand is present. There are two tyrosine kinase domains that become autophosphorylated on receptor activation. Once phosphorylated, they activate a variety of downstream intracellular signaling pathways. Modified from Fig. 2—Postow MA, Carvajal RD (2012) Therapeutic implications of KIT in melanoma. Cancer J 18(2):137–41

intracellular tyrosine kinase domains. Phosphorylation of the tyrosine kinase domains enables KIT to recruit and bind to downstream signaling proteins and initiate signaling in a variety of downstream pathways including the MAPK, PI3K/AKT, JAK/STAT pathways [22]. The downstream effects, however, differ depending upon whether signaling is initiated by soluble or membrane-bound SCF. Binding of membrane-bound SCF to KIT results in prolonged KIT activation, whereas soluble SCF results in KIT activation, internalization, and degradation [23].

Signaling through KIT is critical for the development and maintenance of a variety of cells including hematopoietic progenitor cells [24], primordial germ cells [25, 26], mast cells [27], and the interstitial cells of Cajal [28]. Both KIT and SCF are also critical for normal melanocyte development, proliferation, migration, and survival, in part via KIT-mediated regulation of the melanocyte master regulator Microphthalmia-associated transcription factor (Mitf) [29–31]. Loss-of-function mutations in murine *KIT* or *SCF* results in impaired melanocyte migration and loss of normal pigmentation, and can lead to developmental pigmentary diseases such as piebaldism and Waardenburgs syndrome [32–37]. Loss-of-function mutations of Mitf similarly result in phenotypic defects in pigmentation.

1.2 KIT Alterations in Melanoma

Although KIT function is critical in normal melanocyte development, it was initially thought to function as a tumor suppressor in melanoma. Huang et al. demonstrated that the highly metastatic melanoma cell line A375SM had a reduced ability to form metastases and increased apoptotic sensitivity after transfection with the *KIT* gene [38]. Additionally, immunohistochemical (IHC) studies showed that loss of KIT correlated with more advanced disease (Table 1) [39–42]. Three clinical trials of imatinib mesylate, a small molecule inhibitor of the Abelson (Abl), Arg (abl-related gene), stem cell factor receptor (Kit), and platelet-derived growth factor receptor-α and -β (PDGFR-α and PDGFR-β) tyrosine kinases, were conducted in patients with advanced melanoma in part because of the critical role of KIT in melanocyte survival and the finding of KIT expression on melanoma [43–45]. Consistent with

Table 1
KIT expression by immunohistochemistry and melanoma progression

	Benign melanocytes	Primary melanoma	Metastatic melanoma
Natali et. al. [39]	63 % (19/30)	74 % (34/46)	31 % (10/32)
Montone et. al. [40]	100 % (65/65)	74 % (25/31)	30 % (6/20)
Shen et. al. [42]	59 % (10/17)	96 % (22/23)	45 % (14/31)

the hypothesis that KIT is not a relevant driver of melanoma progression and survival, these studies were negative, with only one radiographic response observed out of 62 patients treated across the three trials.

Despite these negative results, the experience of KIT inhibition in other tumor models such as gastrointestinal stromal tumor (GIST) suggested that incorrect patient selection may have been responsible for the negative clinical results. GIST is a tumor type characterized by activating mutations in *KIT* in 80 % of cases and *PDGFRA* in up to 10 % of cases, and is a disease which is highly responsive to inhibition with agents such as imatinib [46, 47]; however, response to imatinib is dependent upon the presence of a mutation in *KIT* or *PDGFRA* that drives tumor progression. This paradigm indicates that KIT inhibition in melanoma may only be effective if KIT activity was truly driving tumor growth.

Evidence of aberrant KIT function in melanoma arose as early as 1998 when Bastian et al. reported the presence of an amplification on chromosome 4q12 in acral melanoma which includes the *KIT* locus [48]. Went et al. subsequently reported on the first case of a *KIT* mutation identified in melanoma which resulted in an L576P transition mutation (Fig. 2) [49]. A number of investigators have

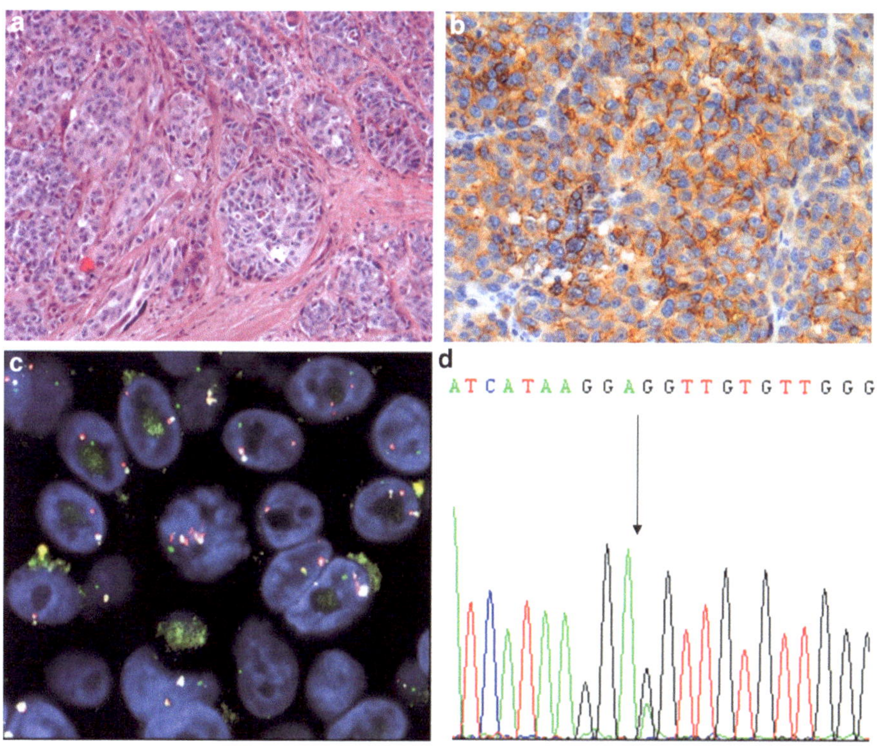

Fig. 2 Melanoma specimen harboring both increased KIT copy number as well as an L576P mutation in KIT. (**a**) Hematoxylin and eosin stain. (**b**) Diffuse (4+) KIT expression by immunohistochemistry. (**c**) Fluorescent in situ hybridization shows increased KIT copy number. (**d**) ABI demonstrating a L576P KIT mutation

subsequently screened additional melanoma samples for the presence of such mutations [7, 17, 50–57].

Work performed by Curtin et. al. demonstrated that the prevalence of mutations in key melanoma genes including *BRAF*, *NRAS*, and *KIT* differed between distinct clinical subgroups of melanoma which included melanomas arising from chronically sun-damaged skin, melanomas arising from nonchronically sun-damaged skin, melanomas arising from acral sites, and melanomas arising from mucosal sites [7]. Mutations in *BRAF* or *NRAS* were very common in melanomas arising from skin without evidence of chronic sun-damage, found in 59 % and 22 % cases, respectively, but were less common in the other melanoma subtypes. A subsequent analysis of 102 melanomas using comparative genomic hybridization identified frequent copy number increases of chromosomal region 4q12 in melanomas arising from mucosal, acral, or chronically sun-damaged surfaces, which correlated with strong expression of the KIT protein and point mutations in the *KIT* gene [16]. Analysis of *KIT* in the full set of melanoma samples revealed *KIT* mutations in 17 % of melanomas arising from chronically sun-damaged skin, 11 % arising from acral surfaces, and 21 % arising from mucosal sites. These alterations in *KIT* were mutually exclusive with *BRAF* and *NRAS* alterations. No mutations in *KIT* were found in melanoma arising from skin that was not chronically sun-damaged. The KIT mutations identified included activating mutations in the juxtamembrane domain, a region of the protein frequently in GIST, a disease known to be dependent upon KIT activation. Since the juxtamembrane domain is involved in autoinhibition of the receptor when not bound with ligand, mutations in this region are expected to enhance ligand-independent receptor dimerization and activation [58]. Unlike in GIST, however, where the majority of mutations identified are deletions or insertions, the majority of KIT alterations identified in melanoma are substitution mutations [59].

In addition to the presence of *KIT* mutations identified in select clinical subsets of melanoma, *KIT* gene amplification was identified in 7 % of acral melanoma, 8 % of mucosal melanomas, and 6 % of melanomas arising from chronically sun-damaged skin [16]. A significant number of cases harbored an increased copy number of *KIT* but did not meet the definition of amplification. A number of other investigators have shown similar findings in other series [17, 51, 52, 55, 57].

Interestingly, the frequency of *KIT* mutations in mucosal melanomas may differ depending upon site of origin [18]. Although the number of cases available for analysis is limited, pooling of the currently available data suggests that the *KIT* mutational frequency is 12 % (10/81) in mucosal melanomas arising from the head and neck and 20 % (18/92) in mucosal melanomas arising from the anorectal or vulvovaginal regions [17, 52–54, 56]. Pooled analysis of series which separated vulvovaginal from anorectal mucosal melanomas demonstrated that *KIT* mutations were present in 27 % (7/26) of vulvovaginal and 12 % (7/57) of anorectal cases [52, 54, 56].

Similarly, the frequency of *KIT* alterations may differ depending upon ethnicity. The majority of series have assessed tumors arising largely from a Caucasian population. In Asian populations, acral and mucosal melanomas constitute more than two thirds of the incidence of melanoma; however, the prevalence of KIT alterations in melanomas arising from this patient population may be lower than that observed in Caucasians [60]. In a series of 92 mucosal and acral melanoma tumor samples from a Korean population, increased copy number of *KIT* was identified in approximately 30 % of cases, with 7.2 % harboring *KIT* mutations [61]. A series of 502 tumor samples from a Chinese population demonstrated an overall *KIT* mutation frequency of 10.8 %, with a frequency of 21 % in melanomas arising from chronically sun-damaged skin, 12 % in melanomas arising from acral surfaces, and 10 % of melanomas arising from mucosal surfaces. Interestingly, 8 % of melanomas arising from nonchronically sun-damaged skin also harbored *KIT* mutations in this series. In Australia, more than 40 % of melanomas are associated with chronically sun-damaged skin; however, unlike the 10–20 % prevalence of *KIT* mutations in this subset of melanoma in the US population, the prevalence of *KIT* mutations in an Australian population is 2 % [62].

1.3 Aberrant KIT Function in Melanoma

Initial work assessing the cellular response to ligand-independent activation of KIT in melanocytes which were altered to express an endogenous constitutively active D814Y KIT receptor suggested that activation of KIT is primarily responsible for the promotion of pro-migratory signals, with no stimulation of melanogenesis or proliferation [35]. The introduction in melanocytes of the L576P and K642E KIT mutations, the two most common KIT mutations identified in melanoma, did result in the transformation melanocytes, but only when grown under hypoxic conditions or following the introduction of exogenous HIF-1α [63]. Introduction of the KIT mutation alone led to activation of PI3K/AKT signaling, but not MEK/ERK signaling. The combination of both hypoxia and KIT activation, however, resulted in activation of both pathways and stimulation of proliferation. Such proliferation was inhibited by exposure to imatinib. Sensitivity of additional *KIT* mutant cell line models to KIT inhibitors has been demonstrated. Antonescu et al. demonstrated sensitivity of a stable transformant Ba/F3 KIT L576P mutant cell line to dasatinib (Sprycel®, Bristol-Myers Squibb, Princeton, NJ) as well as imatinib [52].

Preclinical work using human melanoma cells harboring *KIT* mutations have also been instructive. Jiang et al. characterized three low passage primary cell cultures derived from mucosal melanomas and identified one which harbored an exon 11 V559D mutation in KIT with 12-fold amplification of the *KIT* locus [64]. Treatment of these cells with imatinib resulted in G1 cell cycle arrest and apoptosis that was not observed in the cell lines characterized by a wild-type *KIT*. Furthermore, treatment of the *KIT* mutant cells, but not the wild-type cells, was associated with inhibition of JAK/STAT, PI3K/AKT, and MAPK signaling, as well as inhibition of Bcl-2, survivin, and Mcl-1 expression. Woodman et al. utilized the WM3211 non-mucosal/non-acral melanoma cell line that harbors an L576P KIT mutation and demonstrated sensitivity to dasatinib, with no effects observed with imatinib, nilotinib, or sorafenib [65]. Ashida et al. utilized a mucosal melanoma cell line harboring an exon 17 D820Y KIT mutation which is frequently associated with imatinib resistance in GIST and demonstrated KIT phosphorylation in the absence of SCF, consistent with constitutive activation, not observed in cell lines without *KIT* mutations [55]. Treatment of the mutant cell lines, but not the wild-type cells, with sunitinib resulted in decreased proliferation.

Together, these investigators have demonstrated the constitutive activation of KIT kinase activity in mutant cells which is not observed in *KIT* wild-type cells. Furthermore, exposure of mutant, but not wild-type cells, to clinically available KIT inhibitors result in down-regulation of multiple downstream mediators, cell cycle arrest, decrease in cell proliferation, and induction of apoptosis.

1.4 KIT Inhibition in Melanoma

As noted above, three clinical trials of imatinib were conducted in molecularly unselected patients with advanced melanoma and were negative, with only one radiographic response observed out of 62 patients treated across the three trials (Table 2) [43–45]. Interestingly, the one case who responded had an acral melanoma harboring alternative splicing of exon 15 of unclear significance [45]. Several subsequent case reports demonstrated additional dramatic responses to imatinib in patients with melanoma harboring *KIT* mutations, suggesting the need for ongoing evaluation of targeted therapy for this molecular subgroup of melanoma. A 79-year-old woman with metastatic mucosal melanoma arising

Table 2
Summary of phase II clinical trial results of imatinib in a molecularly unselected metastatic melanoma patient population

	n	Clinical melanoma subtypes	Response rate
Ugurel et al. [43]	18	11 non-CSD, 1 acral, 1 mucosal, 1 ocular, 4 unk	0 % (0/16)
Wyman et al. [44]	26	23 cutaneous, 1 mucosal, 1 ocular	0 % (0/25)
Kim et al. [45]	21	20 non-CSD, 1 acral	5 % (1/21)

Abbreviations: *non-CSD* nonchronically sun-damaged skin, *unk* unknow

from the anorectal mucosal harboring a 7-codon duplication (PYDHKWE) in *KIT* exon 11 achieved a rapid clinical and radiographic response after therapy with imatinib 400 mg daily [66]. A second report described another 79 year-old woman with mucosal melanoma arising from the anorectal mucosal harboring an L576P exon 11 *KIT* mutation who also achieved a significant response to imatinib therapy [67]. A third case of a 69-year-old woman with mucosal melanoma arising from the anorectal mucosal harboring a K642E exon 13 *KIT* mutation suggested that the dose of imatinib may be important in terms of response [68]. Four weeks after beginning therapy with imatinib 400 mg daily, she achieved complete resolution of all recurrent subcutaneous nodules in the anogenital and inguinal region, confirmed by positron emission tomography (PET). Dose reduction was necessary for hematologic toxicity resulting in neutropenia and fever. After being treated for several months at the lower dose, her melanoma recurred, but then responded to a dose increase of imatinib to 600 mg daily, with complete disappearance of disease.

Given the preclinical and available clinical data suggesting that imatinib may be an effective therapeutic strategy specifically in patients whose melanoma was driven by KIT activation, three additional trials of imatinib were conducted in patients molecularly selected based upon the presence of somatic alterations in *KIT* within the tumor (Table 3). These studies have completed accrual, with final results published for two of these studies.

A multicenter clinical trial led by Memorial Sloan-Kettering Cancer Center enrolled 25 evaluable patients with advanced melanoma harboring either a *KIT* mutation or amplification [57]. Patients received imatinib 400 mg PO BID on a continual basis. Six patients achieved a radiographic response, with two patients achieving durable complete responses and two with durable partial responses. Each of these four durable responses persisted for over 1 year. Notably, all six patients who responded had tumor harboring an L576P (exon 11) or K642E (exon 13) *KIT* mutation, with both patients achieving durable complete responses having tumor harboring L576P mutations with concurrent amplification.

Table 3
Summary of phase II clinical trial results of imatinib in a molecularly selected metastatic melanoma patient population

	n	Response rate
Carvajal et al., 2011 [57]	25	16 % (4/25)
Guo et al., 2011 [76]	43	23 % (10/43)
Hodi et al., 2008 [66]	20	25 % (5/20)

A number of previously unreported mutations of unclear functional relevance were identified in this study, suggesting a need to develop a method to separate functionally active driver mutations from functionally irrelevant passenger mutations. In this study, the presence of a mutant to wild-type *KIT* allelic ratio greater than one as determined by their respective electropherogram peak heights appeared to indicate a greater likelihood of benefit from imatinib and is one potential method to separate driver from passenger mutations.

A second trial conducted by Guo et al. treated 43 evaluable patients with imatinib 400 mg daily [60]. Of these 43 patients, 10 (23 %) achieved a partial response, with a total of 18 patients demonstrating tumor regression. Tumor regression or stability was demonstrated to result in a progression-free survival (PFS) and overall survival (OS) superior to that observed in the progressing cases (9.0 vs. 1.5 months PFS, $p < .001$; 15.0 vs. 9.0 months OS, $p = .036$). One patient with a *KIT* amplification without a mutation responded. Interestingly, as observed in the MSKCC trial, each of the responding patients with *KIT* mutations in this trial had mutations in exons 11 and 13.

Finally, interim results from a third trial involving 20 patients treated with imatinib were reported at the 2009 International Melanoma Congress by Hodi et al. [69]. In this trial, 5 responses out of 20 evaluable patients treated at that time were seen (25 %). No responses were observed in the ten patients enrolled whose tumors harbored *KIT* amplification alone, although two achieved stable disease for 6–7 months. The response rate observed in those whose tumors harbored *KIT* mutations, however, was 50 %, with three of the five responders having tumor harboring a concurrent *KIT* amplification.

Responses in *KIT* mutant melanoma are not limited to imatinib therapy. Patients with *KIT* mutant melanoma have been reported to respond to other targeted inhibitors of KIT such as sorafenib [70], dasatinib [65], and sunitinib [71]. Notably all of these patients have had *KIT* mutations involving exon 11 or 13.

Sunitinib: Although several trials investigating KIT inhibitors other than imatinib have been initiated, none have yet successfully fully completed the planned total accrual. Such experiences illustrate the challenge inherent in successfully conducting clinical trials in rare molecular subsets of disease. Minor et al. reported on their experience of sunitinib 50 mg daily, 4 weeks on and 2 weeks off, in ten evaluable patients with tumor harboring mutations, amplification, or overexpression of KIT [72]. Sunitinib is a potent inhibitor of KIT with additional inhibitory effects upon PDGFR-α, PDGFR-β, and the VEGF receptors. This study differed from the three trials of imatinib described above in that protein overexpression was sufficient for eligibility. Of the ten evaluable patients, one achieved a complete response, two achieved durable partial responses, and one achieved a transient partial response. Of the four evaluable patients with tumor harboring a *KIT* mutation, three achieved radiographic responses. Two responders had tumor harboring L576P mutations and one had tumor harboring an exon 11 W557G mutation. Of the four evaluable patients with tumor characterized by *KIT* amplification, no responses were observed. One of the two patients enrolled because of KIT overexpression by immunohistochemistry, one achieved an unconfirmed partial response.

Dasatinib: Dasatinib is an orally active inhibitor of Src, Abl, KIT, PDGFR, FAK, and other kinases. A phase II clinical trial of dasatinib in 36 evaluable molecularly unselected patients with advanced melanoma was conducted by Kluger et al. [73]. In this single-arm, two institution trial, two confirmed partial responses were observed: one response was seen in a patient with a subungual melanoma harboring an exon 13 *KIT* mutation and the other was observed in a patient whose tumor did not harbor a *KIT* mutation. Interestingly, one patient whose tumor harbored an exon 11 mutation did not respond to dasatinib.

Woodman et al. reported on two patients with tumor harboring L576P KIT mutations who responded to dasatinib, lending further support for the potential efficacy of this agent in KIT mutant melanoma [65]. One of these patients was a 55-year-old female with metastatic mucosal melanoma arising from the vulvovaginal mucosal who received approximately 11 months of imatinib in the adjuvant setting prior to developing recurrent disease. After progression to several lines of standard and experimental regimens, one of which included the combination of sorafenib and temsirolimus, she was treated with dasatinib 70 mg BID and achieved a clinical and radiographic response to therapy despite prior therapy with two other inhibitors of KIT.

Although no trial of dasatinib in molecularly selected melanoma patients has been completed, an ongoing phase II study of dasatinib being conducted by the Eastern Cooperative Oncology Group (EGOG 2607) that was initially open to patients with metastatic melanoma arising from sites known to harbor *KIT* mutations was recently amended to require the presence of a *KIT* mutation for eligibility. This revised study will provide important information regarding the efficacy of dasatinib in this patient population.

Nilotinib: Nilotinib is a small molecule multitargeted tyrosine kinase inhibitor that is structurally derived from imatinib and was initially developed for the treatment of imatinib-resistant chronic myelogenous leukemia. It binds to and inhibits the kinase domain of ABL, KIT, and PDGF receptor kinases with greater potency than imatinib. Cho et al. reported on the interim results of their phase II study of nilotinib 400 mg twice daily in nine evaluable patients from South Korea with melanoma harboring *KIT* alterations [74]. Of the nine evaluable patients, three had tumor harboring exon 11 KIT mutations. Six had tumor with *KIT* amplification. Of the three patients with *KIT* mutations, two achieved durable partial responses lasting 8.4 and 10+ months. One patient with *KIT* amplification alone had disease stability for 6 months. Accrual to this study is ongoing.

The only phase III trial to be initiated specifically for *KIT* mutant melanoma is a randomized, phase III, registration trial of nilotinib versus DTIC (TEAM Trial: Tasigna Efficacy in Advanced Melanoma). Unfortunately, since study initiation in 2010, accrual has been challenging, and the study was subsequently modified to a single-arm phase II trial of nilotinib. Accrual to this revised study is anticipated to complete in late 2012; however, the implications of altering the trial from its original design in terms of potential agent registration are unclear.

1.5 Selection of Patients for KIT Inhibition

It has become clear based upon currently available clinical experience that the efficacy of KIT inhibition in melanoma is dependent upon the presence of a driving genetic alteration in *KIT*. The mere presence of KIT as determined by immunohistochemistry is not sufficient to predict response. Furthermore, not all melanomas harboring *KIT* alterations will be susceptible to KIT inhibition, as it is only the tumors dependent upon KIT, or the KIT-driven melanomas, which are likely to be sensitive. The question remains, however, as to how best to differentiate driving genetic alterations predictive of susceptibility to KIT inhibition versus passenger alterations which are irrelevant to tumor progression.

A comparison of the experience of BRAF inhibition and KIT inhibition in melanoma highlights the challenges posed when attempting to properly select patients for KIT inhibition. While 74 % of BRAF mutant melanomas harbor a V600E mutation, mutations in KIT are more widely distributed over the coding region (Table 4) [75]. The V600E BRAF mutation has been demonstrated to be pathologically relevant, resulting in RAS-independent activation of the MAPK pathway and increased tumor proliferation. The relative homogeneity of the genetic alterations in BRAF observed in BRAF mutant melanoma coupled with the clinical availability of inhibitory agents with specificity for V600E BRAF has lead to dramatic improvements in the management of patients with BRAF-mutant melanoma [4]. The more modest results observed with KIT inhibition in KIT-mutant melanoma suggest that only select KIT alterations are truly oncogenic and indicative of an effective therapeutic target.

A review of the patients who have achieved significant radiographic responses to KIT inhibition demonstrates that all most such responses have occurred in patients whose tumors harbored mutations affecting either exons 11 or 13 of KIT (Table 5).

Table 4
Distribution of KIT mutations identified upon analysis of tumor samples tested as part of a phase II trial of imatinib in patients with melanoma harboring somatic alterations of KIT [57]

KIT exon	Associated protein domain	% of Mutations (n=48)	Mutations identified
Exon 9	Extracellular domain	6 % (n=3)	N463S (n=1) G466E (n=1) G466R (n=1)
Exon 11	Juxtamembrane domain	46 % (n=22)	Y553C (n=1) E554K (n=2) W557R (n=2) V559A (n=1) V559C (n=1) V559G (n=1) V560D (n=2) Y570H (n=1) L576P (n=11)
Exon 13	Proximal kinase domain	19 % (n=9)	K642E (n=4) L647F (n=1) G648D (n=2) I653T (n=1) V654A (n=1)
Exon 17	Distal kinase domain	10 % (n=5)	L813P (n=1) K818Q (n=1) D820Y (n=1) N822K (n=1) N822Y (n=1)
Exon 18	Distal kinase domain	19 % (n=9)	A829P (n=1) L831P (n=1) P838L (n=1) S840I (n=1) Y846C (n=1) S850G (n=1) V852I (n=1) L859P (n=1) L862P (n=1)

Furthermore, the majority of these responses occurred in cases harboring either an L576P (exon 11) or K642E (exon 13) mutation, the two most commonly observed KIT mutations in melanoma. The question arises as to whether amplification of KIT in the absence of a mutation in melanoma is a sufficient marker of sensitivity to KIT inhibition. Based upon the limited available data from reported clinical trials, the likelihood of response in a melanoma harboring *KIT* amplification without a mutation appears to be low, but not impossible, with one such event reported thus far [60].

Table 5
KIT alterations identified in patients with radiographic responses by RECIST criteria to KIT inhibition

Study	Agent	*n*	RR (mutant only)	RR (amplified only)	RR (mut + amp)	Responsive mutations
Imatinb	Hodi et al. [66]	1	1/1	n/a	n/a	Exon 11 7 codon duplication (*n* = 1)
Imatinib	Lutzky et al. [68]	1	n/a	n/a	1/1	Exon 13 K642E (*n* = 1)
Imatinib	Salzger et al. [67]	1	1/1	n/a	n/a	Exon 11 L576P (*n* = 1)
Imatinib	Handolias et al. [82]	3	2/3	n/a	n/a	Exon 11 7 codon duplication (*n* = 1) Exon 11 L576P (*n* = 1) Exon 13 K642E (*n* = 1)
Imatinib	Carvajal et al. [57]	25	2/10	0/4	4/11	Exon 11 L576P (*n* = 4) Exon 13 K642E (*n* = 2)
Imatinib	Guo et al. [76]	43	9/40	1/3	NR	Exon 11 (*n* = 6) Exon 13 (*n* = 3)
Nilotinib	Cho et al. [74]	9	2/3	0/9	0/0	Exon 11 L576P (*n* = 1) Exon 11 V559A (*n* = 1)
Dasatinib	Woodman et al. [65]	2	2/2	n/a	n/a	Exon 11 L576P (*n* = 2)
Dasatinib	Kluger et al. [73]	39	1/2	n/a	n/a	Exon 13
Sunitinib	Zhu et al. [71]	1	1/1	n/a	n/a	Exon 11 V559A (*n* = 1)
Sunitinib	Minor et al. [72]	10	3/4	0/4	0/0	Exon 11 L576P (*n* = 2) Exon 11 W557G (*n* = 1)
Sorafenib	Quintas-Cardama et al. [70]	1	1/1	n/a	n/a	Exon 11 V560A (*n* = 1)
Sorafenib	Handolias et al. [82]	1	0/1 (27 % reduction)	n/a	n/a	Exon 13 K642E (*n* = 1)

Abbreviations: *n/a* not assessed, *NR* not reported

Thus, a simplistic but useful model for appropriate patient selection for KIT inhibitor therapy would be to limit treatment to those with disease harboring either a KIT exon 11 or exon 13 mutation.

The presence of an exon 11 or 13 mutation or even an L576P or K642E mutation, however, is not a guarantee of response. Indeed, in the MSKCC-led trial of imatinib in patients with melanoma harboring somatic alterations of KIT, of the 11 patients with tumors harboring either an L576P mutation (n =7) or a K642E mutation (n =4), six radiographic responses were observed, for a response rate in this subset of patients of 54 % [57]. Thus, more refined methods for proper identification of KIT-driven tumors are still required.

Our group used two methods to investigate whether the relative abundance of mutant KIT influenced response to imatinib [57]. First, we assessed whether treated patients with tumors harboring KIT that was both mutated and amplified were more likely to achieve tumor response than those patients whose tumors harbored either alteration alone. Although a greater likelihood of response was observed in these cases, the difference was not statistically significant. We then evaluated whether the ratio of the mutant to wild-type *KIT* allele influenced response to imatinib, as mutations associated with a mutant to wild-type allele ratio of more than one are likely to be pathogenetically relevant. Allelic ratios of more than one indicate the presence of an independent genetic event, such as amplification of the mutant allele, deletion of the wild-type allele, or loss of heterozygosity, which shifts the ratio in favor of the mutant allele and suggests that the mutation is a functionally relevant event. Analysis of this subgroup revealed a higher response rate in cases with an allelic ratio of more than one (71 % vs. 6 %; p= .002), with a longer median time to progression (p= .01) and extended median survival (p= .03). Although this finding must be replicated in a larger series prior to broader application, it may serve as an indicator of a genetic event relevant to oncogenesis and should be investigated further.

Another important consideration is that the sensitivity of specific *KIT* mutations to clinically available inhibitors can differ. The response of KIT-driven melanoma to a small molecule inhibitor of KIT is predicted to be dependent on the region of the protein affected by a mutation. Some mutations affect the binding affinity of specific inhibitor KIT as previously demonstrated in in vitro and clinical studies of GIST [76–78]. Trials have been initiated to evaluate imatinib, sunitinib, sorafenib, nilotinib, dasatinib, and masatinib as single agents in KIT-mutant melanoma and it will be important to attempt to correlate specific mutation to response with particular agents. As the clinically available inhibitors of KIT have varying inhibitory profiles against a range of KIT mutations, it may ultimately be possible to match an individual KIT mutation to a particular drug.

2 Conclusion and Future Directions

With our increasing knowledge of the biological heterogeneity of melanoma, we are making significant strides in developing effective therapies for this disease; however, this success is dependent upon prospective tumor genotyping. Such testing is now standard of care and commercially available for BRAF. Assessment of KIT should additionally be conducted in select clinical subsets of melanoma, including those arising from mucosal, acral, and chronically sun-damaged surfaces.

Despite the significant clinical benefit achieved in select patients with melanoma harboring KIT mutations, such benefit is not observed in all patients and more work is required to optimize the use of KIT inhibitors in melanoma. The generation of KIT mutant cell lines has been difficult; however, the development of additional KIT mutant cell lines, as well as murine models of KIT mutant melanoma will ultimately be necessary to advance our understanding of the biology of this genetic subset of melanoma. Furthermore, while it appears that melanomas harboring mutations in exons 11 or 13 of KIT are more sensitive to KIT inhibition, further work is required to more accurately separate KIT-driven melanomas from the KIT-mutant melanomas harboring passenger mutations unlikely to respond to KIT inhibition.

As with other developmental programs for targeted therapy, further work is necessary to elucidate mechanisms of resistance to KIT inhibition. Primary resistance refers to initial refractoriness of tumors to treatment and may be caused by mutations in portions of the gene not inhibited by the drug. Secondary or acquired resistance refers to ultimate tumor progression following an initial period of response. Our current knowledge of the development of secondary resistance to KIT inhibition in melanoma is limited, but does suggest that melanoma resistance mechanisms differ significantly from that observed in GIST. In GIST, secondary resistance frequently occurs at the level of KIT due to the development of secondary *KIT* mutations that typically affect the tyrosine kinase domains in exons 13 and 17 [77, 79, 80]. Thus far, no such secondary mutations have been observed in melanoma. The development of a previously undetected NRAS Q61K mutation in addition to a previously detected W557G KIT mutation has been described in a secondarily resistant tumor after a 7 month course of sunitinib [72]. Although this finding may be due to genetic heterogeneity in the primary tumor or other technical factors, the true development of a secondary NRAS mutation would be expected to bypass the effects of upstream KIT inhibition and is a plausible mechanism of sunitinib resistance.

A case reported by Si et al. suggests that activation of the mTOR pathway may be another mechanism of secondary resistance to KIT inhibition in melanoma [81]. Pre-imatinib and imatinib-resistant tumor samples were obtained from a 57-year-old female with a mucosal melanoma arising from the nasal cavity harboring an L576P KIT mutation who achieved durable disease control for 8.5 months imatinib prior to the development of tumor resistance. Analysis of a progressive tumor sample revealed no secondary mutations in KIT, PDGFR-α, BRAF, NRAS, PTEN, tuberous sclerosis protein 1, p110alpha subunit of PI3K, and AKT1. Immunohistochemistry, however, revealed increased phosphorylation of S6BP and 4E-BP1, as well as increased phosphorylation of Akt and ERK1/2 in the progressive tumor when compared to pre-imatinib samples. No expression of cyclinD1 or phosphorylated MEK1/2 was detected. Given the evidence of selective activation of the mTOR signaling pathway, the patient was treated with everolimus, an mTOR inhibitor, and achieved a partial response to therapy. Although the mechanism of pathway activation in this case was not fully elucidated, the dramatic clinical efficacy of mTOR inhibition in this case supports the clinical relevance of this finding and requires further evaluation.

Based upon the promising data presented above, the use of imatinib for KIT-mutant melanoma has been added to the National Comprehensive Cancer Network Clinical Practice Guidelines for Melanoma (Version 1.2013). Such therapy represents a major therapeutic advance for those patients with melanoma harboring select *KIT* alterations. The definitive demonstration of efficacy of KIT inhibition over standard therapy in patients with KIT-driven melanoma in a randomized fashion would be optimal; however, given the rarity of this genetic subset of disease, the successful conduct of such a definitive study is challenging, and international collaboration to further assess the optimization of KIT inhibition is required. Such optimization may include the combination of KIT inhibitors with chemotherapy, immunotherapy, and other "targeted" agents. Such combination concepts are beginning to be assessed in clinical trials and hold the potential to enhance the efficacy of KIT inhibition in this molecular subset of disease.

3 Materials

1. DNeasy™ Tissue Kit for genomic DNA extraction from formalin-fixed, paraffin-embedded (FFPE) tumor specimens (contains Buffers ATL, AL, and AW1, Proteinase K, and DNeasy mini-columns) (Qiagen).

2. Microcentrifuge tubes (2.0 ml, 1.5 ml, 0.2 ml) (Life Technologies).
3. Xylene, Ethanol (Fisher Chemicals).
4. Polymerase Chain Reaction (PCR) Reagents: 10× Buffer, $MgCl_2$ solution, Deoxyribonucleotide triphosphate (dNTP) mix (Invitrogen). Platinum TaqDNA Polymerase High Fidelity (Life Technologies).
5. PCR primers for KIT exons 9, 11, 13, 17, and 18 amplification (Table 6).
6. MetaPhor™ agarose for identification of PCR products (BioWhittaker Applications, Rockland, ME).
7. Tris–Acetate EDTA (TAE) Buffer (1×, 40 mM Tris–Acetate pH 8.3, 1 mM EDTA).
8. QIAquickTM PCR Kit for purification of PCR products (Qiagen).
9. Heating block.
10. Microcentrifuge.
11. Thermocycler, GeneAmp PCR System 2700 (Applied Biosystems) or similar.
12. Applied Biosystems 3730 capillary DNA analyzer for direct sequencing (Applied Biosystems).

Table 6
***KIT* exon 9, 11, 13, 17, and 18 primer sequences**

Exon Number	Primers	Primer sequences
9	Ex9-F	AGCCAGGGCTTTTGTTTTCT
	Ex9-R	ACAGAGCCTAAACATCCCCTTA
11	Ex11-F	TGTTCTCTCTCCAGAGTGCTCTAA
	Ex11-R	AAACAAAGGAAGCCACTGGA
13	Ex13-F	CATCAGTTTGCCAGTTGTGC
	Ex13-R	AGCAAGAGAGAACAACAGTCTGG
17	Ex17-F	TCATTCAAGGCGTACTTTTG
	Ex17-R	TCGAAAGTTGAAACTAAAAATCC
18	Ex18-F	CATTTCAGCAACAGCAGCAT
	Ex18-R	CAAGGAAGCAGGACACCAAT

4 Methods

4.1 DNA Extraction from Paraffin-Embedded Tissue

4.1.1 Day 1

1. Add 1.2 ml of Xylene to paraffin curls obtained by scraping H&E stained slides or representative blocks into a microfuge tube.
2. Vortex vigorously for 1 min.
3. Incubate at room temperature for 80 min and vortex 1–2 times while incubating.
4. Spin at 13,000 × *g* for 5 min.
5. Repeat **steps 1** and **2** (*see* **Note 1**).
6. Decant the supernatant; add 1.2 ml of 100 % Ethanol to microfuge tube (*see* **Note 2**).
7. Vortex vigorously for 1 min and spin at 13,000 × *g* for 5 min.
8. Repeat Ethanol wash (**steps 6** and 7).
9. Remove most Ethanol, and leave 200–300 μl in the tube.
10. Leave at room temperature overnight or at 37 °C (heating block) all day, with the microfuge tube uncapped. The next day, one should have just dry tissue.

4.1.2 Day 2

1. Genomic DNA for mutation analysis is extracted from FFPE using the DNeasyTM Tissue Kit.
2. Add 180 μl Buffer ATL to tissue in the microfuge tube.
3. Add 20 μl of Proteinase K solution, mix by vortexing and incubate at 55 °C overnight in heating block. Vortex samples every 2 h until you have a broken pellet. One should see floating pieces, not a pellet.

4.1.3 Day 3

1. Vortex the sample for 15 s. Add 200 μl Buffer AL to the sample. You should see a ring of precipitation. Mix thoroughly by vortexing and incubate at 70 °C for 10 min on a heating block.
2. Add 200 μl of 100 % Ethanol to the sample and mix thoroughly by vortexing.
3. Pipet the mixture from **step 2** into the DNeasy mini-column sitting in 2 ml collection tube. Centrifuge at 6,000 × *g* for 1 min. Discard the flow-through and collection tube.
4. Place the DNeasy mini-column in a new 2 ml collection tube, add 500 μl Buffer AW1, and centrifuge for 1 min at 6,000 × *g*. Discard the flow-through and collection tube.
5. Place the DNeasy mini-column in a 2 ml collection tube, add 500 μl Buffer AW2, and centrifuge for 3 min at full speed to dry the DNeasy membrane. Discard the flow-through and collection tube.

6. Place the DNeasy mini-column in a clean 1.5 ml Microfuge tube and pipet 100 μl Buffer AE directly onto the DNeasy membrane. Incubate at room temperature for 1 min and then centrifuge for 1 min at 6,000 × *g* to elute DNA.
7. Discard the DNeasy mini-column and label microfuge tube containing eluate (DNA).
8. Store the DNA at 4 °C in a paraffin DNA box.

4.2 Make the Primer Stock Solution for PCR Reaction

1. Prepare 1 μg/ul stock solution, e.g., add 672 μl of H_2O to total micrograms of lyophilized primer = 671.71 μg.
2. (1,000 ng/μl)/(0.33)(# of nucleotides) = μM concentration of the above stock. For example, CAGGTAACCATTTATTTGT has 19 nucleotides, so the concentration of this solution is (1,000 ng/μl)/(0.33)(19 nucleotides) = 159 μM.
3. Make 100 μM stock from the present μM stock.

   V1 = (Volume wanted V2)(Concentration wanted C2)/(Concentration have C1)

$$V1 = \left[(V2)(C2)\right] / C1.$$

   In order to make 100 μM stock from present 159 μM stock:

$$V1 = \left[(100\mu l)(100\mu M)\right] / 159\mu M = 63\mu l.$$

   Take 63 μl of 159 μM stock and add 37 μl of ddH_2O to bring it up to 100 μl.
4. Make 10 μM stock from present 100 μM stock for PCR.

   In order to make 10 μM stock from the present 100 μM stock:

$$V1 = \left[(500\mu l)(10\mu M)\right] / 10\mu M = 50\mu l.$$

   Take 50 μl of 100 mM stock and add 450 ml of ddH2) to bring it up to 500 μl.
5. Make 4 μM stock from the present 10 μM stock for sequencing reactions.

   To make 10 μM stock from the present 100 μM stock:

$$V1 = \left[(500\mu l)(4\mu M)\right] / 10\mu M = 200\mu l.$$

   Take 200 μl of 10 mM stock and add 300 ml of ddH2) to bring it up to 500 μl.

4.3 Agarose Gel Preparation for PCR Products (See Note 3)

1. Analytical agarose gel is used to estimate the concentration of PCR samples.

2. Heat up a mixture of 2 g agarose (for 2 % gel) or 1.2 g agarose (for 1.2 % gel) and 100 mL 1× TAE buffer using microwave oven until the agarose dissolves well.
3. Cool the mixture at room temperature until it is 50–60 °C.
4. Shake well.
5. Pour the gel.

4.4 Polymerase Chain Reaction

1. One microgram of genomic DNA is subjected to PCR using Platinum TaqDNA Polymerase High Fidelity. DNA PCR Master Mix:

H_2O	39 µl
10× Buffer	5 µl
$MgCl_2$	1.5 µl
DNA 1 µg	1 µl
10 µM (+ Foward) primer	1 µl
10 µM (– Reverse) primer	1 µl
dNTPs	1 µl
Platinum Taq	.5 µl
Total Rxn volume	50 µl

2. The PCR conditions are as follows: (1) pre-denaturation 94 °C for 4 min; (2) denaturation 94 °C for 30 s, (3) the relevant annealing temperature for each primer set for 30 s (*see* **Note 4**), (4) elongation 72 °C for 30 s (35 cycles); and (5) termination 72 °C for 3 min.
3. Perform polymerase chain reaction assays using primers specific for KIT exons 9, 11, 13, 17, and 18 (Table 6).
4. The PCR products are identified by agarose gel electrophoresis using a 2 % MetaPhor™ agarose gel following Ethidium Bromide staining.
5. Use the QIAquickTM PCR Purification Kit for purification of PCR products and removal of residual primers. Dilute the purified PCR product in a 1:8 ratio with ddH_2O (usually 50 µl of ddH_2O). Load 4 µl DNA density marker as a reference with loading dye. Then, load 4 µl of the PCR product in each lane with loading dye. Read the gel and calculate the DNA concentration according to the density marker. Bring the concentration to ~2 ng/µl for small products. Bring the concentration to ~4 ng/µl for large products.

4.5 KIT Mutation Sequencing

1. Prepare two tubes for each sample, one for Forward sequencing and another for Reverse sequencing, and label them as such. Use a total volume of 12 μl composed of 10 μl of purified PCR product per reaction and 2 μl of primer. Use 8 pmol of primer per reaction (8 ρmol = 2 μl of 4 μM dilution). Always sequence both DNA strands (Forward and Reverse directions).
2. Direct sequencing of the purified PCR product with fluorescently labeled dideoxy chain-terminating nucleotides is then performed at the DNA Sequencing Core Facility, using the Applied Biosystems 3730 capillary DNA analyzer (Applied Biosystems, Foster City, CA). Recommended amounts of PCR products for sequencing:

Template PCR product	Recommended quantity provided for sequencing
100–200 bp	1–3 ng
200–500 bp	3–10 ng
500–1,000 bp	5–20 ng
1,000–2,000 bp	10–40 ng
>2000 bp	40–100 ng

3. Every ABI sequence is compared to a NCBI Human KIT gene nucleotide sequence and blasted using a NCBI Standard Nucleotide Blast Search to determine the presence of mutation.

5 Notes

1. When performing DNA extraction from paraffin-embedded tissue, if you cannot remove all of the xylene, then add up to 1.5 mL of fresh material and retry.
2. If tissue is floating while decanting the supernatant during DNA extraction and one cannot remove xylene without removing tissue, then add 300 μl 100 % ethanol to the tube and spin for 5 min; this will help to tighten the pellet.
3. 2 % Agarose Gel is used for small PCR products, e.g., 200 or 300 bp products whereas 1.2 % Agarose Gel should be used for bigger products, e.g., 800 bp products.
4. Annealing temperature is specific to each primer but ranges from 50 to 60 °C.

References

1. Chapman PB, Einhorn LH, Meyers ML, Saxman S, Destro AN, Panageas KS et al (1999) Phase III multicenter randomized trial of the Dartmouth regimen versus dacarbazine in patients with metastatic melanoma. J Clin Oncol 17(9):2745–2751
2. Atkins MB, Lotze MT, Dutcher JP, Fisher RI, Weiss G, Margolin K et al (1999) High-dose recombinant interleukin 2 therapy for patients with metastatic melanoma: analysis of 270 patients treated between 1985 and 1993. J Clin Oncol 17(7):2105–2116
3. Davies H, Bignell GR, Cox C, Stephens P, Edkins S, Clegg S et al (2002) Mutations of the BRAF gene in human cancer. Nature 417(6892):949–954
4. Chapman PB, Hauschild A, Robert C, Haanen JB, Ascierto P, Larkin J et al (2011) Improved survival with vemurafenib in melanoma with BRAF V600E mutation. N Engl J Med 364(26):2507–2516
5. Hauschild A, Grob JJ, Demidov LV, Jouary T, Gutzmer R, Millward M et al (2012) Dabrafenib in BRAF-mutated metastatic melanoma: a multicentre, open-label, phase 3 randomised controlled trial. Lancet 380(9839): 358–365
6. Robert C, Flaherty K, Hersey P, Nathan P, CGarbe C, Milhem M, et al (2012) METRIC phase III study: efficacy of trametinib (T), a potent and selective MEK inhibitor (MEKi), in progression-free survival (PFS) and overall survival (OS), compared with chemotherapy (C) in patients (pts) with BRAFV600E/K mutant advanced or metastatic melanoma (MM). J Clin Oncol 30(suppl):(abstr LBA8509)
7. Curtin JA, Fridlyand J, Kageshita T, Patel HN, Busam KJ, Kutzner H et al (2005) Distinct sets of genetic alterations in melanoma. N Engl J Med 353(20):2135–2147
8. Onken MD, Worley LA, Long MD, Duan S, Council ML, Bowcock AM et al (2008) Oncogenic mutations in GNAQ occur early in uveal melanoma. Invest Ophthalmol Vis Sci 49(12):5230–5234, PMCID: 2634606
9. Van Raamsdonk CD, Bezrookove V, Green G, Bauer J, Gaugler L, O'Brien JM et al (2009) Frequent somatic mutations of GNAQ in uveal melanoma and blue naevi. Nature 457(7229): 599–602, PMCID: 2696133
10. Van Raamsdonk CD, Griewank KG, Crosby MB, Garrido MC, Vemula S, Wiesner T et al (2010) Mutations in GNA11 in uveal melanoma. N Engl J Med 363(23):2191–2199
11. Harbour JW, Onken MD, Roberson ED, Duan S, Cao L, Worley LA et al (2010) Frequent mutation of BAP1 in metastasizing uveal melanomas. Science 330(6009):1410–1413
12. Rimoldi D, Salvi S, Lienard D, Lejeune FJ, Speiser D, Zografos L et al (2003) Lack of BRAF mutations in uveal melanoma. Cancer Res 63(18):5712–5715
13. Cohen Y, Goldenberg-Cohen N, Parrella P, Chowers I, Merbs SL, Pe'er J et al (2003) Lack of BRAF mutation in primary uveal melanoma. Invest Ophthalmol Vis Sci 44(7):2876–2878
14. Edmunds SC, Cree IA, Di Nicolantonio F, Hungerford JL, Hurren JS, Kelsell DP (2003) Absence of BRAF gene mutations in uveal melanomas in contrast to cutaneous melanomas. Br J Cancer 88(9):1403–1405, PMCID: 2741050
15. Maat W, Kilic E, Luyten GP, de Klein A, Jager MJ, Gruis NA et al (2008) Pyrophosphorolysis detects B-RAF mutations in primary uveal melanoma. Invest Ophthalmol Vis Sci 49(1): 23–27
16. Curtin JA, Busam K, Pinkel D, Bastian BC (2006) Somatic activation of KIT in distinct subtypes of melanoma. J Clin Oncol 24(26): 4340–4346
17. Beadling C, Jacobson-Dunlop E, Hodi FS, Le C, Warrick A, Patterson J et al (2008) KIT gene mutations and copy number in melanoma subtypes. Clin Cancer Res 14(21):6821–6828
18. Besmer P, Murphy JE, George PC, Qiu FH, Bergold PJ, Lederman L et al (1986) A new acute transforming feline retrovirus and relationship of its oncogene v-kit with the protein kinase gene family. Nature 320(6061): 415–421
19. Yarden Y, Kuang WJ, Yang-Feng T, Coussens L, Munemitsu S, Dull TJ et al (1987) Human proto-oncogene c-kit: a new cell surface receptor tyrosine kinase for an unidentified ligand. EMBO J 6(11):3341–3351, PMCID: 553789
20. Woodman SE, Davies MA (2010) Targeting KIT in melanoma: a paradigm of molecular medicine and targeted therapeutics. Biochem Pharmacol 80(5):568–574
21. Huang EJ, Nocka KH, Buck J, Besmer P (1992) Differential expression and processing of two cell associated forms of the kit-ligand: KL-1 and KL-2. Mol Biol Cell 3(3):349–362, PMCID: 275535
22. Ronnstrand L (2004) Signal transduction via the stem cell factor receptor/c-Kit. Cell Mol Life Sci 61(19–20):2535–2548
23. Miyazawa K, Williams DA, Gotoh A, Nishimaki J, Broxmeyer HE, Toyama K (1995) Membrane-bound steel factor induces more persistent tyrosine kinase activation and longer life span of c-kit gene-encoded protein than its soluble form. Blood 85(3):641–649
24. Russell ES (1979) Hereditary anemias of the mouse: a review for geneticists. Adv Genet 20: 357–459

25. Vincent S, Segretain D, Nishikawa S, Nishikawa SI, Sage J, Cuzin F et al (1998) Stage-specific expression of the Kit receptor and its ligand (KL) during male gametogenesis in the mouse: a Kit-KL interaction critical for meiosis. Development 125(22):4585–4593
26. Tian Q, Frierson HF Jr, Krystal GW, Moskaluk CA (1999) Activating c-kit gene mutations in human germ cell tumors. Am J Pathol 154(6):1643–1647, PMCID: 1876773
27. Okayama Y, Kawakami T (2006) Development, migration, and survival of mast cells. Immunol Res 34(2):97–115, PMCID: 1490026
28. Huizinga JD, Thuneberg L, Kluppel M, Malysz J, Mikkelsen HB, Bernstein A (1995) W/kit gene required for interstitial cells of Cajal and for intestinal pacemaker activity. Nature 373(6512):347–349
29. Phung B, Sun J, Schepsky A, Steingrimsson E, Ronnstrand L (2011) C-KIT signaling depends on microphthalmia-associated transcription factor for effects on cell proliferation. PLoS One 6(8):e24064, PMCID: 3161112
30. Hou L, Pavan WJ (2008) Transcriptional and signaling regulation in neural crest stem cell-derived melanocyte development: do all roads lead to Mitf? Cell Res 18(12):1163–1176
31. Cable J, Jackson IJ, Steel KP (1995) Mutations at the W locus affect survival of neural crest-derived melanocytes in the mouse. Mech Dev 50(2–3):139–150
32. Chabot B, Stephenson DA, Chapman VM, Besmer P, Bernstein A (1988) The proto-oncogene c-kit encoding a transmembrane tyrosine kinase receptor maps to the mouse W locus. Nature 335(6185):88–89
33. Spritz RA, Giebel LB, Holmes SA (1992) Dominant negative and loss of function mutations of the c-kit (mast/stem cell growth factor receptor) proto-oncogene in human piebaldism. Am J Hum Genet 50(2):261–269, PMCID: 1682440
34. Geissler EN, Ryan MA, Housman DE (1988) The dominant-white spotting (W) locus of the mouse encodes the c-kit proto-oncogene. Cell 55(1):185–192
35. Alexeev V, Yoon K (2006) Distinctive role of the cKit receptor tyrosine kinase signaling in mammalian melanocytes. J Invest Dermatol 126(5):1102–1110
36. Hachiya A, Sriwiriyanont P, Kobayashi T, Nagasawa A, Yoshida H, Ohuchi A et al (2009) Stem cell factor-KIT signalling plays a pivotal role in regulating pigmentation in mammalian hair. J Pathol 218(1):30–39
37. Wang ZQ, Si L, Tang Q, Lin D, Fu Z, Zhang J et al (2009) Gain-of-function mutation of KIT ligand on melanin synthesis causes familial progressive hyperpigmentation. Am J Hum Genet 84(5):672–677, PMCID: 2680999
38. Huang S, Luca M, Gutman M, McConkey DJ, Langley KE, Lyman SD et al (1996) Enforced c-KIT expression renders highly metastatic human melanoma cells susceptible to stem cell factor-induced apoptosis and inhibits their tumorigenic and metastatic potential. Oncogene 13(11):2339–2347
39. Natali PG, Nicotra MR, Winkler AB, Cavaliere R, Bigotti A, Ullrich A (1992) Progression of human cutaneous melanoma is associated with loss of expression of c-kit proto-oncogene receptor. Int J Cancer 52(2):197–201
40. Montone KT, van Belle P, Elenitsas R, Elder DE (1997) Proto-oncogene c-kit expression in malignant melanoma: protein loss with tumor progression. Mod Pathol 10(9):939–944
41. Lassam N, Bickford S (1992) Loss of c-kit expression in cultured melanoma cells. Oncogene 7(1):51–56
42. Shen SS, Zhang PS, Eton O, Prieto VG (2003) Analysis of protein tyrosine kinase expression in melanocytic lesions by tissue array. J Cutan Pathol 30(9):539–547
43. Ugurel S, Hildenbrand R, Zimpfer A, La Rosee P, Paschka P, Sucker A et al (2005) Lack of clinical efficacy of imatinib in metastatic melanoma. Br J Cancer 92(8):1398–1405, PMCID: 2362005
44. Wyman K, Atkins MB, Prieto V, Eton O, McDermott DF, Hubbard F et al (2006) Multicenter phase II trial of high-dose imatinib mesylate in metastatic melanoma: significant toxicity with no clinical efficacy. Cancer 106(9): 2005–2011
45. Kim KB, Eton O, Davis DW, Frazier ML, McConkey DJ, Diwan AH et al (2008) Phase II trial of imatinib mesylate in patients with metastatic melanoma. Br J Cancer 99(5):734–740, PMCID: 2528157
46. Rubin BP, Heinrich MC, Corless CL (2007) Gastrointestinal stromal tumour. Lancet 369(9574):1731–1741
47. Verweij J, Casali PG, Zalcberg J, LeCesne A, Reichardt P, Blay JY et al (2004) Progression-free survival in gastrointestinal stromal tumours with high-dose imatinib: randomised trial. Lancet 364(9440):1127–1134
48. Bastian BC, LeBoit PE, Hamm H, Brocker EB, Pinkel D (1998) Chromosomal gains and losses in primary cutaneous melanomas detected by comparative genomic hybridization. Cancer Res 58(10):2170–2175
49. Went PT, Dirnhofer S, Bundi M, Mirlacher M, Schraml P, Mangialaio S et al (2004) Prevalence of KIT expression in human tumors. J Clin Oncol 22(22):4514–4522
50. Willmore C, Holden JA, Zhou L, Tripp S, Wittwer CT, Layfield LJ (2004) Detection of c-kit-activating mutations in gastrointestinal stromal tumors by high-resolution amplicon

melting analysis. Am J Clin Pathol 122(2): 206–216
51. Willmore-Payne C, Holden JA, Hirschowitz S, Layfield LJ (2006) BRAF and c-kit gene copy number in mutation-positive malignant melanoma. Hum Pathol 37(5):520–527
52. Antonescu CR, Busam KJ, Francone TD, Wong GC, Guo T, Agaram NP et al (2007) L576P KIT mutation in anal melanomas correlates with KIT protein expression and is sensitive to specific kinase inhibition. Int J Cancer 121(2):257–264
53. Rivera RS, Nagatsuka H, Gunduz M, Cengiz B, Gunduz E, Siar CH et al (2008) C-kit protein expression correlated with activating mutations in KIT gene in oral mucosal melanoma. Virchows Arch 452(1):27–32
54. Satzger I, Schaefer T, Kuettler U, Broecker V, Voelker B, Ostertag H et al (2008) Analysis of c-KIT expression and KIT gene mutation in human mucosal melanomas. Br J Cancer 99(12):2065–2069, PMCID: 2607233
55. Ashida A, Takata M, Murata H, Kido K, Saida T (2009) Pathological activation of KIT in metastatic tumors of acral and mucosal melanomas. Int J Cancer 124(4):862–868
56. Torres-Cabala CA, Wang WL, Trent J, Yang D, Chen S, Galbincea J et al (2009) Correlation between KIT expression and KIT mutation in melanoma: a study of 173 cases with emphasis on the acral-lentiginous/mucosal type. Mod Pathol 22(11):1446–1456
57. Carvajal RD, Antonescu CR, Wolchok JD, Chapman PB, Roman RA, Teitcher J et al (2011) KIT as a therapeutic target in metastatic melanoma. JAMA 305(22):2327–2334
58. Lennartsson J, Blume-Jensen P, Hermanson M, Ponten E, Carlberg M, Ronnstrand L (1999) Phosphorylation of Shc by Src family kinases is necessary for stem cell factor receptor/c-kit mediated activation of the Ras/MAP kinase pathway and c-fos induction. Oncogene 18(40):5546–5553
59. Corless CL, Heinrich MC (2008) Molecular pathobiology of gastrointestinal stromal sarcomas. Annu Rev Pathol 3:557–586
60. Kong Y, Si L, Zhu Y, Xu X, Corless CL, Flaherty KT et al (2011) Large-scale analysis of KIT aberrations in Chinese patients with melanoma. Clin Cancer Res 17(7):1684–1691
61. Yun J, Lee J, Jang J, Lee EJ, Jang KT, Kim JH et al (2011) KIT amplification and gene mutations in acral/mucosal melanoma in Korea. APMIS 119(6):330–335
62. Handolias D, Salemi R, Murray W, Tan A, Liu W, Viros A et al (2010) Mutations in KIT occur at low frequency in melanomas arising from anatomical sites associated with chronic and intermittent sun exposure. Pigment Cell Melanoma Res 23(2):210–215
63. Monsel G, Ortonne N, Bagot M, Bensussan A, Dumaz N (2010) c-Kit mutants require hypoxia-inducible factor 1alpha to transform melanocytes. Oncogene 29(2):227–236
64. Jiang X, Zhou J, Yuen NK, Corless CL, Heinrich MC, Fletcher JA et al (2008) Imatinib targeting of KIT-mutant oncoprotein in melanoma. Clin Cancer Res 14(23):7726–7732
65. Woodman SE, Trent JC, Stemke-Hale K, Lazar AJ, Pricl S, Pavan GM et al (2009) Activity of dasatinib against L576P KIT mutant melanoma: molecular, cellular, and clinical correlates. Mol Cancer Ther 8(8):2079–2085
66. Hodi FS, Friedlander P, Corless CL, Heinrich MC, Mac Rae S, Kruse A et al (2008) Major response to imatinib mesylate in KIT-mutated melanoma. J Clin Oncol 26(12):2046–2051
67. Satzger I, Kuttler U, Volker B, Schenck F, Kapp A, Gutzmer R (2010) Anal mucosal melanoma with KIT-activating mutation and response to imatinib therapy–case report and review of the literature. Dermatology 220(1):77–81
68. Lutzky J, Bauer J, Bastian BC (2008) Dose-dependent, complete response to imatinib of a metastatic mucosal melanoma with a K642E KIT mutation. Pigment Cell Melanoma Res 21(4):492–493
69. Fisher DE, Barnhill R, Hodi FS, Herlyn M, Merlino G, Medrano E et al (2010) Melanoma from bench to bedside: meeting report from the 6th international melanoma congress. Pigment Cell Melanoma Res 23:14–26
70. Quintas-Cardama A, Lazar AJ, Woodman SE, Kim K, Ross M, Hwu P (2008) Complete response of stage IV anal mucosal melanoma expressing KIT Val560Asp to the multikinase inhibitor sorafenib. Nat Clin Pract Oncol 5(12):737–740
71. Zhu Y, Si L, Kong Y, Chi Z, Yuan X, Cui C, et al. (2009) Response to sunitinib in Chinese KIT – mutated metastatic mucosal melanoma. J Clin Oncol 27(abstract):e20017
72. Minor DR, Kashani-Sabet M, Garrido M, O'Day SJ, Hamid O, Bastian BC (2012) Sunitinib therapy for melanoma patients with KIT mutations. Clin Cancer Res 18(5): 1457–1463
73. Kluger HM, Dudek AZ, McCann C, Ritacco J, Southard N, Jilaveanu LB et al (2011) A phase 2 trial of dasatinib in advanced melanoma. Cancer 117(10):2202–2208
74. Cho JH, Kim KM, Kwon M, Kim JH, Lee J (2011) Nilotinib in patients with metastatic melanoma harboring KIT gene aberration. Invest New Drugs 30(5):2008–2014
75. Long GV, Menzies AM, Nagrial AM, Haydu LE, Hamilton AL, Mann GJ et al (2011) Prognostic and clinicopathologic associations of oncogenic BRAF in metastatic melanoma. J Clin Oncol 29(10):1239–1246

76. Guo T, Hajdu M, Agaram NP, Shinoda H, Veach D, Clarkson BD et al (2009) Mechanisms of sunitinib resistance in gastrointestinal stromal tumors harboring KITAY502-3ins mutation: an in vitro mutagenesis screen for drug resistance. Clin Cancer Res 15(22):6862–6870, PMCID: 2783687
77. Heinrich MC, Corless CL, Blanke CD, Demetri GD, Joensuu H, Roberts PJ et al (2006) Molecular correlates of imatinib resistance in gastrointestinal stromal tumors. J Clin Oncol 24(29):4764–4774
78. Heinrich MC, Corless CL, Demetri GD, Blanke CD, von Mehren M, Joensuu H et al (2003) Kinase mutations and imatinib response in patients with metastatic gastrointestinal stromal tumor. J Clin Oncol 21(23): 4342–4349
79. Lasota J, Corless CL, Heinrich MC, Debiec-Rychter M, Sciot R, Wardelmann E et al (2008) Clinicopathologic profile of gastrointestinal stromal tumors (GISTs) with primary KIT exon 13 or exon 17 mutations: a multicenter study on 54 cases. Mod Pathol 21(4):476–484
80. Fletcher JA, Rubin BP (2007) KIT mutations in GIST. Curr Opin Genet Dev 17(1):3–7
81. Si L, Xu X, Kong Y, Flaherty KT, Chi Z, Cui C et al (2012) Major response to everolimus in melanoma with acquired imatinib resistance. J Clin Oncol 30(4):e37–e40
82. Handolias D, Hamilton AL, Salemi R, Tan A, Moodie K, Kerr L et al (2010) Clinical responses observed with imatinib or sorafenib in melanoma patients expressing mutations in KIT. Br J Cancer 102(8):1219–1223, PMCID: 2856012

Chapter 10

Detecting Mechanisms of Acquired BRAF Inhibitor Resistance in Melanoma

Roger S. Lo and Hubing Shi

Abstract

V^{600}BRAF mutation was identified as an ideal target for clinical therapy due to its indispensable roles in supporting melanoma initiation and progression. Despite the fact that BRAF inhibitors (BRAFi) can elicit anti-tumor responses in the majority of treated patients and confer overall survival benefits, acquired drug resistance is a formidable obstacle to long-term management of the disease. Several aberrant events including RTK upregulation, *NRAS* mutation, mutant *BRAF* amplification or alternative splicing, and *MEK* mutation have been reported as acquired BRAFi resistance mechanisms. Clinially, detection of these resistance mechanisms help understand drug response patterns and help guide combinatorial therapeutic strategies. Therefore, quick and accurate diagnosis of the resistant mechanisms in tumor biopsies has become an important starting point for personalized therapy. In this chapter, we review the major acquired BRAFi resistance mechanisms, highlight their therapeutic implications, and provide the diagnostic methods from clinical samples.

Key words BRAF, RTK, NRAS, MEK, MAPK, Drug resistance, Molecular diagnosis

1 Introduction

V^{600}BRAF mutations drive melanoma development in ~50 % melanoma and have become a target for clinical therapy [1]. BRAFi, already approved (vemurafenib/PLX4032) or in advanced clinical development (dabrafenib/GSK2118436) reproducibly elicit anti-tumor responses in melanomas harboring $^{V600E/K}$BRAF, typically shrinking tumors rapidly and bringing quick symptomatic relief to patients [2–6]. This rapid anti-tumor activity is strongly associated with early metabolic and on-target (MAPK) pathway inhibition. However, limited durability of response and almost universal disease progression (DP, acquired drug resistance) present a formidable obstacle to long-term survival benefits [4]. Understanding, detecting, and overcoming BRAFi resistance in melanoma has thus been a major focus of the cancer research community. The reported mechanisms could be

Magdalena Thurin and Francesco M. Marincola (eds.), *Molecular Diagnostics for Melanoma: Methods and Protocols*, Methods in Molecular Biology, vol. 1102, DOI 10.1007/978-1-62703-727-3_10,

categorized as: (1) the reactivation of RAF-MEK-ERK MAPK signaling and (2) the rebound activation of MAPK-redundant signaling via the receptor tyrosine kinase (RTK)-PI3K-AKT pathway, which is parallel but interconnected to the MAPK pathway. MAPK reactivation can occur via *NRAS* activating mutations [7], COT overexpression [8], *^{V600E}BRAF* alternative splicing [9], *^{V600E}BRAF* amplification [10], and *MEK1* activating mutation [11]. MAPK-redundant signaling via RTK overexpression has been shown to result in AKT activation and RAS-CRAF-MEK signaling, bypassing mutant BRAF inhibition [7, 12].

2 Upregulation of RTKs in BRAFi-Resistant Melanoma

Since the first RTK was reported around 27 years ago, about 90 unique RTKs that fall into 20 subfamilies have been identified in human. Mutations or aberrant activations in RTKs and their adaptor components have been linked to many pathological disorders such as diabetes, inflammation, angiogenesis, as well as cancer. The upregulation of RTKs contributes to BRAFi resistance in various human malignancies which harbor *^{V600E}BRAF* mutations, such as colorectal, thyroid, and mammary carcinoma, as well as melanoma [13, 14]. In *^{V600E}BRAF* mutant melanomas, the upregulation of RTKs including PDGFRβ, EGFR, KIT, MET, IGF1R, and FGFR3 has been associated with BRAFi resistance and demonstrated to be functionally relevant to melanoma cell survival in response to BRAF inhibition [7, 12, 15]. Duncan and colleagues provided an explanation for this RTKs dysregulation by showing that ERK inactivation induces c-Myc destabilization, resulting in transcriptional upregulation of many RTKs including PDGFRβ [16]. The upregulation of multiple RTKs then activate two major signaling pathways relevant to cell survival and metabolism: (1) the PI3K/AKT/mTOR pathway and (2) RAS/CRAF/MEK MAPK which accelerates MAPK pathway recovery in response to BRAF inhibition [7, 13]. However, several critical questions remain unaddressed: (1) what is the full-spectrum, combination and timing of RTKs upregulation during BRAFi or combined BRAFi and MEKi therapy (2) how is the dynamic programming of RTKs coupled with the recruitment of adaptor proteins; (3) what are the key signal feedback, transcriptional, and/or epigenetic events that drive RTK reprogramming?

2.1 Clinical Therapeutic Implication

Combined targeting both MAPK and PI3K/AKT/mTOR pathways have been shown to overcome BRAFi-resistance with RTK upregulation. We have shown that inhibiting both mTORC1 and mTORC2 complexes sensitizes resistant melanoma cells to BRAFi treatment, and further blockade of PI3K on top of dual mTORC1/mTORC2 inhibition delays compensatory signaling at AKT, augmenting synergy with BRAFi [17]. RTK upregulation in BRAFi-resistant melanoma can be detected at mRNA/cDNA and protein levels by qPCR and immunohistochemistry (IHC), respectively. This chapter focuses only on DNA-based methods since several other chapters describe the IHC methods in detail.

3 NRAS Mutations in BRAF Inhibitor-Resistant Melanomas

Three canonical small GTPase superfamily members, HRAS, KRAS, and NRAS, play central roles in driving the MAPK pathway [18]. Upon activation of RTKs, RAS proteins switch from an inactive guanosine diphosphate (GDP)-bound to an active guanosine triphosphate (GTP)-bound conformation. Under physiological conditions, the transition between these two states is subtly regulated by guanine nucleotide exchange factors (GEFs), which promote the activation of RAS proteins by stimulating GDP for GTP exchange, and by GTPase-activating proteins (GAPs), which accelerate RAS-mediated GTP hydrolysis. The most frequent mechanism that drives oncogenic transformation involves point mutations affecting the interaction of RAS with these guanine nucleotides. The hot spot for the naturally occurring *RAS* mutations are detected at codons 12, 13, 59, and 61. These mutations result in inhibition of GTP hydrolysis, either by diminishing GTPase activity (for mutations at codons 12, 13, and 61) or by modulating the rate of guanine nucleotide exchange (for mutations at codon 59). The oncogenic functions of canonical RAS genes are tissue specific. Although *HRAS* (2 %) and *KRAS* (1 %) mutants have occasionally been reported, *NRAS* mutants (15–20 %) are most frequently observed, implying a predominant role in melanoma [19]. Usually, *NRAS* mutations and ^{V600E}*BRAF* are mutually exclusive which is thought to be due to the redundancy in hyperactivating the MAPK pathway. However, when ^{V600E}BRAF is blocked by an inhibitor, melanomas can reactivate the MAPK pathway by acquiring activating mutations in NRAS. Oncogenic NRAS mutants bypass BRAF inhibition by signaling through CRAF. To date, we have identified single-nucleotide missense substitutions in three NRAS hot spots (G12, G13, and Q61) in a DP-specific manner. Further investigation is crucial to determine whether or not other oncogenic mutants in NRAS or other RAS members contribute to BRAFi resistance. In this chapter, we provided a protocol to detect NRAS hot spot mutations in BRAFi-resistant melanomas by sequencing exons 1 and 2.

3.1 Clinical Therapeutic Implication

The MAPK reactivation by acquiring NRAS mutations can potentially be blocked by combinatorial treatment with MEK or ERK inhibitors, but this approach may be further complicated by MAPK rebound due to release of negative feedbacks or by further genetic alterations. In this context, the combination of dabrafenib (BRAFi) and trametinib (MEKi) has recently been shown in early clinical data to increase the median progression-free survival from 5.8 to 9.4 months compared to BRAFi monotherapy. Thus, it is again critical to understand the determinants of resistance among patients treated by dual MAPK inhibition. Interestingly, coinhibition of BRAF and MEK has the added benefit of blocking BRAFi-induced paradoxical MAPK activation in the skin, which leads to cutaneous squamous-cell carcinomas [20].

4 Mutant BRAF Alterations in BRAFi-Resistant Melanoma

A common mechanism of resistance in targeting therapy is alteration of the targeted oncogenes. About 50 % lung cancers with EGFR dysregulation develop resistance to gefitinib/erlotinib by acquiring a gatekeeper mutation T790M, which reduces drug binding to EGFR kinase domain [21]. However, our published and unpublished work undertaken to deep sequence *BRAF* has ***not*** identified secondary BRAF mutations in DP tumors. Instead, two types of alterations, *BRAF* alternative splicing and copy number gain, have been detected. Four *BRAF* alternative splice forms (exon 2–9; exon 2–11; exon 4–9; exon 4–11) have been reported which are associated with BRAFi DP tumors. The truncated protein products are thought to confer BRAFi resistance by enhancing RAF dimerization [9]. Preferential mutant (over WT) *BRAF* amplification results in mRNA level increase as well as protein overexpression [10]. Mutant BRAF overexpression can augment both its kinase and regulatory roles in MAPK activation.

4.1 Clinical Therapeutic Implication

Identification of ^{V600E}BRAF truncation and overexpression as mechanisms of acquired BRAFi resistance provides rationale for the testing of CRAF, omni-RAF, and MEK inhibitors in BRAFi-based combinations and dosing schedules. The mechanisms (splicing, gene copy number gain) that drive mutant BRAF truncation and over-expression, however, suggest that further augmentation of these mechanisms will ultimately resist therapeutic strategies solely focused on the MAPK pathway or targets. BRAF amplification and splicing can be detected by genomic DNA copy number analysis and cDNA sequencing, respectively.

5 MEK1 Mutations in BRAF Inhibitor-Resistant Melanoma

MEK1 and MEK2 are highly conserved dual-specificity protein kinases which play critical roles in the canonical mitogen-activated protein kinase (MAPK) cascade. Early clinical data on an allosteric MEK inhibitor showed a low objective response rate (~14 %) and quick disease progression [22]. A saturating mutagenesis screen with an allosteric MEK inhibitor using a ^{V600E}*BRAF* melanoma cell line has shown that many MEK mutants confer MEKi resistance as well as cross resistance to BRAFi by either disrupting inhibitor binding to MEK or improving intrinsic MEK kinase activities [23]. Recently, a novel MEK1(F129L) mutation was reported which leads to MEKi resistance by improving MEK-C-RAF interaction. Some MEK1 mutants (e.g., Q56P, K57E, C121S, and E203K) have been detected specifically in DP tumors, while other MEK1 mutants (e.g., I111S, P124S) have been observed in both pre and post-relapsed melanomas and these weak alleles do not preclude clinical responses to BRAFi [24]. Detailed structural analyses are needed to further understand the specific functional consequences of these MEK mutations occurring spontaneously and under BRAFi selection. We provide here a protocol on detecting MEK1 mutants, including Q56P, K59del (in frame deletion), C121S, and F129L.

5.1 Clinical Therapeutic Implication

One potential strategy to overcome MEK mutant-mediated BRAFi resistance is the combined use of an ERK inhibitor. Because most resistance-associated MEK1 hot spot mutations fall into alpha helix A and C as well as part of C-lobe, melanomas harboring MEK mutations could be detected by sequencing exons 2, 3, and 6.

6 Materials

6.1 Quantitative PCR

1. UV trans-illuminator, CCD (Cambridge, BioDoc-It™ Imaging System).
2. qPCR thermocycler (Bio-Rad, MyiQ™ single-color Real-Time PCR Detection system).
3. iCycler iQ™ PCR 96-well plate (Bio-Rad).
4. RNA and DNA isolation: RNAlater isolation kit (Ambion); miRNeasy FFPE Kit (Qiagne); mirVana™ miRNA Isolation Kit (Invitrogen); All Prep DNA/RNA Mini Kit (Qiagen); QIAamp DNA FFPE Tissue Kit (Qiagen).
5. qPCR reagents: iQ™ SYBR® Green Supermix (Bio-Rad); 10 mM dNTP Mix (Invitrogen); Oligo(dT)$_{12\text{–}18}$ Primer (Invitrogen); SuperScrip™ II Reverse Transcriptase (Invitrogen); RNaseOUT™ Recombinant Ribonuclease Inhibitor (40 units/μL, Invitrogen).
6. Primers for qPCR detection of RTK: (*see* Table 1).

6.2 PCR Amplification and Mutational Analysis for NRAS, BRAF, and MEK1

1. PCR thermocycler (Bio-Rad, iCycler).
2. Electrophoresis apparatus for agarose gel (Invitrogen, Mini ReadySub-Cell™ GT Cell).
3. PowerPac Basic Power Supply (Bio-Rad).

Table 1
Primers for qPCR

No.	Name	Sequence	Description
1	q-PDGFRβ-F	5′-TTCCATGCCGAGTAACAGAC-3′	qPCR primers for PDGFRβ
2	q-PDGFRβ-R	5′-CGTTGGTGATCATAGGGGAC-3′	
3	q-EGFR-F	5′-TCAGCCTCCAGAGGATGTTC-3′	qPCR primers for EGFR
4	q-EGFR-R	5′-CTGTGTTGAGGGCAATGAGG-3′	
5	q-IGF1R-F	5′-CCGCAGACACCTACAACATC-3′	qPCR primers for IGF1R
6	q-IGF1R-R	5′-CAATGTGAAAGGCCGAAGGT-3′	
7	q-COT-F	5′-CCCCTGGAAGCTGACTTACA-3′	qPCR primers for COT
8	q-COT-R	5′-CTGGGATCAGTTTACACGCC-3′	
9	q-BRAF-F	5′-ATGTTGAATGTGACAGCACC-3′	qPCR primers for BRAF
10	q-BRAF-R	5′-CTCACACCACTGGGTAACAA-3′	
11	q-Tubulin-F	5′-GACAGCTCTTCCACCCAGAG-3′	qPCR primers for Tubulin
12	q-Tubulin-R	5′-TGAAGTCCTGTGCACTGGTC-3′	
13	q-GAPDH-F	5′-CAATGACCCCTTCATTGACC-3′	qPCR primers for GAPDH
14	q-GAPDH-R	5′-GACAAGCTTCCCGTTCTCAG-3′	
15	q-KIT-F	5′-AAAAGTGTGAAACGCGCCTA-3′	qPCR primers for KIT
16	q-KIT-R	5′-AGCTTGCTTTGGACACAGAC-3′	
17	q-MET-F	5′-CTGCAGTCAATGCCTCTCTG-3′	qPCR primers for MET
18	q-MET-R	5′-CAAGGGGTGCACTATTTGGG-3′	

4. Biosystems 3730 Capillary DNA Analyzers.
5. PCR Reagents: Platinum® Taq DNA Polymerase High Fidelity (Invitrogen); 10 mM dNTP Mix (Invitrogen).
6. Polyacrylamide gel electrophoresis reagents: Agarose gel (Ambion); 1 kb Plus DNA Ladder (Invitrogen); BlueJuice™ Gel Loading Buffer (Invitrogen); UltraPure™ 10× TAE Buffer (Invitrogen).
7. RNA and DNA isolation: RNAlater isolation kit (Ambion); miRNeasy FFPE Kit (Qiagne); mirVana™ miRNA Isolation Kit (Invitrogen); All Prep DNA/RNA Mini Kit (Qiagen); QIAamp DNA FFPE Tissue Kit (Qiagen).
8. PCR products isolation: QIAquick Gel Extraction Kit (Qiagen); QIAquick® PCR purification kit (Qiagen).
9. Primers for hotspot *NRAS* and MEK1 mutants sequencing and truncated *BRAF* sequencing (t-BRAF-F/R) are listed in Table 2.

Table 2
Primer for sequencing

No.	Name	Sequence	Description
1	NRASE1-F	5′-TAAAGTACTGTAGATGTGGCTCGCC-3′	Primer for NRAS exon1
2	NRASE1-R	5′-ACAGAATATGGGTAAAGATGATCCGAC-3′	
3	NRASE2-F	5′-GGCTTGAATAGTTAGATGCTTATTTAACCT TGGC-3′	Primer for NRAS exon2
4	NRASE2-R	5′-GCTCTATCTTCCCTAGTGTGGTAACCTC-3′	
5	MEK1E2-F	5′-GCTTTCTTTCCATGATAGGAGTAC-3′	Primer for MEK1 exon2
6	MEK1E2-R	5′-ATCAGTCTTCCTTCTACCCTGG-3′	
7	MEK1E3-F	5′-CCTGTTTCTCCTCCCTCTACC-3′	Primer for MEK1 exon3
8	MEK1E3-R	5′- ACACCCACCAGGAATACTGC-3′	
9	MEK1E6-F	5′-AGGGCCTTGGTGTACAGTGTT-3′	Primer for MEK1 exon6
10	MEK1E6-R	5′-TCATCTCCTCAGGGCAGAGC-3′	
11	t-BRAF-F	5′-GCCAGGCTCTGTTCAACGGG-3′	Primer for BRAF truncation
12	t-BRAF-R	5′-TGCTGAGGTGTAGGTGCTGTCA-3′	

7 Methods

7.1 Detection of RTK Expression Level by qPCR

1. Extract mRNA from tumor samples: mRNA could be extracted from paraffin-embedded tissue block or frozen tissue in RNA later by using miRNeasy FFPE Kit or mirVana™ miRNA Isolation Kit, respectively (*see* **Notes 1–4**).
2. Reverse transcription (First-Strand cDNA Synthesis): Set up a 20 μL reaction system in a 200 μL nuclease-free PCR tube: Mix 1 μL of Oligo$(dT)_{12\text{–}18}$ Primer (500 μg/mL), 1 μL of dNTP Mix (10 mM each), 100–200 ng of total RNA or mRNA, and ddH_2O to 12 μL. Heat the mixture to 65 °C for 5 min and quick chill on ice.
3. Collect the contents of the tube by brief centrifugation and add 4 μL of 5× First-Strand Buffer (250 mM Tris–HCl, pH 8.3; 375 mM KCl; 15 mM $MgCl_2$), 2 μL of 0.1 M DTT, and 1 μL RNaseOUT™. Mix contents of the tube gently and incubate at 42 °C for 2 min. Add 1 μL (200 units) of SuperScript™ II RT and mix by pipetting up and down gently.
4. Incubate the mixture at 42 °C for 50 min, and then inactivate the reaction by heating at 70 °C for 15 min.
5. qPCR quantification: Normalize the template concentrations, and mix gene-specific primer pair (*see* Table 1) with qPCR detection reagents: 12.5 μL of iQ™ SYBR® Green Supermix (2×), 1 μL of template cDNA, 0.5 μL of forward primer (10 μM), 0.5 μL of reverse primer (10 μM), 10.5 μL of ddH_2O.

Load reaction replicates into iCycler iQ™ PCR 96-well plate, and seal the reaction vessels (*see* **Notes 5–7**).

6. Place the sealed reaction plate in the MyiQ™ single-color Real-Time PCR thermal cycler block, and start running the PCR protocol: 95 °C for 3 min, 40 cycles of amplification (95 °C for 30 s, 55 °C for 30 s, and 72 °C for 30 s). Melting curve analysis was performed as follow program: from 55 to 95 °C with 0.5 °C increment steps, 10 s/step.

7.2 Identification of Hotspot Mutations in NRAS, BRAF, and MEK1

1. Extract genomic DNA from tumor samples: Genomic DNA could be extracted from paraffin-embedded tissue block or fresh frozen tissue by using QIAamp DNA FFPE Tissue Kit or All Prep DNA/RNA Mini Kit, respectively (*see* **Notes 1–4**).
2. Amplify *NRAS* (exons 1 and 2); *BRAF* cDNA (exon 1–11) or MEK1 (exons 2, 3, and 6) (*see* **Notes 8** and **9**). Create 50 μL PCR reaction mixture by adding the following reagents: 5 μL of 10× High Fidelity PCR Buffer; 1 μL of 10 mM dNTP mixture; 2 μL of 50 mM $MgSO_4$; 1 μL of forward primer (10 μM); 1 μL of reverse primer (10 μM) (*see* Table 2); template DNA 1 μL (30 ng); Platinum® Taq DNA Polymerase High Fidelity 0.2 μL; ddH_2O to 50 μL.
3. Amplify exons by the following program: 3 cycles of 1 min at 95 °C, 1 min at 55 °C, 1 min at 72 °C; then 30 cycles of 30 s at 95 °C, 30 s at 55 °C, 1 min at 72 °C; 10 min at 72 °C; hold at 4 °C.
4. Check the PCR products: PCR products were mixed with BlueJuice™ Gel loading buffer and resolved by 1 % agarose gel. BRAF exon 15 migrates at 370 bp (see Fig. 1, lane 1) *NRAS* exons 1 and 2 migrate at 250 bp and 380 bp, respectively (*see* Fig. 1, lanes 2, 3). PCR products of wild type *BRAF* and truncated *BRAF* should migrate between 263 bp and 1,438 bp (*see* Fig. 3a), respectively. PCR products of MEK1 exons 2, 3, and 6 should migrate at 377 bp, 494 bp, and 439 bp, respectively (*see* Fig. 1 lanes 4–6).
5. PCR products purification and sequencing: PCR products were separated by agarose gel Electrophoresis. Target bands were cut and purified by QIAquick Gel Extraction Kit. Purified PCR products were applied to sequencing by Biosystems 3730 Capillary DNA Analyzers. Sequence was analyzed by sequence scanner version 1.0 (ABI) (NRAS *see* Fig. 2; BRAF *see* Fig. 3b, c; and MEK1 *see* Fig. 4).

8 Notes

1. The quality of the sample for DNA and RNA analysis is critical to yield reliable and accurate results. First and foremost, the purity of tumor tissue is essential for the following studies.

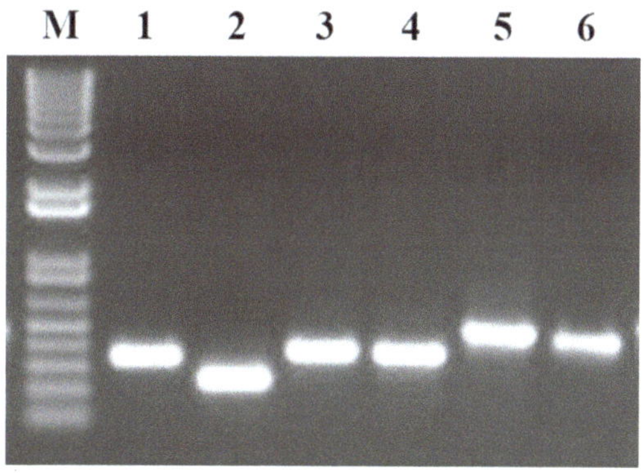

Fig. 1 PCR products of amplified exons. *Lane 1*: *BRAF* exon 15; *lanes 2, 3*: *NRAS* exons 1 and 2; *lanes 4–6*: *MEK1* exons 2, 3, and 6; *M*: DNA ladder (1 kb Plus DNA Ladder, Invitrogen)

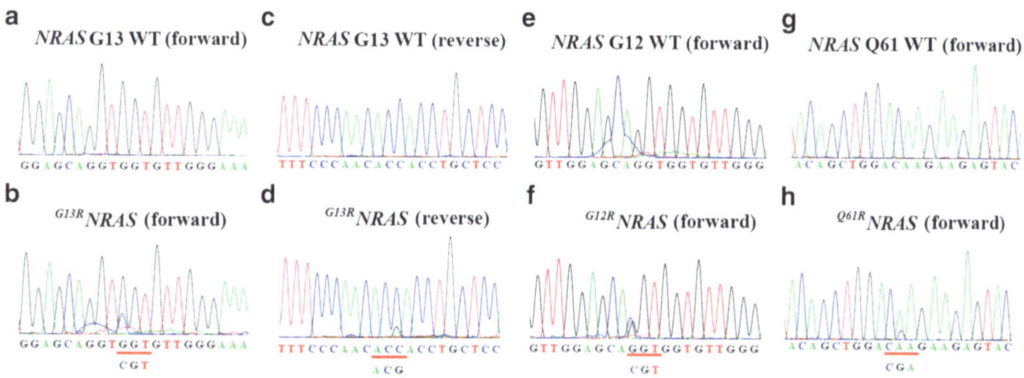

Fig. 2 Detection of *NRAS* hotspot mutations by Sanger sequencing. (**a**–**d**) Examples of wild type (WT) and ^{G13R}*NRAS* Sanger sequencing (forward and reverse). Forward and reverse sequencing can confirm each other which is desirable, especially when one of them looks ambiguous. (**e**, **f**) Examples of WT and ^{G12R}*NRAS* Sanger sequencing (forward). (**g**, **h**) Examples of WT and ^{Q61R}*NRAS* Sanger sequencing (forward). Hotspot mutations are *underlined*, and mutant triplet codons are *labeled* under them

Visible normal tissue, such as fat, should be removed from the tumor mass before extracting and processing for the nucleic acid. Histopathological image analysis by H&E staining of the FFPE or frozen sections is recommended to confirm the purity and isolation of the tumor biopsy.

2. One critical issue when running PCR assays with melanoma samples comes from the pigmentation in the melanoma tissues which is caused by melanin. Melanin is retained during the extractions and interferes with subsequent analysis of the polymerase reactions. Here, we recommend two protocols that can efficiently remove melanin by using ion-exchange column [25] or CTAB-urea reagents [26].

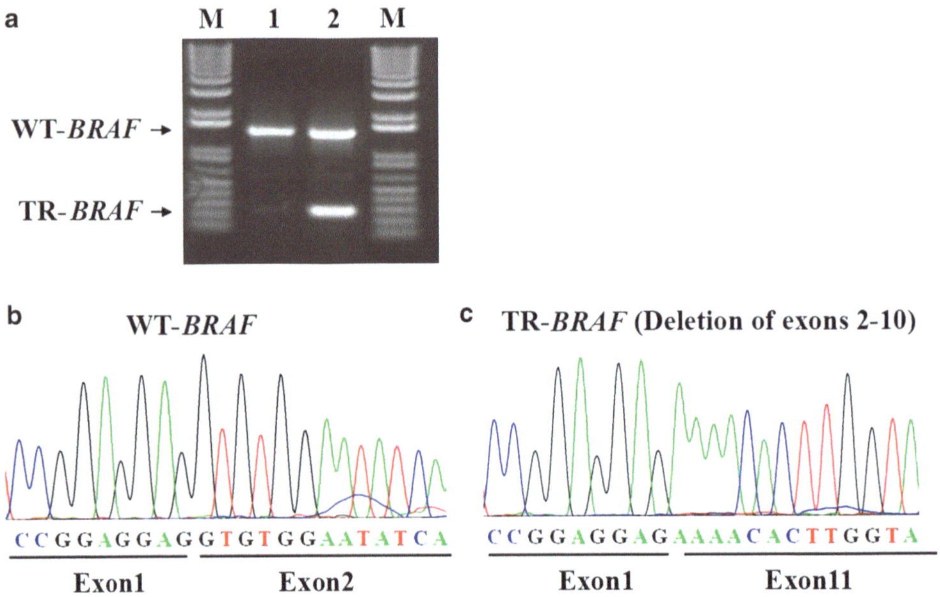

Fig. 3 Detection of *BRAF* alterations. (**a**) PCR products of amplified *BRAF* cDNA. *Lane 1*: WT *BRAF*; *lane 2*: truncated (TR) *BRAF*; *M*: DNA ladder (1 kb Plus DNA Ladder, Invitrogen). (**b**, **c**) Chromatograms from WT and truncated *BRAF* cDNA Sanger sequencing. Exons are *labeled* under the chromatograms

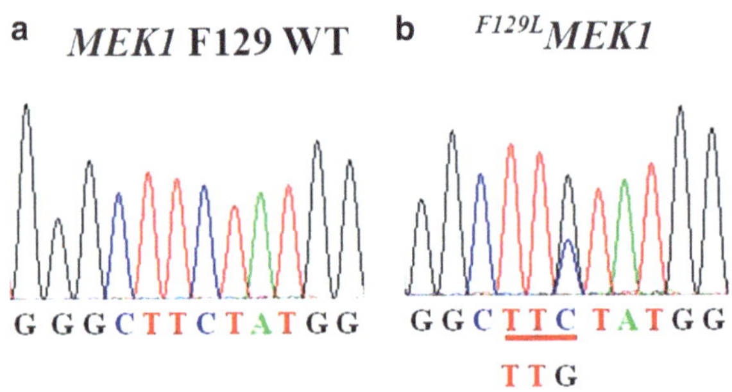

Fig. 4 Detection of *MEK1* mutations by Sanger sequencing. (**a**, **b**) Examples of WT and ^{F129L}*MEK1* Sanger sequencing (forward). Hotspot mutations are *underlined*, and mutant triplet codons are *labeled* under them

3. RNA quality, including the integrity and purity, is crucial for qPCR quantification and sequencing. RNAlater®, which prevents degradation of tissue RNA, is highly recommended before further processing. When extracting RNA, clean all surfaces, equipments such as centrifuges, and materials such as gloves and pipettes with RNaseZap treatment. It is important to use RNase-free tubes and tips to avoid contamination.
4. DNA samples could be kept at 4 °C for short-term storage and at −20 °C for long-term storage. RNA samples should be snap-frozen with liquid nitrogen and kept in −80 °C until further use.

5. The optimal target gene amplicon size is between 90 and 150 bp for qPCR detection. Our primers are designed to amplify an amplicon size around 150 bp to maximize the specificity of amplification.
6. Due to the sensitivity of qPCR, results can be easily altered by pipetting errors. It is advisable to prepare a master mix of iQ™ SYBR® Green Supermix containing the primers and probe. Add the template DNA sample to aliquots of the master mix. Using a master mix and fewer individual pipetting allows for tighter replicability and reproducibility in samples.
7. Checking the melting curve after qPCR data collection is another method to confirm the specificity of the amplified target gene and is highly recommended.
8. Control of contamination associated with PCR amplification and sequencing reactions can eliminate false positives and inaccurate data. Be careful to avoid using the same pipette to set up reactions and load products on a gel or using the same water for PCR and other activities such as restriction digests. Filtered tips should be used to pipette PCR reagents to reduce contamination. Making and using fresh aliquots of reagents are highly recommended to minimize and prevent cross-contamination.
9. Sanger sequencing occasionally produce false positive results, especially when the mutant peak in chromatograms is ambiguous (In our hands, the false peak looks small and take on a strange shape in chromatogram). To rule out false positives, reverse sequencing is advised to confirm the forward results.

References

1. Davies H, Bignell GR et al (2002) Mutations of the BRAF gene in human cancer. Nature 417:949–954
2. Bollag G, Hirth P et al (2010) Clinical efficacy of a RAF inhibitor needs broad target blockade in BRAF-mutant melanoma. Nature 467: 596–599
3. Flaherty KT, Puzanov I et al (2010) Inhibition of mutated, activated BRAF in metastatic melanoma. N Engl J Med 363:809–819
4. Chapman PB, Hauschild A et al (2011) Improved survival with vemurafenib in melanoma with BRAF V600E mutation. N Engl J Med 364:2507–2516
5. Hauschild A, Grob J-J et al (2012) Dabrafenib in BRAF-mutated metastatic melanoma: a multicentre, open-label, phase 3 randomised controlled trial. Lancet 380:358–365
6. Falchook GS, Long GV et al (2012) Dabrafenib in patients with melanoma, untreated brain metastases, and other solid tumours: a phase 1 dose-escalation trial. Lancet 379:1893–1901
7. Nazarian R, Shi H et al (2010) Melanomas acquire resistance to B-RAF(V600E) inhibition by RTK or N-RAS upregulation. Nature 468:973–977
8. Johannessen CM, Boehm JS et al (2010) COT drives resistance to RAF inhibition through MAP kinase pathway reactivation. Nature 468: 968–972
9. Poulikakos PI, Persaud Y et al (2011) RAF inhibitor resistance is mediated by dimerization of aberrantly spliced BRAF(V600E). Nature 480:387–390
10. Shi H, Moriceau G et al (2012) Melanoma whole-exome sequencing identifies

V600EB-RAF amplification-mediated acquired B-RAF inhibitor resistance. Nat Commun 3:724
11. Wagle N, Emery C et al (2011) Dissecting therapeutic resistance to RAF inhibition in melanoma by tumor genomic profiling. J Clin Oncol 29:3085–3096
12. Villanueva J, Vultur A et al (2010) Acquired resistance to BRAF inhibitors mediated by a RAF kinase switch in melanoma can be overcome by cotargeting MEK and IGF-1R/PI3K. Cancer Cell 18:683–695
13. Prahallad A, Sun C et al (2012) Unresponsiveness of colon cancer to BRAF(V600E) inhibition through feedback activation of EGFR. Nature 483:100–103
14. Corcoran RB, Ebi H et al (2012) EGFR-mediated reactivation of MAPK signaling contributes to insensitivity of BRAF-mutant colorectal cancers to RAF inhibition with vemurafenib. Cancer Discov 2:227–235
15. Yadav V, Zhang X et al (2012) Reactivation of mitogen-activated protein kinase (MAPK) pathway by FGF receptor 3 (FGFR3)/ras mediates resistance to vemurafenib in human B-RAF V600E mutant melanoma. J Biol Chem 287:28087–28098
16. Duncan JS, Whittle MC et al (2012) Dynamic reprogramming of the kinome in response to targeted MEK inhibition in triple-negative breast cancer. Cell 149:307–321
17. Shi H, Kong X et al (2011) Combinatorial treatments that overcome PDGFRβ-driven resistance of melanoma cells to V600EB-RAF inhibition. Cancer Res 71:5067–5074
18. Vigil D, Cherfils J et al (2010) Ras superfamily GEFs and GAPs: validated and tractable targets for cancer therapy? Nat Rev Cancer 10: 842–857
19. Fedorenko IV, Gibney GT et al (2013) NRAS mutant melanoma: biological behavior and future strategies for therapeutic management. Oncogene 32(25):3009–3018
20. Flaherty KT, Infante JR et al (2012) Combined BRAF and MEK inhibition in melanoma with BRAF V600 mutations. N Engl J Med 367: 1694–1703
21. Kobayashi S, Boggon TJ et al (2005) EGFR mutation and resistance of non–small-cell lung cancer to gefitinib. N Engl J Med 352: 786–792
22. Patel SP, Kim KB (2012) Selumetinib (AZD6244; ARRY-142886) in the treatment of metastatic melanoma. Expert Opin Investig Drugs 21:531–539
23. Emery CM, Vijayendran KG et al (2009) MEK1 mutations confer resistance to MEK and B-RAF inhibition. Proc Natl Acad Sci 106:20411–20416
24. Shi H, Moriceau G et al (2012) Preexisting MEK1 exon 3 mutations in V600E/KBRAF melanomas do not confer resistance to BRAF inhibitors. Cancer Discov 2:414–424
25. Dörrie J, Wellner V et al (2006) An improved method for RNA isolation and removal of melanin contamination from melanoma tissue: implications for tumor antigen detection and amplification. J Immunol Method 313: 119–128
26. Lagonigro MS, De Cecco L et al (2004) CTAB-urea method purifies RNA from melanin for cDNA microarray analysis. Pigment Cell Res 17:312–315

Part III

Biomarkers for Classification, Diagnosis, and Prognosis

Chapter 11

Current Status of Diagnostic and Prognostic Markers in Melanoma

Danielle Levine and David E. Fisher

Abstract

Melanoma is the most life-threatening common form of skin cancer. While most cutaneous melanomas are cured by surgical resection, a minority will relapse locally, regionally, or distantly. Biomarkers have represented a focal point for research aimed at improving diagnostic accuracy as well as providing prognostic information that may help to guide therapeutic decisions. While systemic melanoma therapies were of extremely limited utility for patients with advanced disease in the past, two drugs have been approved the FDA within the past several years, and it is possible that they may provide even greater impact if employed earlier in the disease process. To optimally employ these therapies, prognostic biomarkers may offer significant value. This article reviews methodologies for both discovery and routine testing of melanoma biomarkers. It also focuses on specific commonly used markers, as well as approaches to studying their applications to specific clinical settings. As the armamentarium of melanoma drugs grows, it is hoped that specific biomarkers will aid in guiding the use of these agents for patients in the clinic.

Key words Melanoma, Biomarker, Prognosis, Epigenetic, Proteomic

1 Introduction

Melanoma is the fifth most common cancer in men and the seventh in women and comprises 4 % of all cancers in the United States [1]. It is estimated that 68,700 people in the United States were diagnosed with melanoma in 2009, of which 8,650 would have died [2]. The mortality rate from melanoma has risen as well, possibly reflecting earlier detection and improved surgical excision [3]. The rate of metastatic relapse among patients with early stage melanoma varies depending on key prognostic factors, such as Breslow depth, presence of ulceration, mitotic rate, and lymph node involvement, which make up the current AJCC (American Joint Committee on Cancer) system [4, 5]. The likelihood of death from stage I to III melanoma is between 10 % and 80 %, depending on these prognostic variables. Within each staging group, we have

Magdalena Thurin and Francesco M. Marincola (eds.), *Molecular Diagnostics for Melanoma: Methods and Protocols*, Methods in Molecular Biology, vol. 1102, DOI 10.1007/978-1-62703-727-3_11, © Springer Science+Business Media New York 2014

no means of determining who will relapse, who will remain disease free, and when they will relapse; therefore, patients are monitored for recurrence by physical examinations, blood tests, and imaging studies. There is no clear consensus regarding selection and timing of laboratory and imaging studies when following patients with resected melanoma. The National Comprehensive Cancer Network (NCCN) recommends imaging for stage I patients only if they have symptoms. For stage II patients, a chest radiograph is optional and for stage IIB and IIC, and III, computed tomography (CT) scans, positron emission tomography (PET) scans, and MRI are recommended as clinically indicated; however, these indications are not defined. Other imaging modalities that have been recommended for staging but are not necessarily widely used include PET scans and ultrasound to assess lymph node involvement [2]. The frequency of laboratory tests and physical examinations is similarly controversial.

2 In-Practice Monitoring Census

Surveillance patterns adopted in other countries are also variable. For example, the U.K. guidelines for surveillance of stage IIB, IIC, or III melanoma include chest radiography, liver ultrasonography, or CT scan of the chest, abdomen, and pelvis, LDH, liver function tests, and CBC count at baseline and frequent clinical follow-up thereafter, but do not recommend subsequent imaging [2]. The consensus-based German guidelines recommend lymph node sonography and serum S100B as part of the routine surveillance every 3–6 months for thicker primary melanomas, and if these studies detect regional lymph node involvement, whole body imaging is recommended [4]. The European Society of Medical Oncology has specific guidelines for frequency of clinical examinations but has no consensus regarding blood tests or imaging technique [6]. The Sydney Melanoma Group recommends scheduled follow-up but does not make recommendations on blood tests or imaging [7].

In other malignancies, tumor markers have been shown to be useful in surveillance of patients at risk for metastatic relapse and might be used instead of periodic imaging in asymptomatic patients. This practice is widely incorporated in the management of resected colon, prostate, liver, ovarian, testicular cancer, and other malignancies. The hope is that melanoma biomarkers will ultimately predict course of disease and allow earlier interventions for patients.

3 Classification of Biomarkers

Tumor profiling has become an important goal in the treatment of many types of cancers, as it allows for individualized therapy based on the unique biomolecular behaviors of the involved tumor cells.

Genomic profiling, which requires fresh tissue from a large number of primary tumors, presents a challenge in melanoma, where the primary tumor is only a few millimeters in size with no residual tissue after the initial diagnosis [8]. Furthermore, genes can result in several different protein isoforms, which in turn might undergo posttranslational modifications that ultimately determine the behavior of the tumor cell. For these reasons, proteomics—screening methods for changes in protein expression—has emerged as an important approach in identifying valuable biomarkers in the prognosis and treatment of melanoma. Although we describe some notable genetic and epigenetic markers of disease progression, the most promising biomarkers identified to date have been proteins, assayed with proteomic methodologies.

Melanoma biomarkers can be classified according to the stage of melanoma that they are presumed to predict. In this classification scheme, growth biomarkers predict progression from normal skin to melanoma, metastatic biomarkers are associated with stage IV disease, and recurrent disease biomarkers correlate with recurrent melanoma. Biomarkers can also be classified based on gene or protein function, regardless of their proven clinical predictive potential. Needless to say, each type of biomarker has the potential to play a critical role in the management of melanoma. Using biomarkers allows for earlier detection of metastases, which not only improves morbidity and mortality but also provides more time to try newer therapies for advanced disease. In this review, we describe some approaches toward biomarker isolation and identify the most frequently described biomarkers based on basic, translational, and clinical studies of melanoma tissue samples, employing a functional classification for the purposes of this review. We then note that despite its potential use for determining prognosis and thus the management of local, metastatic, or recurrent disease, biomarker monitoring has not yet become the standard of care in the clinical management of melanoma. We explore why this may be and review some newer data on the potential applicability of melanoma biomarkers to clinical practice.

4 Identification Methods

Investigational teams have employed functional proteomic approaches using various biochemical and molecular biological methodologies conducted in melanoma cell lines or in tissue or serum samples in an effort to identify, propose, and validate such biomarkers. In this section, we outline the most common approaches, which include immunohistochemistry, tissue microarrays, Enzyme-Linked ImmunoSorbant Assay, reverse-transcription polymerase chain reaction, 2-dimensional gel electrophoresis, and matrix-assisted desorption/ionization time of flight mass spectrometry.

Immunohistochemistry (IHC)—the localization of antigens in tissue ("histo") with antibodies ("immuno") tagged by a fluorescent or color-producing marker—is a well-documented method used to characterize patterns of protein expression while preserving tissue and cellular architecture [9]. Albert H. Coons and his colleagues [10] were the first to label antibodies with a fluorescent dye and to use this approach to identify antigens in tissue sections. IHC staining is widely used to detect the presence of abnormal cells known to harbor molecules that are characteristic of particular cellular events, such as proliferation or apoptosis. Once specific biomarkers are sought based on the stage of disease, IHC can help delineate the distribution and localization of these biomarkers in various tissues, thus in turn providing treatment-guiding information. The tissue type and estimated concentration of the target molecule determine the optimal IHC approach.

Tissue microarrays (TMAs) consist of paraffin blocks in which up to 1,000 separate tissue cores are assembled in array fashion on a single glass slide to allow multiplex histological analysis [11]. First introduced with the so-called multitumor (sausage) tissue block preparation, the current technique requires procurement of tissue cores as small as 0.6 mm in diameter from regions of interest in paraffin-embedded tissues such as clinical biopsies or tumor samples [12]. These tissue cores are then inserted in a recipient paraffin block in a precisely spaced array pattern. Each microarray block can be cut into hundreds of sections that can be subjected to independent tests, such as IHC and in situ hybridization. The high-throughput analysis requires identification of potential proteins in these tissue cores to which the selective tests can be applied [13].

To determine the quantity of a particular protein in a sample, ELISA (Enzyme-Linked ImmunoSorbant Assay) can be applied. ELISAs are performed in 96-well plates coated with a protein to which the target protein will bind. The samples are subject to IHC via conjugated secondary antibodies. When the enzyme reaction is complete, the entire plate is placed into a plate reader and the optical density (colored product) is determined for each well. The amount of color produced is proportional to the amount of primary antibody bound to the proteins in the ELISA wells.

Another high-throughput approach that has been applied toward identification of biomarker genes is reverse-transcription polymerase chain reaction (RT-PCR). This technique involves reverse transcription of a candidate RNA into its DNA complement using the enzyme reverse transcriptase, and amplifying the resultant cDNA using PCR. The exponential amplification provides for a highly sensitive technique in which a very low copy number of RNA molecules can be detected. RT-PCR can also quantitatively determine the abundance of specific RNA molecules within a tissue as a measure of gene expression.

The newest approach used for high-throughput screening of candidate proteins involves separation of proteins using 2-dimensional gel electrophoresis (2DE) and identification of these proteins with matrix-assisted desorption/ionization time of flight mass spectrometry (MALDI-TOF-MS). After candidate protein separation on a 2D gel, the proteins are cleaved by proteolytic enzymes into peptides and are then concentrated and purified for high-sensitivity analysis. A sample peptide mixture is combined with a matrix molecule ("matrix-assisted") and is then subject to mass spectrometric (MS) analysis. MS involves pulsed laser transfer of energy to the mixture, promoting transition of solid particles to gas particles and acceleration of the gas particles to a degree ("time of flight") that is proportional to the mass of the particles. Repeating this process for many peptides derived from the candidate proteins is known as peptide mass mapping or peptide mass fingerprinting; the spectrum of identified peptide masses (known as the mass fingerprint) is unique for a specific protein and can be compared with similar profiles on publicly available online databases. Because of its high sensitivity and specificity—and wide mass range (from 1 to 300 kDa)—MALDI-TOF-MS has become a promising method for the identification of biomarkers in complex samples [14].

5 Specific Biomarkers (*See* Table 1)

As noted above, a variety of both tissue- and serum-based biomarkers have been noted to correlate with various stages of melanoma. The tissue antigens S100β, MART-1, and gp100/HMB45 have been identified as potential histologic markers for the presence of melanoma and play an important role in differentiating normal from malignant skin samples [15]. Biomarkers that have been identified as significantly correlating with histopathologic and clinical prognosis in various stages of melanoma include lactate dehydrogenase (LDH), C-reactive protein (CRP), tumor suppressors/signal transducers (p16, PTEN, EGFR, c-KIT, c-myc, bcl-6, HER3), cell-cycle-associated proteins (Ki-67, proliferating cell nuclear antigen [PCNA], cyclins A, B, D, E, p21, survivin), regulators of apoptosis (bcl-2, bax, Bak, ING3, ING4), proteins involved with cell adhesion and motility (P, E, and N-cadherin, β-catenin, β1 and β3 integrins, matrix metalloproteinases [MMPs]), and others (Hsp90, RGS1, NCOA3, MCM4, MCM6) [16, 17]. The serologic markers associated with poor prognosis in particular include LDH and CRP, proangiogenic factors (vascular endothelial growth factor [VEGF], basic fibroblast growth factor [BFGF], IL-8, MMPs), differentiation antigens (S100β, melanoma inhibitory activity [MIA], tyrosinase), cell adhesion and motility molecules (soluble intracellular adhesion molecule 1 [sICAM-1], soluble vascular cell adhesion molecule 1 [sVCAM], MMP-1, MMP-9),

Table 1
Biomarker trends with progression of disease and method of extraction

Angiogenesis	Trend	Method of isolation
Function		
Vascular endothelial growth factor-A (VEGF-A)	Increase trend with progression [31, 33, 34]	Serum, ELISA
Fibroblast growth factor-2 (FGF-2)	No specific trend [34]	Serum, ELISA
Matrix Metalloproteinases (MMP)	Increase trend with progression [38–40]	Serum, ELISA
Invasion and metastasis		
S100B	Increased with diagnosis (stage I, II), Increase trend with progression (stage III, IV); decrease with treatment efficacy [26]	Serum
LDH	Increase trend with metastasis [19–21]	Serum
CRP	Increased in stage IV vs. nonstage IV [22, 23]	Serum
Intercellular adhesion molecule-1 (ICAM-1)	Increase trend with progression [63–65]	Serum
Carcinoembryonic antigen-related cell adhesion molecule (CEACAM-1)	Increase trend with progression [63–65]	Serum
Melanocyte-specific melanoma cell adhesion molecule (MCAM, cell surface glycoprotein MUC18)	Increase with progression [36, 66–68]	Serum, ELISA
Galectin-3 (gal-3)	No trend seen [60, 61]	Serum, ELISA
Melastatin/TRPM1	Decrease trend with progression [54–66]	mRNA
Signal transduction		
Cytokines	Increase trend with progression, decrease trend on treatments [32, 46, 47]	Serum

cytokines (IL-6, IL-10, soluble IL-2 receptor [sIL-2R]), and others (TA90 immune complex, YKL-40) [16, 18]. In the coming section we focus on those markers that have been most closely linked with melanoma progression in the literature to date.

5.1 Lactate Dehydrogenase and C-Reactive Protein

Despite its low sensitivity and specificity as a predictor of metastatic relapse, LDH is known to correlate with advanced disease and is readily available in most clinical laboratories; it thus remains an important tool in estimating the prognosis of melanoma. Because it correlates with tumor load in stage IV disease, LDH is often used to stratify patients for randomized trials in advanced disease and remains the only marker included in the AJCC staging system of melanoma [19]. Society guidelines differ in their specific recommendations but many do include LDH as a component of prognostic management. For example, the NCCN recommends checking an LDH every 6–12 months for stage II disease, and the United Kingdom guidelines for surveillance of stage IIB, IIC, or III melanoma include baseline and follow-up LDH monitoring alongside imaging and other blood work [20]. By contrast, neither the European Society of Medical Oncology nor the Sydney Melanoma Group currently includes a consensus statement on baseline or follow-up LDH monitoring [21].

Like LDH, CRP is also readily available and has also been linked with poor prognosis in advanced melanoma. In patients with advanced disease, Deichmann et al. found that when using a cut-off value of 3 mg/dl, CRP discriminated between stage IV and non-stage IV melanoma patients with a sensitivity of 76.9 % and a specificity of 90.4 % [22]. Needless to say, however, LDH and CRP alone are clearly insufficient to document progressive disease; detailed information incorporating the history and physical, complete blood counts, imaging, and histopathology must be considered alongside the information provided by these markers. In a recent report, LDH represented the sole indicator of recurrence in only one patient out of 373 where patients were followed for metastatic relapse [23].

5.2 S100β

Whereas both LDH and CRP have been validated in many other types of cancers and inflammatory conditions, the S100β protein appears somewhat more specific for melanoma. Initially isolated from bovine brain in the 1960s, S100β is a 21-kD dimeric protein consisting of two subunits; the *β* subunit is expressed by both glial cells and melanocytes. Although its predominant mechanism in melanogenesis remains incompletely understood, S100β is known to interact with the p53 tumor suppressor gene in a calcium-dependent manner [24]. It is often used as an immunohistochemical marker for histological diagnosis of melanoma. Importantly, it has also been identified as a prognostic biomarker, particularly in patients with advanced disease [25]. Some investigators have argued that time-dependent evaluation of serial blood measurements of

S100β is useful in order to follow melanoma patients in helping to predict the clinical stage of disease and monitoring the effectiveness of antitumoral treatment and probability of relapse, whatever the type of the treatment [26].

Although more specific than LDH and CRP, S100β levels can still be elevated in healthy patients or in patients with nonmelanoma skin cancer, brain tumors, neurological disease, or AIDS. Furthermore, many experts note that it plays a limited prognostic role in patients with stage I and II disease beyond initial histopathologic diagnosis [27]. Despite these shortcomings, S100β remains an important prognostic marker with emerging clinical availability. Indeed, the consensus-based German guidelines recommend lymph node ultrasonography and serum S100β as part of the routine surveillance every 3–6 months for thicker primary melanomas [28, 29]. Retsas et al. have even suggested the use of S100β instead of LDH in the AJCC staging system [30]. Further studies correlating S100β levels with melanoma progression and relapse are underway.

5.3 Vascular Endothelial Growth Factor

As noted above, a number of proangiogenic proteins have been associated with poor prognosis in melanoma. Among its other roles, VEGF is known to be a potent mitogen of endothelial cells and a chemotactic factor for monocytes and tumor-associated macrophages; it is also a vasopermeability stimulant in many cell systems whose expression correlates with tumor progression, particularly under hypoxic conditions [31]. In a multiplex analysis of the serum of 179 patients with high-risk melanoma and 378 healthy patients, Yurkovetsky et al. found that serum cytokine profiles in the melanoma patients consisted of higher levels of VEGF (average concentration of 215 pg/ml in melanoma patients, versus 76.6 pg/ml in healthy patients) alongside higher levels of multiple other cytokines, including interleukins, macrophage inflammatory protein, and tumor necrosis factor. Furthermore, treatment with high-dose interferon (IFN)-α2b therapy resulted in significantly lower levels of angiogenic and growth factors, including VEGF [32].

VEGF isoform levels appear to correlate with severity of disease, as well. Vihinen et al. reported lower serum VEGF-C levels in metastatic patients with skin or subcutaneous metastasis compared to metastatic patients with other distant sites [31]. Using automated quantitative analysis of VEGF and VEGF receptor expression in melanoma tissue microarrays, Mehnert et al. noted higher expression of VEGF receptor 2 (VEGF-R2, or flk2/kdr) in metastases versus primaries and hypothesized that selection for an angiogenic phenotype in metastatic melanoma is conferred via upregulation of VEGF-R2 [33]. Other studies have also showed an overall trend toward increased expression of VEGF or its receptors with progression of disease [34], in contrast to levels of other growth factors such as FGF-2.

5.4 Matrix Metalloproteinases

Because of their association with angiogenesis and other angiogenic factors, MMPs have also been identified as potential markers of melanoma. MMPs comprise a family of 24 structurally related zinc-dependent endopeptidases that have been shown to lyse components of the extracellular membrane, thereby promoting cell turnover and angiogenesis; they can also cleave other proteinases, growth factors, and adhesion molecules, resulting in modulation of various growth processes required for tumor invasion and metastasis independent of angiogenesis [35]. Disturbing the balance between MMP and tissue inhibitors metalloproteinases (TIMP) can result in the acquisition of a malignant phenotype by promoting enhanced tumor growth and invasion and accelerated angiogenesis [36]; in fact, synthetic MMP inhibitors like Batimastat, are currently being studied in murine models of metastatic hepatocellular carcinoma [37]. MMP expression has been reported during melanoma progression as well, and high serum levels of MMP-1, MMP-2, and MMP-14 have been correlated with poor survival [38–40].

A number of MMP modulators have also been linked to melanoma progression, though many of these results have not been corroborated in vivo. The MMP-inducer EMMPRIN/CD147 has been shown to upregulate the VEGF receptor-2 in primary melanoma cell lines, resulting in increased migration and proliferation of these cells [41]. CD147 has also been shown to enhance cellular proliferation and VEGF production by melanoma cells and promote tumor cell invasion by inducing MMP expression in neighboring fibroblasts [42, 43]. In cell biological experiments using a metastatic melanoma cell line, Wang et al. recently found that galectin-3 (gal-3) facilitates cell migration and invasion in melanoma in part by promoting upregulation of MMP-1 expression [44]. In a translational study involving immunohistochemical staining of primary cutaneous malignant melanoma samples from 150 patients, Chen found that higher positive rates of both EMMPRIN and MMP-2 expression were significantly correlated with increased tumor thickness, higher Clark level, and higher AJCC stage; in fact, patients with EMMPRIN+/MMP-2+ expression had a significantly decreased 3-year disease-free survival and 5-year overall survival [45].

5.5 Chemokines and Their Receptors

Chemokines are small signaling polypeptides that can bind to and activate G protein-coupled receptors, a family of seven transmembrane molecules involved in signal transduction. Chemokines are known to play a role in the malignant transformation of many tumors and in the metastatic process. In the multiplex analysis referenced above, Yurkovetsky et al. identified a specific serum cytokine profile comprised of higher serum concentrations of IL-1, IL-6, IL-8, IL-12p40, IL-13, granulocyte colony-stimulating factor, monocyte chemoattractant protein 1 (MCP-1), macrophage inflammatory protein (MIP)-1alpha, MIP-1beta, IFN-alpha, tumor necrosis factor

(TNF)-alpha, epidermal growth factor, and TNF receptor II—in addition to higher concentrations of VEGF—in the patients with melanoma compared with the control group. IFN-alpha2b therapy resulted in a significant decrease of serum levels of immunosuppressive and growth stimulatory factor levels. Importantly, the pretreatment levels of IL-1, IL-6, TNF-alpha, MIP-1alpha, and MIP-1beta in particular were found to be significantly higher in the serum of patients with longer relapse-free survival values, implicating these cytokines as potential molecular targets of IFN therapy in patients with stage IIB-III melanoma [32].

A number of other studies have identified specific chemokines as poor prognostic markers linked with advanced disease. In a retrospective analysis of 90 patients with metastatic melanoma who were enrolled in a phase III study comparing chemotherapy and biochemotherapy, Guida et al. found that higher levels of sIL-2R were correlated with a worse survival. Importantly, a progressive increase of IL-12 and sIL-2R was observed during treatment in patients with a better survival, suggesting that these cytokines might be particularly effective therapeutic targets in metastatic melanoma [46]. Both CXCL8/IL-8 and IL-10 have been correlated with poor outcome as well [47, 48].

5.6 Cell Cycle Proteins

Proteins that effect DNA replication and repair would appear to be good prognostic markers, and recent data suggest that this may be the case. Alonso et al. retrospectively evaluated 175 human melanoma specimens at various stages of disease and found that upregulation of both cyclin A and cyclin D1 was frequently detected in radial growth phase melanomas relative to nevi [49]. Furthermore, upregulation of cyclin D1 and cyclin D3 was noted in metastatic melanomas relative to vertical growth phase (VGP) melanomas. The authors argue that an increasing degree of cyclin and cyclin-dependent kinase expression facilitates progression to advanced clinical and histological stages. As a regulator of aberrant melanocyte proliferation, p16 was not detected in metastatic melanomas relative to VGP melanomas [50]. Both Ki-67 and PCNA, which are involved with DNA-damage checkpoint and repair, have also been statistically linked to disease-free survival (DFS) and all-cause mortality (ACM) in a number of studies [49, 51–53]. Similarly, effectors of DNA replication such as metallothionein play regulatory roles in the cell cycle and have been associated with disease free survival as well [51].

Initially identified as a target whose expression was markedly reduced in the most aggressive melanoma cell lines, melastatin—which encodes the putative calcium channel protein transient receptor potential cation channel, subfamily M, member 1 (TRPM1)—has been proposed as another important tumor suppressor that may be prognostically useful in determining stage of disease [54]. In human samples, all benign nevi reported to date have been shown to uniformly express TRPM1 mRNA, in contrast to primary melanomas, which show variable expression, and melanoma metastases, which invariably show at least regional loss of expression [55]. In a study of 150 patients with localized cutaneous melanoma, Duncan et al. subsequently showed that decreased expression of TRPM1 mRNA in primary cutaneous tumors correlated with an increased risk of developing metastatic disease. In fact, multivariate analysis of TRPM1 mRNA expression and other known clinical and pathological prognostic factors implicated TRPM1 alongside tumor thickness and mitotic activity as independent and interactive predictors of disease-free melanoma survival [56, 57].

The expression of melastatin/TRPM1 itself is tightly controlled by the essential melanocyte transcription factor microphthalmia-associated transcription factor (MITF) [58, 59]. MITF is the master regulator of melanocyte development, differentiation, and pigmentation, and amplification of MITF has been identified in approximately 15 % of melanomas [60]. Indeed, disruption of MITF and its target cyclin-dependent kinase-2 has been shown to suppress growth and cell cycle progression in melanoma, but not other cancers [61], and a recurrent activating point mutation in MITF has recently been discovered in certain cases of familial melanoma [62]. In addition to its role as a potential therapeutic target [63], MITF is clinically useful in identifying melanocytes under certain clinical conditions [64] and has been proposed as an independent prognostic factor for predicting both malignancy [65] and progression-free survival [66].

6 Novel Biomarkers

6.1 Melanoma Inhibitory Activity Protein

MIA is a 12 kDa cell growth inhibitor peptide that decreases cell attachment to extracellular matrix and promotes tumor metastasis [67]. MIA has been noted to be elevated in the serum of relapsing melanoma and has been described as a useful marker to monitor progression of melanoma after surgery [68], especially when considered alongside other markers such as LDH or S100β [36]. In a retrospective study of the serum levels of S100β and MIA in 110 patients with at least stage IIIB melanoma, 66 disease-free patients, and 65 healthy controls, Diaz-Lagares et al. observed that although MIA was an independent prognostic factor of overall survival, the combination of S100β plus MIA had the best diagnostic sensitivity for advanced disease. Patients with both S100β and MIA elevations had a significantly shorter survival than those with normal levels of these markers [69].

6.2 Galectin-3

Galectin-3 (gal-3), the member of the lectin family that selectively binds β-galactosidase residues, has been shown to play important roles in cell proliferation, cell differentiation, cell adhesion, cell migration, angiogenesis, and metastasis [70]. In melanoma, gal-3 has been shown to be overexpressed in malignant melanocytic lesions and preferentially released by both melanoma and inflammatory cells. Gal-3 may induce MMP-1 expression in some cells as noted above [44]. Clinical data remain conflicted, however, with regard to relative gal-3 expression in tissue samples from progressive disease. In a recent translational study evaluating the expression of gal-3 in tissue samples from patients with various stages of melanoma, Brown et al. observed an increase in gal-3 expression between benign nevi and thin primary melanomas, and a progressive decrease in expression between thin primary melanomas and thicker melanomas or metastatic melanoma. Importantly, strong gal-3 expression was associated with both improved overall survival and melanoma-specific survival [71]. By contrast, Buljan et al. found an association between increased expression of gal-3 and increased Breslow thickness in tissue samples from 104 cases of primary melanoma [72]. These conflicting data highlight the need for well-designed prospective trials incorporating novel biomarkers in order to confirm which markers are the most reliable indicators of melanoma progression or prognosis.

6.3 Integrins

Integrins, which are heterodimeric cell adhesion receptors composed of two subunits α and β, help insure cell-cell adhesion and maintenance of tissue structure. The integrins that have been implicated in melanoma progression include αvβ3 (receptor for vitronectin and fibronectin), α2β1 (collagen), α4β1 (fibronectin), and α6β1 (laminin). Some reports have shown that increased serum levels of β integrins have been associated with shorter survival. As noted below, there is increasing evidence for the role of osteopontin, a secreted integrin-binding-protein, in melanoma progression as well [73].

6.4 Intracellular Adhesion Molecules (CAMs)

A number of intracellular adhesion molecules have emerged as promising biomarkers of melanoma progression. Binding of the intracellular adhesion molecule-1 (ICAM-1) to lymphocytes function-associated antigen-1 promotes leukocyte migration and is an early first step in cell motility [74]. Another adhesion molecule, the glandular tissue-associated carcinoembryonic antigen-related cell adhesion molecule 1 (CEACAM-1), is an important cell-cell adhesion molecule detected on leukocytes, epithelia, and endothelia [75]. Both ICAM-1 and CEACAM-1 have been implicated in diverse cellular processes such as cells motility, linkage of cell complexes to the cytoskeleon, ion channel formation, and cell-matrix interactions that have important implications for many cancers including melanoma. Indeed, in a translational analysis of serum from 108 patients with metastatic melanoma matched with serum from age- and gender-matched healthy donors, Kluger et al. employed whole genome expression microarrays to identify of a number of abundantly expressed genes in the blood of melanoma patients, and quantified the differences in protein expression using ELISA. In their analysis, both ICAM-1 and CEACAM-1 were noted to be expressed at significantly higher levels in unresected stage IV patients compared with age- and gender-matched patients with resected, early stage disease. Along with five other proteins (osteopontin, MIA, growth differentiation factor-15 [GDF-15], tissue inhibitor metalloproteinase-1 [TIMP-1], and S100β), ICAM-1 and CEACAM-1 were clearly superior to serum LDH in differentiating between advanced stage patient populations [36].

Other studies have identified melanocyte-specific melanoma cell adhesion molecule (MCAM, also known as the cell surface glycoprotein MUC18) as a marker of worse disease-free survival [76]; this protein can interact with β3 integrins and have been shown to be overexpressed at the leading edge of tumors [77]. Increased expression of MCAM/MUC18 in particular has been linked with significantly worse DFS and ACM in a number of studies [78]. In fact, this protein has been singled out as one of the most promising biomarkers in the field based on a recent meta-analysis as discussed below [51].

7 Melanin-Related Metabolites

7.1 5-S-Cysteinyldopa

A precursor of phaeomelanin, 5-S-cysteinyldopa (5SCD) is produced by both melanocytes and melanoma cells and has been shown to correlate with disease progression [79]. 5SCD may play a role in protecting melanocyte membranes from oxidative damage due to ultraviolet radiation [80], but the clinical implications of this protective role remain poorly defined. As appears to be the case with gal-3, 5SCD's prognostic role becomes more important when considered alongside other biomarkers. For example, Banfalvi et al. found that 5SCD had similar sensitivity but lower specificity for survival than S100β in a cohort of tissue samples from 179 patients with stage III-IV disease, and suggested a biomarker model incorporating 5SCD alongside S100β and LDH in similar patients [81].

7.2 L-Dihydroxyphenylalanine and L-Tyrosine

3, 4-Dihydroxyphenylalanine (L-DOPA) was the first metabolite implicated in melanogenesis and its plasma levels have been correlated with melanoma progression and tumor burden. Along with L-tyrosine, L-DOPA is an intermediate and regulator of melanogenesis that acts via receptor- or non-receptor-mediated mechanisms. The substrate induced L-DOPA or L-tyrosine melanogenic pathway is thought to serve as an autoregulatory pathway in various melanoma subtypes [82]. Some authors have proposed that the

L-DOPA/L-tyrosine ratio, which represents an index of tyrosinase and tyrosine hydroxylase activity, may be particularly predictive of melanoma progression, particularly in stage III patients [68].

8 Other Metabolites

A recent report has identified potentially promising metabolic signatures of melanoma. Metabolites are low molecular weight intermediates that are context dependent and vary according to the physiological or pathological state of the cell, tissue, or organ. Abaffy identified three volatiles—4-methyl decane (a methylated alkane previously linked with lung cancer progression), dodecane, and undecane (associated with membrane lipid peroxidation and oxidative stress)—that were preferentially expressed in both fresh and frozen melanoma, indicating that they were candidate biomarkers and suggesting a potential role for diagnostic and treatment strategies based on altered metabolism [83].

9 Epigenetic Biomarkers

Epigentics refers to heritable changes in gene expression that occur independent of the genomic DNA sequence. Epigenetic aberrations have been associated with melanoma progression including dysregulated DNA promoter methylation, histone modification, and microRNA, and as such some investigators have detected epigenetic biomarkers in the tissue or serum of melanoma patients [84]. Nguyen recently assessed tissue specimens from 15 primary cutaneous melanomas, 15 lymph node metastases, and 31 distant metastases to determine the significance of microRNA-29 isoform C and DNA methyltransferase 3A and 3B (DNMT3A and B, which catalyse DNA methylation) expression in melanoma progression and clinical outcome and noted that downregulation of microRNA-29c inversely correlated with DNMTsA and B expression in metastatic tumors [85]. By contrast, expression of microRNA-29c was noted to be a significant prognostic factor predicting overall survival in patients with lymph node metastases. These findings suggest that microRNA-29c might serve as a potential tumor suppressor who expression provides prognostic information regarding disease progression [50].

10 Clinical Applicability of Molecular Biomarkers

Although many studies have sought to identify potentially valuable prognostic biomarkers in predicting the course of melanoma, few molecular methods have been incorporated into mainstream clinical practice and expert opinion recommendations. The most important reason for this disconnect is that many of the clinical biomarker studies have not consistently designed or analyzed data according to what are now referred to as REMARK criteria, a set of National Cancer Institute-published guidelines aimed at providing relevant information about the study design, preplanned hypotheses, patient and specimen characteristics, assay methods, and statistical analysis methods of tumor marker studies in clinical oncology [86]. The REMARK effort aimed at standardizing the general methodologic differences, poor study designs, atypical biochemical assays, and inappropriate or overreaching statistical analyses characteristic of many biomarker studies. In these criteria, recommended biomarker reporting studies were encouraged to state a focused introduction; incorporate materials and methods that clearly outline the patients, biomarker characteristics, assay methods, study design, and statistical methods used; present data that includes all patients in the study and univariate and multivariate analyses to clearly define the relation between the marker and outcome; and interpret the results within the context of the prespecified hypotheses and other relevant studies. While acknowledging that guidelines may evolve to address new study paradigms and new assay technologies, the multidisciplinary REMARK team established an important paradigm that, at the very least, has led to a new standard of rigor in the analysis of tumor marker studies. Reports that do not meet these criteria may have been designed as translational or basic science studies, or may have methodological flaws that preclude generalizability.

Indeed, a number of systematic reviews have attempted to integrate biomolecular, histopathological, and clinical data in an effort to identify candidate biomarkers differentially linked to various stages of melanoma. In a meta-analytic study aimed at distilling clinical applicability from nearly 1,800 published melanoma biomarker studies, Rothberg et al. identified 102 cohort studies that reported associations between immunohistochemical expression and survival outcomes in melanoma that conformed to the REMARK criteria, as applied by the authors to melanoma studies [51]. Many reports had been initially excluded from the analysis because of inappropriate methods (such as not performing immunohistochemistry), inappropriate study design (such as cross-sectional analysis), or incomplete statistical analysis. The authors identified 37 studies incorporating 62 unique proteins that met their criteria by avoiding these shortcomings and presenting multivariable survival estimates for differential levels of candidate protein expression on melanoma samples. Proteins that facilitate tissue invasion and metastasis (for example, members of the CAM family and MMPs) were most likely associated with melanoma prognosis, with increased expression of many of these proteins statistically significant for either worse disease free survival or mortality outcomes. Overall, the most promising prognostic biomarkers that emerged from this analysis including MCAM/MUC18

(ACM HR 16.34, MMP-2 (melanoma-specific mortality HR 2.6), Ki-67 (combined ACM HR 2.66), PCNA (ACM HR 2.27, and p16 (ACM HR 0.29). Importantly, many reports regarding growth factors or signal transduction proteins such as VEGF and VEGF receptors, ephrins, or hypoxia-inducible transcription factors as melanoma biomarkers, some of which we reference above, did not meet the authors' inclusion criteria.

In another recent analysis, Schramm and Mann applied REMARK-derived criteria to identify high-quality studies from among 617 studies analyzing protein expression by IHC and 45 gene expression microarray studies. Among REMARK-compliant literature (which was noted to be less than 15 % of published peer-reviewed studies), 41 proteins were noted to share a significant relationship with prognosis in primary melanoma [87]. In this study, only two eligible gene microarray-based studies were identified, as most such studies appeared to use samples that were not primary melanoma. However, there were two candidate biomarkers—PCNA and survivin—with evidence for an association with clinical outcome at both gene and protein levels.

This review also highlighted the potential value of using multimarker prognostic discriminators (MPDs), factors that incorporate the combined effect of three of more biomarkers in a multivariate setting [88, 89]. For example, Kashani-Sabet et al. assessed expression of three previously derived markers (NCOA3, a member of the steroid receptor coactivator family; the integrin-binding protein SPP1 or osteopontin, discussed above; and RGS1, a GTPase-activating protein) using IHC analysis in a TMA cohort of 395 patients [89]. The cumulative overexpression of all three markers was embodied in a multimarker index or MPD score, whose prognostic effect on melanoma-specific survival and sentinel lymph node status was assessed. The authors found that higher MPD scores were significantly predictive of reduced melanoma-specific survival and increased sentinel lymph node metastasis in this cohort. Indeed, in their analysis, Schramm and Mann found that when ranked by *p*-value and compared with single-molecule predictors of outcome, MPDs better predict outcome.

The quest for melanoma biomarkers is a young field that still lacks a unifying in-practice surveillance consensus. Larger prospective studies are needed to examine the most promising biomarkers individually and in combination.

References

1. Jemal A, Siegel R, Ward E, Hao Y, Xu J, Thun MJ (2009) Cancer statistics, 2009. CA Cancer J Clin 59:225–249
2. Ak I, Stokkel MP, Bergman W, Pauwels EK (2000) Cutaneous malignant melanoma: clinical aspects, imaging modalities and treatment. Eur J Nucl Med 27:447–458
3. Balch CM, Gershenwald JE, Soong SJ, Thompson JF, Atkins MB, Byrd DR et al (2009) Final version of 2009 AJCC melanoma

staging and classification. J Clin Oncol 27: 6199–6206
4. Garbe C, Hauschild A, Volkenandt M, Schadendorf D, Stolz W, Reinhold U et al (2007) Evidence and interdisciplinary consense-based German guidelines: diagnosis and surveillance of melanoma. Melanoma Res 17:393–399
5. Bishop JA, Corrie PG, Evans J, Gore ME, Hall PN, Kirkham N et al (2002) UK guidelines for the management of cutaneous melanoma. Br J Plast Surg 55:46–54
6. Dummer R, Hauschild A (2008) Jost L Cutaneous malignant melanoma: ESMO clinical recommendations for diagnosis, treatment and follow-up. Ann Oncol 19(Suppl 2):ii86–ii88
7. Francken AB, Accortt NA, Shaw HM, Colman MH, Wiener M, Soong SJ et al (2008) Follow-up schedules after treatment for malignant melanoma. Br J Surg 95:1401–1407
8. Sabel MS, Liu Y, Lubman DM (2011) Proteomics in melanoma biomarker discovery: great potential, many obstacles. Int J Proteomics 2011:181890
9. Shi SR, Liu C, Taylor CR (2007) Standardization of immunohistochemistry for formalin-fixed, paraffin-embedded tissue sections based on the antigen-retrieval technique: from experiments to hypothesis. J Histochem Cytochem 55(2):105–109
10. Coons AH (1791) The development of immunohistochemistry. NY Acad Sci 177:5–9
11. Kononen J, Bubendorf L, Kallioniemi A, Bärlund M, Schraml P, Leighton S, Torhorst J, Mihatsch MJ, Sauter G, Kallioniemi OP (1998) Tissue microarrays for high-throughput molecular profiling of tumor specimens. Nat Med 4(7):844–847
12. Battifora H, Skacel M, Skilton B, Pettay JD, Tubbs RR (2002) Tissue microarrays: a powerful tool for high-throughput analysis of clinical specimens. Appl Immunohistochem Mol Morphol 10:1–6
13. Horne BD, Carlquist JF, Cannon-Albright LA, Muhlestein JB, McKinney JT, Kolek MJ, Clarke JL, Anderson JL, Camp NJ (2006) High-resolution characterization of linkage disequilibrium structure and selection of tagging single nucleotide polymorphisms: application to the cholesteryl ester transfer protein gene. Ann Hum Genet 70(Pt 4):524–534
14. Marvin LF, Roberts MA, Fay LB (2003) Matrix-assisted laser desorption/ionization time-of-flight mass spectrometry in clinical chemistry. Clin Chim Acta 337(1–2):11–21
15. de Vries TJ, Smeets M, de Graaf R, Hou-Jensen K, Bröcker EB, Renard N, Eggermont AM, van Muijen GN, Ruiter DJ (2001) Expression of gp100, MART-1, tyrosinase, and S100 in paraffin-embedded primary melanomas and locoregional, lymph node, and visceral metastases: implications for diagnosis and immunotherapy. A study conducted by the EORTC Melanoma Cooperative Group. J Pathol 193(1):13–20
16. Utikal J, Schadendorf D, Ugurel S (2007) Serologic and immunohistochemical prognostic biomarkers of cutaneous malignancies. Arch Dermatol Res 298(10):469–477
17. Gogas H, Eggermont AM, Hauschild A, Hersey P, Mohr P, Schadendorf D, Spatz A, Dummer R (2009) Biomarkers in melanoma. Ann Oncol 20(Suppl 6):vi8–vi13
18. Liu S, Kirschmeier P, Simon J, Seidel-Dugan C, Puhlmann M (2008) Prognostic and predictive molecular markers in cutaneous malignant melanoma: the first step toward personalized medicine. Curr Pharmacogenomics Person Med 6(4):272–294
19. Deichmann M, Benner A, Bock M, Jäckel A, Uhl K, Waldmann V, Näher H (1999) S100-Beta, melanoma-inhibiting activity, and lactate dehydrogenase discriminate progressive from nonprogressive American Joint Committee on Cancer stage IV melanoma. J Clin Oncol 17(6):1891–1896
20. Coit DG, Andtbacka R, Bichakjian CK, Dilawari RA, Dimaio D, Guild V, Halpern AC, Hodi FS, Kashani-Sabet M, Lange JR, Lind A, Martin L, Martini MC, Pruitt SK, Ross MI, Sener SF, Swetter SM, Tanabe KK, Thompson JA, Trisal V, Urist MM, Weber J, Wong MK, NCCN melanoma panel (2009) Melanoma. J Natl Compr Canc Netw 7(3):250–275
21. Thompson JF, Shaw HM, Stretch JR, McCarthy WH, Milton GW (2003) The Sydney melanoma unit—a multidisciplinary melanoma treatment center. Surg Clin North Am 83(2):431–451
22. Deichmann M, Kahle B, Moser K, Wacker J, Wüst K (2004) Diagnosing melanoma patients entering American Joint Committee on Cancer stage IV, C-reactive protein in serum is superior to lactate dehydrogenase. Br J Cancer 91(4):699–702
23. Moore Dalal K, Zhou Q, Panageas KS, Brady MS, Jaques DP, Coit DG (2008) Methods of detection of first recurrence in patients with stage I/II primary cutaneous melanoma after sentinel lymph node biopsy. Ann Surg Oncol 15(8):2206–2214
24. Lin J, Yang Q, Wilder PT, Carrier F, Weber DJ (2010) The calcium-binding protein S100B down-regulates p53 and apoptosis in malignant melanoma. J Biol Chem 285(35): 27487–27498

25. Kruijff S, Hoekstra HJ (2012) The current status of S-100B as a biomarker in melanoma. Eur J Surg Oncol 38(4):281–285
26. Bouwhuis MG, Suciu S, Kruit W, Salès F, Stoitchkov K, Patel P, Cocquyt V, Thomas J, Liénard D, Eggermont AM, Ghanem G (2011) Prognostic value of serial blood S100B determinations in stage IIB-III melanoma patients: a corollary study to EORTC trial 18952. European Organisation for Research and Treatment of Cancer Melanoma Group. Eur J Cancer 47(3):361–368
27. Vereecken P, Cornelis F, Van Baren N, Vandersleyen V, Baurain JF (2012) A synopsis of serum biomarkers in cutaneous melanoma patients. Dermatol Res Pract 2012:260643
28. Dummer R, Panizzon R, Bloch PH, Burg G (2005) Updated Swiss guidelines for the treatment and follow-up of cutaneous melanoma. Dermatology 210(1):39–44
29. Garbe C, Schadendorf D, Stolz W, Volkenandt M, Reinhold U, Kortmann RD, Kettelhack C, Frerich B, Keilholz U, Dummer R, Sebastian G, Tilgen W, Schuler G, Mackensen A, Kaufmann R, Hauschild A (2008) Short German guidelines: malignant melanoma. J Dtsch Dermatol Ges 6(Suppl 1):S9–S14
30. Retsas S, Mastrangelo MJ (2007) Reflecting on the 2001 American Joint Committee on Cancer Staging System for melanoma. Semin Oncol 34(6):491–497
31. Vihinen PP, Hilli J, Vuoristo MS, Syrjänen KJ, Kähäri VM, Pyrhönen SO (2007) Serum VEGF-C is associated with metastatic site in patients with malignant melanoma. Acta Oncol 46(5):678–684
32. Yurkovetsky ZR, Kirkwood JM, Edington HD, Marrangoni AM, Velikokhatnaya L, Winans MT, Gorelik E, Lokshin AE (2007) Multiplex analysis of serum cytokines in melanoma patients treated with interferon-alpha2b. Clin Cancer Res 13(8):2422–2428
33. Mehnert JM, McCarthy MM, Jilaveanu L, Flaherty KT, Aziz S, Camp RL, Rimm DL, Kluger HM (2010) Quantitative expression of VEGF, VEGF-R1, VEGF-R2, and VEGF-R3 in melanoma tissue microarrays. Hum Pathol 41(3):375–384, Epub 2009 Dec 11
34. Osella-Abate S, Quaglino P, Savoia P, Leporati C, Comessatti A, Comessatti MG (2002) VEGF-165 serum levels and tyrosinase expression in melanoma patients: correlation with the clinical course. Melanoma Res 12(4):325–334
35. Väisänen A, Kuvaja P, Kallioinen M, Turpeenniemi-Hujanen T (2011) A prognostic index in skin melanoma through the combination of matrix metalloproteinase-2, Ki67, and p53. Hum Pathol 42(8):1103–1111
36. Kluger HM, Hoyt K, Bacchiocchi A, Mayer T, Kirsch J, Kluger Y, Sznol M, Ariyan S, Molinaro A, Halaban R (2011) Plasma markers for identifying patients with metastatic melanoma. Clin Cancer Res 17(8):2417–2425
37. Bu W, Tang ZY, Sun FX, Ye SL, Liu KD, Xue Q, Chen J, Gao DM (1998) Effects of matrix metalloproteinase inhibitor BB-94 on liver cancer growth and metastasis in a patient-like orthotopic model LCI-D20. Hepatogastroenterology 45(22):1056–1061
38. Rey MC, Bonamigo RR, Cartell A, Furian R, Bonfá R, Bonfá R (2011) MMP-2 and TIMP-2 in cutaneous melanoma: association with prognostic factors and description in cutaneous metastases. Am J Dermatopathol 33(4):413–414
39. Kurschat P, Wickenhauser C, Groth W, Krieg T, Mauch C (2002) Identification of activated matrix metalloproteinase-2 (MMP-2) as the main gelatinolytic enzyme in malignant melanoma by in situ zymography. J Pathol 197(2): 179–187
40. Djukanovic D, Hofmann U, Sucker A, Rittgen W, Schadendorf D (2000) Comparison of S100 protein and MIA protein as serum marker for malignant melanoma. Anticancer Res 20(3B):2203–2207
41. Bougatef F, Menashi S, Khayati F, Naïmi B, Porcher R, Podgorniak MP, Millot G, Janin A, Calvo F, Lebbé C, Mourah S (2010) EMMPRIN promotes melanoma cells malignant properties through a HIF-2alpha mediated up-regulation of VEGF-receptor-2. PLoS One 5(8):e12265
42. Kanekura T, Chen X (2010) CD147/basigin promotes progression of malignant melanoma and other cancers. J Dermatol Sci 57(3): 149–154
43. van den Oord JJ, Paemen L, Opdenakker G, de Wolf-Peeters C (1997) Expression of gelatinase B and the extracellular matrix metalloproteinase inducer EMMPRIN in benign and malignant pigment cell lesions of the skin. Am J Pathol 151(3):665–670
44. Wang YG, Kim SJ, Baek JH, Lee HW, Jeong SY, Chun KH (2012) Galectin-3 increases the motility of mouse melanoma cells by regulating MMP-1 expression. Exp Mol Med 44(6): 387–393
45. Chen T, Zhu J (2010) Evaluation of EMMPRIN and MMP-2 in the prognosis of primary cutaneous malignant melanoma. Med Oncol 27(4):1185–1191
46. Guida M, Riccobon A, Biasco G, Ravaioli A, Casamassima A, Freschi A, Palma MD, Galligioni E, Nortilli R, Chiarion-Sileni V, Picozzo J, Romanini A, Nanni O, Ridolfi R, Italian Melanoma Intergroup (IMI) (2006)

Basal level and behaviour of cytokines in a randomized outpatient trial comparing chemotherapy and biochemotherapy in metastatic melanoma. Melanoma Res 16(4):317–323

47. Boyano MD, Garcia-Vázquez MD, López-Michelena T, Gardeazabal J, Bilbao J, Cañavate ML, Galdeano AG, Izu R, Díaz-Ramón L, Raton JA, Díaz-Pérez JL (2000) Soluble interleukin-2 receptor, intercellular adhesion molecule-1 and interleukin-10 serum levels in patients with melanoma. Br J Cancer 83(7): 847–852
48. Vuoristo MS, Laine S, Huhtala H, Parvinen LM, Hahka-Kemppinen M, Korpela M, Kumpulainen E, Kellokumpu-Lehtinen P (2001) Serum adhesion molecules and interleukin-2 receptor as markers of tumour load and prognosis in advanced cutaneous melanoma. Eur J Cancer 37(13):1629–1634
49. Alonso SR, Ortiz P, Pollán M, Pérez-Gómez B, Sánchez L, Acuña MJ, Pajares R, Martínez-Tello FJ, Hortelano CM, Piris MA, Rodríguez-Peralto JL (2004) Progression in cutaneous malignant melanoma is associated with distinct expression profiles: a tissue microarray-based study. Am J Pathol 164(1):193–203
50. de Souza CF, Morais AS, Jasiulionis MG (2012) Biomarkers as key contributors in treating malignant melanoma metastases. Dermatol Res Pract 2012:156068. Epub 2011 Oct 31
51. Gould Rothberg BE, Bracken MB, Rimm DL (2009) Tissue biomarkers for prognosis in cutaneous melanoma: a systematic review and meta-analysis. J Natl Cancer Inst 101(7):452–474
52. Florenes VA, Maelandsmo GM, Faye R, Nesland JM, Holm R (2001) Cyclin A expression in superficial spreading malignant melanomas correlates with clinical outcome. J Pathol 195(5):530–536
53. Niezabitowski A, Czajecki K, Rys J (1999) Prognostic evaluation of cutaneous malignant melanoma: a clinicopathologic and immunohistochemical study. J Surg Oncol 70(3): 150–160
54. Duncan LM, Deeds J, Hunter J, Shao J, Holmgren LM, Woolf EA, Tepper RI, Shyjan AW (1998) Down-regulation of the novel gene melastatin correlates with potential for melanoma metastasis. Cancer Res 58:1515
55. Deeds J, Cronin F, Duncan LM (2000) Patterns of melastatin mRNA expression in melanocytic tumors. Hum Pathol 31:1346
56. Erickson LA, Letts GA, Shah SM, Shackelton JB, Duncan LM (2009) TRPM1 (Melastatin-1/MLSN1) mRNA expression in Spitz nevi and nodular melanomas. Mod Pathol 22(7): 969–976
57. Duncan LM, Deeds J, Cronin FE, Donovan M, Sober AJ, Kauffman M, McCarthy JJ (2001) Melastatin expression and prognosis in cutaneous malignant melanoma. J Clin Oncol 19:568–576
58. Miller AJ, Du J, Rowan S, Hershey CL, Widlund HR, Fisher DE (2004) Transcriptional regulation of the melanoma prognostic marker melastatin (TRPM1) by MITF in melanocytes and melanoma. Cancer Res 64:509
59. Hoek KS, Schlegel NC, Eichhoff OM, Widmer DS, Praetorius C, Einarsson SO, Valgeirsdottir S, Bergsteinsdottir K, Schepsky A, Dummer R, Steingrimsson E (2008) Novel MITF targets identified using a two-step DNA microarray strategy. Pigment Cell Melanoma Res 21:665
60. Garraway LA, Widlund HR, Rubin MA, Getz G, Berger AJ, Ramaswamy S, Beroukhim R, Milner DA, Granter SR, Du J, Lee C, Wagner SN, Li C, Golub TR, Rimm DL, Meyerson ML, Fisher DE, Sellers WR (2005) Integrative genomic analyses identify MITF as a lineage survival oncogene amplified in malignant melanoma. Nature 436:117–122
61. Du J, Widlund HR, Horstmann MA, Ramaswamy S, Ross K, Huber WE, Nishimura EK, Golub TR, Fisher DE (2004) Critical role of CDK2 for melanoma growth linked to its melanocyte-specific transcriptional regulation by MITF. Cancer Cell 6:565–576
62. Yokoyama S, Woods SL, Boyle GM, Aoude LG, MacGregor S, Zismann V, Gartside M, Cust AE, Haq R, Harland M, Taylor JC, Duffy DL, Holohan K, Dutton-Regester K, Palmer JM, Bonazzi V, Stark MS, Symmons J, Law MH, Schmidt C, Lanagan C, O'Connor L, Holland EA, Schmid H, Maskiell JA, Jetann J, Ferguson M, Jenkins MA, Kefford RF, Giles GG, Armstrong BK, Aitken JF, Hopper JL, Whiteman DC, Pharoah PD, Easton DF, Dunning AM, Newton-Bishop JA, Montgomery GW, Martin NG, Mann GJ, Bishop DT, Tsao H, Trent JM, Fisher DE, Hayward NK, Brown KM (2011) A novel recurrent mutation in *MITF* predisposes to familial and sporadic melanoma. Nature 480:99–103
63. Flaherty KT, Hodi FS, Fisher DE (2012) From genes to drugs: targeted strategies for melanoma. Nat Rev Cancer 12(5):349–361
64. Hillesheim PB, Slone S, Kelley D, Malone J, Bahrami S (2011) An immunohistochemical comparison between MiTF and MART-1 with Azure blue counterstaining in the setting of solar lentigo and melanoma in situ. J Cutan Pathol 38(7):565–569

65. Nielsen PS, Riber-Hansen R, Steiniche T (2011) Immunohistochemical double stains against Ki67/MART1 and HMB45/MITF: promising diagnostic tools in melanocytic lesions. Am J Dermatopathol 33(4):361–370
66. Samija I, Lukac J, Marić-Brozić J, Buljan M, Alajbeg I, Kovacević D, Situm M, Kusić Z (2010) Prognostic value of microphthalmia-associated transcription factor and tyrosinase as markers for circulating tumor cells detection in patients with melanoma. Melanoma Res 20(4):293–302
67. Bosserhoff AK, Hein R, Bogdahn U, Buettner R (1996) Structure and promoter analysis of the gene encoding the human melanoma-inhibiting protein MIA. J Biol Chem 271(1):490–495
68. Garnier JP, Letellier S, Cassinat B, Lebbé C, Kerob D, Baccard M, Morel P, Basset-Seguin N, Dubertret L, Bousquet B, Stoitchkov K, Le Bricon T (2007) Clinical value of combined determination of plasma L-DOPA/tyrosine ratio, S100B, MIA and LDH in melanoma. Eur J Cancer 43(4):816–821
69. Díaz-Lagares A, Alegre E, Arroyo A, González-Cao M, Zudaire ME, Viteri S, Martín-Algarra S, González A (2011) Evaluation of multiple serum markers in advanced melanoma. Tumour Biol 32(6):1155–1161
70. Nakahara S, Oka N, Raz A (2005) On the role of galectin-3 in cancer apoptosis. Apoptosis 10(2):267–275
71. Brown ER, Doig T, Anderson N, Brenn T, Doherty V, Xu Y, Bartlett JM, Smyth JF, Melton DW (2012) Association of galectin-3 expression with melanoma progression and prognosis. Eur J Cancer 48(6):865–874
72. Buljan M, Šitum M, Tomas D, Milošević M, Krušlin B (2011) Prognostic value of galectin-3 in primary cutaneous melanoma. J Eur Acad Dermatol Venereol 25(10):1174–1181
73. Rangel J, Nosrati M, Torabian S, Shaikh L, Leong SP, Haqq C, Miller JR 3rd, Sagebiel RW, Kashani-Sabet M (2008) Osteopontin as a molecular prognostic marker for melanoma. Cancer 112(1):144–150
74. Klein WM, Wu BP, Zhao S, Wu H, Klein-Szanto AJ, Tahan SR (2007) Increased expression of stem cell markers in malignant melanoma. Mod Pathol 20(1):102–107
75. Ebrahimnejad A, Streichert T, Nollau P, Horst AK, Wagener C, Bamberger AM, Brümmer J (2004) CEACAM1 enhances invasion and migration of melanocytic and melanoma cells. Am J Pathol 165(5):1781–1787
76. Thies A, Moll I, Berger J, Wagener C, Brümmer J, Schulze HJ, Brunner G, Schumacher U (2002) CEACAM1 expression in cutaneous malignant melanoma predicts the development of metastatic disease. J Clin Oncol 20(10):2530–2536
77. Watson-Hurst K, Becker D (2006) The role of N-cadherin, MCAM and beta3 integrin in melanoma progression, proliferation, migration and invasion. Cancer Biol Ther 5(10):1375–1382
78. Pacifico MD, Grover R, Richman PI, Daley FM, Buffa F, Wilson G (2005) Development of a tissue array for primary melanoma with long-term follow-up: discovering melanoma cell adhesion molecule as an important prognostic marker. Plast Reconstr Surg 115(2):367–375
79. Kärnell R, Kågedal B, Lindholm C, Nilsson B, Arstrand K, Ringborg U (2000) The value of cysteinyldopa in the follow-up of disseminated malignant melanoma. Melanoma Res 10(4): 363–369
80. Kvam E, Dahle J (2005) The pheomelanin precursor 5-S-cysteinyldopa protects melanocytes from membrane damage induced by ultraviolet A radiation. Cancer Lett 221(2):131–134
81. Bánfalvi T, Boldizsár M, Gergye M, Gilde K, Kremmer T, Ottó S (2002) Comparison of prognostic significance of serum 5-S-Cysteinyldopa, LDH and S-100B protein in Stage III-IV malignant melanoma. Pathol Oncol Res 8(3):183–187
82. Slominski A, Zmijewski MA, Pawelek J (2012) L-tyrosine and L-dihydroxyphenylalanine as hormone-like regulators of melanocyte functions. Pigment Cell Melanoma Res 25(1): 14–27
83. Abaffy T, Duncan R, Riemer DD, Tietje O, Elgart G, Milikowski C, DeFazio RA (2010) Differential volatile signatures from skin, naevi and melanoma: a novel approach to detect a pathological process. PLoS One 5(11):e13813
84. Greenberg ES, Chong KK, Huynh KT, Tanaka R, Hoon DS (2012) Epigenetic biomarkers in skin cancer. Cancer Lett
85. Nguyen T, Kuo C, Nicholl MB, Sim MS, Turner RR, Morton DL, Hoon DS (2011) Downregulation of microRNA-29c is associated with hypermethylation of tumor-related genes and disease outcome in cutaneous melanoma. Epigenetics 6(3):388–394
86. McShane LM, Altman DG, Gion M, Clark GM, Statistics Subcommittee of NCI-EORTC Working Group on Cancer Diagnostics (2006) Reporting recommendations for tumor MARKer prognostic studies (REMARK). Breast Cancer Res Treat 100(2):229–235
87. Schramm SJ, Mann GJ (2011) Melanoma prognosis: a REMARK-based systematic review and bioinformatic analysis of immunohistochemical and gene microarray studies. Mol Cancer Ther 10(8):1520–1528, Epub 2011 Jun 9. Review

88. Pras F, Perra MT, Murtas D, Minerba L, Floris C, Maxia C (2008) Combinations of apoptosis and cell-cycle control biomarkers predict the outcome of human melanoma. Oncol Rep 20:271–277

89. Kashani-Sabet M, Venna S, Nosrati M, Rangel J, Sucker A, Egberts F (2009) A multimarker prognostic assay for primary cutaneous melanoma. Clin Cancer Res 15: 6987–6992

Chapter 12

Chromosomal Copy Number Analysis in Melanoma Diagnostics

Jeffrey P. North, Swapna S. Vemula, and Boris C. Bastian

Abstract

The majority of melanocytic neoplasms can be correctly diagnosed using routine histopathologic analysis. However, a significant minority of tumors have ambiguous histopathologic attributes that overlap between melanocytic nevi and melanoma. Ancillary tests that assist in distinguishing potentially lethal melanomas from benign melanocytic nevi with atypical histopathologic features are available, but still need refining.

Most melanomas have chromosomal copy number aberrations, frequently involving multiple chromosomes. With rare exceptions, such anomalies are not found in melanocytic nevi. This difference formed the basis to develop assays that can help distinguish melanoma from nevi by fluorescence in situ hybridization (FISH) and comparative genomic hybridization (CGH). FISH can detect chromosomal copy number changes of a limited number of loci within individual cells. By contrast, CGH assesses copy number across the entire genome, but typically is performed on bulk cell populations so that copy number changes in individual cells or subpopulations of cells can go undetected. Both FISH and CGH have been used to provide genomic information in histopathologically ambiguous melanocytic tumors that can assist pathologists make correct diagnoses.

Key words Fluorescence in situ hybridization, FISH, Comparative genomic hybridization, CGH, Molecular diagnostics, Ambiguous melanocytic tumors, Copy number changes

1 Introduction

1.1 Chromosomal Copy Number Changes in Melanocytic Tumors

Testing for chromosomal aberrations in melanoma began with karyotyping of cultured melanocytes from various types of tumors. An initial study showed normal karyotypes for common nevi, single karyotypic abnormalities in a minority of dysplastic nevi (2/6), and multiple aberrations in 37 melanomas [1]. Subsequent studies confirmed abnormal chromosomal copy numbers among melanomas, while the vast majority of melanocytic nevi had normal karyotypes [2]. Loss of one copy of chromosome 9 was reported to occur in both dysplastic nevi (2/26) and melanoma cell cultures (2/11). Most of these preliminary studies found melanomas had multiple chromosomal rearrangements or deletions which were not present

Magdalena Thurin and Francesco M. Marincola (eds.), *Molecular Diagnostics for Melanoma: Methods and Protocols*, Methods in Molecular Biology, vol. 1102, DOI 10.1007/978-1-62703-727-3_12, © Springer Science+Business Media New York 2014

in nevi. Small studies found chromosomal rearrangements in some dysplastic nevi [3] and single reciprocal translocations in 50 % (4/8) of cultured nevi [4].

1.2 Comparative Genomic Hybridization (CGH) in Melanoma Diagnostics

In 1992, comparative genomic hybridization (CGH) was introduced as a method for analyzing DNA copy number changes in neoplasms and organisms [5]. CGH determines DNA copy number by the competitive hybridization of two differentially labeled DNA populations, e.g., tumor DNA and normal control DNA, hybridized to a substrate representing the genome. Initially the hybridization was performed on metaphase chromosomes, but refinement of the technique led to replacement of metaphase chromosomes with printed microarrays of genomic DNA. The ratio of the two fluorescent signals is used to determine copy number at each locus, where increased signal intensity from the tumor DNA over control DNA at a given genomic coordinate indicates a copy number increase, whereas the opposite scenario indicates a copy number decrease (Fig. 1). The first studies with CGH in melanoma were performed on uveal melanomas, revealing multiple chromosomal gains and losses [6]. Further studies demonstrated that CGH could reliably be used on formalin-fixed paraffin-embedded (FFPE) tissue of uveal melanomas, expanding the use of this

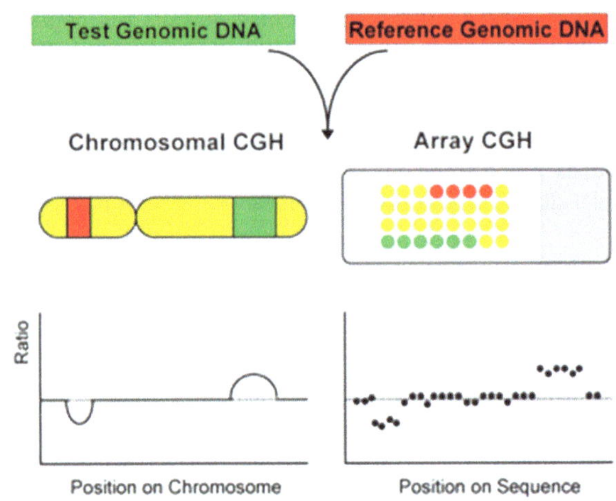

Fig. 1 Comparative genomic hybridization (CGH). DNA from the test sample and a normal reference DNA are labeled with different fluorophores (e.g., *green* and *red*) and then simultaneously hybridized to a third DNA attached to a solid substrate, such as a glass slide. Originally, hybridizations were carried out on metaphase spreads, which represent the genome in an orientated state (*left panel*). This method has become replaced by microarrays of printed DNA fragments, representing the genome or genomic region of interest at a specific resolution that depends on the spacing of the DNA fragments (*right panel*). DNA copy number increase in the *green-labeled* test DNA will manifest as increased test-to-reference fluorescence intensity ratio, whereas copy number decreases result in a lower ratio. A ratio of 1 indicates a balanced copy number

technique to the vast libraries of archived FFPE specimens stored at pathology labs [7].

The first study of CGH in cutaneous melanoma detected chromosomal gains and/or losses in 94 % (30/32) of melanomas [8]. A subsequent study of CGH on cutaneous melanomas and melanocytic nevi showed chromosomal gains or losses in 96 % (127/132) of melanomas, while such aberrations were detected in only 13 % (7/54) of melanocytic nevi [9]. All nevi with aberrations were Spitz nevi and 6 of the 7 had isolated 11p gain, a distinct chromosomal gain not seen in any of the melanomas. Sites commonly gained among melanomas included chromosomes 6p (37.1 %), 1q (32.6 %), 7p (31.8 %), 7q (31.8 %), 8q (25.0 %), 17q (24.2 %), and 20q (22.0 %). The most frequent losses were 9p (64.4 %), 9q (36.4 %), 10q (36.4 %), 10p (29.5 %), 6q (25.8 %), and 11q (21.2 %). Additional gains at chromosomes 1p, 4q12 were reported in a smaller analysis of 28 melanomas [10]. The differential pattern of chromosomal aberrations observed in melanomas and not in nevi served as the basis for developing tests to assist in the diagnosis of melanocytic neoplasms with ambiguous histopathologic features.

In 2001, microarrays utilizing bacterial artificial chromosomes (BACs) spanning all 24 chromosomes were introduced [11]. Depending on the spacing of probes, microarrays provide a higher resolution of the genome compared to CGH on metaphase chromosomes, which due to the dense packing of the DNA, practically restricts the resolution to 10–20 megabases. The initial CGH arrays offered approximately 1.4 megabase resolution, with subsequent generations of microarrays tiling the entire genome. Commercial oligonucleotide arrays offer theoretical resolution in the low kilobase range, but practically have a lower resolution, as the signals have to be averaged over several adjacent probes. Array-based CGH (aCGH) has dramatically increased the precision and usability of CGH for clinical diagnostics, permitting detection of smaller regions of chromosomal gains and losses (Fig. 1, right panel). A first aCGH study of 126 primary melanomas by Curtin et al. showed common, recurrent copy number changes of several chromosomes and revealed differences in the pattern of copy number changes depending on the anatomic site of the primary tumor and the degree of sun-exposure as detailed below. An analysis of 101 short-term cultures and melanoma cell lines with aCGH for copy number changes and LOH alterations showed a largely similar pattern of aberrations [12].

1.2.1 Melanomas on Chronically and Intermittently Sun-Damaged Skin

The aCGH study by Curtin et al. found increased copy numbers of chromosomes 1q, 6p, 7, 8q, 17q, and 20q and loss of 9p, 6q, 10 in melanomas associated with intermittent sun damage. Melanomas occurring in areas with chronic sun exposure had similar chromosomal aberrations but in addition, showed gain of 11q13 and loss 13, while chromosome 10 was infrequently lost [13].

1.2.2 Acral Melanoma

Melanomas on acral skin exhibit a high grade of genomic instability early in development, with 89–100 % exhibiting focal chromosomal amplifications (>3-fold copy number increase) [9, 13, 14]. The most common sites of amplification include chromosome 11q13 (CCND1-cyclin D1 gene), 12q14 (CDK4 gene), 22q11-13, and 5p15 (hTERT-telomerase gene). Such amplifications have been observed in acral melanoma in situ and even in melanocytes in the histologically normal-appearing skin surrounding acral melanoma (field cells) [14, 15]. Other chromosomal regions commonly gained in acral melanoma include 4q, 6p, 7, 8q, 17q, 20q. Reported areas of loss include 6q, 9p, 10, 11q, 15q, 16q, 21q [9, 13].

1.2.3 Mucosal Melanoma

Like acral melanoma, melanomas occurring at mucosal sites frequently exhibit marked genomic instability with numerous focal amplifications and deletions [13]. In contrast to the regions of amplification in acral melanoma, 1q31, 4q12, and 12q14 (CDK4 gene) are the most common sites of amplification in mucosal melanomas. Chromosomes 1q, 6p, 7, 8q, 11q13, 17q, and 20q are often gained, while 3q, 4q, 6q, 8p, 9p, 10, 11p, 11q, 21q are often lost. A study of 14 sinonasal melanomas with CGH showed repetitive chromosomal gains on 1q (14/14 cases), 6p (13/14), and 8q (8/14) [16].

1.2.4 Blue Nevus and Blue Nevus-Like Melanoma

CGH analysis of 10 unambiguous cellular blue nevi, one deep penetrating nevus, 11 histopathologically ambiguous blue nevus-like proliferations, and 7 unambiguous blue nevus-like melanomas found all 11 nevi and 8 of the 11 ambiguous tumors had no chromosomal aberrations [17]. Three of the ambiguous tumors showed one to three chromosomal aberrations, two of which showed loss of chromosome 3. Other abnormalities included 15q loss, and gain of 6p, 8, and 9q. The one ambiguous tumor with the most aberrations (3) displayed the greatest degree of cytologic atypia, focal necrosis and had a mitotic rate of 3 mitoses/HPF. All 7 blue nevus-like melanomas had at least three chromosomal aberrations (average 8 per case) with chromosome 9 loss and chromosome 20 gain representing the most common aberrations. Gain of chromosome 2p, 4p, 6p, 8q, 16p, 17, 22q and loss of 1p, 5q, 6q, 10p, 16 was seen in at least two of the malignant tumors. In addition to the two ambiguous tumors, chromosome 3 loss was also seen in one blue nevus-like melanoma.

Another diagnostic challenge in blue nevi involves the formation of large, hypercellular nodules in preexisting plaque type blue nevi, raising concern for the possibility of melanoma arising in a blue nevus. Initial report of two such cases labeled plaque type blue nevus with subcutaneous cellular nodules did not have molecular analysis, but had benign clinical follow-up [18]. Subsequent reports of three similar lesions that had more concerning histopathologic features (e.g., focal necrosis or nuclear atypia) found multiple chromosomal aberrations consistent with melanoma [19, 20]. Loss of 6q and gain of 6p was found in all three cases, and 8q and 17q gain, along with 9p and 11q loss, were seen in two of the three. Chromosome 6p gain and 6q loss has also been reported in a blue nevus-like melanoma arising in a Nevus of Ota [21]. Other aberrations in that case included gains of chromosome 1q, 8q, and 9q.

1.2.5 Spitz Nevus and Spitzoid Melanoma

Spitzoid melanocytic proliferations can frequently have conflicting benign and malignant features on routine histopathologic exam. Molecular assessment for genomic aberrations can provide additional valuable diagnostic information. The majority of Spitz nevi have a normal chromosomal complement, while a minority (12–26 %) have chromosome 11p gains [9, 22, 23]. Tumors with11p gain frequently (67 %) harbor HRAS mutations and histopathologically tend to be larger in size, predominantly intradermal, markedly desmoplastic, infiltrative in architecture, and have increased nuclear pleomorphism when compared with Spitz nevi with no chromosomal aberrations [23]. Rarely, Spitz nevi with an isolated 7q21-7qter gain have been reported [22, 24]. Two Spitz nevi with 9p loss of heterozygosity have been reported as well [25].

In a study of 8 unambiguous Spitz nevi, 16 atypical Spitz tumors (ASTs), and 2 unambiguous spitzoid melanomas, aCGH showed no chromosomal aberrations in 88 % (7/8) of Spitz nevi (one Spitz nevus had an isolated 11p gain) and 56 % (9/16) of atypical Spitz tumors [26]. No difference was found in the number of chromosomal aberrations in ASTs with a positive sentinel lymph node biopsy (SLNB) versus those with a negative SLNB. The number of aberrations in ASTs ranged from 1 to 8. Three cases had a gain at chromosome 1p. Loss of chromosome 9 and 1q was seen in two cases each. The only patient with an AST that metastasized causing death had a CGH pattern typical of melanoma with aberrations including loss of 3p, 7q, 8p and 9, and gain of 8q. The one spitzoid melanoma that metastasized widely had multiple chromosomal aberrations including gain of chromosome 8p, 9q, and 11q13. The other spitzoid melanoma had a positive SLNB, but no further recurrence. Only a single aberration (chromosome 9 loss) was found on aCGH. Gain of chromosome 19p in an AST and gain of 6p and 17q, with loss of 1p and 15p in a spitzoid melanoma has also been reported [24].

Deletions of chromosome 3p21 have been identified in a subset of Spitz nevi. The deletions target the BAP1 gene and bi-allelic loss of BAP1 together with BRAF mutation accounts for a type of Spitz nevus with characteristic histopathologic findings [27, 28].

1.2.6 Uveal Melanoma

Uveal melanomas were among the first to be analyzed with CGH, with initial studies showing chromosome 3 and 6q loss and chromosome 6p and 8q gain [6]. Further studies found loss of chromosome 3 had prognostic significance and was found in 73 % of metastasizing uveal melanomas versus 21 % of nonmetastasizing tumors [29]. Chromosome 6q loss and 8q gain were seen more often in metastasizing tumors, and loss of 1p was seen only in metastasizing tumors (33 %) in one study. Another analysis of 100 uveal melanomas reported gain of chromosome 18q11 and loss of 1p33 were the most powerful predictors of poor prognosis [30]. Gains at chromosomes 6q16, 21q11.2, 9q12, and 3q12 were also poor prognostic indicators in that cohort. However, subsequent studies have not found 18q11 or 21q11 to be a significant prognostic marker [31]. In another study gain of 8q, and losses of 3, 8p, and 16q were associated with metastasis [32]. Other reported aberrations in studies of uveal melanoma include losses at chromosomes 8p, 13q and 18, and gains of chromosomes 1q, 6p, 16p, 20q, and 22.

1.2.7 Congenital Melanocytic Nevi

CGH analysis of congenital nevi typically has not revealed any chromosomal aberrations. So called benign nodular proliferations ("proliferative nodules") within congenital melanocytic nevi frequently show gain or loss of entire chromosomes, particularly loss of chromosome 7, 9, or 10 [33]. Despite the presence of hypercellularity, nuclear atypia and an increased proliferation rate, these lesions behave in a benign fashion. The CGH pattern observed in these nodules is distinct from melanoma, which features multiple gains or losses of chromosome fragments. Loss or gain of entire chromosomes does occur in melanomas, including melanomas arising within congenital nevi, but typically occurs with other aberrations involving fragments of chromosomes.

1.2.8 Metastatic Melanoma

Comparison of genetic aberrations present in metastatic melanoma and absent in the corresponding primary tumors can provide insight into tumor progression and the genetic changes associated with metastasis. One study of 16 primary melanomas and 12 metastatic lesions showed gain of chromosome 1q, 2q25, 6q25, 7, 8, 10q, 11q13, 11q21, 13q21, 14q, 15q, 17q, and loss of chromosome 1p33, 2p21, 9q34, 9p21, 12q24, 16p, 16q, 17, 19q, 20, 21, 22, and Y in metastatic lesions that were not present in the corresponding primary melanoma. Loss of chromosome 4, 9p21, and 10p were associated with a metastatic phenotype in one cell line [34].

By substituting normal control DNA with some other type of test DNA, the CGH technique can be modified to provide comparative genetic information between two tumors. For example, to characterize a more invasive phenotype in a melanoma cell line, CGH directly comparing DNA from a highly invasive clone and a weakly invasive clone derived from the same melanoma cell line was performed. This modified CGH showed many similarities in the CGH profiles supporting a common derivation, but the more invasive cells featured additional losses at 1q, 4q, 11p, 19q, and 20p [35].

1.3 Fluorescence In Situ Hybridization (FISH) in Melanoma Diagnostics

Multi-probe FISH assays are currently used as ancillary tests in the diagnosis of ambiguous melanocytic neoplasms. The most widespread method combines three probes to loci on chromosome 6 (6p25, 6q23, and CEP6) and one to chromosome 11q13. This 4-probe combination was determined as useful for discriminating melanomas from nevi in a study which used existing CGH data to select and validate various probe combinations in melanocytic neoplasms divided into training and validation cohorts [36]. Among the 14 probes tested, the combination of the four aforementioned probes showed the greatest sensitivity and specificity in differentiating melanomas and nevi in an initial cohort of 192 unambiguous melanomas and nevi, with gain of 6p25, gain of 11q13, or loss of 6q23 indicating a malignant diagnosis. The centromeric probe for chromosome 6 served as a reference to calculate gain or loss of 6p25 and 6q23. A second cohort of 109 melanomas and nevi was tested to optimize thresholds for FISH probe counts to discriminate between melanomas and nevi. The assay was then validated on a third cohort yielding a diagnostic sensitivity and specificity of 87 % and 95 % respectively. In a fourth group consisting of 27 ambiguous neoplasms for which long-term clinical follow up was available, all six cases that developed either bulky regional metastasis or distant metastasis tested positive (100 % sensitivity).

Multiple studies using the same 4 probe FISH set reported similar sensitivity and specificity values in differentiating melanomas from nevi [37–39]. Prior to this 2009 FISH study, FISH had been used in small studies of melanocytic tumors for detecting homozygous deletions at the CDKN2 9p21 locus in melanoma cell lines [40], detecting monosomy 3 in uveal melanomas [41], confirming chromosomal aberrations found in CGH studies [42, 43], detection of 17p11 (*TP53* gene) loss in melanoma metastases [44], identifying increased telomere length in invasive and metastatic melanoma [45], identification of 11p gain in 12 % (12/102) of Spitz nevi [23], detecting increased copy number of 8q24 (c-Myc) and 7p12 (EGFR) in metastatic melanoma [46, 47], and to differentiate melanoma from clear cell sarcoma by testing for the t(12;22)(q13;q13) translocation typical of clear cell sarcoma [48]. FISH has also been used in acral melanoma to characterize the evolution of histopathologically normal-appearing melanocytes with chromosomal aberrations surrounding primary melanomas (field cells) [15]. Field cells extended significantly beyond the in situ component in the majority of acral melanoma (average 6 mm for melanoma in situ, 4.5 mm for invasive melanoma), and FISH could be used to assess surgical margins at the genetic level in such cases.

After the 2009 4 probe FISH study, FISH has been increasingly used in both the research and clinical settings. Small scale studies with this probe set targeting chromosomes 6 and 11 have yielded similar or better sensitivities and specificities compared to the original study in the following settings:

- Distinguishing "lentiginous junctional melanoma of the elderly" from lentiginous nevi [49]
- Distinguishing blue nevi from blue nevus-like melanoma [50, 51]
- Distinguishing nodal nevi from metastatic melanoma in lymph nodes [52]
- Distinguishing conjunctival nevi from conjunctival melanomas [53]
- Distinguishing nevoid melanoma from mitotically active nevi [54]
- Differentiating intraepidermal melanocytic proliferations with prominent pagetoid scatter (e.g., junctional Spitz nevi, "de novo epithelioid melanocytic dysplasia", melanoma in situ) [55]

A lower sensitivity (73 %) was reported for this 4 probe FISH test in differentiating 22 pigmented spindle cell nevi from 24 spindle cell melanomas, with a specificity of 93 % [56]. Results from a study of desmoplastic melanoma and sclerosing nevi showed a sensitivity of 47 % (7/15) for detecting desmoplastic melanoma with a specificity of 100 % (0/15 sclerosing nevi) [57].

1.3.1 FISH in Spitzoid Melanocytic Neoplasms

Use of the chromosome 6 and 11 FISH assay in spitzoid melanocytic proliferations has generated mixed results. FISH testing in a cohort of 25 atypical Spitz tumors (AST) was positive in 24 % (6/25), with the only case with a fatal outcome testing positive [58]. In another study of 16 ASTs and 2 spitzoid melanomas with both FISH and aCGH, FISH was negative in all 16 ASTs, including one case that metastasized and six cases that by aCGH had chromosomal aberrations at loci not covered by the FISH assay [26]. As no adverse outcomes were reported in the latter six cases, it is not clear if these were benign or malignant. FISH was positive in 50 % (1/2) of spitzoid melanomas tested.

In a cohort of 90 ambiguous melanocytic tumors (50 % spitzoid) tested with the 4 probe FISH test, 43 % (9/21) of cases with lymph node involvement or distant metastasis tested positive [59]. The sensitivity in the spitzoid group was slightly higher at 55 % (6/11). This sensitivity is considerably lower than in the other studies of unambiguous neoplasms. However, while this report does raise concern about the utility of FISH in ambiguous melanocytic tumors, the inclusion of regional lymph node involvement as an endpoint in this study is controversial. While atypical Spitz tumors appear to have an increased frequency of regional lymph node involvement, progression to metastatic disease appears to be much less frequent than in bona fide melanomas [60]. One possible confounding problem contributing to the divergent results is the fact that several of the studies used different thresholds and evaluation criteria. In summary, while a positive FISH test seems to identify melanomas with metastatic potential with high specificity, the sensitivity in specific settings needs to be improved to make a negative test more clinically useful.

The CDKN2A gene on chromosome 9p21 encoding the tumor suppressor proteins p16 and p14ARF is the most commonly deleted locus in melanoma. FISH testing for 9p21 loss in 28 ASTs and 13 Spitz nevi showed 9p21 loss in 29 % (8/28) of ASTs and in the one congenital Spitz nevus tested, while all 12 conventional Spitz nevi were normal [61]. However, 9p21 loss did not correlate with progression to metastatic disease in the group of ASTs. Addition of a chromosome 9p21 probe to the 4 probe FISH set targeting chromosomes 6 and 11 has been reported to improve sensitivity of FISH in detecting spitzoid melanomas [62]. The sensitivity for the standard 4 probe FISH test alone for unambiguous spitzoid melanoma was 70 % (30/43) [62]. Detection of homozygous 9p21 loss in >33 % of cells increased the sensitivity to 85 %. No homozygous 9p21 loss was seen in a training cohort of 146 nevi, including 16 Spitz nevi. A study of a 4 probe FISH set testing for homozygous 9p21 loss along with gain of 6p25, 11q13, or 8q24 has yielded a sensitivity and specificity of 94 % and 98 % respectively in a validation cohort of 51 unambiguous melanomas and 51 unambiguous nevi [63]. Additional studies are needed to confirm these findings and to determine the utility in ambiguous tumors.

1.3.2 FISH and Prognosis

While data for FISH in the prognosis of histopathologically ambiguous melanocytic tumors are mixed and few in number, studies evaluating the prognostic ability of the FISH in unambiguous melanomas have shown positive results. FISH detection of topoisomerase 1 amplification on 20q12 has been associated with a poor prognosis in one study [64]. A retrospective analysis of the 4 probe FISH set targeting chromosomes 6 and 11 on 144 primary melanomas with a tumor thickness >2 mm showed that melanomas that tested positive had a worse disease-specific survival than melanomas that were negative with FISH [65]. 82 % of the melanomas tested positive, similar to the sensitivity reported in other studies. However, the sensitivity for melanomas that progressed to stage IV disease was 93 % (40/43), with a 97 % sensitivity for melanoma-specific mortality (26/27) [65]. A second study of the same 4 probe FISH set and an additional probe set containing 8q24, 9p21, cent9, and 20q13 in 55 metastasizing melanomas and 42 nonmetastasizing melanomas found that copy number gains in 11q13 and 8q24 are highly linked to metastatic potential [66].

A subsequent study of 40 melanomas with 8q24 gain by the same research group confirmed the prognostic value of 8q24 gain [67]. Additionally, the melanomas with 8q24 gain were noted to preferentially occur in skin with intermittent sun exposure, to be clinically and histologically amelanotic, to have a nodular or primary dermal architecture, and were infrequently associated with a precursor nevus. Amplification of chromosome 11q13 gain was also proposed as an indicator of poor prognosis based on a study of seven patients [68].

1.4 Pitfalls of CGH and FISH

The main pitfall of CGH is that aberrations can remain undetected in the presence of a significant proportion of cells that do not share the aberrations. This can happen due to heterogeneity of the neoplastic cell population or due to an excess of normal cells in the sample. The quality of the measurement is dependent on DNA quality, which depends on sample age and fixation time. Suboptimal DNA quality can manifest itself as "noisy" profiles with jitters or waves that may simulate copy number changes.

The strength of FISH is that it can be applied to single cells of a neoplastic population. It therefore has a higher potential sensitivity to detect cancerous growth in cases in which the neoplastic population is small, or if the growth is heterogeneous and only contains a small proportion of cells that harbor the aberrations of interest. A disadvantage compared to CGH is that it can only assess a comparatively minor portion of the genome for copy number alterations. Pitfalls include observer bias in how cells are selected for copy number analysis. This can be a significant source of error in finding aberrations that are not present, at least not in a clone of cells. A clone of cells is defined as a collection of cells that share a common ancestor from which they recently derived (ultimately all cells in an organism are clonally related). For that reason they are expected to reside in close proximity to each other. Benign neoplasms can have random, i.e., nonclonal, chromosomal aberrations and, furthermore, individual nuclei are subject to truncation by sectioning and thereby to loss of FISH signals. For these reasons, it is important that a large enough sample of random cells in a given region of interest is analyzed to avoid observer selection bias.

As the goal is to identify a clonal population of cells that share common chromosomal aberrations, the regions from which the nuclei are enumerated should be carefully selected after screening the entire neoplasm for possible imbalances in number. After an area with potential aberrations has been located, a random sample of at least ten nuclei within that area should be enumerated. Other pitfalls of FISH are those that result from polyploidy of tumor cells, which results in a copy number increase of the loci interrogated, but in a balanced way, as the entire genome is present at increased copy number. This can lead to false positive results. Elevated signal counts for all probes in all or most cells (single signals may be lost due to truncation of nuclei in cutting tissue sections) is indicative of polyploidy. Tetraploidy has been seen in 10 % (4/41) of Spitz nevi in one study [69]. Similarly, tetraploidy was seen in the epithelioid/spitzoid portion of 14 % (4/28) of biphasic melanocytic nevi with an "atypical epithelioid cell component" with benign clinical follow up [70]. Tetraploidy can also be seen in melanoma [71].

Finally it can also be difficult to find the neoplastic population in samples that are small or heterogeneous, as, with a fluorescent microscope, components of normal tissue can be misidentified as

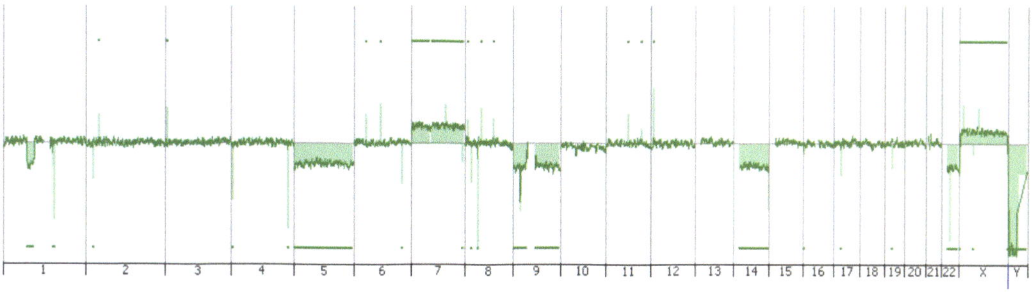

Fig. 2 CGH analysis of an archival sample of a primary melanoma. The *x* axis represents the genome from the short arm of chromosome 1 to the Y chromosome at the very *right*. The *y* axis shows the smoothed log2 ratio of tumor to reference signal for each array element. The test DNA stems from archival tissue, which due to its suboptimal quality introduces jitter. The ratio changes indicate copy number increase of chromosome 7 and loss of parts of chromosome 1p, as well as chromosomes 5, 9, 14, and 22. There also is a narrow homozygous deletion encompassing the CDKN2A locus on chromosome 9p.21. The *narrow vertical lines* showing positive and negative log2 ratios represent narrow regions of constitutional copy number variation and are irrelevant for the assessment of tumor-specific copy number changes

tumor components. Familiarity with the use of immunofluorescent microscopy and the microanatomy of the skin helps minimize this problem.

1.5 Conclusions

Molecular techniques such as CGH and FISH can provide valuable diagnostic and prognostic information in melanocytic tumors. Each technique has its own strengths and weaknesses. CGH provides an overview of the entire genome (Fig. 2), but requires a relatively pure sample of tumor DNA and cannot visualize genetic heterogeneity within a tumor. FISH allows resolution of genomic aberrations at the single cell level (Fig. 3), but provides only a small glimpse of the tumor genome. FISH can also be utilized to detect structural aberrations such as translocations in the absence of copy number changes, e.g., differentiating melanoma from clear cell sarcoma by detection of the clear cell sarcoma t(12:22) translocation.

2 Materials

2.1 Fluorescence In Situ Hybridization (FISH)

1. HYBrite temperature control platform (Vysis, we use Model #30-102720).
2. VP 2000 tissue processor (Vysis) (optional—*see* **Note 1**).
3. Zeiss Imager. M1 fluorescence microscope with appropriate filter sets.
4. Two water baths.

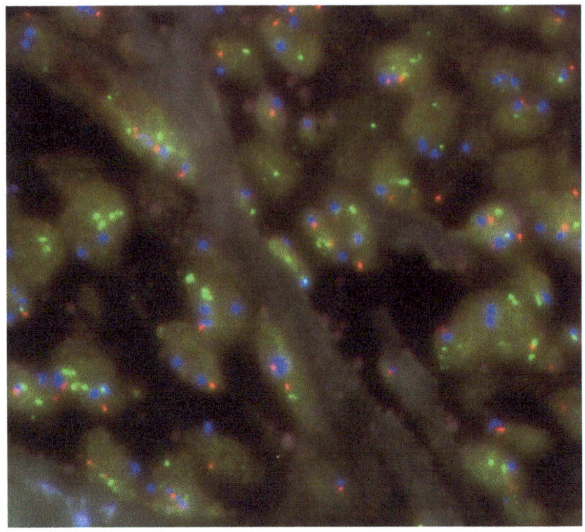

Fig. 3 FISH Analysis of a primary melanoma. The image shows three channels of the four-color hybridization with a copy number increase of the green probe (CCND1) compared to the blue probe (centromere of chromosome 6), and relative loss of the red probe (MYB) compared to the blue probe

5. Melanoma FISH probe mix (Vysis): Make probe mix according to Vysis probe instructions, RREB1(6p25) (SpRed): (#04N32-020), CEP6 (centromere 6, 6p11.1-q11.1) (SpAqua):(#06J54-016), MYB1(6q23) (SpGold):(#04N33-020), CCND1 (11q13)(SpGreen):(#01N88-020). Each slide requires approximately 10 μL, comprised of 7 μL of hybridization buffer (Vysis LSI/WCP hybridization mix) per 1 μL equivalent of FISH probe. Add water to bring to 10 μL if needed. If more than 3 μL of DNA probes, the mix of DNA probes need to be precipitated to 3 μL before adding the hybridization buffer.
6. DAPI I (1 μg/ml) (4,6-Diamidino-2-Phenylindole in phenylene diamine dihydrochloride), glycerol, and buffer (Vysis).
7. Pretreatment solution (0.150 M sodium chloride, 0.015 M sodium citrate (1× SSC), pH 6.3): 50 ml 20× SSC, dH_2O to final volume of 1,000 ml, add few drops of 2 N HCl to pH 6.3. Store at room temperature.
8. Protease Solution: Protease I (Pepsin) (Vysis) 200 mg dissolved in 50 ml 0.2 N HCl (4 mg/ml) (*see* **Note 2**).
9. 100 % ethanol (use dH_2O to make various dilutions), Xylene or SafeClear II (ThermoFisher Scientific) for deparaffinization.

10. Post-Hybridization Wash Buffer (2× SSC/0.3 % NP-40): 100 ml 20× SSC, 897 ml H_2O, 3 ml NP 40. Adjust pH to 7.0–7.5. Store at room temperature.
11. White Rubber cement, glass slides and coverslips, microtubes (0.2 ml), pipet, Coplin jars (50 ml).

2.2 Comparative Genomic Hybridization (CGH)

1. Dissecting microscope.
2. Incubating shaker (quantity 2).
3. Centrifuge and microcentrifuge.
4. Vortex mixer.
5. Magnetic stir plate.
6. DNA120 Speed Vac (Fisher Scientific).
7. Wheaton slide washing units.
8. 180K CGH microarray (or equivalent) (Agilent).
9. Gasket slides, slide holders, and Ozone covers (Agilent).
10. SureHyb chamber base (Agilent).
11. DNA Microarray Scanner (Agilent).
12. Hybridization oven.
13. Computer with array data analysis software (we use Feature Extraction 10.7.3.1 and Genomic Workbench 6.0 lite).
14. Nanodrop nucleic acid analyzer (Thermo Scientific).
15. Qubit DNA fluorometric analyzer (Qiagen).
16. Quan-iT dsDNA BR kit (Qiagen).
17. CGH Digestion Buffer (50 ml): 2.5 ml 10 % SDS, 47.5 ml 1× Tris EDTA (TE) (10 mM Tris–HCl, pH 7.4, 1 mM EDTA).
18. 10× Blocking Agent (Agilent): Add 1,350 μL of nuclease free water to the vial containing lyophilized 10× CGH blocking agent (supplied with Agilent Oligo aCGH Hybridization kit), mix on vortex mixer and leave at room temp for 60 min.
19. 2× Hi-RPM Hybridization Buffer, Wash buffer 1 and 2 (Agilent).
20. Proteinase K, Cot1 DNA.
21. QIAmp DNA FFPE Tissue kit (contains buffers AW1 and AL).
22. Phenol:Chloroform:Isoamyl alcohol (25:24:1), Chloroform:Isoamyl alcohol (24:1), 7.5 M Ammonium acetate, Ethanol, Safeclear II, Sodium dodoceyl sulfate (SDS), Glycogen 20 mg/ml, TE buffer.
23. BioPrime® Total FFPE Genomic Labeling System.
24. Microfuge tubes, pipet/tips (2, 20, 200, 1000 μL), scalpel with 11 blade.

3 Methods

3.1 FISH for Formalin-Fixed, Paraffin-Embedded Tissue (FFPE)

3.1.1 Digestion and Denaturation of FFPE Sections

1. Obtain 5 micron-thick sections on charged glass slides (*see* **Note 3**).
2. Bake the slides at 60 °C for 30–60 min.
3. Using a VP 2000 or 50 ml Coplin jars, place the slides through the following steps (*see* **Note 1**).
4. Deparaffinize slides:
   (a) Place slides in Safeclear II, 3 times for 5 min each.
   (b) Place slides in 100 % ethanol, twice for 2 min each.
   (c) Rinse in water for 3 min.
   (d) Place slides in Pretreatment solution 1× SSC pH 6.3 at 80 °C for 35 min.
   (e) Rinse with water for 3 min.
   (f) Treat slides in Protease solution (4.0 mg/ml Pepsin in 0.2 N HCl) at 37 °C for 5–15 min (*see* **Note 8**).
   (g) Rinse in water for 3 min and in 70 % Ethanol, 85 % Ethanol and 100 % Ethanol for 2 min each.
   (h) Allow slides to air dry (28 °C) for at least 5 min before proceeding.

3.1.2 Hybridization on Vysis HYBrite Instrument

1. Place 10 μL of Vysis Melanoma FISH probe mix on target area of sample and cover with a glass coverslip (*see* **Note 4**).
2. Seal the edges of the coverslip with rubber cement (*see* **Note 5**).
3. Place slides in HYBrite chamber. Moisten humidity strips on the top of the chamber with distilled water. Choose appropriate HYBrite program to denature sample and probe at 73 °C for 5 min, followed by a hybridization period of 16–20 h at 37 °C.

3.1.3 Post-hybridization Wash

1. Heat Coplin jar(s) containing 50 ml of Post-Hybridization Wash Buffer to 73 °C in a water bath.
2. Remove rubber cement from coverslip (*see* **Note 6**).
3. Soak slide with intermittent agitation in room temperature Post-Hybridization Wash Buffer 5–10 min until coverslip is easily removed.
4. Immerse slides in Wash Buffer at 73 °C for 2 min.
5. Air dry slide in the dark.
6. Mount in Vysis DAPI I antifade and place coverslip on slide.
7. Incubate slides at −20 °C for 30 min.

3.1.4 Slide Analysis

1. Using the DAPI filter on a fluorescent microscope, scan the slide with the 2.5×, and 10× objective to determine the area to be analyzed. Correlate with H&E-stained sections to ensure

presence of tumor tissue following hybridization and wash procedures (*see* **Note 7**).

2. Scan with the 40× objective to determine quality of hybridization and DAPI staining. Keratinocytes can be used as a positive control to ensure adequate hybridization of FISH probes.
3. If nuclei appear overdigested or FISH signals are too few/faint, repeat the above steps and increase/decrease the pepsin digestion time accordingly (*see* **Note 8**).
4. Using a high power objective, scan the entire tumor for abnormalities in each of the 4 FISH probes in the tumor cells.
5. A minimum of three regions with the most abnormal FISH signal ratios are selected (*see* **Note 9**). From these areas, FISH signals from ≥10 nonoverlapping nuclei are counted either manually or via a software system such as Metasystems Metafer program. Truncated nuclei in which 0 signals are present for ≥2 probes are not counted.
6. The test is considered positive if one of the following four criteria are met: (1) 55 % or more nuclei have higher 6p25 signal counts than CEP6 counts (relative 6p gain), (2) 40 % of nuclei have lower 6q23 signal counts than CEP6 counts (6q loss), (3) 29 % or more nuclei have more than two signals for 6p25 (6p gain), or (4) 38 % or more nuclei have more than two signals for 11q13 (11q gain) (*see* **Note 10**).

3.2 aCGH on FFPE Tissue Samples

3.2.1 Digestion and Denaturation with Paraffin Sections

1. Cut 5–15 thick sections (25 μm) per case and place on glass slides (*see* **Note 11**).
2. Label one 1.5 ml microcentrifuge tube per sample.
3. Preheat shaking incubator block to 56 °C.
4. Prepare CGH Digestion Buffer.
5. Deparaffinize slides:
   (a) Place slides 3–5 min in Safeclear II, 3 times.
   (b) Place slides 3–5 min in 100 % ethanol, twice.
   (c) Place slides 3–5 min in 70 % ethanol, once.
   (d) Allow slides to air dry for at least 30 min before proceeding.

3.2.2 Microdissect Tumor Cells from Slides

1. Using an H&E-stained slide as a guide for tumor cells and a #11 scalpel with a dissecting microscope, remove tumor regions from the slides and place into the prelabeled 1.5 ml microcentrifuge tube (*see* **Note 12**).
2. Add 500 μl of CGH Digestion Buffer.
3. Incubate using a shaking incubator at 56 °C and 550 rpm.
4. Add 20 μl of Proteinase K each day for 3–4 days or until all the tissue is completely digested.

3.2.3 DNA Isolation from FFPE Tissue Using Phenol:Chloroform:Isoamyl Alcohol (See **Note 13**)

1. Label one 1.5 ml and one 2.0 ml microcentrifuge tube per sample.
2. Thaw glycogen vial.
3. Bring Phenol:Chloroform:Isoamyl alcohol to room temperature.
4. After the tissue is completely digested, add 500 μL of Phenol:Chloroform:Isoamyl Alcohol, mix gently by shaking and incubate for 10 min at room temperature.
5. Spin for 5 min at 20,000 × *g*. Collect the top aqueous phase into a new 1.5 ml tube.
6. Add 500 μl of Chloroform:Isoamyl Alcohol (24:1) to the aqueous phase, mix gently by shaking and incubate at room temperature for 10 min.
7. Spin at 20,000 × *g* for 5 min. Collect the top aqueous phase into a new 2.0 ml tube.
8. Add 1 ml of cold absolute Ethanol, 300 μL of 7.5 M ammonium acetate and 5 μL of Glycogen to the 2.0 ml tube and incubate at −20 °C for 2 h or overnight.
9. Spin down, at 20,000 × *g* at 4 °C for 30 min. Discard the supernatant.
10. Wash the pellet with 300 μl of 70 % ethanol, air dry the pellet, and dissolve in 30 μL of water.

3.2.4 Alternate Method of DNA Isolation Using QIAmp DNA FFPE Tissue Kit (See **Note 14**)

1. Add Ethanol to buffer AW1 according to directions on the bottle. Mark bottle as ethanol added.
2. Prepare 80 % Ethanol using 100 % ethanol and milli-Q water.
3. Label one 1.5 ml microcentrifuge tube and one spin column per sample.
4. Preheat TE buffer in a 37 °C water bath.
5. If buffer AL contains precipitates dissolve by incubating at 70 °C with agitation.
6. Add 200 μL of Buffer AL to the sample and mix by vortexing.
7. Add 200 μL 100 % Ethanol and mix by vortexing.
8. Transfer entire volume to the QIAmp MiniElute column. Be careful not to wet the rim of the spin column. Spin at 6,000 × *g* for 1 min. Discard flow-through.
9. Add 500 μL Buffer AW1. Spin at 8,000 × *g* for 1 min. Discard flow-through.
10. Add 500 μL 80 % ethanol. Spin at 8,000 × *g* for 1 min. Discard flow-through and replace collection tube with a clean tube.
11. Centrifuge at full speed (20,000 × *g*) for 3 min to dry the membrane.

12. Remove collection tube and place the spin column in a clean, labeled 1.5 ml tube. Apply 30 μL of TE to the membrane.
13. Incubate at room temperature for 5 min.
14. Centrifuge at full speed (20,000 × *g*) for 1 min.

3.2.5 Quantitation of DNA by Qubit Fluorometer (See **Note 15***)*

1. Label two tubes for the required standards and label one tube for each test sample. Use only thin-wall, clear 0.5 ml PCR tubes.
2. Make the Quant-iT™ working solution by diluting the Quant-iT™ dsDNA BR reagent 1:200 in Quant-iT™ dsDNA BR buffer.
3. Use a clean plastic tube each time you make Quant-iT™ working solution. Do not mix the working solution in a glass container.
4. Load 190 μL of Quant-iT™ working solution into each of the tubes used for standards. Add 10 μL of each Quant-iT™ standard to the appropriate tube and mix by vortexing 2–3 s, being careful not to create bubbles.
5. Load 195 μL of Quant-iT™ working solution into each of the tubes used for test samples. Load 5 μL of your test sample into its respective tube and mix by vortexing 2–3 s, being careful not to create bubbles.
6. Allow all tubes to incubate at room temperature for 2 min.
7. Turn on the Qubit™ fluorometer.
8. Press HOME and use the arrow keys to select Qunait-iT DNA, BR. Press GO. Select Run New Calibration.
9. Insert the tube for standard one, close the lid, and press Go. Remove the tube and insert the tube for standard two, close the lid, and press Go.
10. Once the calibration is complete, place your test sample tube in the Qubit, close the lid, and Press go.
11. After reading all of your samples use the following equation to calculate DNA concentration. Concentration of your sample = QF value × (200)/X where: QF value = the value given by the Qubit™ fluorometer. x = the number of microliters of sample you added to the assay tube.

3.2.6 Fluorescent Labeling of Samples, Bioprime Total FFPE DNA Labeling Module (See **Note 16***)*

1. Thaw 2.5× Random Primer and Alexa Fluor 10× Nucleotide mixes at room temperature. Keep on ice after thawing and protect Alexa Fluor mixes from light.
2. Heat fragment reference DNA by incubating at 95 °C for 10 min followed by a 4 °C incubation for 3 min. Do not heat fragment FFPE samples.
3. Set preamplification heat block to 95 °C.
4. Using the data generated from the Qubit, add 1 μg of DNA to the appropriately labeled tube. The volume added will vary

based on the concentration of each sample. For example, if the concentration of the sample is 100 ng/μL you would add 10 μL for a total of 1 microgram.

5. Bring volume up to 22 μL with nuclease-free water. Following the above example add 12 μL of water.
6. Repeat this process with the control sample, creating one control tube for each sample. Control sample could be normal DNA from the same sample or commercially available normal DNA.
7. Place all tubes in ice prior to adding primers and fluorophores.
8. Add 20 μL of 2.5× Random Primers Solution to each tube.
9. Add 5 μL of Alexa Fluor 3 to each commercial control tube.
10. Add 5 μL of Alexa Fluor 5 to each unknown sample tube.
11. Vortex and briefly spin tubes.
12. Incubate tubes at 95 °C, protected from light, for 5 min.
13. Immediately cool samples on ice for 5 min.
14. On ice, add 3 μL of Exo-Klenow Fragment to each tube.
15. Vortex and briefly spin tubes.
16. Move to post-amplification room and incubate samples at 37 °C, protected from light, for 2 h.
17. Proceed immediately to the purification module or follow the optional stop step listed below.
18. *Optional Stopping Point*: After incubation you may stop the reaction by adding 5uL of Stop Buffer to each tube and storing the samples overnight at −20 °C.

3.2.7 Bioprime Total FFPE DNA Purification Module (See **Note 17***)*

1. Prepare the binding buffer and Wash buffer W1 by adding isopropanol and ethanol respectively according to the directions on the bottle.
2. Label 1 PureLink Spin column and 1 Amber-colored tube for each sample.
3. Preset two heat blocks one at 37 °C and the other at 95 °C.
4. Add 200 μL of Binding Buffer to each tube from the labeling module. Vortex and briefly spin.
5. Load each sample into a labeled PureLink Spin Column.
6. Centrifuge at 10,000 ×*g* for 1 min. Discard flow-through.
7. Add 650 μL of Wash Buffer W1 to each column.
8. Centrifuge at 10,000 ×*g* for 1 min. Discard flow-through.
9. Spin columns at maximum speed (20,000 ×*g*) for 3 min to remove any residual wash buffer.
10. Place spin column in a labeled amber tube. Add 30 μL of Elution Buffer directly to the membrane.

Table 1
Expected yield and specific activity after labeling

Input gDNA (μg)	Yield (μg)	Specific activity of cyanine-3-labeled sample (pmol/μg)	Specific activity of cyanine-5-labeled sample (pmol/μg)
0.2–0.5	2.5–3.0	15–25	15–20
0.5	5–7	25–40	25–35
3	7–10	35–55	25–40

11. Incubate at room temperature for 5 min.
12. Centrifuge tubes at maximum speed (20,000 × *g*) for 2 min.
13. Pipet out the Elution Buffer and reapply it to the membrane. Incubate at room temperature for 5 min.
14. Centrifuge tubes at maximum speed (20,000 × *g*) for 2 min to collect DNA.

3.2.8 Measuring the Degree of Labeling Using Nanodrop

1. Turn on Nanodrop software and select the Microarray option.
2. Check the box on the upper right-hand corner of the window to make sure you are reading DNA-50 (double stranded DNA).
3. Load 1.5 μL of Qiagen Elution Buffer onto the pedestal and lower the arm. Choose "Initialize Instrument".
4. Using the same aliquot of buffer click the "Blank" button on the upper left-hand corner of the window.
5. After blanking wipe pedestal and arm with a KimWipe.
6. Load 1.5 μL of sample, lower the arm, and click the "Measure" button.
7. After measuring wipe pedestal and arm with a KimWipe.
8. Repeat the above steps until you have quantitated all of your samples. Calculate the labeling efficiency using the following formula: Labeling efficiency = Dye (pmole)/(ng/μL) × 1,000.
9. Specific activity = (pmol per μL dye)/(μg per μL genomic DNA) (Table 1).

3.2.9 Array Assembly and Preparation (Agilent 180K Microarray)

1. The microarray is printed on the side of the glass slide containing the Agilent barcode. This side is called the active side. The other side containing the numerical barcode is the inactive side.
2. The hybridization mixture is applied on the gasket slide and the active side of the array is placed on top of the gasket slide.
3. Ensure that the hybridization chamber is screwed together very tightly. This will prevent leakage from one array to the next.

Table 2
Hybridization master mix

Component	Volume (μL) per hybridization	×4 rxns (μL) including excess
Cot-1 DNA (1.0 mg/ml)	5	22.5
Agilent 10× blocking agent	11	49.5
Agilent 2× Hi-RPM buffer	55	247.5
Final volume of hybridization master mix	71	319.5

4. Make sure to use an ozone barrier, if appropriate. Alexa Flour 5 is known to degrade when exposed to ozone for extended periods of time.
5. Clean SureHyb chamber base with water.
6. Set the Hybridization oven to 65 °C.

3.2.10 Preparation of Labeled Genomic DNA for Hybridization

1. Turn on heat blocks. One is set at 95 °C and the other is set at 37 °C.
2. Prepare the 10× Blocking Agent.
3. Combine Cy5 and Cy3-labeled gDNA mixture and check the total volume.
4. Use a Speed Vac to concentrate the combine Cy5- and Cy3-labeled gDNA.
5. Place tubes inside the DNA 120 Speed Vac with the tops open. Close the lid and turn on heat to Medium and drying rate to Medium. Dry samples for about 6–8 min. Be careful not to over-dry the samples.
6. Measure the volume and add TE, if necessary, to bring the total volume to 39 μL.
7. Make the hybridization master mix according to the Table 2. Agilent 2× Hi RPM buffer is viscous, pipette it gently to avoid making bubbles.
8. Add 71 μL of the hybridization master mix to each sample. Total volume of each sample is now 110 μL. Mix sample by gently pipetting up and down and briefly spin tubes to collect contents.
9. Incubate samples at 95 °C for 3 min.
10. Incubate samples at 37 °C for 30 min.
11. Briefly spin tubes to collect contents.

3.2.11 Microarray Hybridization

1. Set the Hybridization oven to 65 °C.
2. The microarray is printed on the side of the glass slide containing the Agilent barcode. This side is called the active side. The other side containing the numerical barcode is the inactive side.
3. Place a clean gasket slide gasket-side up inside the bottom portion of the SureHyb chamber base. Pipet 100 μL of sample one into the square well closest to the Agilent barcode. Be careful not to introduce bubbles by pipetting very slowly. Pipet sample two into the next well and so forth until all four samples are loaded on to the gasket slide.
4. Very carefully, in one smooth motion, lay the array active-side down (Agilent barcode side) on top of the gasket slide.
5. Place the SureHyb chamber cover on top of the sandwiched slides.
6. Slide the clamp over the entire assembly and hand-tighten the screw tightly.
7. Ensure that the hybridization chamber is screwed together very tightly. This will prevent leakage from one array to the next.
8. Rotate chamber to ensure that the air bubble moves freely around the well. If the air bubble does not move freely, tap the entire chamber very firmly on the bench and check again to make sure the liquid is moving freely around the entire well.
9. Place the chamber inside the prewarmed Hybridization Oven. Close the door and turn the knob to activate rotation. If hybridizing an odd number of slides, balance with an empty SureHyb chamber. Allow array to incubate at 65 °C in the Hybridization Oven for 40–42 h.

3.2.12 Preparing the Array for Scanning (See **Notes 18** and **19**)

1. Place a tupperware container filled with distilled tap water and the bag of Agilent Wash Buffer 2 in a 37 °C incubator at least 2 h before washing slides.
2. Wash three Wheaton slide washing units and one slide holder very well with milli-Q water. It is important not to use any detergents on these Wheaton units.
3. Using gloves, take the SureHyb chamber out of the Hybridization oven. *CAUTION!!! Chamber will be VERY HOT.*
4. The active side of the array contains all of the features. This side is the labeled with a barcode reading AGILENT.
5. Once the array is open take every precaution not to touch the active side of the array.
6. Wash two Wheaton slide washing units and one slide holder with Agilent Wash Buffer 1. Wash the third Wheaton slide washing unit with Agilent Wash Buffer 2.

7. Fill two Wheaton units with Agilent Wash Buffer 1. Place one on the bench and the other on the stir plate. Place a small stir bar in the bottom of the Wheaton unit.
8. Open the SureHyb chamber base by turning the knob counterclockwise. Slide the top off and carefully take the array out. Make sure to touch only the very ends of the array.
9. Holding one end of the array slowly submerge the slides into the Wheaton unit on the bench top. Using the plastic forceps insert one edge of the forceps in between the array and the gasket slide. Slowly turn the forceps until the array and the gasket slide separate.
10. Quickly take the array out and place into the Wheaton slide unit containing the slide holder and stir bar on the stir-plate. Wash in Agilent Wash Buffer 1 for 5 min.
11. Slowly and evenly pull the slide holder out of the buffer. This will pull most of the wash buffer off the slides and the slide holder. Scrap the bottom of the slide holder against the edge of the Wheaton unit to remove any excess Wash Buffer 1.
12. Quickly submerge the slide holder into the third Wheaton container filled with warm Agilent Wash Buffer 2. Wash for 2 min.

3.2.13 Assemble the Cassette and Scan the Array (See **Note 19***)*

1. Turn on the computer, then the scanner, and then open the Agilent Scan Control software. The lasers need about 15 min to warm up.
2. Very carefully take the array out of the slide holder and dab the top and bottom edges on the paper towel to remove any residual buffer.
3. Carefully set the array in the Agilent Slide Holder with the active side (Agilent Barcode side) facing up. Carefully set an Ozone barrier over the array.
4. Close the Agilent Slide Holder by pressing the top down and sliding it back at the same time.
5. Place the Agilent Slide Holder into slot one in the DNA Microarray scanner. Close the lid of the scanner.
6. Using the protocol for the type of slide scanner used, scan the slide and generate the data and image files. For 180K arrays scan at 3 μm.

4 Notes

1. A VP 2000 processor (Abbott) can be programmed with the protocol steps for a large number of cases (>10). Less than ten cases can be done using two 50 ml Coplin jars to avoid wasting reagents.

2. For reliable digestion times, the protease solution should be made fresh daily.
3. Do not use standard 3 μm sections or excessive truncation of nuclei can occur.
4. Photobleaching of FISH probes can occur with excessive exposure to light. Once probe has been applied, take care to protect the slides from light. Foil wrapping of Coplin jars works nicely.
5. Rubber cement can be easily applied around the coverslip using a 3–5 ml syringe with a plastic pipet tip. Cut the distal 1/3 of the pipet tip to allow a larger hole for drawing up and pushing out the rubber cement.
6. Do not use excessive upward force when removing rubber cement or tissue fragmentation will occur.
7. Cut a routine H&E section at the same time 5 μm FISH sections are cut to serve as a guide when viewing under the fluorescent microscope.
8. Optimal pepsin incubation times for tissue can vary. In general, pepsin treatment is the most crucial stage in tissue processing. If there are no FISH signals and nuclei are faint or hollow on the DAPI filter, the DNA has been overdigested. Repeat the protocol with a reduced pepsin digestion time, e.g., decrease the digestion time in pepsin by 1/2. If the problems persist, repeat and reduce the pepsin time again. If DAPI signals are bright and there is no (or very weak) hybridization signal, use longer pepsin digestion conditions on a fresh slide, e.g., increase digestion time in pepsin to 15–20 min. If no signals are detectable after multiple (3–4) attempts with varied digestion conditions or if there is only diffuse autofluorescence repeatedly in all fluorochromes, we designate the case as unreadable.
9. Melanomas can be genetically heterogeneous within the same tumor. It is important to scan the entire tumor for aberrations and select the most atypical areas for enumeration.
10. Caution should be taken in cases of polyploidy. If all FISH signals are gained in equal proportions, a state of polyploidy exists and can yield a false positive result. Polyploidy can be seen in both melanoma and nevi (particularly Spitz nevi).
11. The number of sections depends on the size of the lesional tissue. A total area of approximately 10 mm^2 is needed to get sufficient DNA for CGH. For example, in case of a small lesion with only one square millimeter area with a relatively pure tumor cell population, 10 unstained sections of 25 μm thickness would be needed.
12. Accurate assessment of genomic DNA quantity and quality are crucial to the success of an aCGH experiment. High quality genomic DNA should be free of contaminants such as proteins,

and traces of organic solvents, and should also be intact with minimal degradation. Minimize the amount of nontumor DNA dissected from slides by circling the area of tumor to be analyzed on an H&E-stained section for guidance during microdissection.

13. In the preamplification steps, all reagents and consumables (scalpels, TE, tubes, etc.) should be PCR-clean to avoid contamination of tumor DNA.
14. If the DNA isolated using the Phenol:Chloroform method has a lot of protein including melanin, use the QIAmp DNA FFPE tissue kit for further purification.
15. The minimum amount of DNA required for aCGH is 500 ng. Whenever possible use 1,000 ng to ensure high quality data.
16. Protect fluorescently labeled reagents (e.g., Cy3, Cy5 reagents) from prolonged exposure to light. Store in the dark and do not leave out longer than needed unless covered in foil.
17. Accidental contamination of work areas or reagents with amplified DNA products may interfere with this test. Maintain a unidirectional workflow at all times, handling material containing amplified products in a designated post-amplification area only.
18. Take caution not to touch the active side of the array. Handle the array by its edges and wear powder free gloves while handling the array. Never allow the microarray surface to dry out during the process of hybridization and washing.
19. Cy5 has been shown to be sensitive to ozone degradation. Ozone levels as low as 5 ppb can affect Cy5 signal and compromise microarray results. Once the washing is done, minimize the exposure of the array to the atmosphere and try to work as fast as possible during slide assembly.

References

1. Balaban GB, Herlyn M, Clark WH Jr, Nowell PC (1986) Karyotypic evolution in human malignant melanoma. Cancer Genet Cytogenet 19(1–2):113–122
2. Cowan JM, Halaban R, Francke U (1988) Cytogenetic analysis of melanocytes from premalignant nevi and melanomas. J Natl Cancer Inst 80(14):1159–1164
3. Hecht F, Hecht BK (1988) Chromosome rearrangements in dysplastic nevus syndrome predisposing to malignant melanoma. Cancer Genet Cytogenet 35(1):73–78
4. Richmond A, Fine R, Murray D, Lawson DH, Priest JH (1986) Growth factor and cytogenetic abnormalities in cultured nevi and malignant melanomas. J Invest Dermatol 86(3):295–302
5. Kallioniemi A, Kallioniemi OP, Sudar D, Rutovitz D, Gray JW, Waldman F, Pinkel D (1992) Comparative genomic hybridization for molecular cytogenetic analysis of solid tumors. Science 258(5083):818–821
6. Speicher MR, Prescher G, du Manoir S, Jauch A, Horsthemke B, Bornfeld N, Becher R, Cremer T (1994) Chromosomal gains and losses in uveal melanomas detected by comparative genomic hybridization. Cancer Res 54(14):3817–3823
7. Ghazvini S, Char DH, Kroll S, Waldman FM, Pinkel D (1996) Comparative genomic hybridization analysis of archival formalin-fixed paraffin-embedded uveal melanomas. Cancer Genet Cytogenet 90(2):95–101

8. Bastian BC, LeBoit PE, Hamm H, Bröcker E-B, Pinkel D (1998) Chromosomal gains and losses in primary cutaneous melanomas detected by comparative genomic hybridization. Cancer Res 58(10):2170–2175
9. Bastian BC, Olshen AB, LeBoit PE, Pinkel D (2003) Classifying melanocytic tumors based on DNA copy number changes. Am J Pathol 163(5):1765–1770
10. Balázs M, Adám Z, Treszl A, Bégány A, Hunyadi J, Adány R (2001) Chromosomal imbalances in primary and metastatic melanomas revealed by comparative genomic hybridization. Cytometry 46(4):222–232
11. Snijders AM, Nowak N, Segraves R, Blackwood S, Brown N, Conroy J, Hamilton G, Hindle AK, Huey B, Kimura K, Law S, Myambo K, Palmer J, Ylstra B, Yue JP, Gray JW, Jain AN, Pinkel D, Albertson DG (2001) Assembly of microarrays for genome-wide measurement of DNA copy number. Nat Genet 29(3): 263–264
12. Lin WM, Baker AC, Beroukhim R, Winckler W, Feng W, Marmion JM, Laine E, Greulich H, Tseng H, Gates C, Hodi FS, Dranoff G, Sellers WR, Thomas RK, Meyerson M, Golub TR, Dummer R, Herlyn M, Getz G, Garraway LA (2008) Modeling genomic diversity and tumor dependency in malignant melanoma. Cancer Res 68(3):664–673
13. Curtin JA, Fridlyand J, Kageshita T, Patel HN, Busam KJ, Kutzner H, Cho K-H, Aiba S, Bröcker E-B, LeBoit PE, Pinkel D, Bastian BC (2005) Distinct sets of genetic alterations in melanoma. N Engl J Med 353(20): 2135–2147
14. Bastian BC, Kashani-Sabet M, Hamm H, Godfrey T, Moore DH 2nd, Bröcker EB, LeBoit PE, Pinkel D (2000) Gene amplifications characterize acral melanoma and permit the detection of occult tumor cells in the surrounding skin. Cancer Res 60(7):1968–1973
15. North JP, Kageshita T, Pinkel D, LeBoit PE, Bastian BC (2008) Distribution and significance of occult intraepidermal tumor cells surrounding primary melanoma. J Invest Dermatol 128(8):2024–2030
16. van Dijk M, Sprenger S, Rombout P, Marres H, Kaanders J, Jeuken J, Ruiter D (2003) Distinct chromosomal aberrations in sinonasal mucosal melanoma as detected by comparative genomic hybridization. Genes Chromosomes Cancer 36(2):151–158
17. Maize JC Jr, McCalmont TH, Carlson JA, Busam KJ, Kutzner H, Bastian BC (2005) Genomic analysis of blue nevi and related dermal melanocytic proliferations. Am J Surg Pathol 29(9):1214–1220
18. Busam KJ, Woodruff JM, Erlandson RA, Brady MS (2000) Large plaque-type blue nevus with subcutaneous cellular nodules. Am J Surg Pathol 24(1):92–99
19. Yeh I, Fang Y, Busam KJ (2012) Melanoma arising in a large plaque-type blue nevus with subcutaneous cellular nodules. Am J Surg Pathol 36(8):1258–1263
20. North JP, Yeh I, McCalmont TH, LeBoit PE (2012) Melanoma ex blue nevus: two cases resembling large plaque-type blue nevus with subcutaneous cellular nodules. J Cutan Pathol 39(12):1094–1099
21. Gerami P, Pouryazdanparast P, Vemula S, Bastian BC (2010) Molecular analysis of a case of nevus of ota showing progressive evolution to melanoma with intermediate stages resembling cellular blue nevus. Am J Dermatopathol 32(3):301–305
22. Bastian BC, Wesselmann U, Pinkel D, Leboit PE (1999) Molecular cytogenetic analysis of Spitz nevi shows clear differences to melanoma. J Invest Dermatol 113(6):1065–1069
23. Bastian BC, LeBoit PE, Pinkel D (2000) Mutations and copy number increase of HRAS in Spitz nevi with distinctive histopathological features. Am J Pathol 157(3):967–972
24. Ali L, Helm T, Cheney R, Conroy J, Sait S, Guitart J, Gerami P (2010) Correlating array comparative genomic hybridization findings with histology and outcome in spitzoid melanocytic neoplasms. Int J Clin Exp Pathol 3(6):593–599
25. Healy E, Belgaid CE, Takata M, Vahlquist A, Rehman I, Rigby H, Rees JL (1996) Allelotypes of primary cutaneous melanoma and benign melanocytic nevi. Cancer Res 56(3):589–593
26. Raskin L, Ludgate M, Iyer RK, Ackley TE, Bradford CR, Johnson TM, Fullen DR (2011) Copy number variations and clinical outcome in atypical spitz tumors. Am J Surg Pathol 35(2):243–252
27. Wiesner T, Obenauf AC, Murali R, Fried I, Griewank KG, Ulz P, Windpassinger C, Wackernagel W, Loy S, Wolf I, Viale A, Lash AE, Pirun M, Socci ND, Rütten A, Palmedo G, Abramson D, Offit K, Ott A, Becker JC, Cerroni L, Kutzner H, Bastian BC, Speicher MR (2011) Germline mutations in BAP1 predispose to melanocytic tumors. Nat Genet 43(10):1018–1021
28. Busam KJ, Sung J, Wiesner T, von Deimling A, Jungbluth A (2013) Combined BRAFV600E-positive melanocytic lesions with large epithelioid cells lacking BAP1 expression and conventional nevomelanocytes. Am J Surg Pathol 37:193–199
29. Aalto Y, Eriksson L, Seregard S, Larsson O, Knuutila S (2001) Concomitant loss of chromosome 3 and whole arm losses and gains of

chromosome 1, 6, or 8 in metastasizing primary uveal melanoma. Invest Ophthalmol Vis Sci 42(2):313–317
30. White JS, McLean IW, Becker RL, Director-Myska AE, Nath J (2006) Correlation of comparative genomic hybridization results of 100 archival uveal melanomas with patient survival. Cancer Genet Cytogenet 170(1):29–39
31. Mensink HW, Kiliç E, Vaarwater J, Douben H, Paridaens D, de Klein A (2008) Molecular cytogenetic analysis of archival uveal melanoma with known clinical outcome. Cancer Genet Cytogenet 181(2):108–111
32. Trolet J, Hupé P, Huon I, Lebigot I, Decraene C, Delattre O, Sastre-Garau X, Saule S, Thiéry J-P, Plancher C, Asselain B, Desjardins L, Mariani P, Piperno-Neumann S, Barillot E, Couturier J (2009) Genomic profiling and identification of high-risk uveal melanoma by array CGH analysis of primary tumors and liver metastases. Invest Ophthalmol Vis Sci 50(6): 2572–2580
33. Bastian BC, Xiong J, Frieden IJ, Williams ML, Chou P, Busam K, Pinkel D, LeBoit PE (2002) Genetic changes in neoplasms arising in congenital melanocytic nevi: differences between nodular proliferations and melanomas. Am J Pathol 161(4):1163–1169
34. Adám Z, Adány R, Ladányi A, Tímár J, Balázs M (2000) Liver metastatic ability of human melanoma cell line is associated with losses of chromosomes 4, 9p21-pter and 10p. Clin Exp Metastasis 18(4):295–302
35. Günther K, Fleischer A, Buettner R, Bosserhoff AK (2001) Detection of invasion-related chromosomal changes in highly and weakly invasive melanoma cell clones by a modified comparative genomic hybridization approach. Melanoma Res 11(2):105–115
36. Gerami P, Jewell SS, Morrison LE, Blondin B, Schulz J, Ruffalo T, Matushek P 4th, Legator M, Jacobson K, Dalton SR, Charzan S, Kolaitis NA, Guitart J, Lertsbarapa T, Boone S, LeBoit PE, Bastian BC (2009) Fluorescence in situ hybridization (FISH) as an ancillary diagnostic tool in the diagnosis of melanoma. Am J Surg Pathol 33(8):1146–1156
37. Clemente C, Bettio D, Venci A, Scopsi L, Rao S, Ferrari A, Piris A, Mihm MC Jr (2009) A fluorescence in situ hybridization (FISH) procedure to assist in differentiating benign from malignant melanocytic lesions. Pathologica 101(5):169–174
38. Morey AL, Murali R, McCarthy SW, Mann GJ, Scolyer RA (2009) Diagnosis of cutaneous melanocytic tumours by four-colour fluorescence in situ hybridisation. Pathology 41(4): 383–387
39. Newman MD, Lertsburapa T, Mirzabeigi M, Mafee M, Guitart J, Gerami P (2009) Fluorescence in situ hybridization as a tool for microstaging in malignant melanoma. Mod Pathol 22(8):989–995
40. Dreyling MH, Bohlander SK, Adeyanju MO, Olopade OI (1995) Detection of CDKN2 deletions in tumor cell lines and primary glioma by interphase fluorescence in situ hybridization. Cancer Res 55(5):984–988
41. Becher R, Korn WM, Prescher G (1997) Use of fluorescence in situ hybridization and comparative genomic hybridization in the cytogenetic analysis of testicular germ cell tumors and uveal melanomas. Cancer Genet Cytogenet 93(1):22–28
42. Barks JH, Thompson FH, Taetle R, Yang JM, Stone JF, Wymer JA, Khavari R, Guan XY, Trent JM, Pinkel D, Nelson MA (1997) Increased chromosome 20 copy number detected by fluorescence in situ hybridization (FISH) in malignant melanoma. Genes Chromosomes Cancer 19(4):278–285
43. Guan XY, Zhang H, Yang JM, Wang J, Taetle R, Meltzer PS, Trent JM (1998) Detection of chromosome 6 abnormalities in melanoma cell lines by chromosome arm painting probes. Cancer Genet Cytogenet 107(2):89–92
44. Okamoto I, Pirc-Danoewinata H, Ackermann J, Drach J, Schlagbauer Wadl H, Jansen B, Wolff K, Pehamberger H, Marosi C (1999) Deletions of the region 17p11-13 in advanced melanoma revealed by cytogenetic analysis and fluorescence in situ hybridization. Br J Cancer 79(1):131–137
45. Multani AS, Ozen M, Sen S, Mandal AK, Price JE, Fan D, Radinsky R, Ali-Osman F, Von Eschenbach AC, Fidler IJ, Pathak S (1999) Amplification of telomeric DNA directly correlates with metastatic potential of human and murine cancers of various histological origin. Int J Oncol 15(3):423–429
46. Kraehn GM, Utikal J, Udart M, Greulich KM, Bezold G, Kaskel P, Leiter U, Peter RU (2001) Extra c-myc oncogene copies in high risk cutaneous malignant melanoma and melanoma metastases. Br J Cancer 84(1):72–79
47. Rákosy Z, Vízkeleti L, Ecsedi S, Vokó Z, Bégány A, Barok M, Krekk Z, Gallai M, Szentirmay Z, Adány R, Balázs M (2007) EGFR gene copy number alterations in primary cutaneous malignant melanomas are associated with poor prognosis. Int J Cancer 121(8):1729–1737
48. Langezaal SM, Graadt van Roggen JF, Cleton-Jansen AM, Baelde JJ, Hogendoorn PC (2001) Malignant melanoma is genetically distinct from clear cell sarcoma of tendons and

aponeurosis (malignant melanoma of soft parts). Br J Cancer 84(4):535–538
49. Newman MD, Mirzabeigi M, Gerami P (2009) Chromosomal copy number changes supporting the classification of lentiginous junctional melanoma of the elderly as a subtype of melanoma. Mod Pathol 22(9):1258–1262
50. Pouryazdanparast P, Newman M, Mafee M, Haghighat Z, Guitart J, Gerami P (2009) Distinguishing epithelioid blue nevus from blue nevus-like cutaneous melanoma metastasis using fluorescence in situ hybridization. Am J Surg Pathol 33(9):1396–1400
51. Gammon B, Beilfuss B, Guitart J, Busam KJ, Gerami P (2011) Fluorescence in situ hybridization for distinguishing cellular blue nevi from blue nevus-like melanoma. J Cutan Pathol 38(4):335–341
52. Dalton SR, Gerami P, Kolaitis NA, Charzan S, Werling R, LeBoit PE, Bastian BC (2010) Use of fluorescence in situ hybridization (FISH) to distinguish intranodal nevus from metastatic melanoma. Am J Surg Pathol 34(2):231–237
53. Busam KJ, Fang Y, Jhanwar SC, Pulitzer MP, Marr B, Abramson DH (2010) Distinction of conjunctival melanocytic nevi from melanomas by fluorescence in situ hybridization. J Cutan Pathol 37(2):196–203
54. Gerami P, Wass A, Mafee M, Fang Y, Pulitzer MP, Busam KJ (2009) Fluorescence in situ hybridization for distinguishing nevoid melanomas from mitotically active nevi. Am J Surg Pathol 33(12):1783–1788
55. Gerami P, Barnhill RL, Beilfuss BA, LeBoit P, Schneider P, Guitart J (2010) Superficial melanocytic neoplasms with pagetoid melanocytosis: a study of interobserver concordance and correlation with FISH. Am J Surg Pathol 34(6):816–821
56. Díaz A, Valera A, Carrera C, Hakim S, Aguilera P, García A, Palou J, Puig S, Malvehy J, Alos L (2011) Pigmented spindle cell nevus: clues for differentiating it from spindle cell malignant melanoma. A comprehensive survey including clinicopathologic, immunohistochemical, and FISH studies. Am J Surg Pathol 35(11): 1733–1742
57. Gerami P, Beilfuss B, Haghighat Z, Fang Y, Jhanwar S, Busam KJ (2011) Fluorescence in situ hybridization as an ancillary method for the distinction of desmoplastic melanomas from sclerosing melanocytic nevi. J Cutan Pathol 38(4):329–334
58. Massi D, Cesinaro AM, Tomasini C, Paglierani M, Bettelli S, Dal Maso L, Simi L, Salvianti F, Pinzani P, Orlando C, De Giorgi V, Lukic S, Maiorana A, Santucci M, Canzonieri V (2011) Atypical Spitzoid melanocytic tumors: a morphological, mutational, and FISH analysis. J Am Acad Dermatol 64(5):919–935
59. Vergier B, Prochazkova-Carlotti M, de la Fouchardière A, Cerroni L, Massi D, De Giorgi V, Bailly C, Wesselmann U, Karlseladze A, Avril M-F, Jouary T, Merlio J-P (2011) Fluorescence in situ hybridization, a diagnostic aid in ambiguous melanocytic tumors: European study of 113 cases. Mod Pathol 24(5):613–623
60. Hung T, Piris A, Lobo A, Mihm MC Jr, Sober AJ, Tsao H, Tanabe KK, Duncan LM (2013) Sentinel lymph node metastasis is not predictive of poor outcome in patients with problematic spitzoid melanocytic tumors. Hum Pathol 44:87–94
61. Cesinaro AM, Schirosi L, Bettelli S, Migaldi M, Maiorana A (2010) Alterations of 9p21 analysed by FISH and MLPA distinguish atypical spitzoid melanocytic tumours from conventional Spitz's nevi but do not predict their biological behaviour. Histopathology 57(4):515–527
62. Gammon B, Beilfuss B, Guitart J, Gerami P (2012) Enhanced detection of spitzoid melanomas using fluorescence in situ hybridization with 9p21 as an adjunctive probe. Am J Surg Pathol 36(1):81–88
63. Gerami P, Li G, Pouryazdanparast P, Blondin B, Beilfuss B, Slenk C, Du J, Guitart J, Jewell S, Pestova K (2012) A highly specific and discriminatory FISH assay for distinguishing between benign and malignant melanocytic neoplasms. Am J Surg Pathol 36(6):808–817
64. Ryan D, Rafferty M, Hegarty S, O'Leary P, Faller W, Gremel G, Bergqvist M, Agnarsdottir M, Strömberg S, Kampf C, Pontén F, Millikan RC, Dervan PA, Gallagher WM (2010) Topoisomerase I amplification in melanoma is associated with more advanced tumours and poor prognosis. Pigment Cell Melanoma Res 23(4):542–553
65. North JP, Vetto JT, Murali R, White KP, White CR Jr, Bastian BC (2011) Assessment of copy number status of chromosomes 6 and 11 by FISH provides independent prognostic information in primary melanoma. Am J Surg Pathol 35(8):1146–1150
66. Gerami P, Jewell SS, Pouryazdanparast P, Wayne JD, Haghighat Z, Busam KJ, Rademaker A, Morrison L (2011) Copy number gains in 11q13 and 8q24 [corrected] are highly linked to prognosis in cutaneous malignant melanoma. J Mol Diagn 13(3):352–358
67. Pouryazdanparast P, Cowen DP, Beilfuss BA, Haghighat Z, Guitart J, Rademaker A, Gerami P (2012) Distinctive clinical and histologic features in cutaneous melanoma with copy number gains in 8q24. Am J Surg Pathol 36(2): 253–264

68. Gammon B, Ali L, Guitart J, Gerami P (2012) Homogeneous staining regions for cyclin D1, a marker of poor prognosis in malignant melanoma. Am J Dermatopathol 34(5):487–490
69. Isaac AK, Lertsburapa T, Pathria Mundi J, Martini M, Guitart J, Gerami P (2010) Polyploidy in spitz nevi: a not uncommon karyotypic abnormality identifiable by fluorescence in situ hybridization. Am J Dermatopathol 32(2):144–148
70. Pouryazdanparast P, Haghighat Z, Beilfuss BA, Guitart J, Gerami P (2011) Melanocytic nevi with an atypical epithelioid cell component: clinical, histopathologic, and fluorescence in situ hybridization findings. Am J Surg Pathol 35(9):1405–1412
71. Satoh S, Hashimoto-Tamaoki T, Furuyama J, Mihara K, Namba M, Kitano Y (2000) High frequency of tetraploidy detected in malignant melanoma of Japanese patients by fluorescence in situ hybridization. Int J Oncol 17(4):707–715

Chapter 13

Construction and Analysis of Multiparameter Prognostic Models for Melanoma Outcome

Bonnie E. Gould Rothberg and David L. Rimm

Abstract

The outcome of Stage II melanoma is uncertain. Despite that 10-year melanoma-specific survival can approach 50 % following curative-intent wide local excision and negative sentinel lymph node biopsy, the adverse risk–benefit ratio of interferon-based adjuvant regimens precludes their use in most patients. The discovery and translation of protein-based prognostic biomarkers into the clinic offers the promise for residual risk stratification of Stage II melanoma patients beyond conventional clinicopathologic criteria to identify an additional subset of patients who, based upon tumor molecular profiles, might also derive benefit from adjuvant regimens. Despite incorporation of Ki-67 assays into clinical practice, systematic review of REMARK-compliant, immunostain-based prognostic biomarker assays in melanoma suggests that residual risk of recurrence might be best explained by a composite score derived from a small panel of proteins representing independent features of melanoma biology. Reflecting this trend, to date, five such multiparameter melanoma prognostic models have been published. Here, we review these five models and provide detailed protocols for discovering and validating multiparameter models including: appropriate cohort recruitment strategies, comprehensive laboratory protocols supporting fully quantitative chromogenic or fluorescent immunostaining platforms, statistical approaches to create composite prognostic indices recommended steps for model validation in independent cohorts.

Key words Multiparameter models, Prognosis, Systematic review, Multivariate statistical modeling, Immunohistochemistry, Quantitative immunofluorescence, Tissue microarray

1 Introduction

The prognosis for Stage II melanoma is uncertain. Despite curative-intent wide local excision and negative sentinel lymph node dissection, the 10-year melanoma-specific survival ranges from 65 % in Stage IIA to 40 % for Stage IIC [1]. Yet, due to the morbidity associated with currently approved interferon-based therapeutic regimens, adjuvant therapy is only recommended for Stage IIB/C patients with "*high-risk*" features such as ulceration and/or in-transit metastases [2] with active surveillance as the standard of care for the remaining patients. To maximize the potential benefit of adjuvant treatment among Stage II melanoma patients, current

Magdalena Thurin and Francesco M. Marincola (eds.), *Molecular Diagnostics for Melanoma: Methods and Protocols*, Methods in Molecular Biology, vol. 1102, DOI 10.1007/978-1-62703-727-3_13, © Springer Science+Business Media New York 2014

melanoma research priorities include the identification of complementary biomarkers that can stratify additional Stage II patients as high-risk with the overall goal of reducing melanoma mortality among patients for whom cure is possible. In addition to the consideration of mitotic index, which has recently been shown to be independently prognostic among Stage II melanomas [3], a significant focus surrounds the adjudication of in situ expression of candidate proteins, as assessed by immunostaining on paraffin-embedded tissues, to identify signatures corresponding to melanomas with poor melanoma-specific survival.

To identify those protein candidates with potential for translation into the clinic as prognostic indicators from among the vast literature of evaluated candidates, we published a systematic review and meta-analysis critically evaluating the body of published melanoma immunostaining data through January 2008 [4]. Of the 455 identified manuscripts that reported immunostaining data on melanoma samples, only 37 manuscripts reported multivariable survival estimates across either prospective or retrospective cohorts while meeting REMARK criteria [5] for immunostaining assay rigor for 62 unique individual protein candidates. Schramm and Mann updated our review through December 2009, identifying an additional eligible 14 studies and bringing the total number of rigorously evaluated proteins to 86 [6]. For this report, we extended our systematic review search criteria through August 15th, 2012 and identified an additional 15 eligible manuscripts collectively evaluating 12 proteins including 9 candidates not previously considered in prior reports [7–21].

The incremental value of molecular markers added to clinicopathologic prognostic models is dependent on both the magnitude of the effect size and the inverse of the correlation with the clinicopathologic parameters already in the model [22]. Altogether, across the 66 included studies, statistically significant ($p<0.05$) multivariable adjusted Cox Proportional Hazards results were reported for 14/49 protein associations with overall survival, 25/47 for melanoma-specific survival, and 20/31 for melanoma-free survival [4, 6–21]. Interestingly, of the 58 significant associations, only 20 results representing 17 markers, including Ki-67, achieved a hazard ratio $\geq$3.0 with 13 of these based upon total sample sizes of <100 (Table 1). Furthermore, only metallothionein was independently validated with just the disease-free survival association repeated in an independent cohort [23, 24]. None of the other extreme values were independently recapitulated. By comparison, individual proteins whose significant prognostic hazard ratios were independently recapitulated across multiple cohorts (e.g., p16/INK4A, Matrix metalloproteinase-2) displayed more modest, but consistent, *p*-values in each of these studies (Table 2).

Table 1

Significant, multivariable-adjusted individual protein melanoma-related prognostic hazard ratios ≥3.0 (≤0.33)

Protein	Total *n*	Reference group	Hazard ratio (95 % confidence interval)	*p*-value	References
Overall survival					
Bcl-xL	60	<10 % cells positive	8.07 (1.77–36.89)	$p=0.007$	[83]
Bcl-6	60	No immunostain	3.98 (1.37–11.60)	$p=0.01$	[83]
p16/INK4A	60	<50 % cells positive	0.29 (0.10–0.83)	$p=0.02$	[83]
p27/KIP1	60	<10 % cells positive	3.08 (1.20–7.91)	$p=0.02$	[83]
Matrix metallo-proteinase-2	50	<34 % cells positive	4.5 (1.5–13.0)	$p=0.006$	[84]
Melanoma cell adhesion molecule/MUC18	76	No immunostain	16.34 (3.80–70.28)	$p<0.001$	[85]
SNF5	88	No immunostain	5.15 (1.48–17.89)	$p=0.01$	[86]
Melanoma-specific survival					
iNOS	132	<5 % cells positive	4.63 (2.60–8.25)	$p<0.001$	[87]
Ki-67	187	<16 % cells positive	3.7 (1.6–8.9)	$p=0.003$	[88]
MCM3	255	Nuclear H score ≤3 (of 9)	4.96 (1.77–13.87)	$p=0.002$	[9]
Metallothionein	1,428	<10 % cells positive	3.08 (2.02–4.68)	$p<0.001$	[23, 24]
p53	187	No immunostain	8.9 (2.7–29.0)	$p<0.001$	[88]
SNF5	88	No immunostain	4.64 (1.15–18.63)	$p=0.03$	[86]
Disease-free survival					
CEACAM-1	100	<20 % cells positive	7.17 (3.22–15.95)	$p<0.001$	[89]
Cyclin A	172	<5 % cells positive	3.7 (3.4–4.1)	$p=0.001$	[90]
L1-CAM	100	<20 % cells positive	4.38 (2.08–9.23)	$p<0.001$	[91]
Melanoma cell adhesion molecule/MUC18	76	No immunostain	14.83 (5.20–42.24)	$p=0.01$	[75]
Metallothionein	1,428	<10 % cells positive	3.77 (2.73–5.22)	$p<0.001$	[23, 24]
Microtubule-associated protein-2	37	<70 % cells positive	0.18 (0.06–0.56)	$p=0.003$	[92]
Proliferating cell nuclear antigen	93	≤15 % cells positive	4.00 (2.05–7.81)	$p=0.039$	[93]
Survivin	50	No nuclear immunostain	7.32 (1.43–37.38)	$p=0.017$	[94]

Table 2
Individual proteins with multivariable hazard ratios independently assayed across multiple cohorts

Protein	Study	Total *n*	Reference group	Hazard Ratio (95 % confidence iinterval)	*p*-value	References
Overall survival						
Cyclin A						
	Tran 1998	66	<5 % cells positive	5.00 (0.56–44.69)	$p=0.15$	[95]
	Florenes 2001	172	<5 % cells positive	0.80 (0.40–1.60)	$p=0.43$	[90]
	Alonso 2004	60	<5 % cells positive	0.76 (0.27–2.14)	$p=0.60$	[83]
Ki-67						
	Niezabitowski 1999	93	<20 % cells positive	5.17 (2.17–12.29)	$p=0.0002$	[93]
	Alonso 2004	60	<20 % cells positive	1.24 (0.49–3.14)	$p=0.65$	[83]
Cyclin D3						
	Florenes 2000	172	<5 % cells positive	1.00 (0.60–1.67)	$p>0.99$	[96]
	Alonso 2004	59	<5 % cells positive	3.63 (0.81–16.27)	$p=0.09$	[83]
Cyclin D1						
	Florenes 2000	172	<5 % cells positive	1.00 (0.40–2.50)	$p>0.99$	[96]
	Alonso 2004	60	<5 % cells positive	1.22 (0.35–4.25)	$p=0.75$	[83]
nm23						
	McDermott 2000	145	Weak/moderate immunostain	0.79 (0.41–1.51)	$p=0.48$	[97]
	Pacifico 2005a	76	Weak/moderate immunostain	0.44 (0.10–1.99)	$p=0.29$	[98]

skp2						
	Alonso 2004	59	<5 % cells positive	1.04 (0.38–2.85)	$p=0.94$	[83]
	Li 2004	104	<5 % cells positive	1.07 (0.55–2.08)	$p=0.84$	[99]
Melanoma-specific survival						
Metallothionein						
	Weinlich 2006	1,270	<10 % cells positive	3.49 (2.25–5.41)	$p<0.0001$	[23]
	Weinlich 2007	158	<10 % cells positive	0.85 (0.21–3.45)	$p=0.82$	[24]
Matrix metalloproteinase-2						
	Vaisanen 2008	157	≤20 % cells positive	2.60 (1.32–5.07)	$p=0.006$	[84]
	Rotte 2012	330	≤Moderate immunostaining	2.38 (1.39–4.09)	$p=0.002$	[19]
p16/INK4A						
	Straume 2000	187	Weak stain	0.4 (0.24–0.67)	$p=0.007$	[88]
	Gould Rothberg 2009	187	Weak nuclear immunostain (1st quartile AQUA score)	2nd quartile: 0.46 (0.27–0.88)		
				3rd quartile: 0.42 (0.22–0.81)		
				4th quartile: 0.60 (0.32–1.15)	$p=0.04$	[32]
Galectin-3						
	Bulijan 2011	104	Weak/moderate immunostain	3.54 (0.57–22.00)	$p=0.18$	[21]
	Brown 2012	314	Weak/moderate nuclear immunostain	0.74 (0.55-1.00)	$p=0.06$	[20]
Disease-free survival						
Metallothionein						
	Weinlich 2006	1270	<10 % cells positive	3.94 (2.77–5.60)	$p<0.0001$	[23]
	Weinlich 2007	158	<10 % cells positive	2.98 (1.31–6.78)	$p=0.009$	[24]

Taken together, these data suggest that the independent marginal gain in risk prediction over the base clinicopathologic prognostic models for most independent markers might not be of substantial clinical benefit to warrant further translation.

Consequently, one alternate strategy with the potential for augmenting the clinical relevance of melanoma-related molecular predictors is to assemble a portfolio of orthogonally prognostic proteins that, when combined as a single parameter, yield a high-magnitude independently prognostic measure. Creation of multi-marker prognostic models from differential transcriptome profiling is well-established with both the Oncotype DX [25, 26] and MammaPrint [27, 28] tests approved for breast cancer prognostic stratification and, similarly, the Oncotype Dx Colon Cancer [29] and ColoPrint [30] offer risk stratification for patients with Stage II colorectal cancer. Moreover, the immunohistochemistry-based 5-protein Mammostrat panel to identify estrogen receptor-positive breast cancer patients at high risk for relapse despite estrogen-modulating adjuvant therapy has recently been validated in a prospective, randomized clinical trial [31]. Similarly, in melanoma, multiparameter-based approaches for prognostic biomarkers are beginning to emerge as our updated systematic review identified five manuscripts that each proposes a prognostic index based upon the combination of 3–7 individual biomarkers with the potential for translation into the clinic (Table 3) [7, 8, 32–34]. Eighteen unique proteins were included across the five models with only three proteins—p16/INK4A, p53, and β-catenin—included in multiple models. Altogether, the five models highlight the diversity of both laboratory and statistical methodologies as well as the breadth of protein combinations. Although the most straightforward approaches leverage standard semi-quantitative chromogenic immunostaining, build a composite model from the subset of protein candidates that yield significant univariate survival relationships and create an index score reflecting the number of markers that exceed a specified threshold, more objective approaches that integrate fully quantitative measures of protein expression or more complex, parameterized statistical models are beginning to emerge.

In this review, we present a stepwise approach for discovering and validating novel multiparameter biomarker-based prognostic models. We outline appropriate cohort recruitment strategies, comprehensively describe laboratory protocols supporting fully quantitative assessment of protein expression using either chromogenic or immunofluorescent platforms and present a suite of innovative statistical approaches for combining the assayed markers. Finally, we present recommended steps for validating the model in an independent cohort, necessary to support potential generalizability to the greater melanoma population.

Table 3
Published melanoma multiparameter prognostic models

Study	Assay method	Parameter triage method	Selected markers and cut-points	Prognostic index categories	Discovery cohort Hazard ratios (95 % CI)	*p*-value	Validation cohort hazard ratio (95 % CI)	*p*-value
Piras 2008 [34]	Qualitative chromogenic immunostaining	Significance in univariate log-rank analysis	Total p53: any + Nuclear p16: any + Nuclear survivin: any +	0–1 altered 2–3 altered	1.00 4.77 (2.14–10.59)	$p<0.0001$	NA	–
Kashani-Sabet 2009 [33]	Semi-quantitative chromogenic immunostaining	Independent significance in multivariable models	Osteopontin[a] NCOA3/AIB-1 RGS1	Score of −3 to 0 Score of 1–3	1.00 1.29 (1.19–1.40)	$p=0.002$	1.00 1.34 (1.22–1.47)	$p=0.001$
Gould Rothberg 2009 [32]	Quantitative immunofluorescence	Genetic algorithms	ln(ATF2 ratio) > -0.052 β-catenin > 38.68 Fibronectin ≤ 57.93 ln(p16 ratio) ≤ −0.083 Nuclear p21 > 12.98	≤3 markers + 4–5 markers +	1.00 2.84 (1.46–5.49)	$p=0.002$	1.00 2.72 (1.12–6.58)	$p=0.027$
Vaisanen 2011 [8]	Semi-quantitative chromogenic immunostaining	Significance in univariate log-rank analysis	Ki-67: >40 % cells + p53: any + MMP-2: >20 % cells +	0 altered 1 altered 2 altered 3 altered	NA[b]	–	NA	–
Meyer 2012 [7]	Semi-quantitative chromogenic immunostaining	Significance in univariate log-rank analysis	Bax[c] Bcl-X β-catenin CD20 Cox-2 MTAP PTEN	0th–50th percentile 51st–100th percentile	1.00 5.1 (1.4–18.2)	$p=0.012$	1.00 14.45 (1.68–124.49)	$p=0.015$

[a]Selected cut-points were not defined in the published manuscript
[b]The multiparameter assay was developed but assessed only as a univariate parameter. The reported multivariable Cox proportional hazards model simultaneously included MMP-2 and Ki-67 as independent parameters, which were both independently significant
[c]Cut-points were not used. Each marker was scored as a 5-level semi-quantitative variable (0–4) and this value was used to calculate the summary score

2 Materials

2.1 Tissue Microarray (TMA) Construction

1. Paraffin blocks from each of the index primary melanomas of all eligible individuals accessioned in the Discovery and Validation cohorts.
2. Paraffin blocks from tissue reference controls and cell line reference controls.
3. Stainless steel coring needle (Estigen OÜ, Tartu, Estonia).
4. Tape transfer system (Leica Microsystems, Buffalo Grove, IL).
5. Nitrogen chamber/dessicator (Terra Universal, Fullerton, CA).

2.2 Antigen Retrieval

1. 60 °C hybridization oven (we use an HB-1000 hybridization oven—UVP, Upland, CA).
2. Stainless steel, 30-slide staining dish (500 mL) and racks (Mopec, Oak Park, MI).
3. Xylene.
4. 100 % ethanol and 75 % ethanol.
5. Antigen Retrieval Buffer: (6.5 mM sodium citrate (3.84 g sodium citrate in 2 L ddH_2O)), pH 6.0 or 1.3 mM EDTA (0.76 g EDTA in 2 L ddH_2O), pH = 8.0.
6. Pre-Treatment (PT) Module automated dewaxing and epitope recovery device (Lab Vision, Fremont, CA).
7. 0.75 % hydrogen peroxide in absolute methanol.
8. Tris-buffered saline (TBS, 1×, 8.76 g sodium chloride and 2.42 g trizma base/L, pH = 8.0).
9. TBS with 0.5 % Tween-20.
10. 0.3 % bovine serum albumin (BSA) in TBS/0.5 % Tween-20 (1.5 g BSA dissolved in 500 mL 1× TBS with 0.5 % TWEEN-20).

2.3 Quantitative Chromogenic Immunohistochemistry (IHC) Using the Aperio Scan Scope™ CS Brightfield Platform

1. Anti-target primary mouse/rabbit monoclonal antibodies.
2. PAP pen (Kiyota International, Elk Grove Village, IL).
3. EnVision™-HRP anti-target species (mouse/rabbit) secondary antibody (DAKO, Carpenteria, CA).
4. 3,3′-diaminobenzidine (DAB) or3-amino-9-ethylcarbazole (AEC+) substrate chromogens and Substrate Buffer (DAKO, Carpenteria, CA).
5. TACHA hematoxylin (Biocare Medical, Concord, CA).
6. Cytoseal 60™ mounting medium (Richard-Allan Scientific, Kalamazoo, MI).
7. Aperio ScanScope® CS digital light microscope platform with *Console* and *Spectrum* software platforms (Aperio, Vista, CA).

2.4 Quantitative Immunofluorescence (QIF) Using the AQUA® Technique

1. Anti-target primary mouse/rabbit monoclonal antibodies.
2. Mask antibodies: Rabbit anti-S100 polyclonal antibody (DAKO, Carpenteria, CA) and anti-gp100 polyclonal antibody (Abcam, Cambridge, MA) or Mouse anti-S100B monoclonal antibody (clone 15E2E2, Abcam, Cambridge, MA) and HMB45 monoclonal antibody (Abcam, Cambridge, MA).
3. PAP pen (Kiyota International, Elk Grove Village, IL).
4. AlexaFluor 546-conjugated goat anti-mask species secondary antibody (Life Technologies, Carlsbad, CA).
5. EnVision™-HRP anti-target species (mouse/rabbit) secondary antibody (DAKO, Carpenteria, CA).
6. 10× Cy5-tyramide and Amplification Buffer (Perkin-Elmer Life Sciences, Waltham, MA).
7. Prolong Gold mounting medium with 4′6-diamidino-2-phenylindole (DAPI) (Life Technologies, Carlsbad, CA).
8. Digital fluorescent image capture platform—Caliper Life Sciences Vectra® 2 (Caliper Life Sciences, Hopkinton, MA) or Aperio ScanScope® FL (Aperio, Vista, CA).
9. *AQUAsition*™ image capture and *AQUAnalysis*™ image analysis software packages (HistoRx, Branford, CT).

3 Methods

3.1 Selection of Cases for Discovery and Validation Cohorts (See Note 1)

1. Obtain institutional review board approval for the use of human tissue specimens and to obtain their corresponding clinicopathological data and melanoma-related outcomes.
2. Define the sampling frame for each of the *Discovery* and *Validation* cohorts.
3. Define the study inclusion/exclusion criteria (e.g., Stage II melanoma cases only, exclusion of all new diagnoses in children <18 years of age).
4. Query the appropriate hospital records or population-based tumor registry to ascertain the complete list of all potentially eligible melanoma cases according to the defined inclusion/exclusion criteria.
5. Query the appropriate surgical/dermatopathological tissue repositories to identify the subset of eligible patients with available residual tissue.
6. Review diagnostic H&E sections and complete medical record abstraction for all eligible cases, whether residual tissue is available or not.
7. Within each of the Discovery and Validation cohorts, to rule out the potential for selection bias due to availability of residual

tissue, compare the distribution of clinicopathologic criteria between those cases with and without available tissue.

8. To ensure the comparability of the *Discovery* and *Validation* cohorts, compare their respective distributions of the conventional clinicopathologic parameters planned for inclusion in multivariable modeling.

3.2 Construction of Tissue Microarrays (See Note 2*)*

TMAs are constructed using the standard method [35] and cut sections are adhered to the glass slides using a tape transfer technique.

1. Retrieve the paraffin blocks and their associated cut H&E slides corresponding to the primary tumors from all eligible *Discovery* and *Validation* cohort members from the tissue archive (*see* **Note 3**).
2. Review the H&E slide to confirm the presence of residual tumor and, using a fine-tip marker, circle on the H&E slide the region most representative of the primary tumor for inclusion onto the TMA.
3. To allow for adequate modeling of intra-tumoral heterogeneity and to guard against missing values, inclusion of 4 0.6 mm histospots per case in melanoma tumors is recommended (*see* **Note 4**).
4. In addition to the cohort histospots, a series of controls must also be included in the TMA.
   (a) *Tissue reference controls.* These controls allow for the normalization of the quantitative scores to a single reference point across multiple builds of a single TMA or between the training and validation TMAs, especially when these experiments were conducted at separate, distinct time points. Specifically, these provide the reference standards allowing correction for any laboratory drift that may occur. These are selected as follows:
   - Three to four benign tissues with anticipated homogeneous expression are selected. Our group selects liver, kidney medulla, and uterine smooth muscle but other tissue choices can be made.
   - Paraffin blocks of each targeted tissue from 8 to 10 individuals are retrieved and included in the TMA for a total of 24–30, 0.6 mm histospots dedicated to these controls.

   (b) *Cell line controls.* Formalin-fixed, paraffin-embedded pellets from 10 to 12 melanoma cell lines representing the diversity of known somatic mutation subtypes (e.g., BRAF mutants, NRAS mutants, RAC1 mutants, and BRAF/NRAS/RAC1 wild type cell lines) are prepared (*see* [36] for complete method) in parallel with a series of cell lysates. Cores from these pellets are included in duplicate on the TMA to both serve as known internal positive and negative controls (*see* Subheading 3.3.1: Primary anti-biomarker antibody selection and validation) for the primary antibody and, among those positively expressing the antigen, to verify within-sample heterogeneity of expression.

5. To ensure an unbiased array of the tumor samples and random admixture of all the control samples, TMA row and column location are assigned using a random number generator. Each planned core is randomly assigned a number between 0 and 1, rank ordered according to that number assignment and then row/column addresses are sequentially given.
6. Donor blocks are aligned according to row/column assignment and 0.6 mm cores, created with a stainless steel coring needle are arrayed into the recipient paraffin block to create the microarray [35].
7. The completed TMA block is then faced and cut using the tape-transfer method. Tape-transfer substantially reduces the number of lost histospots and distortion of the histospot array that can occur during sectioning [37] and, in our experience, does not interfere with immunostain quality or readability.
   (a) Place an adhesive Tape Window to the block face. The tape supports and captures the section.
   (b) The Tape Window is placed section-side-down on corresponding, complimentary adhesive-coated slides and laminated to the slide using the included hand roller.
   (c) Expose the slide to 30–60 s of 360 nm ultraviolet light to polymerize the slide adhesive layer into a hard, solvent-resistant plastic that anchors the section to the slide.
   (d) Remove the Tape Window by immersing the section in TPC solvent for 3 min.
   (e) Dip slide briefly in Xylene to dry and then coat the slide in paraffin and store in a desiccator maintained at 10.5 % relative humidity using nitrogen gas until use to preserve tissue antigenicity by reducing exposure of the cut face to ambient oxygen and relative humidity [38].

3.3 Methods for Biomarker Quantification

Diverse commercial quantitative immunostaining platforms with capabilities for brightfield, chromogenic immunostaining or quantitative immunofluorescence are available (Table 1). Brightfield platforms are based upon the visualization of chromogenic stains (e.g., DAB or AEC) against a hematoxylin counterstain. Machine-learning-based feature extraction algorithms or other more simple size-based methods can resolve relevant cellular (e.g., tumor, stroma, vasculature, inflammatory infiltrates) and subcellular (e.g., nuclear vs. cytoplasmic) compartments. The definition of these compartments may be dependent on the counterstain or other methods. Protein expression is then quantified by measuring the levels of white light absorbance by the chromogenic stain, typically operationalized as the average intensity of the stain's color (hue and saturation) across all pixels included in a selected compartment [39–41]. By comparison, QIF multiplexes the target antibody fluorophore (typically at or above 650 nm to avoid contamination with tissue autofluorescence) with fluorophores directed against relevant cellular and subcellular features. In this manner, cellular and subcellular compartments are resolved through colocalization with the selected fluorescent signal and protein expression is quantified by measuring the level of light emission at the appropriate wavelength corresponding to the target fluorophore within the compartment(s) of interest [42]. Multiplexing of targets can be executed by selecting fluorophores with nonoverlapping emission spectra [43]. By example, we provide detailed methodologic protocols for quantitative chromogenic IHC optimized for the Aperio ScanScope CS brightfield platform and its associated Positive Pixel Count Algorithm as well as QIF using the AQUA® technique.

3.3.1 Primary Anti-Biomarker Antibody Selection and Validation

Prior to initiating any immunostaining assays to assess levels of the candidate biomarker, advance consideration must be given towards choice of the primary anti-biomarker antibody. First, where possible, assay development with a monoclonal antibody is preferred. Once established, monoclonal antibody reagents are synthesized in vitro from an immortalized lymphocyte cell line which not only ensures a steady, consistent supply of quality reagent over the complete life cycle of assay development but also, if translation into the clinic is warranted, the antibody reagent quality and consistency can be validated according to Clinical Laboratory Improvement Amendments (CLIA) standards to support necessary clinical trial work. In contrast, while use of polyclonal antibodies can indeed uncover novel significant and biologically relevant biomarkers for melanoma prognosis, translating their use into the clinic is less straightforward and uncertain at best. The most striking consideration is that, unlike an immortalized, clonal cell line capable of scalable monoclonal antibody production that is potentially unlimited, the availability of any polyclonal reagent is limited at any one time by the amount of blood obtained from host organism during the lifespan of the individual animal. The specific polyclonal mixture is exhausted upon the host's death and may never be regenerated in an identical manner due to variability in the immune systems in the host species, even when challenged with identical antigen. Although QC metrics for creating similarly effective polyclonal reagents for molecular techniques such as chromatin immunoprecipitation from across a population of immunized rabbits are routinely used [44], antibody-based projects requiring a high degree of standardization such as the prognostic biomarker assays described here, are best served with monoclonal antibodies [45].

Next, all selected antibodies must undergo comprehensive validation procedures to verify that the antibody is both sensitive and specific for its presumed target. The method preferred by our lab has been recently published [46]. One simple method of antibody validation is to conduct a Western blot on a spectrum of cell lines including one with previously confirmed expression of the target protein and one where protein expression is known to be absent. In this assay, the goal is to verify specific band(s) at the confirmed expected molecular weight(s) for the target and to rule out visualization of any additional electrophoretic signals at spurious molecular weights. While a Western blot can eliminate an antibody due to cross-reactivity, absence of signal does not necessarily mean the antibody will not work in IHC or QIF applications. When the Western Blot is noninformative due to lack of antibody reactivity with the denatured antigen, it may still be valuable and specific in the less denatured conditions seen in tissue sections, so in situ validation methods are recommended. "Blocking peptide" methods where a soluble peptide expected to adsorb to the antibody are not recommended since they cannot confirm specificity as they do not rule out binding to off-target sites on the tissue sections. Rigorous in situ antibody validation is best achieved using small interfering-RNA (si-RNA) in vitro knockdown experiments on positively expressing cell lines or progressive induction of target antigen in nonexpressing lines. Here, levels of protein expression on the selected cell line(s) are assayed by IHC or QIF in the presence/absence of siRNAs. If levels of the protein do not decrease with target knockdown, cross-reactivity with alternate antigens is suspected and the antibody should be abandoned. Alternatively, transfection and progressively increased induced expression can also show in situ specificity [47].

3.3.2 Antigen Retrieval

The initial steps of the immunostaining protocol through application of the primary antibodies are identical for both brightfield and immunofluorescent techniques as described below:

1. Align slides in a metal slide rack and place the rack in a 60 °C oven for 20 min to overnight to melt off excess paraffin. For sections not adhered to the glass slides using an ultraviolet crosslinked tape-transfer method, overnight incubation at 60 °C is necessary to cure the slides.
2. Deparaffinize the tissues using two exchanges of 400 ml xylene for 20 min each.

3. Rehydrate the tissues through two exchanges of 400 ml 100 % ethanol and one exchange of 75 % ethanol for 1 min each and then place the slides under running water for 10 min.
4. Pour 2 L of Antigen Retrieval Buffer (6.5 mM sodium citrate, pH 6.0 or 1.3 mM EDTA pH = 8.0) in the PT Module vessel and preheat the unit to 85 °C.
5. Once the buffer has reached the preheating temperature, place the slides in the Module using the accompanying slide rack, seal the device, and set antigen retrieval at 97 °C for 20 min.
6. Following antigen retrieval, once the PT Module has cooled down to 75 °C, remove the slides from the Module, place them under cold running water for 10 min and then submerge the slides in 400 ml absolute methanol containing 0.75 % hydrogen peroxide for 30 min to quench endogenous peroxidase activity.
7. Wash the slides in two exchanges of water for 30 s and in 1× TBS for 5 min.
8. Blot each slide dry and apply 1 mL of TBS-Tween/0.3 % BSA solution to the exposed tissue section for 30 min to adsorb nonspecific binding sites.
9. Blot off the TBS-Tween/BSA and proceed to **step 1** of Subheading 3.3.3 (chromogenic immunostaining for brightfield platforms) or **step 2** of Subheading 3.3.3 (quantitative immunofluorescence) to begin with primary antibody application for the desired platforms.

3.3.3 Quantitative Chromogenic IHC Using the Aperio Scanscope™ CS brightfield platform (See ***Note 5****)*

1. Prepare the desired titer of the validated primary target antibody by diluting it into TBS-Tween/0.3 % BSA to create a final volume of 1 mL.
2. Place the TMA slide in a level humid chamber and pipette the full 1 mL volume of the primary antibody cocktail onto the TMA section, ensuring that the full surface of the section is evenly covered with fluid. To create a hydrophobic barrier that ensures retention of the antibody cocktail on the section, outline the TMA boundary with a PAP pen.
3. Set the slide to incubate at 4 °C overnight.
4. Wash off the excess primary antibody by placing in two 10-min exchanges of TBS-Tween followed by one 10-min exchange of TBS.
5. Apply 1 mL of species-appropriate EnVision™ HRP-labeled polymer secondary antibody and incubate at room temperature for 1 h.
6. Wash the EnVision™ by placing in two 5-min exchanges of TBS followed by one 5-min exchange of distilled water.
7. Apply 1 mL of the diluted AEC + substrate chromogen (20 μL chromagen diluted into 980 μL Substrate Buffer), incubate for

5 min and then wash off by applying two 5-min exchanges of TBS and one 5-min exchange of distilled water.

8. Apply 1 mL TACHA hematoxylin to the TMA and incubate at room temperature for 1 min. In our experience, as the TACHA hematoxylin does not require a bluing step, it yields a more consistent color and reduces measurement error during automated assessment of staining intensity.
9. Rinse the slide in two exchanges of distilled water, dehydrate through an ethanol gradient of 1-min exchanges at 70, 85, 95, and 100 % then place in a final 100 % ethanol exchange for 5 min.
10. Transfer the slides into xylene for 5 min then remove each slide one at a time from the xylene, blot dry, apply 1–2 drops of CytoSeal 60™ mounting medium, coverslip each slide, and allow the mounting medium to set.
11. Automated image capture is accomplished on the Aperio ScanScope CS using the *Console* application installed with the machine. Briefly, 1–5 stained slides are loaded into the tray and a photomicrograph snapshot of each slide covering all magnifications from 10× to 200× is captured.
12. The region of the slide containing the stained tissue is identified and each histospot is identified within the TMA by engaging the *Find focus points* algorithm. At this step, histospots not automatically identified can be marked by the user and slide artifacts erroneously tagged can be manually removed.
13. Automated quantification of levels of staining is then executed using the provided *Spectrum* software package. The "*area of interest*," or the region containing the tumor cells is identified using a two-step process where first a single, closed polygon is drawn around the entire tumor-containing region of the histospot using the freehand "*Pen Tool*" and then the "*Negative Pen Tool*" is used to exclude smaller regions of nontumor areas within the larger encircled region. This step introduces a level of subjectivity into the analysis. Other software tools like the Definiens software (Definiens, Parsippany, NJ) or the Genie software (Flagship Biosciences, Flagstaff, AZ) may be used to make this step more objective.
14. With the tumor region now defined, application of available algorithms allows for quantitation of immunostain intensity and percent coverage.
    (a) The *Nuclear Algorithm* defines included nuclei according to light absorption according to the counterstain colorization with the subsequent ability to define levels of chromogen intensity within this segregated region. Outputted values include: total area covered in the nuclear analysis, average nuclear size, percent of nuclei with any

positive stain and the average intensity of stain across all included nuclei.

(b) The *Positive Pixel Count Algorithm* identifies all pixels within the Annotated region and assigns to them a score ranging from 0 to 255 reflecting the chromagen intensity at the preselected color. Three user-defined arbitrary cut-offs along this continuum are then selected to define the boundaries separating "no stain (0)," "weak positive (+1)," "moderate positive (+2)", and "strong positive (+3)". Outputted metrics then include: Average intensity ([**Σ**pixel intensity scores (0–255)]/total number of included pixels), number of weak positive, moderate positive, and strong positive pixels and percent pixel positivity (number of pixels with any positivity/total number of pixels). Users may define methods to produce a continuous scale if desired.

15. Histospot-level data describing all measured parameters are then exported through the *Spectrum* software platform into Excel for further integration with the clinicopathologic and outcomes measures as described below (Subheading 3.4).

3.3.4 Quantitative Immunofluorescence Using the AQUA® technique (See **Note 6***)*

The methods for conducting QIF/AQUA® are provided, highlighting its similarities and differences with the brightfield chromogenic methods outlined above (**step 1** of Subheading 3.3.3).

1. For each TMA slide, prepare 1 mL primary antibody solution in TBS-Tween/0.3 % BSA by adding the desired titer of the validated primary target antibody in addition to the melanoma "mask" cocktail of S100/gp100 antibodies that will allow for the discrimination of melanoma cells from surrounding nonmelanoma stromal elements in the absence of counterstain. When non-rabbit anti-target primary antibodies are selected (e.g., mouse, rat), the preferred rabbit-based mask includes 5 μL (1:200) anti-S100 polyclonal antibody and 40 μL (1:25) anti-gp100 polyclonal antibody. Using rabbit anti-target primary antibodies necessitates a mouse-based mask of 10 μL (1:100) anti-S100B clone 15E2E2 and 10 μL (1:100) of HMB45.
2. Place the TMA slide in a level humid chamber and pipette the full 1 mL volume of the primary antibody cocktail onto the TMA section, ensuring that the full surface of the section is evenly covered with fluid. To create a hydrophobic barrier that ensures retention of the antibody cocktail on the section, outline the TMA boundary with a PAP pen.
3. Apply the primary antibody cocktail to each slide and incubate in a humid chamber at 4 °C overnight.
4. Wash off the excess primary antibody by placing in two 10-min exchanges of TBS-TWEEN followed by one 10-min exchange of TBS.

5. Prepare the secondary antibody cocktail by adding 10 μL of AlexaFluor 546-conjugated goat anti-mask species into each 1 mL target species-appropriate EnVision™ HRP-labeled polymer secondary antibody.
6. Apply 1 mL of the secondary antibody cocktail to each TMA and incubate at room temperature for 1 h.
7. Wash the secondary antibody cocktail by placing in two 10-min exchanges of TBS-TWEEN followed by one 5-min exchange of TBS.
8. Dilute 20 μL of concentrated 10× Cy5-tyramide into 980 μL of the accompanying Amplification Buffer and add fluorescent label to the Envision™ by applying 1 mL of 1× Cy5-tyramide to the TMA for 10 min.
9. Wash the excess Cy5 by placing in two 10-min exchanges of TBS-Tween followed by one 5-min exchange of TBS.
10. Apply 120 μL of Prolong Gold mounting medium with DAPI, the latter to visualize the nuclei, and coverslip allowing the mounting medium to set overnight before commencing automated image capture.
11. Automated image capture is compatible with the Caliper Life Sciences Vectra® 2 or the Aperio ScanScope® FL microscopy instrumentation platforms using the respective native software platforms. Image capture on the PM-2000™ is executed with the *AQUAsition*™ platform (HistoRx, Branford, CT), described in detail in ref. [48]. Image analysis is universally executed by the *AQUAnalysis*™ software package (HistoRx). The current version of AQUA® is robust to inter-operator variation [49] and minimizes coefficients of variability through standard instrument calibration procedures (e.g., calibration cube, light source, and Cy5 optical path factors [50]). The AQUA® method is summarized below.
    (a) A 4× low-resolution image of the entire slide in the DAPI channel is captured and used to localize the specific Cartesian coordinates defining each histospot.
    (b) A series of 20× images, one image for each fluorescent channel used (Nuclear (DAPI), Mask (Cy3), Target (Cy5)), is captured for each histospot. To maximize the dynamic range of the target immunofluorescent signal, the exposure time is automated for each channel in each histospot to ensure in yielding only 0.02 % saturated pixels for the selected channel.
    (c) Global TMA quality assessment is executed using the stack of Mask-labeled Cy3 images as a reference. Histospots that are devoid of tumor, where the histospot has fallen off or where the image is substantially out of focus should be eliminated outright. Among the included histospots, specific

regions that contain major artifacts such as folded tissue, air bubbles should be cropped out leaving the remaining, adequately stained histospot regions available for analysis.

(d) The tumor mask is determined as the set of pixels that display a level of Cy3 staining above a prespecified minimal threshold (binary gating) followed by spatial image analysis procedures (e.g., filling holes) to create multiple continuous regions corresponding to the tumor locations.

(e) Subcellular compartments (e.g., nuclear, cytoplasmic) are then defined within the tumor mask using an unsupervised k-means clustering algorithm [49]. Each pixel is plotted on a two-dimensional scatter plot according to the DAPI and Cy3 intensities. The clustering algorithm is then applied according to three fundamental assumptions: (1) background pixels will have low intensities for both channels, (2) nuclear pixels will have high DAPI but low Cy3 intensity and (3) cytoplasmic pixels will have high Cy3 but low DAPI intensity. Pixels are then assigned to each cluster according to Euclidean distance from each of the three cluster centroids.

(f) Levels of target protein expression within the tumor mask and in each subcellular compartment are reported as a continuous value ranging from 0 to 33,000 that represents the mean Cy5 channel intensity across the subset of pixels included in the selected compartment. As high-resolution 8-bit image capture generates 256 discrete intensity values per pixel, raw pixel intensity reflects the mean intensity value across the 256 readings. Next, to account for the spot-to-spot variability in exposure time, pixel *power*, the raw pixel intensity/exposure time is calculated. Raw AQUA score is then calculated as the mean *pixel power* across all pixels included in the selected compartment. Finally, corrections reflecting the instrument calibration standards are applied to yield a *normalized AQUA score* which is the product of the raw AQUA score and each of the calibration cube, light source, and optical path factors.

3.4 Computational Methods for Feature Selection, Model Construction, and Internal Validation

REMARK stipulates adjudication of individual markers using Cox Proportional Hazards. But creating a multimarker model by entering multiple biomarkers into a single Cox model adjusted for clinicopathologic variables is not effective as the sample size required to allow for sufficient power to adequately consider not only the main effects of each protein but also all of their pairwise and higher-order interactions is excessive. An efficient alternative is to create a single multimarker parameter that reflects the composite prognostic impact of all component markers for subsequent evaluation in adjusted survival analyses.

A diversity of statistical approaches exist for *dimension reduction* and *feature selection*, the process of condensing and culling from a larger set of individual protein candidates the subset that best explain the variance observed in the Discovery Cohort and their subsequent parameterization within the multiparameter model including: (1) weighted summation of individual variables, (2) genetic algorithms, (3) classification and regression trees (CART), (4) random forest analysis, (5) k nearest neighbors and learning-based methods such as (6) support vector machines and (7) discriminant analysis. In this section, we provide detailed methods for the first three approaches as each have been used to define multi-parameter models with prognostic potential in melanoma. We also outline the steps required for internal validation of the results on the Discovery Cohort and provide a strategy for evaluating their prognostic potential in the Validation Cohort.

3.4.1 Cox Univariate Regression Coefficient-Derived Summary Estimates

Of the five published multiparameter models in melanoma, four [7, 8, 33, 34] have their composite measures derived from the individual marker univariate Cox Proportional Hazards regression estimate (*see* **Note 7**). Here, candidate proteins are selected for the summary measure based upon their individual univariate prognostic value. The Cox univariate-based method featured in Meyer et al. is presented in detail (*see* **Note 8**) [7].

1. The crude prognostic value of the semi-quantitative score (0–4) captured for each eligible protein was determined using univariate Cox Proportional Hazards.
2. Markers achieving a *p*-value of 0.05 in the setting of a False Discovery Rate [51] of 0.15 were included in the multiparameter model. Altogether, seven markers, were thus included in their final model.
3. The risk score is then calculated by summing up the individual products of the immunostaining score (0–4) and the univariate Cox regression coefficient across all included markers with available data. To account for the situation of each individual, due to missing data, can contribute fewer than seven markers to the summary score, the raw summary score is normalized through dividing by the number of included markers, according to the following equation (*see* **Note 8**):

$$Score(patient\ X) = \left(\sum_{i=1}^{D} \beta_i x_i\right) \Big/ \left(\sum_{i=1}^{D} \alpha_i\right).$$

   Where $\alpha_i = 1$ if x_i immunostaining for marker $\mathrm{x_i}$ was successful or 0 if the experiment failed and the data is missing.
4. High- versus low-risk scores were determined by splitting the normalized scores at the median.

3.4.2 Genetic Algorithm-Derived Summary Estimates

Genetic algorithms represent an iterative, learning-based approach to model building that exploit the working principles evolution and natural genetics to allow for an efficient, but comprehensive search through a large data space to identify the combination of markers from a larger set of available protein candidates that maximally optimizes prognostic stratification [52]. Beginning with a large panel of candidate proteins with (semi-)quantitative measures of expression, the algorithm arbitrarily selects a set of markers from which to construct a prognostic model and uses the product-limit log-rank chi-square statistic returned from this initial assessment as a benchmark. Then, the algorithm attempts to improve on this initial model by iteratively altering a single parameter in the model ("generation") either by modifying the cut-point selected to binarize the (semi-) quantitative expression level variable for any individual component candidate ("mutation") or by swapping out one of the included markers for another choice from the larger dataset ("cross-over"). For each new model thusly created, the product-limit log-rank chi-square statistic is calculated and compared to the previous benchmark. If the resulting chi-square statistic exceeds the benchmark, the model is kept to become the new benchmark; otherwise, this model is discarded. The algorithm is iterated until "convergence" is reached where no new benchmark can be established, typically occurring after over 20 million generations. We employed a genetic algorithm-based approach to generate our 5-marker melanoma prognostic model selected from 20 available candidates [32]. After marker and cut-point selection, binarized markers were scored, by convention, as "1" if they indicated "reduced risk" and "0" if they contrarily indicated "increased risk" with participants tallied according to the sum of "reduced risk" markers (0–5) which was subsequently used to calculate the benchmark log-rank score (*see* **Note 9**). We seeded our genetic algorithm according to the following parameters:

1. Cross-over rate—the rate at which a swap of markers will be introduced in successive generations, selected at 33 %.
2. Mutation rate—the rate at which an alteration in marker cut-points is introduced, selected at 33 %.
3. Minimum size of the eligible population—when missing data are present, this sets a lower bound for the number of individuals with complete data across the selected markers for model nomination. To ensure sufficient power for multivariable analyses, we required that a minimum of 100 of the 192 assayed individuals be included each model.
4. Threshold for the minimum number of individuals to be included in each arm of a binarized protein expression marker after cut-point selection. Our choice of 10 % helped guard against excessive leverage of extreme observations in defining risk profiles.

5. Threshold for the minimum number of individuals to be included in category of the final ordinal score. Our choice of 15 % further reduced the risk of extreme data point leverage and, to further maintain statistical robustness of our final model, we additionally required that no ordinal category enumerate fewer than two melanoma-related deaths.
6. The minimum and maximum number of parameters to be included in the final model. To balance maximizing the number of complementary markers with the desire for simplicity and ease of translation, we constrained our model to include at least three but no more than eight eligible protein candidates.

3.4.3 Classification and Regression Tree (CART)-Derived Summary Estimates

Recursive partitioning is a nonparametric, iterative algorithm that repeatedly splits subsets of the population into two descendant subsets, beginning with the full population itself according to the parameter that best optimizes the desired outcome among the subset X_i [53]. Thus, once the initial population has been split, the optimal variable to subdivide the left branch of the population might differ from the variable selected to further classify the right branch. Nested partitioning continues along each branch until endpoint assessment is no longer statistically feasible, with tree right-sizing accomplished through pruning of terminal branches to optimize experimental feasibility (e.g., no more than five protein assays required per terminal branch). Binary, ordinal, and continuous independent variables can be included with the CART algorithm selecting the optimal cut-point for nondichotomous variables that maximizes the outcome separation between the two sub-classes. Regression trees modify the baseline classification tree algorithm initially developed for binary outcomes (e.g., dead/alive) to accommodate time-to-failure data and right-censoring of observations [54].

While no multiparameter molecular model has, to date, been constructed using this method, Gimotty et al. successfully applied the Segal algorithm [55] that employs the two-sample log-rank test statistic to determine the between-node heterogeneity measures to select each partitioning variable to refine prognostic strata among patients with thin melanomas (<1.0 mm) using clinicopathologic criteria [56]. Although overall SEER data from 1988 to 2001 indicate 97.4 and 90.2 % 10-year survival rates among Stage IA and IB patients, respectively, the refined algorithm identified subsets from within each of these populations (e.g., Stage IA Clark level II/III men with lesions of 0.78–1.00 mm thick; 90.6 % 10-year survival and Stage IB patients with Clark level IV/V, ulcerated melanomas; 69.8 % 10-year survival) with survival estimates outside those generated for the whole population. This classification was subsequently validated on a second independent cohort to serve as a paradigm for a multiparameter model that integrates clinicopathologic and molecular variables.

3.4.4 Confirmation of the Independent Prognostic Value of the Multiparameter Model in Multivariable Models

The REMARK criteria [5] require adjudication of all candidate molecular prognostic markers in a multivariable Cox Proportional Hazards model that includes all routinely assessed clinicopathologic variables to confirm the marker's independent prognostic value. This necessary step recognizes that these clinicopathologic evaluations reflect the current standard of care and that any molecular test must supplement this standard to justify the assay. For locoregional cutaneous melanoma, Breslow thickness (mm), presence of ulceration, number of mitotic figures/mm^2, presence of microsatellite lesions, sentinel lymph node status, age, and gender [1, 3] are validated parameters and should be included in the multivariable assessment. Clark level of invasion, while independently prognostic in the large, multicenter validation of both the 2001 and 2009 AJCC staging systems [1, 57], is typically collinear with Breslow thickness in smaller populations and cannot be included. Additional clinicopathologic characteristics such as growth phase, histopathologic subtype, anatomic location, tumor vascularity and presence of regression, tumor-infiltrating lymphocytes, solar keratosis, vascular mimicry, and lymphovascular invasion have all been associated with melanoma outcome [58–65] are not yet formally validated and their inclusion is optional.

3.4.5 Multi-parameter Model Internal Validation Using Tenfold and Leave-One-Out Cross Validation

Internal validation experiments assess the model's sensitivity to sample outliers and predict the overall likelihood for generalizability to the general locoregional melanoma population and guard against Type III or Procrustean Errors where the proposed model is suggested by the data due to the leverage of selected extreme data points [66]. Two common methods for internal cross-validation, tenfold and leave-one-out cross-validation are presented [7, 67].

Tenfold Cross Validation

1. Divide the entire Discovery Cohort into ten equally sized groups.
2. Create "training set #1" by combining groups 1–9, leaving group 10 as the "test set #1".
3. Using the raw data for "training set #1," rebuild the multiparameter model, following all of the steps exactly.
4. Apply the regression parameters obtained for the "training set #1" to the "test set #1" to obtain their predicted score for the prognostic model.
5. Calculate the univariate and multivariable (if sufficiently powered) melanoma-specific survival hazard ratio and 95 % confidence interval for the individuals in "test set #1".
6. Repeat **steps 2–4** nine more times to create training sets 2–10 and test sets 2–10, each time selecting a different group as the test set to obtain nine more unique sets of hazard ratios and confidence intervals.

7. Calculate an aggregate hazard ratio and 95 % confidence interval using the ten "test set" values according to the general inverse variance method [68] to obtain a cross-validated estimate for the hazard ratio and 95 % confidence interval for the proposed multiparameter model.

Leave-one-out Cross-Validation

1. Starting with the entire Discovery Cohort (total sample size = n), *n* training sets are built that include all but one patient such that each patient is included in its own $n = 1$ "test set" exactly once.
2. For each of the *n* "training sets", apply the raw data for the included $n-1$ individuals to rebuild the multiparameter model accordingly and then calculate the predicted value from the acquired regression parameters for the one individual included in the "test set".
3. Combine the predicted values from all *n* "test set" iterations into a single dataset and use these values to conduct the univariate and Cox multivariable analyses to obtain a cross-validated estimate for the hazard ratio and 95 % confidence interval.

3.5 External Multiparameter Model Validation

Construction concludes with confirmation of model generalizability through demonstrating prognostic relevance in at least one independent *Validation* cohort. This is done in two phases: demonstration of a significant hazard ratio upon multivariable Cox proportional hazards modeling and assessing the model prediction error. The latter step assesses whether the prognostic algorithm can prospectively assign an independent set of new cases (i.e., the *Validation* cohort) into high risk versus low risk better than pure chance which would have a 50 % success rate in randomly categorizing new individuals [67].

3.5.1 Multivariable Cox Proportional Hazards Modeling

1. A TMA or whole-slide sections are prepared from the primary tissue blocks pertaining to the *Validation* cohort participants.
2. All biomarkers are assayed and scored using the exact methods and criteria applied for model discovery. This can be challenging and methods to standardize scoring between assays over time elapsed between discovery and validation set are critical, but beyond the scope of this chapter.
3. To overcome any potential laboratory drift, all quantitative measures must be normalized to a referent standard to ensure comparability between *Discovery* and *Validation* cohort values.
4. Categorize continuous scores using the same cut-points developed during the model discovery phase. For example, if the *Discovery* cohort was dichotomized at the median of the

Discovery cohort scores, the *Validation* cohort should be divided at the score corresponding to the *Discovery* cohort median and not at the median *Validation* cohort score.

5. Calculate the prognostic index score for each individual according to the developed schema.
6. Complete a multivariable Cox proportional hazards model evaluating the *Validation* cohort prognostic index scores adjusting for the same conventional clinicopathologic covariates applied in the *Discovery* multivariable Cox model.

3.5.2 Prediction Error Estimation

1. Calculate the prognostic index score and its 95 % confidence interval for each individual using the developed schema.
2. Divide the *Validation* cohort into "high-risk" and "low-risk" groups according to the index score cut-point selected during model discovery.
3. Binarize the *Validation* cohort based upon their true outcomes at a fixed timepoint (e.g., 5-year recurrence-free survival, 10-year melanoma-specific survival).
4. Create a 2 × 2 cross-tabular display of the data, calculating the sensitivity, specificity, positive predictive value, and negative predictive values for the table.

4 Notes

1. Correct study design is paramount for developing melanoma prognostic models with translational potential. REMARK criteria require that biomarker studies rigorously report the method of case selection, including details regarding methods of ascertainment (prospective or retrospective) and any inclusion/exclusion criteria that lead to stratification or matching as well as the time period from which cases were taken, then end of the follow-up period and the median follow-up time [5]. In our systematic reviews [4, 69], we have further stipulated that study design must conform to the definition of a prospective or retrospective cohort [70]. The sampling frame must be defined with recruitment strategies striving for complete source population enrollment and documenting study nonparticipation. Convenience samples comprised of a subset of eligible cases (e.g., case series), no matter how large, risk introducing bias. We also advocate against conducting case-control studies since they do not support survival analysis. Simon et al. [71] advocate for additional study design rigor, requiring biomarker validation in prospective cohort studies or randomized clinical trials. At a minimum, two independent cohorts must be identified for the initial model development. A *Discovery Cohort* is used to

explore the independent prognostic utility of the component markers, to conduct feature selection and to execute the initial multivariable Cox proportional hazard modeling. A *Validation Cohort* is required to verify the model's robustness through its generalizability across additional cohorts. In anticipation of their synergistic use, it is critical that the Discovery and Validation cohorts have parallel inclusion/exclusion criteria. For example, if the Discovery cohort is restricted to patients with Stage II melanoma, the correct Validation cohort would be similarly restricted to Stage II melanoma cases.

2. Development of multiparameter biomarker assays for melanoma prognosis requires a significant initial investment in candidate protein evaluation. In our experience [32], as well as that of others [7] between six and ten candidates are triaged through the Training set for every marker selected for inclusion in the model. As a result, model discovery is most efficiently conducted using TMAs. Not only do TMAs allow for efficient rationing of small primary melanomas but they also ensure that all tumors are evaluated concurrently using the same batch of laboratory reagents. However, the risk of using TMAs is that they do not directly translate to patient care and require further validation cohorts that use conventional sections prior to introduction into laboratories for clinical usage.
3. For melanoma patients who have multiple independent primary tumors, inclusion of material from multiple lesions is possible. However, these data must be summarized such that each patient enters only once into the survival analyses assessing prognosis.
4. Although the within- and between-sample variance of expression, the principal determinants of optimized histospot number, is variable and marker-dependent [72], melanoma TMA validation experiments have shown over 95 % concordance between 4 randomly selected cores and whole slides [73] and this approach has been successfully applied across a series of candidate proteins [74, 75].
5. Automated quantitative brightfield platforms measure immunostain intensity as the level of white light absorbance in the range of the particular color of the selected chromogen, defined by its hue and saturation. To avoid possible mismeasurement of the selected antigen, the color of the chromogen must be distinct from any naturally occurring cellular melanin-containing inclusion body. Recognizing that the range of browns associated with melanin can overlap with the color produced by the DAB chromogen, we suggest using a red chromogen such as AEC or Vector Red [76, 77] to minimize possible target protein measurement error due to confounding by endogenous melanin pigment.

6. Quantitative immunofluorescence (QIF)/AQUA® measures levels of protein expression by measuring the intensity of light emitted by the target Cyanine (Cy) 5 or Cy7 label across the subset of pixels that colocalize to certain cellular and subcellular architectural compartments, the latter defined by additional, nonoverlapping fluorescent labels (e.g., Cy3, Fluorescein isothiocyanate (FITC)/Cy2, 4′6-diamidino-2-phenylindole (DAPI)) that are required in the absence of hematoxylin counterstain [36, 42].
7. Univariate estimates can be obtained by modeling fully quantitative data as a continuous parameter or after categorization. Splitting the population, a priori, at the median, by tertiles or by quartiles yields unbiased estimates. If semi-quantitative scores are captured, dichotomization according to an a priori convention (e.g., <20 % cells positive versus ≥20 % cells positive) is also acceptable. A third approach of binarizing semi-quantitative or continuous data according to an "optimal cut-point" that maximizes the survival differential requires special consideration. Although optimal cut-points may reflect nonintuitive but biologically driven boundaries, the volume of multiple comparisons required to search the entire space for an optimal cut-point risks selection of falsely positive values that do not validate in independent populations [78]. Strategies for p-value corrections that account for multiple comparisons such as applying Monte-Carlo simulations [79] should be applied in this setting.
8. Meyer et al. applied several compelling statistical techniques during model discovery. First, rather than equally considering all component markers in creating the summary risk score, markers are weighted according to the magnitude of their Cox univariate regression coefficient. Next, component markers are not binarized; their original semi-quantitative immunostaining scores are used when calculating the summary risk score. Third, they account for the possibility of "missing data" due to failed laboratory experiments by adjusting the composite scores according to the number of proteins with available data. Finally, when initially triaging among a 70-gene panel of eligible candidates, they corrected for a false discovery rate of 0.15 to avoid promoting falsely positive markers to the next steps of model construction [7].
9. Genetic algorithms are not robust to missing data. Any individual with missing data for one or more selected markers will be excluded each time that protein is incorporated in a proposed model which can introduce bias if missingness is not completely at random [80]. In particular, as has been shown in melanoma [32] and in breast cancer [81], missing data on a TMA is more likely among smaller tumors that are either more

difficult to sample or become exhausted among serial cuts such that patients with missing data tend to have better prognosis than those with complete data. One strategy to overcome this potential weakness is to impute values for the missing data to create a complete dataset for all available observations and a recent robust simulation study in breast cancer identified that, among available imputation methods including *mean substitution* and *multiple imputation* where survival time was either omitted (MI−) or included (MI+) in the imputation algorithm, the MI+ calculation yielded the most robust survival estimates [81] and multiple imputation has been used to develop a breast cancer prognostic model derived from QIF data [82].

References

1. Balch CM, Gershenwald JE, Soong SJ, Thompson JF, Atkins MB, Byrd DR, Buzaid AC, Cochran AJ, CoitDG DS, Eggermont AM, Flaherty KT, Gimotty PA, Kirkwood JM, McMasters KM, Mihm MC Jr, Morton DL, Ross MI, Sober AJ, Sondak VK (2009) Final version of 2009 AJCC melanoma staging and classification. J Clin Oncol 27(36): 6199–6206
2. Petrella T, Verma S, Spithoff K, Quirt I, McCready D (2012) Adjuvant interferon therapy for patients at high risk for recurrent melanoma: an updated systematic review and practice guideline. Clin Oncol (R Coll Radiol) 24(6):413–423
3. Thompson JF, Soong SJ, Balch CM, Gershenwald JE, Ding S, Coit DG, Flaherty KT, Gimotty PA, Johnson T, Johnson MM, Leong SP, Ross MI, Byrd DR, Cascinelli N, Cochran AJ, Eggermont AM, McMasters KM, Mihm MC Jr, Morton DL, Sondak VK (2011) Prognostic significance of mitotic rate in localized primary cutaneous melanoma: an analysis of patients in the multi-institutional American Joint Committee on Cancer melanoma staging database. J Clin Oncol 29(16):2199–2205
4. Gould Rothberg BE, Bracken MB, Rimm DL (2009) Tissue biomarkers for prognosis in cutaneous melanoma: a systematic review and meta-analysis. J Natl Cancer Inst 101(7): 452–474
5. Altman DG, McShane LM, Sauerbrei W, Taube SE (2012) Reporting recommendations for tumor marker prognostic studies (REMARK): explanation and elaboration. PLoS Med 9(5):e1001216, PMEDICINE-D-11-01220 [pii]
6. Schramm SJ, Mann GJ (2011) Melanoma prognosis: a REMARK-based systematic review and bioinformatic analysis of immunohistochemical and gene microarray studies. Mol Cancer Ther 10(8):1520–1528
7. Meyer S, Fuchs TJ, Bosserhoff AK, Hofstadter F, Pauer A, Roth V, Buhmann JM, Moll I, Anagnostou N, Brandner JM, Ikenberg K, Moch H, Landthaler M, Vogt T, Wild PJ (2012) A seven-marker signature and clinical outcome in malignant melanoma: a large-scale tissue-microarray study with two independent patient cohorts. PLoS One 7(6):e38222. doi:10.1371/journal.pone.0038222
8. Vaisanen A, Kuvaja P, Kallioinen M, Turpeenniemi-Hujanen T (2011) A prognostic index in skin melanoma through the combination of matrix metalloproteinase-2, Ki67, and p53. Hum Pathol 42(8):1103–1111
9. Nodin B, Fridberg M, Jonsson L, Bergman J, Uhlen M, Jirstrom K (2012) High MCM3 expression is an independent biomarker of poor prognosis and correlates with reduced RBM3 expression in a prospective cohort of malignant melanoma. Diagn Pathol 7:82. doi:1746-1596-7-82 [pii]
10. Ladstein RG, Bachmann IM, Straume O, Akslen LA (2010) Ki-67 expression is superior to mitotic count and novel proliferation markers PHH3, MCM4 and mitosin as a prognostic factor in thick cutaneous melanoma. BMC Cancer 10:140. doi:10.1186/1471-2407-10-140
11. Ladstein RG, Bachmann IM, Straume O, Akslen LA (2012) Prognostic importance of the mitotic marker phosphohistone H3 in cutaneous nodular melanoma. J Invest

Dermatol 132(4):1247–1252. doi:10.1038/jid.2011.464, jid2011464 [pii]

12. Jonsson L, Bergman J, Nodin B, Manjer J, Ponten F, Uhlen M, Jirstrom K (2011) Low RBM3 protein expression correlates with tumour progression and poor prognosis in malignant melanoma: an analysis of 215 cases from the Malmo Diet and Cancer Study. J Transl Med 9:114. doi:10.1186/1479-5876-9-114, 1479-5876-9-114 [pii]
13. Gremel G, Ryan D, Rafferty M, Lanigan F, Hegarty S, Lavelle M, Murphy I, Unwin L, Joyce C, Faller W, McDermott EW, Sheahan K, Ponten F, Gallagher WM (2011) Functional and prognostic relevance of the homeobox protein MSX2 in malignant melanoma. Br J Cancer 105(4):565–574. doi:10.1038/bjc.2011.249, bjc2011249 [pii]
14. Zhang Z, Chen G, Cheng Y, Martinka M, Li G (2011) Prognostic significance of RUNX3 expression in human melanoma. Cancer 117(12):2719–2727. doi:10.1002/cncr.25838
15. Chen G, Cheng Y, Zhang Z, Martinka M, Li G (2011) Cytoplasmic Skp2 expression is increased in human melanoma and correlated with patient survival. PLoS One 6(2):e17578. doi:10.1371/journal.pone.0017578
16. Svobodova S, Browning J, MacGregor D, Pollara G, Scolyer RA, Murali R, Thompson JF, Deb S, Azad A, Davis ID, Cebon JS (2011) Cancer-testis antigen expression in primary cutaneous melanoma has independent prognostic value comparable to that of Breslow thickness, ulceration and mitotic rate. Eur J Cancer 47(3):460–469. doi:10.1016/j.ejca.2010.09.042, S0959-8049(10)00963-9 [pii]
17. Jafarnejad SM, Wani AA, Martinka M, Li G (2010) Prognostic significance of Sox4 expression in human cutaneous melanoma and its role in cell migration and invasion. Am J Pathol 177(6):2741–2752. doi:10.2353/ajpath.2010.100377, S0002-9440(10)62903-3 [pii]
18. Li J, Cheng Y, Tai D, Martinka M, Welch DR, Li G (2011) Prognostic significance of BRMS1 expression in human melanoma and its role in tumor angiogenesis. Oncogene 30(8):896–906. doi:10.1038/onc.2010.470, onc 2010470 [pii]
19. Rotte A, Martinka M, Li G (2012) MMP2 expression is a prognostic marker for primary melanoma patients. Cell Oncol (Dordr) 35(3):207–216. doi:10.1007/s13402-012-0080-x
20. Brown ER, Doig T, Anderson N, Brenn T, Doherty V, Xu Y, Bartlett JM, Smyth JF, Melton DW (2012) Association of galectin-3 expression with melanoma progression and prognosis. Eur J Cancer 48(6):865–874. doi:10.1016/j.ejca.2011.09.003, S0959-8049(11)00714-3 [pii]
21. Buljan M, Situm M, Tomas D, Milosevic M, Kruslin B (2011) Prognostic value of galectin-3 in primary cutaneous melanoma. J Eur Acad Dermatol Venereol 25(10):1174–1181. doi:10.1111/j.1468-3083.2010.03943.x
22. Pencina MJ, D'Agostino RB, Pencina KM, Janssens AC, Greenland P (2012) Interpreting incremental value of markers added to risk prediction models. Am J Epidemiol 176(6):473–481. doi:10.1093/aje/kws207, kws207 [pii]
23. Weinlich G, Eisendle K, Hassler E, Baltaci M, Fritsch PO, Zelger B (2006) Metallothionein – overexpression as a highly significant prognostic factor in melanoma: a prospective study on 1270 patients. Br J Cancer 94(6):835–841
24. Weinlich G, Topar G, Eisendle K, Fritsch PO, Zelger B (2007) Comparison of metallothionein-overexpression with sentinel lymph node biopsy as prognostic factors in melanoma. J Eur Acad Dermatol Venereol 21(5):669–677
25. Paik S, Shak S, Tang G, Kim C, Baker J, Cronin M, Baehner FL, Walker MG, Watson D, Park T, Hiller W, Fisher ER, Wickerham DL, Bryant J, Wolmark N (2004) A multigene assay to predict recurrence of tamoxifen-treated, node-negative breast cancer. N Engl J Med 351(27):2817–2826
26. Cronin M, Sangli C, Liu ML, Pho M, Dutta D, Nguyen A, Jeong J, Wu J, Langone KC, Watson D (2007) Analytical validation of the Oncotype DX genomic diagnostic test for recurrence prognosis and therapeutic response prediction in node-negative, estrogen receptor-positive breast cancer. Clin Chem 53(6):1084–1091. doi:10.1373/clinchem.2006.076497, clinchem.2006.076497 [pii]
27. Buyse M, Loi S, Van't Veer L, Viale G, Delorenzi M, Glas AM, d' Assignies MS, Bergh J, Lidereau R, Ellis P, Harris A, Bogaerts J, Therasse P, Floore A, Amakrane M, Piette F, Rutgers E, Sotiriou C, Cardoso F, Piccart MJ (2006) Validation and clinical utility of a 70-gene prognostic signature for women with node-negative breast cancer. J Natl Cancer Inst 98(17):1183–1192. doi:10.1093/jnci/djj329, 98/17/1183 [pii]
28. Glas AM, Floore A, Delahaye LJ, Witteveen AT, Pover RC, Bakx N, Lahti-Domenici JS, Bruinsma TJ, Warmoes MO, Bernards R, Wessels LF, Van;t Veer LJ (2006) Converting a breast cancer microarray signature into a high-throughput diagnostic test. BMC

Genomics 7:278. doi:10.1186/1471-2164-7-278, 1471-2164-7-278 [pii]
29. Gray RG, Quirke P, Handley K, Lopatin M, Magill L, Baehner FL, Beaumont C, Clark-Langone KM, Yoshizawa CN, Lee M, Watson D, Shak S, Kerr DJ (2011) Validation study of a quantitative multigene reverse transcriptase-polymerase chain reaction assay for assessment of recurrence risk in patients with stage II colon cancer. J Clin Oncol 29(35):4611–4619. doi:10.1200/JCO.2010.32.8732, JCO.2010.32.8732 [pii]
30. Salazar R, Roepman P, Capella G, Moreno V, Simon I, Dreezen C, Lopez-Doriga A, Santos C, Marijnen C, Westerga J, Bruin S, Kerr D, Kuppen P, van de Velde C, Morreau H, Van Velthuysen L, Glas AM, Van't Veer LJ, Tollenaar R (2011) Gene expression signature to improve prognosis prediction of stage II and III colorectal cancer. J Clin Oncol 29(1):17–24. doi:10.1200/JCO.2010.30.1077, JCO.2010.30.1077 [pii]
31. Bartlett JM, Bloom KJ, Piper T, Lawton TJ, van de Velde CJ, Ross DT, Ring BZ, Seitz RS, Beck RA, Hasenburg A, Kieback D, Putter H, Markopoulos C, Dirix L, Seynaeve C, Rea D (2012) Mammostrat as an immunohistochemical multigene assay for prediction of early relapse risk in the tamoxifen versus exemestane adjuvant multicenter trial pathology study. J Clin Oncol. doi:10.1200/JCO.2012.42.8896, JCO.2012.42.8896 [pii]
32. Gould Rothberg BE, Berger AJ, Molinaro AM, Subtil A, Krauthammer MO, Camp RL, Bradley WR, Ariyan S, Kluger HM, Rimm DL (2009) A melanoma prognostic model using tissue microarrays and genetic algorithms. J Clin Oncol 27(34):5772–5780
33. Kashani-Sabet M, Venna S, Nosrati M, Rangel J, Sucker A, Egberts F, Baehner FL, Simko J, Leong SP, Haqq C, Hauschild A, Schadendorf D, Miller JR 3rd, Sagebiel RW (2009) A multi-marker prognostic assay for primary cutaneous melanoma. Clin Cancer Res 15(22):6987–6992. doi:10.1158/1078-0432.CCR-09-1777, 1078-0432.CCR-09-1777 [pii]
34. Piras F, Perra MT, Murtas D, Minerba L, Floris C, Maxia C, Demurtas P, Ugalde J, Ribatti D, Sirigu P (2008) Combinations of apoptosis and cell-cycle control biomarkers predict the outcome of human melanoma. Oncol Rep 20(2):271–277
35. Kononen J, Bubendorf L, Kallioniemi A, Barlund M, Schraml P, Leighton S, Torhorst J, Mihatsch MJ, Sauter G, Kallioniemi OP (1998) Tissue microarrays for high-throughput molecular profiling of tumor specimens. Nat Med 4(7):844–847
36. Moeder CB, Giltnane JM, Moulis SP, Rimm DL (2009) Quantitative, fluorescence-based in-situ assessment of protein expression. Methods Mol Biol 520:163–175
37. Rimm DL, Camp RL, Charette LA, Olsen DA, Provost E (2001) Amplification of tissue by construction of tissue microarrays. Exp Mol Pathol 70(3):255–264
38. DiVito KA, Charette LA, Rimm DL, Camp RL (2004) Long-term preservation of antigenicity on tissue microarrays. Lab Invest 84(8):1071–1078
39. Brennan DJ, Rexhepaj E, O'Brien SL, McSherry E, O'Connor DP, Fagan A, Culhane AC, Higgins DG, Jirstrom K, Millikan RC, Landberg G, Duffy MJ, Hewitt SM, Gallagher WM (2008) Altered cytoplasmic-to-nuclear ratio of survivin is a prognostic indicator in breast cancer. Clin Cancer Res 14(9):2681–2689. doi:10.1158/1078-0432.CCR-07-1760, 14/9/2681 [pii]
40. Rexhepaj E, Brennan DJ, Holloway P, Kay EW, McCann AH, Landberg G, Duffy MJ, Jirstrom K, Gallagher WM (2008) Novel image analysis approach for quantifying expression of nuclear proteins assessed by immunohistochemistry: application to measurement of oestrogen and progesterone receptor levels in breast cancer. Breast Cancer Res 10(5):R89. doi:10.1186/bcr2187, bcr2187 [pii]
41. Lloyd MC, Allam-Nandyala P, Purohit CN, Burke N, Coppola D, Bui MM (2010) Using image analysis as a tool for assessment of prognostic and predictive biomarkers for breast cancer: how reliable is it? J Pathol Inform 1:29. doi:10.4103/2153-3539.74186
42. Camp RL, Chung GG, Rimm DL (2002) Automated subcellular localization and quantification of protein expression in tissue microarrays. Nat Med 8(11):1323–1327
43. Neumeister V, Agarwal S, Bordeaux J, Camp RL, Rimm DL (2010) In situ identification of putative cancer stem cells by multiplexing ALDH1, CD44, and cytokeratin identifies breast cancer patients with poor prognosis. Am J Pathol 176(5):2131–2138. doi:10.2353/ajpath.2010.090712, S0002-9440(10)60010-7 [pii]
44. Goens G, Rusu D, Bultot L, Goval JJ, Magdalena J (2009) Characterization and quality control of antibodies used in ChIP assays. Methods Mol Biol 567:27–43. doi:10.1007/978-1-60327-414-2_2
45. Larsson PH (2008) Purification of antibodies. Methods Mol Med 138:197–207. doi:10.1007/978-1-59745-366-0_16
46. Bordeaux J, Welsh A, Agarwal S, Killiam E, Baquero M, Hanna J, Anagnostou V, Rimm D

(2010) Antibody validation. Biotechniques 48(3):197–209. doi:10.2144/000113382, 000113382 [pii]

47. Welsh AW, Moeder CB, Kumar S, Gershkovich P, Alarid ET, Harigopal M, Haffty BG, Rimm DL (2011) Standardization of estrogen receptor measurement in breast cancer suggests false-negative results are a function of threshold intensity rather than percentage of positive cells. J Clin Oncol 29(22):2978–2984. doi:10.1200/JCO.2010.32.9706, JCO.2010.32.9706 [pii]
48. Gustavson M, Dolled-Filhart M, Christiansen J, Pinard R, Rimm D (2009) AQUA technology and molecular pathology. In: Platero JS (ed) Molecular pathology in drug discovery and development. Wiley, Hoboken, NJ, pp 295–333
49. Gustavson MD, Bourke-Martin B, Reilly DM, Cregger M, Williams C, Tedeschi G, Pinard R, Christiansen J (2009) Development of an unsupervised pixel-based clustering algorithm for compartmentalization of immunohistochemical expression using Automated QUantitative Analysis. Appl Immunohistochem Mol Morphol 17(4):329–337. doi:10.1097/PAI.0b013e318195ecaa
50. Gustavson MD, Molinaro AM, Tedeschi G, Camp RL, Rimm DL (2008) AQUA analysis of thymidylate synthase reveals localization to be a key prognostic biomarker in 2 large cohorts of colorectal carcinoma. Arch Pathol Lab Med 132(11):1746–1752. doi:10.1043/1543-2165-132.11.1746, 2007-0718-OA [pii]
51. Benjamini Y, Hochberg Y (1995) Controlling the false discovery rate: a practical and powerful approach to multiple testing. J R Statist Soc B 57(1):289–300
52. Ooi CH, Tan P (2003) Genetic algorithms applied to multi-class prediction for the analysis of gene expression data. Bioinformatics 19(1):37–44
53. Breiman L, Friedman JH, Olshen RA, Stone CJ (1984) Classification and regression trees. CRC Press, Boca Raton, FL
54. Molinaro AM, Dudoit S, van der Laan MJ (2004) Tree-based multivariate regression and density estimation with right-censored data. J Multivar Anal 90:154–177
55. Segal MR, Bloch DA (1989) A comparison of estimated proportional hazards models and regression trees. Stat Med 8(5):539–550
56. Gimotty PA, Elder DE, Fraker DL, Botbyl J, Sellers K, Elenitsas R, Ming ME, Schuchter L, Spitz FR, Czerniecki BJ, Guerry D (2007) Identification of high-risk patients among those diagnosed with thin cutaneous melanomas. J Clin Oncol 25(9):1129–1134
57. Balch CM, Buzaid AC, Soong SJ, Atkins MB, Cascinelli N, Coit DG, Fleming ID, Gershenwald JE, Houghton A Jr, Kirkwood JM, McMasters KM, Mihm MF, Morton DL, Reintgen DS, Ross MI, Sober A, Thompson JA, Thompson JF (2001) Final version of the American Joint Committee on Cancer staging system for cutaneous melanoma. J Clin Oncol 19(16):3635–3648
58. Massi D, Franchi A, Borgognoni L, Paglierani M, Reali UM, Santucci M (2002) Tumor angiogenesis as a prognostic factor in thick cutaneous malignant melanoma. A quantitative morphologic analysis. Virchows Arch 440(1):22–28
59. de Giorgi V, Rossari S, Gori A, Grazzini M, Savarese I, Crocetti E, Cervadoro E, Massi D (2012) The prognostic impact of the anatomical sites in the 'head and neck melanoma': scalp versus face and neck. Melanoma Res 22(5):402–405. doi:10.1097/CMR.0b013e3283577b96
60. Thies A, Mangold U, Moll I, Schumacher U (2001) PAS-positive loops and networks as a prognostic indicator in cutaneous malignant melanoma. J Pathol 195(5):537–542. doi:10.1002/path.988, 10.1002/path.988 [pii]
61. Gimotty PA, Guerry D (2010) Prognostication in thin cutaneous melanomas. Arch Pathol Lab Med 134(12):1758–1763. doi:10.1043/2009-0653-RAR.1, 10.1043/2009-0653-RAR.1 [pii]
62. Lindholm C, Andersson R, Dufmats M, Hansson J, Ingvar C, Moller T, Sjodin H, Stierner U, Wagenius G (2004) Invasive cutaneous malignant melanoma in Sweden, 1990-1999. A prospective, population-based study of survival and prognostic factors. Cancer 101(9):2067–2078. doi:10.1002/cncr.20602
63. Storr SJ, Safuan S, Mitra A, Elliott F, Walker C, Vasko MJ, Ho B, Cook M, Mohammed RA, Patel PM, Ellis IO, Newton-Bishop JA, Martin SG (2012) Objective assessment of blood and lymphatic vessel invasion and association with macrophage infiltration in cutaneous melanoma. Mod Pathol 25(4):493–504. doi:10.1038/modpathol.2011.182, modpathol2011182 [pii]
64. Xu X, Chen L, Guerry D, Dawson PR, Hwang WT, VanBelle P, Elder DE, Zhang PJ, Ming ME, Schuchter L, Gimotty PA (2012) Lymphatic invasion is independently prognostic of metastasis in primary cutaneous melanoma. Clin Cancer Res 18(1):229–237. doi:10.1158/1078-0432.CCR-11-0490, 1078-0432.CCR-11-0490 [pii]
65. Yun SJ, Gimotty PA, Hwang WT, Dawson P, Van Belle P, Elder DE, Elenitsas R, Schuchter L, Zhang PJ, Guerry D, Xu X (2011) High

lymphatic vessel density and lymphatic invasion underlie the adverse prognostic effect of radial growth phase regression in melanoma. Am J Surg Pathol 35(2):235–242. doi:10.1097/PAS.0b013e3182036ccd, 00000478-201102000-00008 [pii]
66. Mills JL (1993) Data torturing. N Engl J Med 329(16):1196–1199
67. Molinaro AM, Simon R, Pfeiffer RM (2005) Prediction error estimation: a comparison of resampling methods. Bioinformatics 21(15): 3301–3307
68. Deeks JJ, Altman DG, Bradburn MJ (2001) Chapter 15: Statistical methods for examining heterogeneity and combining results from several studies in meta-analysis. In: Egger M, Smith GD, Altman DG (eds) Systematic reviews in health care: meta-analysis in context, 2nd edn. BMJ Press, Cornwall, UK, pp 285–312
69. Gould Rothberg BE, Bracken MB (2006) E-cadherin immunohistochemical expression as a prognostic factor in infiltrating ductal carcinoma of the breast: a systematic review and meta-analysis. Breast Cancer Res Treat 100(2):139–148. doi:10.1007/s10549-006-9248-2
70. Rothman KJ, Greenland S (2008) Chapter 7: Cohort studies. In: Rothman KJ, Greenland S, Lash TL (eds) Modern epidemiology, 3rd edn. Lippincott Williams & Wilkins, Philadelphia, PA
71. Simon RM, Paik S, Hayes DF (2009) Use of archived specimens in evaluation of prognostic and predictive biomarkers. J Natl Cancer Inst 101(21):1446–1452. doi:10.1093/jnci/djp335, djp335 [pii]
72. Tolles J, Bai Y, Baquero M, Harris LN, Rimm DL, Molinaro AM (2011) Optimal tumor sampling for immunostaining of biomarkers in breast carcinoma. Breast Cancer Res 13(3):R51. doi:10.1186/bcr2882, bcr2882 [pii]
73. Pacifico MD, Grover R, Richman P, Daley F, Wilson GD (2004) Validation of tissue microarray for the immunohistochemical profiling of melanoma. Melanoma Res 14(1):39–42, 00008390-200402000-00006 [pii]
74. Pacifico MD, Grover R, Richman PI, Buffa F, Daley FM, Wilson GD (2005) Identification of P-cadherin in primary melanoma using a tissue microarrayer: prognostic implications in a patient cohort with long-term follow up. Ann Plast Surg 55(3):316–320
75. Pearl RA, Pacifico MD, Richman PI, Wilson GD, Grover R (2008) Stratification of patients by melanoma cell adhesion molecule (MCAM) expression on the basis of risk: implications for sentinel lymph node biopsy. J Plast Reconstr Aesthet Surg 61:265–271
76. De Jong AS, Van Kessel-van VM, Raap AK (1985) Sensitivity of various visualization methods for peroxidase and alkaline phosphatase activity in immunoenzyme histochemistry. Histochem J 17(10):1119–1130
77. Harlow E, Lane D (2006) Detection of horseradish peroxidase-labeled reagents with aminoethylcarbazole. CSH Protoc 2006(1). doi:2006/1/pdb.prot4334 [pii]10.1101/pdb.prot4334
78. Altman DG, Lausen B, Sauerbrei W, Schumacher M (1994) Dangers of using "optimal" cutpoints in the evaluation of prognostic factors. J Natl Cancer Inst 86(11):829–835
79. Camp RL, Dolled-Filhart M, Rimm DL (2004) X-tile: a new bio-informatics tool for biomarker assessment and outcome-based cutpoint optimization. Clin Cancer Res 10(21):7252–7259
80. Greenland S, Finkle WD (1995) A critical look at methods for handling missing covariates in epidemiologic regression analyses. Am J Epidemiol 142(12):1255–1264
81. Ali AM, Dawson SJ, Blows FM, Provenzano E, Ellis IO, Baglietto L, Huntsman D, Caldas C, Pharoah PD (2011) Comparison of methods for handling missing data on immunohistochemical markers in survival analysis of breast cancer. Br J Cancer 104(4):693–699. doi:10.1038/sj.bjc.6606078, 6606078 [pii]
82. Emerson JW, Dolled-Filhart M, Harris L, Rimm DL, Tuck DP (2009) Quantitative assessment of tissue biomarkers and construction of a model to predict outcome in breast cancer using multiple imputation. Cancer Inform 7:29–40
83. Alonso SR, Ortiz P, Pollan M, Perez-Gomez B, Sanchez L, Acuna MJ, Pajares R, Martinez-Tello FJ, Hortelano CM, Piris MA, Rodriguez-Peralto JL (2004) Progression in cutaneous malignant melanoma is associated with distinct expression profiles: a tissue microarray-based study. Am J Pathol 164(1): 193–203
84. Vaisanen AH, Kallioinen M, Turpeenniemi-Hujanen T (2008) Comparison of the prognostic value of matrix metalloproteinases 2 and 9 in cutaneous melanoma. Hum Pathol 39:377–385
85. Pacifico MD, Grover R, Richman PI, Daley FM, Buffa F, Wilson GD (2005) Development of a tissue array for primary melanoma with long-term follow-up: discovering melanoma cell adhesion molecule as an important prog-

nostic marker. Plast Reconstr Surg 115(2): 367–375
86. Lin H, Wong RP, Martinka M, Li G (2009) Loss of SNF5 expression correlates with poor patient survival in melanoma. Clin Cancer Res 15(20):6404–6411. doi:10.1158/1078-0432.CCR-09-1135, 1078-0432.CCR-09-1135 [pii]
87. Ekmekcioglu S, Ellerhorst JA, Prieto VG, Johnson MM, Broemeling LD, Grimm EA (2006) Tumor iNOS predicts poor survival for stage III melanoma patients. Int J Cancer 119(4):861–866
88. Straume O, Sviland L, Akslen LA (2000) Loss of nuclear p16 protein expression correlates with increased tumor cell proliferation (Ki-67) and poor prognosis in patients with vertical growth phase melanoma. Clin Cancer Res 6(5):1845–1853
89. Thies A, Moll I, Berger J, Wagener C, Brummer J, Schulze HJ, Brunner G, Schumacher U (2002) CEACAM1 expression in cutaneous malignant melanoma predicts the development of metastatic disease. J Clin Oncol 20(10):2530–2536
90. Florenes VA, Maelandsmo GM, Faye R, Nesland JM, Holm R (2001) Cyclin A expression in superficial spreading malignant melanomas correlates with clinical outcome. J Pathol 195(5):530–536
91. Thies A, Schachner M, Moll I, Berger J, Schulze HJ, Brunner G, Schumacher U (2002) Overexpression of the cell adhesion molecule L1 is associated with metastasis in cutaneous malignant melanoma. Eur J Cancer 38(13): 1708–1716
92. Soltani MH, Pichardo R, Song Z, Sangha N, Camacho F, Satyamoorthy K, Sangueza OP, Setaluri V (2005) Microtubule-associated protein 2, a marker of neuronal differentiation, induces mitotic defects, inhibits growth of melanoma cells, and predicts metastatic potential of cutaneous melanoma. Am J Pathol 166(6):1841–1850
93. Niezabitowski A, Czajecki K, Rys J, Kruczak A, Gruchala A, Wasilewska A, Lackowska B, Sokolowski A, Szklarski W (1999) Prognostic evaluation of cutaneous malignant melanoma: a clinicopathologic and immunohistochemical study. J Surg Oncol 70(3):150–160
94. Piras F, Murtas D, Minerba L, Ugalde J, Floris C, Maxia C, Colombari R, Perra MT, Sirigu P (2007) Nuclear survivin is associated with disease recurrence and poor survival in patients with cutaneous malignant melanoma. Histopathology 50(7):835–842
95. Tran TA, Ross JS, Carlson JA, Mihm MC Jr (1998) Mitotic cyclins and cyclin-dependent kinases in melanocytic lesions. Hum Pathol 29(10):1085–1090
96. Florenes VA, Faye RS, Maelandsmo GM, Nesland JM, Holm R (2000) Levels of cyclin D1 and D3 in malignant melanoma: deregulated cyclin D3 expression is associated with poor clinical outcome in superficial melanoma. Clin Cancer Res 6(9):3614–3620
97. McDermott NC, Milburn C, Curran B, Kay EW, Barry Walsh C, Leader MB (2000) Immunohistochemical expression of nm23 in primary invasive malignant melanoma is predictive of survival outcome. J Pathol 190(2):157–162
98. Pacifico MD, Grover R, Richman PI, Buffa F, Daley FM, Wilson GD (2005) nm23 as a prognostic marker in primary cutaneous melanoma: evaluation using tissue microarray in a patient group with long-term follow-up. Melanoma Res 15(5):435–440
99. Li Q, Murphy M, Ross J, Sheehan C, Carlson JA (2004) Skp2 and p27kip1 expression in melanocytic nevi and melanoma: an inverse relationship. J Cutan Pathol 31(10):633–642

Chapter 14

Immunohistochemical Diagnostic and Prognostic Markers for Melanoma

Mehdi Nosrati and Mohammed Kashani-Sabet

Abstract

Recent studies in our laboratory have identified novel molecular diagnostic and prognostic markers based on analyses in large cohorts of melanoma patients. These markers were initially derived from gene expression profiling analyses of distinct stages of melanoma progression. Immunohistochemical analyses confirmed the differential expression of these markers, and immunohistochemistry-based multimarker assays were developed to assess melanoma diagnosis and prognosis at the molecular level. In this chapter we review the development of these assays and the methodologies used to assess marker expression in both nevi and primary melanomas.

Key words Immunohistochemistry, Molecular diagnosis, Prognostic markers, ARPC2, FN1, RGS1, SPP1, WNT2, NCOA3

1 Introduction

1.1 Rationale for Development of Molecular Diagnostic Markers for Melanoma

The diagnosis of primary cutaneous melanoma at the pathological level can represent a daunting task [1]. Several features are used to diagnose melanoma, such as cytologic atypia, maturation with descent, poor circumscription, presence of mitoses, and asymmetry. However, the pathologic diagnosis of melanoma remains challenging, resulting in a high degree of interobserver variability [2–6]. As a result, the misdiagnosis of melanoma is a major cause of inappropriate therapy as well as malpractice claims involving pathologists and dermatologists in the United States [7]. These issues have created an unmet need in the molecular diagnosis of melanoma. While certain molecular aberrations have been described to differentiate benign from malignant melanocytic neoplasms [8, 9], no molecular assays are routinely performed to assist in the differential diagnosis of nevus versus primary melanoma. Moreover, several of these studies may require sophisticated assays (such as comparative genomic hybridization), which may not be

Magdalena Thurin and Francesco M. Marincola (eds.), *Molecular Diagnostics for Melanoma: Methods and Protocols*, Methods in Molecular Biology, vol. 1102, DOI 10.1007/978-1-62703-727-3_14, © Springer Science+Business Media New York 2014

available in routine diagnostic pathology laboratories. In addition, the standard immunohistochemical markers used to determine melanocytic lineage, such as S100, HMB-45, MART-1, and MITF, are unable to distinguish primary melanomas from nevi [10–14]. Thus, the development of a multimarker assay using immunohistochemical methods and reagents would represent an important advance in the pathologist's armamentarium in assisting with this differential diagnosis.

1.2 Development of a Multimarker Diagnostic Assay for Melanoma

cDNA microarray analyses of distinct stages of melanoma progression demonstrated a specific gene expression signature for nevi when compared with that of primary melanomas, and identified several markers that could potentially aid in the diagnosis of melanoma [15]. Five markers [actin-related protein 2/3 complex, subunit 2 (ARPC2), fibronectin (FN1), regulator of G-protein signaling 1(RGS1), osteopontin (SPP1), and wingless-type MMTV integration site family member 2 (WNT2)] derived from this original profiling analysis were incorporated into a multimarker immunohistochemical diagnostic assay using commercially available antibodies and analyzed in a cohort of 693 melanocytic neoplasms, composed of a training set and four validation sets [16]. Each marker was assessed for its staining intensity on a four-point (0–3) scale. In addition, marker expression was assessed at the junctional zone of the lesion (termed the "top") and the base of the lesion (termed the "bottom"), and differences in "top-to-bottom" expression were evaluated for each marker. In this analysis, nevi were observed to lose expression (with the "top" score greater than the "bottom" score), whereas in melanomas, this "top-to-bottom" loss of marker expression was not readily observed. A diagnostic algorithm that combined (a) marker intensity scores with (b) top-to-bottom differences in expression was shown to achieve a specificity of 95 % and a sensitivity of 91 % in melanoma diagnosis in the training set. Applying the same diagnostic algorithm to the validation sets, the multimarker assay achieved 95 % specificity and 97 % sensitivity in melanomas arising in a nevus and correctly identified 95 % (37/39) of dysplastic nevi and 95 % (20/21) of Spitz nevi. Finally, the assay correctly diagnosed 18/24 (75 %) of initially misdiagnosed lesions. These studies established the diagnostic accuracy of this multimarker immunohistochemical assay for melanoma. The assay is undergoing additional validation prior to its commercial application and availability for use in the molecular diagnosis of melanocytic neoplasms.

1.3 Rationale for Development of Molecular Prognostic Markers for Melanoma

The clinical behavior of malignant melanoma can be capricious. Even though the thickness of the primary tumor is an important prognostic factor to determine survival, it is by itself inadequate to accurately predict the outcome of individual melanoma patients. This highlights the need for additional markers to improve predictive algorithms for melanoma patients. The development of molecular prognostic markers for melanoma, based on the identification of the molecular determinants of melanoma tumor progression, would allow further improvements in the prognostic assessment of melanoma patients. Moreover, the development of a molecular prognostic assay for primary melanomas should identify patient subsets at higher risk of relapse and death, as well as those who may benefit from systemic adjuvant therapies. Despite the identification of several prognostic factors that may correlate with melanoma outcome (reviewed in [17]), no molecular factors are routinely used in the prognostic evaluation of melanoma patients.

1.4 Development of a Multimarker Prognostic Assay for Melanoma

We also developed a multimarker immunohistochemical prognostic assay for primary cutaneous melanoma [18] combining the expression levels of three markers (nuclear receptor coactivator 3 (NCOA3), SPP1, and RGS1) in an initial cohort of 395 patients with primary cutaneous melanoma. Each marker was shown to significantly predict sentinel lymph node (SLN) status and disease-specific survival (DSS) [19–21]. The cumulative impact of marker overexpression was assessed using DSS as the primary endpoint. A multimarker index was developed, and reflected the total number of markers overexpressed or under-expressed. Increasing multimarker scores were significantly predictive of SLN metastasis and reduced DSS. Multimarker overexpression was associated with significantly reduced DSS by Kaplan-Meier analysis. Multivariate logistic regression analysis indicated that the multimarker assay was independently predictive of SLN status, and was more significant than tumor thickness. Multivariate Cox regression analyses of DSS identified the multimarker index as the most significant predictor of DSS. Even with the inclusion of SLN status in the model, the multimarker expression level remained the most significant factor predicting DSS. The prognostic role of this immunohistochemical assay was then confirmed using a digital imaging analysis of the stained specimens.

The prognostic impact of this multimarker assay was also demonstrated in tissues from 141 patients collected from Germany. Multivariate Cox regression analysis indicated that the multimarker expression index was independently predictive of DSS in this cohort, confirming the prognostic impact of this assay.

These studies described the first independently predictive molecular assay for primary melanoma. Importantly, the significant prognostic impact of this multimarker assay was demonstrated in a tissue set drawn from a completely different patient population (Germany), across different tissue platforms, and using both pathologist scoring and digital imaging analysis. Based on these results, the prognostic impact of this multimarker assay is undergoing additional evaluation on tissues collected from the Eastern Cooperative Oncology Group (ECOG) E1690 randomized trial of observation versus high-dose and low-dose interferon in the setting of high-risk melanoma.

2 Materials

2.1 Solutions for Immunohistochemical (IHC) Staining

1. 3 % H2O2 in PBS: Add 25 mL 30 % H2O2 to 225 mL 1× PBS (10 mM, pH 7.4).
2. 10 mM Citrate Buffer for steaming or microwave antigen retrieval. Add 1.05 g of Citrate Monohydrate to dH2O and adjust the final volume to 500 mL; then adjust to pH 6.0 using 1 N NaOH.
3. Diluent for antibody solutions-1 % Bovine Serum Albumin (BSA) in PBS: Add 1 g of BSA to 100 mL of 1× PBS.
4. Avidin/biotinylated enzyme staining complex-Horseradish peroxidase(ABC-HRP) (1:100 Dilution): Add 30 μL Avidin to 30 μL Biotin-HRP and 2,940 μL Diluent. Prepare the ABC-HRP reagent 30 min before use.
5. 3,3′-Diaminobenzidine(DAB)/H2O2 HRP substrate: Add 10 mg DAB tablet to 20 mL PBS and 20 μL 30 % H2O2. Add 30 % H2O2 just before use.
6. PBS Tween-20 (PBST): Add 500 μL Tween-20 to 800 mL of 1× PBS, adjust pH to 7.4, and adjust the final volume to 1 L with PBS for a final concentration of 0.05 % Tween-20. Always prepare freshly before use. PBST is a more stringent wash buffer. Alternatively, it can be used in place of PBS in the protocols in this chapter.

2.2 Antibodies and Dilutions

1. ARPC2 primary Rabbit Polyclonal Antibody (Upstate Cell Signaling). For 1:25 dilution, add 80 μL antibody to 1.92 mL Diluent.
2. Fibronectin primary Rabbit Polyclonal Antibody (Dako): For 1:400 dilution, add 5 μL Fibronectin Antibody to 1.995 mL Diluent.
3. NCOA3 primary Mouse Monoclonal Antibody (Abcam): For 1:10 dilution, add 300 μL NCOA3 to 2.7 mL Diluent.
4. RGS1 primary Chicken Polyclonal Antibody (GeneTex): For 1:50 dilution add 60 μL RGS1 Antibody to 2.94 mL Diluent, and for 1:100 dilution add 30 μL RGS1 Antibody to 2.97 mL Diluent.
5. SPP1/Osteopontin primary Rabbit Polyclonal Antibody (Abcam): For 1:200 dilution add 15 μL SPP1 Antibody to 2,985 mL Diluent.
6. Wnt-2 primary Rabbit Polyclonal Antibody (Biovision): For 1:5 dilution, add 400 μL Wnt-2 Antibody to 1.6 mL Diluent.
7. Normal Goat Serum (Vector Labs; 1:10 Dilution): Add 300 μL Normal Goat Serum to 2.7 mL Diluent.
8. Normal Horse Serum (Vector Labs): For 1:10 dilution, add 300 μL Normal Horse Serum to 2.7 mL Diluent.

9. Biotinylated goat anti-Rabbit secondary antibody (Vector Labs). For 1:200 dilution, add 15 μL Biotinylated Goat Anti-Rabbit to 2,985 mL Diluent.
10. Biotinylated Horse Anti-Mouse secondary antibody (Vector Labs): For 1:200 dilution, add 15 μL Biotinylated Horse Anti-Mouse to 2,985 mL Diluent.
11. Biotinylated Goat anti-Chicken secondary antibody (Vector Labs): For 1:200 dilution, add 15 μL Biotinylated Goat Anti-Chicken to 2,985 mL Diluent.

2.3 Kits

1. ABC-HRP Kit (Vectastain, Vector Labs).
2. Avidin Biotin Blocking Kit (Vector Labs).

3 Methods

3.1 Actin-Related Protein 2/3 Complex, Subunit 2 (ARPC2) (Fig. 1) (See Note 1)

1. Bake slides in oven at 60 °C for 30 min prior to staining.
2. Deparaffinize and rehydrate (Subheading 3.7).
3. Steaming in 10 mM Citrate Buffer: Heat up 1 L Citrate buffer in a 2 L beaker in the microwave at high power for 6 min. Transfer the heated Citrate buffer to the plastic bowl in a steamer and steam the buffer to 97 °C. Place the slide rack in the Citrate buffer and steam at 95–100 °C for 20 min. Check the temperature of the buffer with a thermometer and regulate the temperature by positioning the lid of the steamer. After

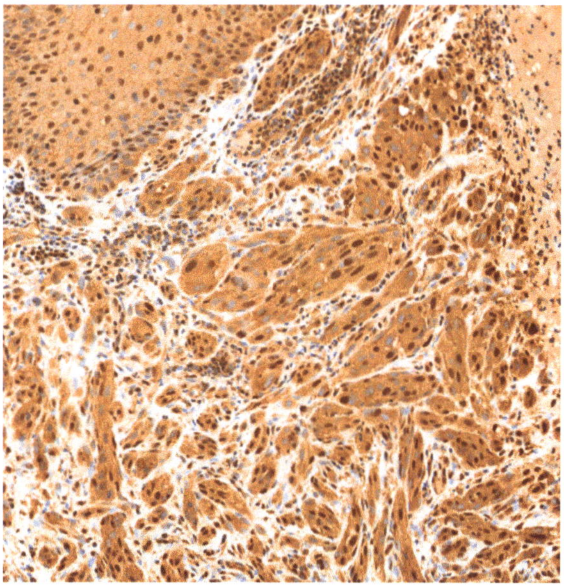

Fig. 1 Photomicrograph of ARPC2 immunostaining in primary melanoma

steaming, allow the slides to cool at room temperature for 20 min. Pressure cooker appears to results in superior antigen retrieval compared to microwave or steamer. The user is encouraged to use pressure cooker in the protocols that were previously optimized with microwave or steamer.

4. Wash in dH2O for 5 min.
5. Wash in PBS for 5 min.
6. Block in 3 % H2O2 in PBS for 15 min.
7. Wash in PBS three times, each for 3.5 min.
8. Incubate with Normal Goat Serum (1:10) at room temperature for 30 min.
9. Incubate with ARPC2 primary antibody (1:25, **item 1** of Subheading 2.2), and coverslip overnight at 4 °C (*see* **Note 1**).
10. Wash off coverslip with PBS for 8 min.
11. Wash in PBS three times, each for 3.5 min.
12. Incubate with Biotinylated Goat anti-Rabbit (1:200) at room temperature for 30 min.
13. Wash in PBS three times, each for 3.5 min.
14. Incubate with ABC reagent at room temperature for 30 min.
15. Wash in PBS three times, each for 3.5 min.
16. Incubate with DAB/H2O2 at room temperature for5 min.
17. Wash in running H2O for 5 min.
18. Counterstain with Hematoxylin Gill #2 for 10 s.
19. Wash in running H2O for 3 min.
20. Blue in Scott's H2O for 1 min.
21. Wash in running H2O for 3 min.
22. Dehydrate through graded alcohols and xylene (Subheading 3.8).
23. Coverslip with permount medium.

3.2 Fibronectin 1 (FN1) (Fig. 2) (*See* Note 2)

1. Bake slides in oven at 60 °C prior to staining for 30 min.
2. Deparaffinize and Rehydrate (Subheading 3.7).
3. Wash in PBST for 5 min.
4. Block in 3 % H2O2 in PBS for 15 min.
5. Wash in PBST for 5 min.
6. Wash in dH2O for 5 min.
7. Steaming in 10 mM Citrate Buffer as in **step 3** of Subheading 3.1.
8. Wash in dH2O for 5 min.
9. Wash in PBST for 5 min.
10. Block in Avidin blocking reagent for 15 min.
11. Wash in PBST three times, each for 3.5 min.

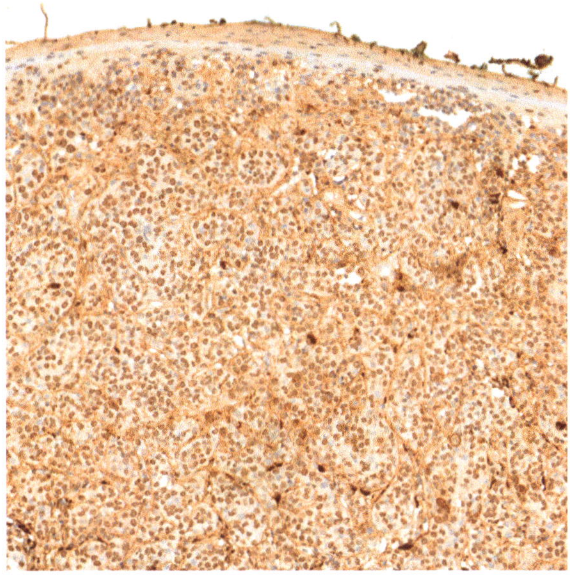

Fig. 2 Photomicrograph of FN1 immunostaining in primary melanoma

12. Block in Biotin blocking reagent for 15 min.
13. Wash in PBST three times, each for 3.5 min.
14. Incubate with Normal Goat Serum (1:10) at room temperature for 30 min.
15. Incubate with Fibronectin primary antibody (1:400, **item 2** of Subheading **2.2**), and coverslip overnight at 4 °C (*see* **Note 2**).
16. Wash off coverslip with PBS for 8 min.
17. Wash in PBST three times, each for 3.5 min.
18. Incubate with Biotinylated Goat anti-Rabbit (1:200) at room temperature for 30 min.
19. Wash in PBST three times, each for 3.5 min.
20. Incubate with ABC reagent at room temperature for 30 min.
21. Wash in PBST three times, each for 3.5 min.
22. Incubate with DAB/H2O2 at room temperature for 5 min.
23. Wash in running H2O for 5 min.
24. Counterstain with Hematoxylin Gill #2 for 10 s.
25. Wash in running H2O for 3 min.
26. Blue in Scott's H2O for 1 min.
27. Wash in running H2O for 3 min.
28. Dehydrate through graded alcohols and xylene (Subheading 3.8).
29. Coverslip with permount medium.

3.3 Nuclear Receptor Coactivator 3 (NCOA3) (Fig. 3) (See Note 3)

1. Bake slides in oven at 60 °C for 30 min prior to staining.
2. Deparaffinize and rehydrate (Subheading 3.7).
3. Microwave in 10 mM Citrate Buffer: Place slides in three plastic coupling jars filled with 10 mM Citrate Buffer; four slides in each jar, filling empty spaces with blank slides. Microwave (900 W, high power) slides in coupling jars for 10 min, stop and check to see if dH2O needs to be replenished. After microwaving, allow the slides to cool for 30 min at room temperature. Pressure cooker appears to results in superior antigen retrieval compared to microwave or steamer. The user is encouraged to use pressure cooker in the protocols that were previously optimized with microwave or steamer.
4. Wash in dH2O for 5 min.
5. Wash in PBST for 5 min.
6. Block in 3 % H2O2 in PBS for 30 min.
7. Wash in PBST three times, each for 3.5 min.
8. Block in Avidin blocking reagent for 15 min.
9. Wash in PBST three times, each for 3.5 min.
10. Block in Biotin blocking reagent for 15 min.
11. Wash in PBST three times, each for 3.5 min.
12. Incubate with Normal Horse Serum at room temperature for 30 min.
13. Incubate with NCOA3 primary antibody (1:10, **item 3** of Subheading 2.2) at room temperature for 60 min (*see* **Note 3**).

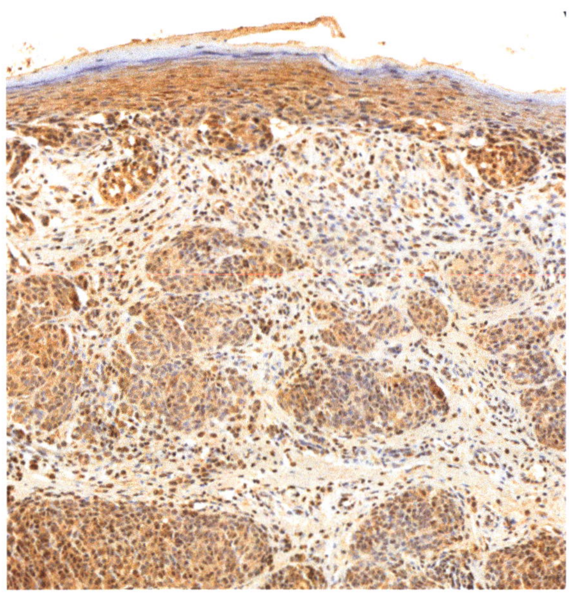

Fig. 3 Photomicrograph of NCOA3 immunostaining in primary melanoma

14. Wash in PBST three times, each for 3.5 min.
15. Incubate with Biotinylated Horse Anti-Mouse (1:200) at room temperature for 30 min.
16. Wash in PBST three times, each for 3.5 min.
17. Incubate with ABC reagent at room temperature for 30 min.
18. Wash in PBST three times, each for 3.5 min.
19. Incubate with DAB/H2O2 at room temperature for 5 min.
20. Wash in running H2O for 5 min.
21. Counterstain with Hematoxylin Gill #2 for 10 s.
22. Wash in running H2O for 3 min.
23. Blue in Scott's H2O for 1 min.
24. Wash in running H2O for 3 min.
25. Dehydrate through graded alcohols and xylene (Subheading 3.8).
26. Coverslip with permount medium.

3.4 Regulator of G-Protein Signaling 1 (RGS1) (Fig. 4) (See Note 4*)*

1. Bake slides in oven at 60 °C for 30 min prior to staining.
2. Deparaffinize and Rehydrate (Subheading 3.7).
3. Pressure Cook with Citrate (Subheading 3.9).
4. Wash in dH2O for 5 min.
5. Wash in PBS for 5 min.
6. Block in 3 % H2O2 in PBST for 15 min.
7. Wash in PBST three times, each for 3.5 min.

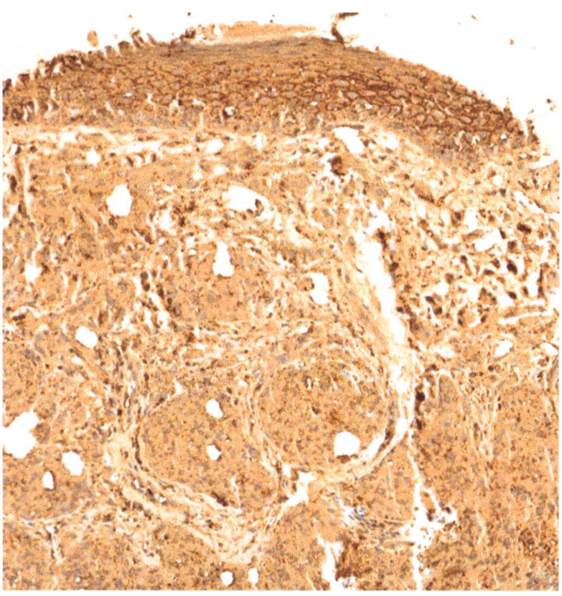

Fig. 4 Photomicrograph of RGS1 immunostaining in primary melanoma

8. Incubate with Normal Goat Serum (1:10) at room temperature for 30 min.
9. Incubate with RGS1 primary antibody (1:50 or 1:100, **item 4** of Subheading 2.2), and coverslip overnight at 4 °C (*see* **Note 4**).
10. Wash off coverslip with PBST for 8 min.
11. Wash in PBST three times, each for 3.5 min.
12. Incubate with Biotinylated Goat anti-Chicken (1:200) at room temperature for 30 min.
13. Wash in PBST three times, each for 3.5 min.
14. Incubate with ABC reagent at room temperature for 30 min.
15. Wash in PBST three times, each for 3.5 min.
16. Incubate with DAB/H2O2 at room temperature for 5 min.
17. Wash in running H2O for 5 min.
18. Counterstain with Hematoxylin Gill #2 10 s.
19. Wash in running H2O for 3 min.
20. Blue in Scott's H2O for 1 min.
21. Wash in running H2O for 3 min.
22. Dehydrate through graded alcohols and xylene (Subheading 3.8).
23. Coverslip with permount medium.

3.5 Secreted Phosphoprotein 1 (SPP1, or Osteopontin) (Fig. 5) (See Note 5)

1. Bake slides in oven at 60 °C for 30 min prior to staining.
2. Deparaffinize and Rehydrate (Subheading 3.7).
3. Microwave in 10 mM Citrate Buffer as in **step 3** of Subheading 3.3).

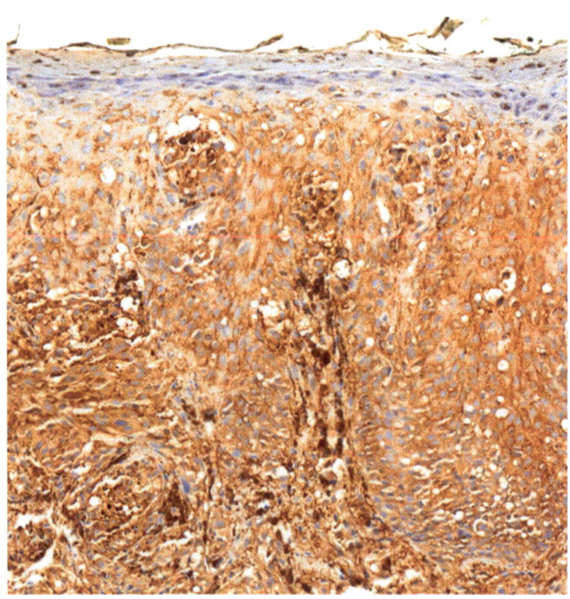

Fig. 5 Photomicrograph of SPP1 immunostaining in primary melanoma

4. Wash in dH2O for 5 min.
5. Wash in PBST for 5 min.
6. Block in 3 % H2O2 in PBS for 30 min.
7. Wash in PBST three times, each for 3.5 min.
8. Incubate with Normal Goat Serum (1:10) at room temperature for 30 min.
9. Incubate with SPP1 primary antibody (1:200, **item 5** of Subheading 2.2), and coverslip overnight at 4 °C (*see* **Note 5**).
10. Wash off coverslip with PBST for 8 min.
11. Wash in PBST three times, each for 3.5 min.
12. Incubate with Biotinylated Goat anti-Rabbit (1:200) at room temperature for 30 min.
13. Wash in PBST three times, each for 3.5 min.
14. Incubate with ABC reagent at room temperature for 30 min.
15. Wash in PBST three times, each for 3.5 min.
16. Incubate with DAB/H2O2 at room temperature for 5 min.
17. Wash in running H2O for 5 min.
18. Counterstain with Hematoxylin Gill #2 10 s.
19. Wash in running H2O for 3 min.
20. Blue in Scott's H2O for 1 min.
21. Wash in running H2O for 3 min.
22. Dehydrate through graded alcohols and xylene (Subheading 3.8).
23. Coverslip with permount medium.

3.6 Wingless-Type MMTV Integration Site Family Member 2 (WNT2) (Fig. 6) (*See* Note 6)

1. Bake slides in incubator at 37 °C for 60 min. Then bake slides in oven at 60 °C for 30 min prior to staining.
2. Deparaffinize and Rehydrate (Subheading 3.7).
3. Pressure Cook with Citrate (Subheading 3.9).
4. Wash in dH2O for 5 min.
5. Wash in PBS for 5 min.
6. Block in 3 % H2O2 in PBST for 15 min.
7. Wash in PBST three times, each for 3.5 min.
8. Incubate with Normal Goat Serum (1:10) at room temperature for 30 min.
9. Incubate with Wnt-2 primary antibody (1:5, **item 6** of Subheading 2.2), and coverslip overnight at 4 °C (*see* **Note 6**).
10. Wash off coverslip with PBS for 8 min.
11. Wash in PBST three times, each for 3.5 min.

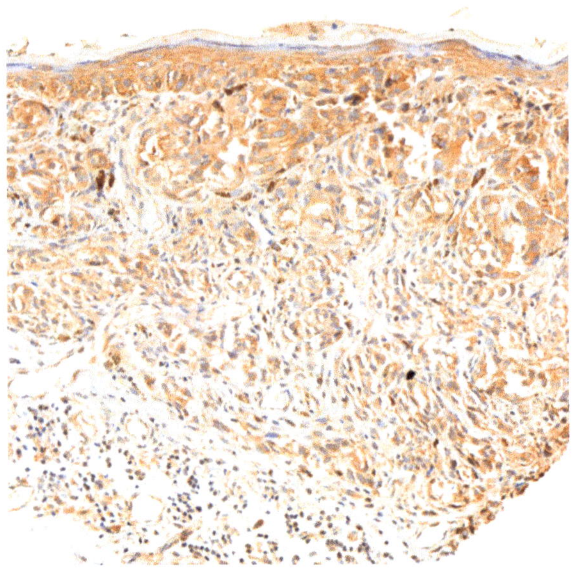

Fig. 6 Photomicrograph of WNT2 immunostaining in primary melanoma. All sections were scanned by using a whole slide high-resolution scanning system, and the digital snapshots represented were captured at the final magnification of 400× (20× objective × 20× software) at a resolution of 0.32 μm per pixel

12. Incubate with Biotinylated Goat anti-Rabbit (1:200) at room temperature for 30 min.
13. Wash in PBST three times, each for 3.5 min.
14. Incubate with ABC reagent at room temperature for 30 min.
15. Wash in PBST three times, each for 3.5 min.
16. Incubate with DAB/H2O2 at room temperature for5 min.
17. Wash in running H2O for 5 min.
18. Counterstain with Hematoxylin Gill #2 10 s.
19. Wash in running H2O for 3 min.
20. Blue in Scott's H2O for 1 min.
21. Wash in running H2O for 3 min.
22. Dehydrate through graded alcohols and xylene (Subheading 3.8).
23. Coverslip with permount medium.

3.7 Deparaffinize and Rehydrate

1. Place the tissue section sequentially in the following solutions for the specified time: xylene twice, each for 5 min; 100 % ethanol twice, each for f5 min; 95 % ethanol twice, each for 5 min 70 % ethanol twice, each for 5 min; deionized water (dH2O) for 5 min.
2. After deparaffination the blocking step (3 % H2O2 in PBS) can be performed before or after the antigen retrieval.

3.8 Dehydrate Through Graded Alcohols

Place the tissue section sequentially in the following solutions for the specified time: deionized water (dH2O) for 5 min; 70 % ethanol twice, each for 5 min; 95 % ethanol twice, each for 5 min; 100 % ethanol twice, each for 5 min; xylene twice, each for 5 min.

3.9 Pressure Cooking for Antigen Retrieval (*See* Note 7)

1. In a Pascal Pressure Cooker (Dako), place 500 mL of dH2O in the chamber, and place the heat shield at the center of the chamber.
2. Place slides in a Coupling Jar or staining container filled with the appropriate buffer (e.g. Trilogy or Citrate Buffer). No need to put on the lid.
3. Place all the jars or containers in the pressure cooker chamber.
4. Place Pascal Quality Strip (Dako) on top rim of the container.
5. The chamber can accommodate a maximum of four staining containers, i.e., 4×24 slides at one time. There is no need to put in blank slides to make up the total number of slides.
6. Place the lid on the chamber and close by aligning “OPEN” on the lid to the “white dot” on the brown handle and close the lid clockwise.
7. Check that there is no gap in the lid and the handles are all lined up.
8. Turn POWER on.
9. Press “start”, SP1 Light will illuminate. The temperature will automatically rise to the preset 125 °C. It will take approximately 15 min.
10. The chamber will hold the temperature (125 °C) for 30 s.
11. The chamber will beep. Record the temperature and pressure for quality control.
12. Press “Stop”, SP2 light will illuminate, the chamber will start cooling off. It takes about 25 min to cool to 90 °C.
13. When the temperature falls to 90 °C, it will hold the temperature for 10 s, and the alarm will sound.
14. Press “Stop” to end the alarm and the program.
15. Confirm the pressure reach 0 psi.
16. Release the pressure of the chamber by pressing on one edge of the brown knob on the lid.
17. Turn the lid anti-clockwise and lift the lid with the concave side facing away from self.
18. Turn POWER off.
19. Check the Temperature/Pressure Quality strip for proper color (dark gray to charcoal black).
20. Cool the slides in the buffer solution by adding room temperature dH2O slowly and in small amounts until the slides reach the room temperature.

21. The slides are done with antigen retrieval and are ready for further processing.
22. The chamber has to be cooled before use for another run.

3.10 Immunohistochemical Scoring System

Prior to scoring, the significance of cellular localization of each specific antibody—cytoplasmic for the above protocols—was assessed based on the pattern and positivity of staining, and biological relevance of the antigen. During the process of scoring all other areas (such as background, nuclear, and membrane staining) were ignored. Each marker was graded on a 4-point scale for cellular intensity using the following scale: no staining (0), weak staining (1), moderate staining (2), and intense staining (3).

4 Notes

1. ARPC2 dilution of 1:25 should be used for both regular section and the tissue microarray (TMA) slides. The positive controls for immunohistochemical staining of ARPC2 in cell lines are LOX, FEM, Jurkat, and HeLa, and in tissues spleen, thymus, and primary melanoma. The histological evaluation of this antibody was assessed based on cytoplasmic localization.
2. FN1 dilution of 1:400 should be used for both regular section and the tissue microarray (TMA) slides. The positive controls for IHC staining of FN1 in tissues are primary melanoma, normal kidney, and tonsil. The histological evaluation of this antibody was assessed based on cytoplasmic localization.
3. NCOA3 dilution of 1:10 should be used for both regular section and the tissue microarray (TMA) slides. The positive controls for IHC staining of NCOA3 in cell lines are melanoma (LOX, FEM), breast (BT474, SKBR3), and in tissues are breast tumor, metastatic melanoma, or ovarian tumor. The histological evaluation of this antibody was assessed based on cytoplasmic localization.
4. RGS1 dilution of 1:50 should be used for regular section and 1:100 for the tissue microarray (TMA) slides. The positive controls for IHC staining of NCOA3 in cell lines is Jurkat, and in tissues are primary or metastatic melanoma, and non-Hodgkin lymphoma. The histological evaluation of this antibody was assessed based on cytoplasmic localization.
5. SPP1 dilution of 1:200 should be used for both regular section and the tissue microarray (TMA) slides. The positive controls for IHC staining of SPP1 in tissues are breast carcinoma or metastatic melanoma. The histological evaluation of this antibody was assessed based on cytoplasmic localization.
6. WNT2 dilution of 1:5 should be used for both regular section and the tissue microarray (TMA) slides. The positive controls for IHC staining of WNT2 in tissues are primary or metastatic

melanoma, and breast tumor. The histological evaluation of this antibody was assessed based on cytoplasmic localization.

7. In the optimization process of RGS1 and WNT2, better antigen retrieval was achieved by using EDTA instead of citrate, but the harsher pH treatment caused tissue wash off in the subsequent steps. This problem was circumvented by fixing the tissue on to the glass slide in a pressure cooker (Subheading 3.9) rather than by microwave. However, after baking the tissue with pressure cooker, switching back to citrate did not result in any difference in antigen retrieval. It is conceivable that stronger treatment in pressure cooker would cause the same level of antigen retrieval for both citrate and EDTA. Hence, these two protocols differ from the rest in this regard.

References

1. Ming ME (2000) The histopathologic misdiagnosis of melanoma: sources and consequences of "false positives" and "false negatives". J Am Acad Dermatol 43:704–706
2. Piepkorn MW et al (1994) A multiobserver, population-based analysis of histologic dysplasia in melanocytic nevi. J Am Acad Dermatol 30:707–714
3. Farmer ER, Gonin R, Hanna MP (1996) Discordance in the histopathologic diagnosis of melanoma and melanocytic nevi between expert pathologists. Hum Pathol 27:528–531
4. Corona R et al (1996) Interobserver variability on the histopathologic diagnosis of cutaneous melanoma and other pigmented skin lesions. J Clin Oncol 14:1218–1223
5. Barnhill RL et al (1999) Atypical Spitz nevi/tumors: lack of consensus for diagnosis, discrimination from melanoma, and prediction of outcome. Hum Pathol 30:1523–1526
6. Brochez L et al (2002) Inter-observer variation in the histopathological diagnosis of clinically suspicious pigmented skin lesions. J Pathol 196: 459–466
7. Troxel DB (2003) Pitfalls in the diagnosis of malignant melanoma: findings of a risk management panel study. Am J Surg Pathol 27: 1278–1283
8. Wettengel GV, Draeger J, Kiesewetter F, Schell H, Neubauer S, Gebhart E (1999) Differentiation between Spitz nevi and malignant melanomas by interphase fluorescence in situ hybridization. Int J Oncol 14:1177–1183
9. Bastian BC, Wesselmann U, Pinkel D, Leboit PE (1999) Molecular cytogenetic analysis of Spitz nevi shows clear differences to melanoma. J Invest Dermatol 11:1065–1069
10. Busam KJ et al (1998) Expression of melan-A (MART1) in benign melanocytic nevi and primary cutaneous malignant melanoma. Am J Surg Pathol 22:976–982
11. King R, Weilbaecher KN, McGill G, Cooley Mihm M, Fisher DE (1999) Microphthalmia transcription factor. A sensitive and specific melanocyte marker for melanoma diagnosis. Am J Pathol 155:731–738
12. Fullen DR, Reed JA, Finnerty B, McNutt NS (2001) S100A6 preferentially labels type C nevus cells and nevic corpuscles: additional support for Schwannian differentiation of intradermal nevi. J Cutan Pathol 28: 393–399
13. King R, Googe PB, Weilbaecher KN, Mihm MC Jr, Fisher DE (2001) Microphthalmia transcription factor expression in cutaneous benign, malignant melanocytic, and nonmelanocytic tumors. Am J Surg Pathol 25:51–57
14. Kucher C et al (2004) Expression of Melan-A and Ki-67 in desmoplastic melanoma and desmoplastic nevi. Am J Dermatopathol 26: 452–457
15. Haqq C et al (2005) The gene expression signatures of melanoma progression. Proc Natl Acad Sci U S A 102:6092–6097
16. Kashani-Sabet M et al (2009) A multi-marker assay to distinguish benign nevi from malignant melanomas. Proc Natl Acad Sci U S A 106: 6268–6272
17. Gogas H et al (2009) Biomarkers in melanoma. Ann Oncol 20(Suppl 6):vi 8–13
18. Kashani-Sabet M et al (2009) A multi-marker prognostic assay for melanoma. Clin Cancer Res 15:6987–6992
19. Rangel J et al (2006) Prognostic significance of NCOA3 overexpression in primary cutaneous melanoma. J Clin Oncol 24:4565–4569
20. Rangel J et al (2008) Osteopontin as a molecular prognostic marker for melanoma. Cancer 112:144–150
21. Rangel J et al (2008) Novel role for RGS1 in melanoma progression. Am J Surg Pathol 32: 1207–1212

Chapter 15

Lymphatic Invasion as a Prognostic Biomarker in Primary Cutaneous Melanoma

Xiaowei Xu, Phyllis A. Gimotty, DuPont Guerry, Giorgos Karakousis, and David E. Elder

Abstract

Melanoma has a propensity for lymph node metastasis. However, the incidence of lymphatic invasion detected by histology alone in primary melanoma is disproportionately low in comparison to the incidence of positive sentinel lymph nodes (SLN). With the discovery of lymphatic endothelial cell markers, such as podoplanin and LYVE-1, lymphatic vessels can be reliably detected in formalin-fixed paraffin-embedded (FFPE) tissues. There is a now consensus that lymphatic invasion detected by immunohistochemical stains in primary melanoma is much more common than previously reported by histological examination alone. Immunohistochemical stains show that lymphangiogenesis and lymphatic invasion in primary melanoma may occur intratumorally or peritumorally, and lymphatic invasion is common across the range of tumor thicknesses in primary vertical growth phase (VGP) melanomas. A number of studies have shown that lymphatic invasion in primary melanoma is associated with a positive sentinel lymph node biopsy and a worse clinical outcome. Although not currently a part of the standard of care for staging of melanoma, the detection of lymphatic invasion in primary melanoma using immunohistochemical markers may be helpful in planning of therapy in some cases and may find a routine role in primary melanoma microscopic attributes in future.

Key words Lymphangiogenesis, Lymphatic invasion, Melanoma, Podoplanin, D2-40, LYVE-1, Prognosis

1 Introduction

Clinically apparent distant metastasis is the cause of most deaths in patients with primary cutaneous melanoma. Tumor dissemination may occur through a number of pathways: (a) local tissue invasion, (b) direct seeding of body cavities or surfaces, (c) hematogenous spread, and (d) lymphatic spread. Melanoma has a propensity for lymph node metastasis and clinical and pathological observations suggest transport of melanoma cells via lymphatics is the most common pathway of initial dissemination, with patterns of spread via afferent lymphatics following routes of natural drainage [1, 2].

Magdalena Thurin and Francesco M. Marincola (eds.), *Molecular Diagnostics for Melanoma: Methods and Protocols*, Methods in Molecular Biology, vol. 1102, DOI 10.1007/978-1-62703-727-3_15,

The growth of new lymphatic vessels, called lymphangiogenesis, is largely absent in normal adult tissues, but can be induced in pathological processes, such as inflammation, wound healing, and cancer [3]. Lymphangiogenesis and lymphatic invasion (LI, defined as melanoma cells in lymphatic vessels) have been under increasing investigation in the lesions of primary melanoma because of the recent availability of antibodies specific for lymphatic endothelial cells, such as antibodies to podoplanin and Lymphatic Vessel Endothelial Receptor 1 (LYVE-1) [4, 5]. Podoplanin, also known as GP36, T1 alpha, and Aggrus, is a mucin-type transmembrane glycoprotein with extensive O-glycosylation. It is specifically expressed by lymphatic endothelial cells but not blood vascular endothelial cells. In addition, a range of non-endothelial cells in numerous normal tissues also express this protein [6]. LYVE-1 is a CD44 homolog found primarily on lymphatic endothelial cells. While LYVE-1 functions continue to be defined, potential roles have been suggested in hyaluronan (HA) transport and turnover, or in promoting HA localization to the surfaces of lymphatic endothelium [7]. Unlike the pan-endothelial cell marker CD31, antibodies against podoplanin (D2-40) and LYVE-1 specifically detect lymphatic endothelial cells, but not blood vascular endothelial cells, making these markers particularly useful to study lymphangiogenesis and LI in tumors.

1.1 Lymphangiogensis and Melanoma Prognosis

Similar to the blood vasculature, lymphatic vessels in most adult tissues and organs are quiescent under physiological conditions. Tumor cells or tumor-infiltrating inflammatory cells secrete growth factors that likely promote lymphangiogenesis, which in turn may promote lymphatic metastasis. Among known lymphangiogenic factors, the VEGFC/VEGFD–VEGFR3 pathway is the best-characterized signalling system. It has a vital role in the budding of initial lymphatics from vein endothelium that expresses PROX1. Recently, several other lymphangiogenic factors have been reported. In addition to members of the VEGF family, these factors include members of the FGF, PDGF, and angiopoietin families, and they seem to have interdependent or collaborative roles with each other or with the members of the VEGF family in the establishment of functional lymphatics [8]. Melanoma cells and activated leukocytes in inflammatory sites produce a broad spectrum of growth factors, including members of the FGF, VEGF, and PDGF families, as well as pro-inflammatory cytokines and chemokines that might stimulate proliferation, migration, and survival of isolated lymphatic endothelial cells [9, 10]. Macrophages have been shown to be a rich source of lymphangiogenic factors such as VEGFC and VEGFD [11]. Indeed, we recently showed that in melanomas with radial growth phase (RGP) regression, which is characterized by a dense lymphocytic and melanophage infiltrate and an absence of melanoma cells, lymphatic vessel density was significantly higher in the areas with complete regression (mean ± SD, 23.7 ± 12.3/mm^2) compared with adjacent normal dermis (7.3 ± 3.5/mm^2) and distant normal dermis (5.5 ± 2.6/mm^2). This observation supports the hypothesis that tumor stromal-infiltrating inflammatory cells contribute to lymphangiogenesis [12].

Dilated lymphatic vessels are commonly observed within or at the periphery of malignant tumors, including melanoma [13]. Valencak et al. showed that those patients whose primary lesions had high lymphatic density had shorter overall and disease-free survival [14]. Dadres et al. noted that intratumoral lymphatics detected by immunohistochemical (IHC) staining of LYVE-1 were more frequent in primary melanomas excised from patients whose sentinel lymph nodes (SLN) had metastases than in those taken from SLN-negative patients [15]. We have previously demonstrated in univariate analyses that higher intratumoral lymphatic density was significantly associated with metastasis and melanoma-related death, whereas peritumoral lymphatic density was associated only with melanoma-specific death [13]. These studies provide evidence that lymphangiogenesis is a potential prognostic marker for sentinel lymph node metastasis and melanoma-related death. Nevertheless, the cohorts used in these studies were relatively small and additional studies are needed to clarify the prognostic role of lymphangiogenesis in melanoma while controlling for other potential explanatory factors.

1.2 Frequency of Lymphatic Invasion in Melanoma

The detection of lymphatic invasion by routine histology alone in primary melanoma is disproportionately low at 0–7.8 % [16, 17], relative to the incidence of sentinel lymph node (SLN) positivity (16–20 %) [18, 19]. Although blood vascular invasion is even more uncommon than lymphatic invasion, ranging from 1 to 3 % [14, 20], it potentially confounds the detection of LI. Thus, routine histology detects lymphovascular invasion (LVI). With the use of markers specific for lymphatic endothelial cells, however, the rate of LI detected by IHC stains increases dramatically. When only a lymphatic endothelial cell marker was used for IHC, the rate of LI in primary invasive melanoma ranged from 16 to 37% [16, 21–27]; whereas when double staining of lymphatic endothelial cells and melanoma cells was used, the rate of LI in primary invasive melanoma ranged from 33 to 43% [13, 28](Table 1). In thin melanomas (Breslow thickness ≤1 mm) with vertical growth phase, we found that the LI rate is 9.6 % (12/125) [28]. The lymphatic invasion rate in thin to intermediate thickness (Breslow thickness ≤2 mm) melanoma was 21.9 % [27]. These results indicate that LI is frequent in primary melanoma and suggest that it occurs early during melanoma progression.

Based on our studies, we have found that double staining of tissue sections with D2-40 and a melanocytic marker is the most sensitive method to detect melanoma LI [12, 13, 28]. On sections

Table 1
Summary of studies using lymphatic endothelial cell markers to detect LI in primary melanoma

Series	Markers	No. cases	LVI by histology (%)	LI by IHC (%)	LI and microstage attributes	LI and SLN status	LI and DFS/OS
Xu et al.	D2-40/ S100	106	5	33	Thickness	N/A	DFS, univariate
Xu et al.	D2-40/ S100	251	4.6	43	Thickness, mitotic rate, ulceration, gender	N/A	OS, multivariate
Sahni et al.	LYVE-1	36	0	16	No associate ions noted	N/A	N/A
Niakosari et al.	D2-40	96	N/A	33	Clark level, thickness	Significant, multivariate	N/A
Doeden et al.	D2-40, LYVE-1, CD31	94	6	16	Stage, histologic subtype	Significant, univariate	No associations noted
Petersson et al.	D2-40	74	0	23	N/A	Significant, univariate	DFS and OS, multivariate
Petitt et al.	D2-40	27	4	37	No associations noted	Not significant	N/A
Rose et al.	D2-40, CD34	246	3	18	Thickness, ulceration, mitotic rate, histologic subtype	Not significant	DFS and OS, multivariate
Storr et al.	D2-40, CD34	202	8	30	Thickness, ulceration, mitotic rate, histologic subtype, microsatellite	Not significant	No assciateions noted
Fohn et al.	D2-40	64	3.1	22	Thickness, Mitotic rate	Significant, multivariate	N/A

stained with D2-40 alone, we occasionally observe single cells in the lymphatic vessels and it is difficult without doing S-100 staining to decide whether some of the single cells are melanoma cells or hematopoietic cells (Fig. 1a, b). A double stain more reliably and accurately detects single or cluster of melanoma cells in the lymphatic space (Fig. 1b, c).

1.3 Lymphatic Invasion, Lymphovascular Invasion, and Sentinel Lymph Status

The most powerful predictor of survival for patients with early-stage melanoma is the presence of regional lymph node metastases, currently assessed by sentinel lymph node (SLN) biopsy. Given that melanoma metastasizes through lymphatic channels to the regional lymph nodes, it is logical to consider invasion into

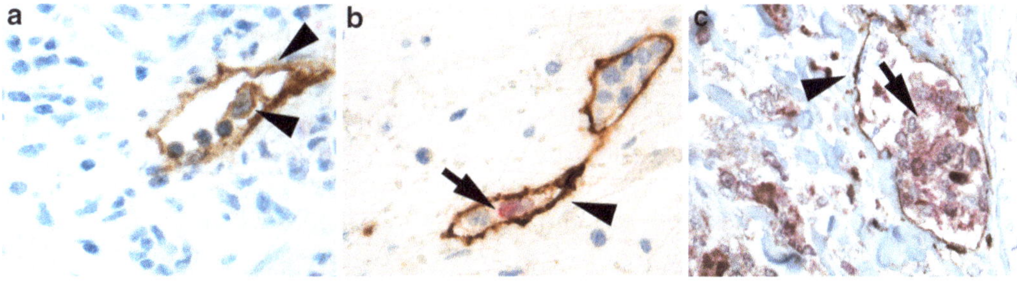

Fig. 1 Lymphatic invasion detected by double S-100 and D2-40 staining using light microscopy. Sections of melanocytic lesions were sequentially stained with D2-40 and S-100. (**a**) A single DAB-positive lymphatic endothelial cell is inside a lymphatic vessel highlighted by staining of endothelial cells with DAB. (**b**) A single Fast Red-positive melanoma cell is inside a lymphatic vessel highlighted by DAB-stained lymphatic endothelial cells. The hematopoietic cells in the lymphatic vessel are negative for Fast Red or DAB staining. (**c**) A cluster of Fast Red positive melanoma cells is inside a lymphatic vessel highlighted by DAB-stained lymphatic endothelial cells. *Arrow heads* point to D2-40 (DAB) positive endothelial cells aligning lymphatic vessel; *arrows* point to S-100 (Fast Red)- positive melanoma cells

lymphatic vessels by the primary tumor a sign of aggressive disease. Investigators have studied whether lymphovascular invasion and LI can predict SLN metastasis, thus identifying higher or lower risk patients to refine our patient selection for sentinel node biopsy.

In the Sunbelt Melanoma trial, 171/2183 (7.8 %) patients had lymphovascular invasion (LVI) identified by routine histology alone, and therefore did not specifically distinguish between LI and LVI [17]. Median follow-up was 68 months. Factors significantly associated with the presence of LVI included tumor thickness, ulceration, and histologic subtype ($P<0.05$). LVI was associated with a greater risk of SLN metastasis ($P<0.05$). In more recent studies, the presence of LI detected by IHC in primary melanoma has been shown to be independently predictive of the presence of SLN metastasis. Fohn et al. estimated the sensitivity, specificity, and predictive value of LI detected by D2-40 staining in patients with thin to intermediate thickness (Breslow thickness: ≤2.0 mm) melanomas [27]. Among the 64 patients in this study, 12 of 14 patients with D2-40 LI were SLN positive (positive predictive value, 85.7 %). D2-40 LI was detected in the primary biopsy specimen of 12 of 18 patients with a positive SLN (sensitivity 66.7 %). Of 50 patients without D2-40 LI, 44 were SLN negative (negative predictive value, 88.0 %), and among the 46 SLN-negative patients, 44 did not have D2-40 LI (specificity, 95.7 %). In their multivariate analysis, D2-40-detected LI was the only significant predictor of SLN status. Niakosari et al. demonstrated that LI identified by D2-40 was present in 15 of 23 SLN-positive cases (sensitivity, 65 %), whereas no lymphatic invasion was present in 56 of 73 SLN-negative cases (specificity 77 %) [21]. In addition, the assessment of LI detected by D2-40 had a positive predictive value of 46.9 % and a negative predictive value of 87.5 %. In their multivariate analysis, LI detected by D2-40 was significantly associated with SLN positivity ($P=0.01$; odds ratio, 6.7; 95 % confidence interval, 1.64–27.5). However, in three other studies LI detected by immunohistochemical staining was found to be not associated with SLN status [23, 25, 26]. Therefore, the impact of LI (or LVI) on SLN metastases remains an area of controversy within the literature.

1.4 Lymphatic Invasion, Lymphovascular Invasion, and DFS/OS in Melanoma

In the initial report of the Sunbelt Melanoma trial where the median follow-up was 68 months and LVI was identified by histology, LVI was reported to be significantly associated with worse OS ($P=0.0009$) by comparing the KM curves [17]. LVI was not an independent predictor of OS in the multivariate analysis. However in a subset analysis of patients with radial growth phase regression, the 5-year OS rate was 49.4 % for patients with LVI compared to 81.1 % those who did not have LVI ($P<0.0001$).

In another study of 251 melanoma patients with at least 10 years of protocol-driven, prospective follow-up and who had paraffin blocks available for immunohistochemical staining, double staining of S-100, and D2-40 identified 43 % of the primary melanomas had LI [28]. Four independent prognostic factors were identified in a multivariate model for 10-year metastasis: tumor thickness, mitotic rate, LI, and anatomic site. Of those who had a first metastasis within 10 years of treatment ($n=72$), 65.2 % had LI (95 % CI = 54.3–76.3); of those without a 10-year metastasis ($n=179$), only 34.0 % had LI (95 % CI = 27.2–41.0). LI was a significant independent prognostic factor (adjusted OR = 2.2). For the group of patients with thin melanomas, LI was also independently associated with 10-year metastasis with an unadjusted OR of 4.3. Interesting, in patients with thin melanoma with dermal mitotic activity (stage IB), LI can further distinguish two groups with different metastasis rates; the 10-year metastasis rate for those with LI was 50 % (95 % CI = 22–78) and it was six-fold higher than the rate of 8.3 % (95 % CI = 0–19) for those without LI (Fig. 2).

In another cohort of 246 melanoma patients with median follow-up time of 6.0 years, Rose et al. found that LI detected using IHC is a significant predictor of reduced DFS and OS in a multivariate model controlling for clinical stage [25]. In the multivariate model controlling for clinical stage at diagnosis (I/II vs. III/IV), LI detected using IHC markers remained a significant predictor of reduced DFS [hazard ratio (HR) 2.01; 95 % CI: 1.27–3.18] and OS (HR 2.08; 95 % CI: 1.25–3.46). Similar association of LI detected by D2-40 with DFS/OS was observed by Petersson et al. [23]. However, two other studies failed to show definitive associations of LI with DFS and OS in multivariate models [22, 26]. Nevertheless, one of the two studies did show a significant association of LI

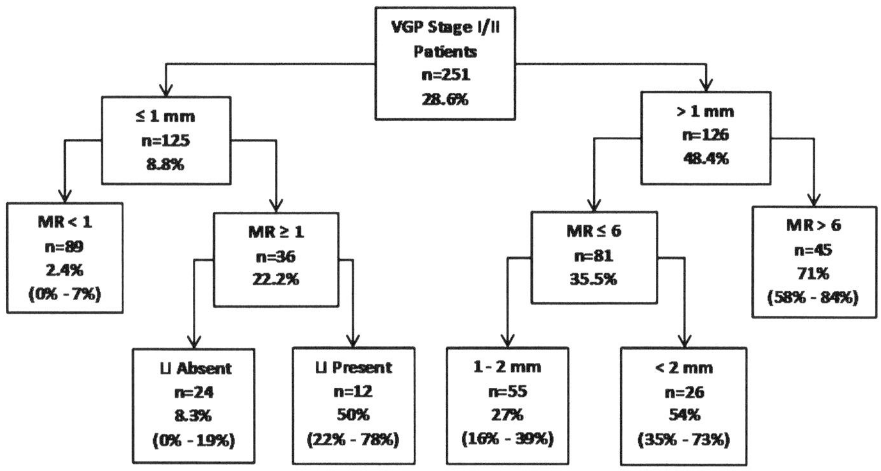

Fig. 2 Prognostic tree developed using recursive partitioning with 10-year metastasis rates and 95 % CIs for each risk group and prognostic value of LI in thin melanoma (≤1 mm)

detected using IHC markers with the presence of microsatellites and with disease stage [26].

In conclusion, IHC-based lymphatic markers can reliably detect lymphatic vessels in formalin-fixed paraffin-embedded (FFPE) tissues. LI is underappreciated using H&E staining alone. LI detected by IHC has been demonstrated to be associated with significantly worse clinical outcome (SLN metastasis and/or DSF/OS) in 7/9 studies (Table 1), and it is likely predictive of regional nodal metastasis and prognostic of poorer measures of survival. In addition to prognostic value, LI detected by IHC may also have diagnostic value in further classifying atypical and ambiguous melanocytic lesions (i.e. melanocytic tumor of uncertain malignant potential). We are currently investigating the predictive value of LI detected by IHC in atypical and ambiguous melanocytic lesions. Some authors have proposed that detection of LI in primary melanoma using IHC markers should be incorporated in routine melanoma biopsy evaluation. Nevertheless, larger studies are needed to confirm the association of LI detected by IHC with SLN status and DFS/OS and to evaluate more precisely the potential contributions of this marker to multivariate predictive and prognostic modeling and to staging.

2 Materials

2.1 Formalin-Fixed Paraffin-Embedded (FFPE) Tissue Sections

Immunohistochemistry (IHC) assays are performed on 5-μm-thick, formalin-fixed, paraffin-embedded sections.

2.2 Reagents for IHC Staining of FFPE Sections with D2-40 Antibody

1. Primary D2-40 antibody specific for podoplanin (mouse monoclonal antibody, to stain lymphatic vessels (Signet Laboratories, Dedham, MA).
2. Secondary antibody for use with mouse primary antibody: HRP-labeled polymer Dako Envision™+System (DakoCytomation).
3. 3,3′-diaminobenzidine (DAB) peroxidase substrate system produces brown reaction product for staining tissue sections. DAB is diluted using Dilution Buffer included in the Dako EnVision™+System (DakoCytomation).
4. EDTA buffer: 1 mM EDTA, 0.05 % Tween 20, pH 8.0, for antigen retrieval.
5. Washing Buffer: 50 mM Tris–HCl, 150 mM NaCl, 0.05 % Tween 20, pH 7.6.
6. Diluted hydrogen peroxide solution for blocking of endogenous peroxidase. Prepare solution by diluting 5 ml of 30 % hydrogen peroxidase in 145 ml of deionized water.
7. Normal mouse serum (Jackson ImmunoResearch) (1:1,000 dilution) was substituted for the primary antibody in a negative control reagent.
8. Hematoxylin solution (Fisher Scientific).
9. Antibody diluent for preparing antibody solutions (DakoCytomation).
10. Coverslips.
11. Permount slide mounting medium (Fisher Scientific).
12. LiCO3 (30 mM, Sigma).

2.2.1 Reagents for IHC S-100 Staining

1. Rabbit polyclonal S-100 antibody, diluted, ready to use (DakoCytomation).
2. Secondary antibody conjugated to HRP-labeled polymer Dako Envision™+System for use with rabbit primary antibody (DakoCytomation).
3. Fast Red chromogen system (Covance, Inc). Fast Red produces bright red reaction product for staining tissue sections. Prepare Fast Red substrate solution immediately before use by dissolving one Fast Red chromogen tablet in 5 ml of substrate buffer which is included in the system.

3 Methods

3.1 D2-40 Staining

1. Bake the slides in 45–50 °C oven overnight and let it cool for 30 min.
2. Deparaffinize sections in xylene, 3×, 5 min each time.
3. Hydrate with 100 % ethanol, 2×, 3 min each time and with 95 % ethanol, 1× for 1 min.

4. Rinse slides in deionized water 2×, 5 min each time.
5. Antigen Retrieval: Bring EDTA buffer to boil at 100 °C using a hot plate, place the slides in boiling buffer for 20 min. Allow them to cool for 20 min on bench top (*see* **Note 1**).
6. Wash sections in deionized water 3×, 5 min each time.
7. Incubate sections in diluted hydrogen peroxide solution for 10 min to quench endogenous peroxidase activity.
8. Wash sections in deionized water 3×, 5 min each time.
9. Wash sections in Washing Buffer 2×, 5 min each time.
10. Remove extra buffer from the slides, dilute primary Antibody D2-40 (1:25 dilution with Antibody Diluent) and incubate sections at room temperature for 1 h (*see* **Note 2**). Normal mouse serum (1:1,000 dilution in Antibody Diluent) is substituted for the primary antibody in negative control reagent.
11. Remove antibody solution by rinsing in Washing Buffer 3×, 5 min each time.
12. Incubate sections with secondary HRP-labeled antibody (anti-mouse) at room temperature for 30 min (*see* **Notes 3** and **4**).
13. Wash sections in Washing Buffer for 3×, 5 min each time.
14. Incubate sections in DAB solution at room temperature for 5–10 min (*see* **Note 5**).
15. Wash sections with Washing Buffer for 5 min.
16. Counterstain sections with Hematoxylin (not diluted) for exactly 30 s, dip in tap water, then in 30 mM LiCO3 solution for 10 s, and dip in tap water.
17. Dehydrate slides in ethanol (100 %) 3×, 3 min each time and then in xylene 3×, 3 min each time.
18. Coverslip mounting with Permount for permanent sealing. Apply 1–2 drops of Permount onto the tissue section and gently place the coverslip eliminating any air bubbles.
19. Examine the slides microscopically to identify tumor cells in D2-40 antibody-stained lymphatic vessels (brown) (*see* **Note 6**).

3.2 Double Staining with D2-40 and S-100 Antibodies

For the second color staining for detection of S-100 antigen please follow exactly the steps for the first color staining with D2-40 antibody using DAB peroxidase substrate described above in the Subheading 3.1 **steps 1–15**. After these steps are completed continue second color staining to visualize S-100 antigen using Fast Red peroxidase substrate as chromogen with the following **steps** (1–9) described below:

1. Remove extra buffer from the slides, apply diluted primary antibody S-100 to slides and incubate at room temperature for 30 min.

2. Remove antibody solution by rinsing in Washing Buffer 3×, 5 min each time.
3. Incubate the sections in secondary HRP-labeled antibody (anti-rabbit) in room temperature for 30 min.
4. Rinse sections in Washing Buffer 3×, 5 min each time.
5. Add Fast Red solution and let it incubate at room temperature for 10–20 min. Stop the reaction by immersing in deionized water.
6. Counterstain sections with Hematoxylin (no dilution) for exactly 30 s, dip in tap water, then in 30 mM LiCO3 solution for 10 s, and dip in tap water.
7. Dehydrate slides in ethanol (100 %) 3×, 3 min each time and then in xylene 3×, 3 min each time.
8. Coverslip with Permount as described above.
9. Examine the slides microscopically to identify melanoma cells (red) in lymphatic vessels (brown) (*see* **Notes 6** and 7).

4 Notes

1. Antigenic determinants masked by formalin fixation and paraffin embedding often may be exposed by heat-induced epitope retrieval, epitope unmasking using enzymatic digestion (e.g., trypsin) or saponin, etc. Different antigens may require different antigen unmasking methods. Do not use EDTA buffer boiling as antigen unmasking method with frozen sections or cultured cells that are not paraffin-embedded.
2. It is critical to keep the sections wet during the staining process. Drying at any stage will lead to nonspecific binding and ultimately nonspecific background staining. If staining is performed manually, placing wet tissue paper in the bottom of slide tray helps to prevent slides from drying.
3. Reducing of nonspecific binding by incubating sections with serum or immunoglobulin from the same species may be helpful to decrease background staining. However, we found that this step is unnecessary in the protocol that we use.
4. Incubation time with DAB, Fast Red, or other chromogens varies depending on the amount of tissue antigen expression and the antibody used. The optimal developing time should be determined empirically for each chromogen, each antigen and antibody, and the type of tissue immunohistochemically stained. In general DAB usually requires less time to develop than other chromogens such as Nova Red or Fast Red. Because melanomas often contain abundant melanin pigment which may be difficult to separate from DAB staining histologically,

Nova red, Fast Red, or AEC (3-amino-9-ethylcarbazole) may be used as a chromogen when only one antibody is needed. The advantage of using DAB is that it is very stable and does not dissolved in alcohols or other organic liquids.

5. D2-40 (DAB) staining allows for rapid identification of endothelial cells and S-100 (Fast Red) allows for rapid identification of melanoma cells. With double staining, it is easy to identify a cluster of melanoma cells in the lymphatic vessels (Fig. 1c). However, single cell metastases are difficult to observe even with double staining (Fig. 1b). Therefore, it is critical to examine the slides carefully and thoroughly. Based on our experience we recommend that at least two well-trained observers assess slides to reach consensus regarding for lymphatic invasion.
6. Currently, LI is reported by pathologists as a binary variable (present or absent) based on light microscopy observation. Ability to assess the level of LI quantitatively (number of vessels containing melanoma cells and number of melanoma cells in the lymphatic vessels) might increase the prognostic value of LI in primary melanomas and future studies should consider reading LI quantitatively.
7. *Supported provided by:* Specialized Program of Research Excellence (SPORE) on Skin Cancer (P50-CA-093372).

Acknowledgments

We would like to thank Jie Dai for technical assistance. This work was supported by NIH grant CA-093372.

References

1. Balch CM, Cascinelli N (2006) Sentinel-node biopsy in melanoma. N Engl J Med 355: 1370–1371
2. Balch CM, Soong SJ, Gershenwald JE et al (2001) Prognostic factors analysis of 17,600 melanoma patients: validation of the American Joint Committee on cancer melanoma staging system. J Clin Oncol 19:3622–3634
3. Alitalo K, Tammela T, Petrova TV (2005) Lymphangiogenesis in development and human disease. Nature 438:946–953
4. Dadras SS, Paul T, Bertoncini J et al (2003) Tumor lymphangiogenesis: a novel prognostic indicator for cutaneous melanoma metastasis and survival. Am J Pathol 162:1951–1960
5. Giorgadze TA, Zhang PJ, Pasha T et al (2004) Lymphatic vessel density is significantly increased in melanoma. J Cutan Pathol 31:672–677
6. Al-Rawi MA, Mansel RE, Jiang WG (2005) Molecular and cellular mechanisms of lymphangiogenesis. Eur J Surg Oncol 31: 117–121
7. Banerji S, Ni J, Wang SX et al (1999) LYVE-1, a new homologue of the CD44 glycoprotein, is a lymph-specific receptor for hyaluronan. J Cell Biol 144:789–801
8. Adams RH, Alitalo K (2007) Molecular regulation of angiogenesis and lymphangiogenesis. Nat Rev Mol Cell Biol 8:464–478
9. Rinderknecht M, Detmar M (2008) Tumor lymphangiogenesis and melanoma metastasis. J Cell Physiol 216:347–354
10. Alitalo A, Detmar M (2011) Interaction of tumor cells and lymphatic vessels in cancer progression. Oncogene. doi:10.1038/onc.2011.602

11. Gordon EJ, Rao S, Pollard JW et al (2010) Macrophages define dermal lymphatic vessel calibre during development by regulating lymphatic endothelial cell proliferation. Development 137:3899–3910
12. Yun SJ, Gimotty PA, Hwang WT et al (2011) High lymphatic vessel density and lymphatic invasion underlie the adverse prognostic effect of radial growth phase regression in melanoma. Am J Surg Pathol 35:235
13. Xu X, Gimotty PA, Guerry DP et al (2008) Lymphatic invasion revealed by multispectral imaging is common in primary melanomas and associates with prognosis. Hum Pathol 39:901–909
14. Valencak J, Heere-Ress E, Kopp T et al (2004) Selective immunohistochemical staining shows significant prognostic influence of lymphatic and blood vessels in patients with malignant melanoma. Eur J Cancer 40:358–364
15. Dadras SS, Lange-Asschenfeldt B, Muzikansky A et al (2005) Tumor lymphangiogenesis predicts melanoma metastasis to sentinel lymph nodes. J Cutan Pathol 32:84–84
16. Sahni D, Robson A, Orchard G et al (2005) The use of LYVE-1 antibody for detecting lymphatic involvement in patients with malignant melanoma of known sentinel node status. J Clin Pathol 58:715–721
17. Egger ME, Gilbert JE, Burton AL et al (2011) Lymphovascular invasion as a prognostic factor in melanoma. Am Surg 77:992–997
18. Morton DL, Thompson JF, Cochran AJ et al (2006) Sentinel-node biopsy or nodal observation in melanoma. N Engl J Med 355: 1307–1317
19. Thompson JF, Shaw HM (2007) Sentinel node mapping for melanoma: results of trials and current applications. Surg Oncol Clin N Am 16:35–54
20. Schuchter L, Schultz DJ, Synnestvedt M et al (1996) A prognostic model for predicting 10-year survival in patients with primary melanoma. Ann Intern Med 125:369–375
21. Niakosari F, Kahn HJ, McCready D et al (2008) Lymphatic invasion identified by monoclonal antibody D2-40, younger age, and ulceration: predictors of sentinel lymph node involvement in primary cutaneous melanoma. Arch Dermatol 144:462
22. Doeden K, Ma Z, Narasimhan B et al (2009) Lymphatic invasion in cutaneous melanoma is associated with sentinel lymph node metastasis. J Cutan Pathol 36:772–780
23. Petersson F, Diwan AH, Ivan D et al (2009) Immunohistochemical detection of lymphovascular invasion with D2-40 in melanoma correlates with sentinel lymph node status, metastasis and survival. J Cutan Pathol 36: 1157–1163
24. Petitt M, Allison A, Shimoni T et al (2009) Lymphatic invasion detected by D2-40/S-100 dual immunohistochemistry does not predict sentinel lymph node status in melanoma. J Am Acad Dermatol 61:819–828
25. Rose AE, Christos PJ, Lackaye D et al (2011) Clinical relevance of detection of lymphovascular invasion in primary melanoma using endothelial markers D2-40 and CD34. Am J Surg Pathol 35:1441
26. Storr SJ, Safuan S, Mitra A et al (2012) Objective assessment of blood and lymphatic vessel invasion and association with macrophage infiltration in cutaneous melanoma. Mod Pathol 25:493–504
27. Fohn LE, Rodriguez A, Kelley MC et al (2011) D2–40 lymphatic marker for detecting lymphatic invasion in thin to intermediate thickness melanomas: association with sentinel lymph node status and prognostic value – a retrospective case study. J Am Acad Dermatol 64:336–345
28. Xu X, Chen L, Guerry DP et al (2012) Lymphatic invasion is independently prognostic of metastasis in primary cutaneous melanoma. Clin Cancer Res 18:229–237

Chapter 16

Tumor-Infiltrating Lymphocytes and Their Significance in Melanoma Prognosis

Tobias Schatton, Richard A. Scolyer, John F. Thompson, and Martin C. Mihm Jr.

Abstract

The role of the tumor-infiltrating lymphocyte (TIL) and its relationship to prognosis has been most extensively studied in malignant melanoma. The purpose of this chapter is to discuss in depth the immunobiology and molecular aspects of lymphocyte function in general and particularly TIL function in the context of antimelanoma immunity. Emphasis is placed upon the role of these inflammatory mediators in the enhancement and impairment of progression of this often fatal human cancer. In addition, the analysis of TILs in melanoma and their direct relationship to prognosis as well as their effect on the positivity of the sentinel lymph node will be discussed. Furthermore, details of lymph node responses to metastatic melanomas and their prognostic significance will be clarified. Finally, the importance of TILs for the evaluation of therapeutic response and how TIL immunobiology could critically inform the design of novel melanoma immunotherapeutic protocols will be elucidated.

Key words Tumor-infiltrating lymphocyte, TIL, Melanoma, Prognosis, Tumor immunology, Antitumor immunity, Immune surveillance, Immunologic tolerance, T cell, Regulatory T cell, Treg, Cytotoxic T cell, CTL, Activation, Priming, Anergy, Exhaustion, Antigen presentation, Antigen presenting cell, Dendritic cell, DC, Macrophage, Natural killer cell, Major histocompatibility complex, MHC, Tumor therapy, Outcome, Staging, Progression, Metastasis, Tumor-reactive lymphocyte, Tumor-associated antigen, gp100, Tyrosinase, MART-1, Sentinal lymph node, SNL, CTLA-4, Ipilimumab, PD-1

1 Introduction

In 1863, the German pathologist, Rudolf Virchow, first described the occurrence of leukocytes in malignant tumors [1], which are now broadly referred to as tumor-infiltrating lymphocytes (TILs). Originally, TILs were thought to constitute the cells of origin of cancer occurring at sites of chronic inflammation [1]. Early subsequent findings in experimental animal models and the clinic suggested that TILs may indeed foster tumor progression through protumorigenic inflammatory processes [1]. However, it was soon recognized that TIL frequencies commonly correlate with

Magdalena Thurin and Francesco M. Marincola (eds.), *Molecular Diagnostics for Melanoma: Methods and Protocols*, Methods in Molecular Biology, vol. 1102, DOI 10.1007/978-1-62703-727-3_16, © Springer Science+Business Media New York 2014

favorable prognosis in cancer patients [2, 3]. For instance, dense T cell infiltrates in the vertical growth phase of primary melanomas correlated with prolonged patient survival and reduced risk of metastatic disease [4, 5]. Additionally, the presence of brisk T cell infiltrates in melanomas metastatic to lymph nodes similarly predicted improved survival compared to lesions showing low to absent TIL reactivity [6]. Correlations between TILs and prolonged survival have also been reported in other cancers, including ovarian [7] and colorectal [8] carcinomas. Together, these findings indicate that the presence of TILs could also reflect the immune system's attempt to eliminate cancer.

In further support of this possibility, Clark and colleagues demonstrated many decades ago that the radial growth phase of primary melanomas commonly evokes a dermal lymphocyte infiltration that can cause partial tumor elimination [3]. The initial characterization of cytolytic immune responses against autologous tumors in melanoma patients by Hersey and Rosenberg, among others [9, 10], lent further support to the possibility that TILs might indeed play key roles in facilitating immunologic tumor clearance. Tumor-reactive cytotoxic T lymphocytes (CTLs) have since been identified in the blood, lymph nodes, and among TILs infiltrating primary tumors and metastatic nodules of many cancer patients [11]. Furthermore, clonal CTL expansions have been documented in primary regressing melanomas [12] and in metastatic melanomas undergoing spontaneous regression [13], and these immune effector populations were found capable of cytotoxicity against autologous cancer cells [12]. Remarkably, adoptive transfer of autologous TILs in combination with interleukin-2 (IL-2) treatment resulted in tumor regression in metastatic melanoma patients [14]. These findings underscore the inherent ability of TILs to promote antitumor immunity and, as a result, tumor regression. However, some other studies did not find a significant impact of TILs on patient survival [15, 16] and, as aforementioned, in some instances TILs may even stimulate tumor outgrowth and metastasis [1]. Therefore, understanding the mechanisms regulating TILs and how they influence disease progression and outcome are critical for these mechanisms to be harnessed as successful therapeutic strategies.

Together, the apparent discrepancies between independent investigations aimed at correlating TIL frequencies with patient outcome and the observed opposing (i.e., growth-inhibitory versus tumor-promoting) effects of TILs during the tumorigenic process suggest that the molecular and cellular makeup of tumoral lymphocytes is not homogeneous. TILs may comprise a variety of immune cell subsets and their products, which may positively or negatively affect tumor progression. Indeed, accumulating evidence indicates that not only T cells, but also natural killer (NK) cells, macrophages, and dendritic cells (DCs), among other immune cell types, infiltrate tumor tissues in variable quantities [1]. Additionally, TIL composition and immune effector functions may further vary as a result of the accumulation of immunoregulatory immune cell subsets, including regulatory T (Treg) cells and tolerogenic DCs, or due to alternative immune escape mechanisms operative in the tumor microenvironment. These considerations highlight the necessity to both immunophenotype and functionally characterize TILs, in order to better define TIL subtypes and TIL-specific immunoregulatory pathways responsible for tumor regression versus those that enhance cancer growth. Additionally, the tumor cells themselves have immune regulatory effects, which are also critical to understand. Such research endeavors could yield refined and perhaps more robust correlations between TIL composition, diversity, and/or architecture with patient prognosis and ultimately may be harnessed to improve melanoma patient management.

The emerging literature on TILs and their prognostic significance in melanoma will be the focus of this chapter. In the following sections, we discuss the divergent roles of distinct TIL subtypes in melanomagenesis, primary and metastatic melanoma progression, and review TIL immunobiology in the context of established mechanisms of melanoma immune evasion. In addition, we critically evaluate the potential relevance of TILs as biomarkers for melanoma prognosis and progression, and for predicting and optimizing patient response to biological and immunotherapeutic agents.

2 Antitumor Immunity and Melanoma

2.1 The Tumor Surveillance Hypothesis

Over a century ago, Paul Ehrlich first proposed that the host immune response could eliminate cancerous cells, thereby preventing tumorigenesis and neoplastic progression. In 1957, Sir Francis Macfarlane Burnet and Lewis Thomas formulated the "tumor surveillance" hypothesis, which postulates that malignantly transformed cells might display altered "self-antigens" that enable the immune system to recognize and eradicate them during early phases of tumorigenesis [17]. While the "tumor surveillance" theory remains controversial, a substantial body of evidence now supports pertinent roles for both innate and adaptive immunity in controlling tumor development [18]. For example, several genetically engineered mouse models with deficiencies in prominent immune effector pathways, including NOD/SCID (nonobese diabetic severely combined immunodeficiency), $RAG2^{-/-}$ (recombinant activation gene 2 knockout), $IFN\gamma^{-/-}$ (interferon gamma knockout), and $Pfp^{-/-}$ (perforin knockout) mice, demonstrate markedly increased occurrence of sarcomas, lymphomas, and/or carcinomas [18]. Moreover, tumor take rates in these and other syngeneic mouse tumor models inversely correlate with the degree of host immunocompetence [18], further implying that a functional immune response may restrain cancer onset and progression. A potential importance of the immune system in controlling tumorigenesis is also suggested by epidemiologic meta-analyses of cancer incidence rates in immunocompromised patients [18]. For instance, organ transplant recipients on immunosuppressive regimens and HIV patients have significantly increased risks of developing various types of cancer.

2.2 Immune Recognition of Self and Immunity Against Cancer

Direct evidence supporting immunologic tumor surveillance is provided by the characterization of cytolytic immune responses against autologous tumors and the identification of tumor-reactive CTLs capable of inducing tumor regression in the blood circulation of cancer patients and among TILs infiltrating malignant tissues [9–11, 14]. Furthermore, numerous antigens have been identified that demonstrate selective and/or enhanced expression in tumors compared with normal tissues [19]. Antigen recognition by CTLs requires presentation of antigenic peptides by major histocompatibility complex (MHC) class I (also known as human leukocyte antigen (HLA)-A, -B, or -C) molecules (Fig. 1a), which are polymorphic cell-surface proteins that are principally expressed on all nucleated cells [20]. T-helper (Th) cells recognize antigenic peptides presented by MHC class II (HLA-DR, -DP, -DQ) molecules (Fig. 1a), the expression of which is typically limited to professional antigen presenting cells (APCs). MHC class II orchestrates specific immunity to a particular antigen, and MHC class I thereafter facilitates immunologic destruction of host cells displaying that antigen. The aberrant expression of tumor antigens by MHC class I molecules enables tumor-reactive CTLs to recognize cancer as foreign and subsequently kill autologous tumor cells in an HLA-restricted manner [20] (Fig. 1a). Two distinct categories of tumor antigens can be distinguished, namely tumor-specific antigens (TSAs) and tumor-associated antigens (TAAs) [19]. TSAs are abnormal gene products resulting from mutations or chromosomal rearrangements, such as the leukemia-specific BCR-ABL fusion protein. TAAs result from aberrant transcriptional or translational activation of immunogenic molecules in tumors compared to physiologic tissues [19]. One category of TAAs includes lineage-specific differentiation antigens, also referred to as melanoma differentiation antigens (MDAs), such as melanoma antigen recognized by T cells (MART-1, also known as melan-A), glycoprotein 100 (gp100), tyrosinase (TYR), or tyrosinase-related proteins (TRP) 1 and 2 (TRP2, also known as DCT) [19]. Cancer-germline genes termed cancer testis antigens (CTAs), including NY-ESO-1 and MAGE, represent another category of TAAs.

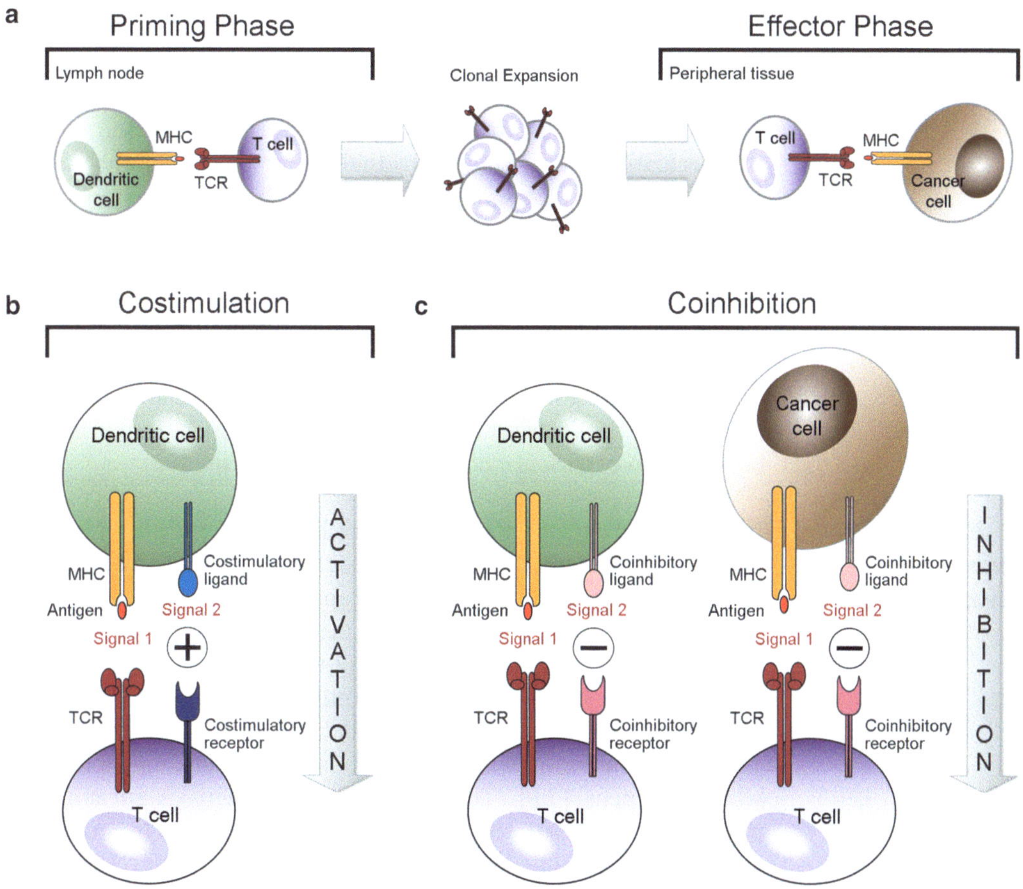

Fig. 1 The "two-signal" paradigm of antigen-dependent T cell activation. (**a**) T cell priming in lymph nodes (LNs) requires information exchange between T cells and dendritic cells (DCs). Specifically, the T cell receptor (TCR) enables T cells to recognize antigenic peptides presented by major histocompatibility complex (MHC) class II molecules displayed by DCs. However, TCR engagement with the MHC/antigenic peptide complex (signal 1) is not enough to elicit a T cell response. Full T cell activation requires a second signal delivered by costimulatory molecules (signal 2; *see* panel (**b**)), leading to clonal expansion of an antigen-specific T effector population. These antigen-reactive T effector cells can subsequently recognize target cells as foreign and launch an immune effector response if these cells present the appropriate antigenic peptide on their MHC class I surface molecules. For instance, the aberrant expression of tumor antigens by MHC class I molecules enables tumor-reactive cytotoxic T lymphocytes (CTLs) to recognize cancer as foreign and subsequently kill autologous tumor cells. (**b**) Upon antigen encounter, naïve T cells receive signal 1 through TCR engagement with the MHC/antigenic peptide complex and signal 2 through ligation of a costimulatory receptor, leading to full T cell activation. (**c**) In contrast, TCR engagement coincident with coinhibitory signaling dampens immune effector responses. Specifically, coinhibitory signaling interactions inhibit T cell expansion and the secretion of proliferative cytokines, induce T cell anergy and apoptosis, and may control the suppressive function of regulatory T (Treg) cells. Importantly, MHC class I and II expression and signal 2 pathway members may not only be expressed by T cells and DCs. Costimulatory and coinhibitory ligand- and/or receptor-mediated signaling interactions have also been documented for other immune cell compartments as well as nonlymphoid tissues, including cancer cells

2.3 Immunogenic Properties of Melanoma

Melanoma is considered a particularly immunogenic cancer, at least in part owing to its exorbitant expression of numerous MAAs that have been characterized as targets of cellular immune responses [19]. Indeed, high levels of melanoma-specific antibodies and large numbers of TAA-reactive immune effector cells are present both in the circulation and within individual tumors of melanoma patients [20]. Additionally, spontaneous and complete regression of primary and metastatic melanomas with concomitant onset of vitiligo have been reported [21], further indicating marked immunogenic properties of melanoma. Finally, immunotherapies with nonspecific immune enhancers, such as IL-2 and IFN-α, have achieved objective responses in some melanoma patients [22, 23]. However, despite the commonly observed induction of melanoma-specific immunity, the overwhelming majority of melanoma patients continue to experience advancement of their disease.

2.4 Immunologic Tolerance and Melanoma

One possible explanation for the inability of the antitumor immune response to fully eradicate cancer is that the degree of tumor cell proliferation might simply exceed the capacity of immunologic tumor clearance [18]. An alternative explanation is that because cancers arise from malignant transformation of the host's own tissues, they express self-antigens to which immune effector cells have been tolerized [18]. Immune tolerance is defined as a mechanism that prevents immune effector populations from attacking a particular set of antigens [24]. Tolerance to self-antigens is sustained by immunologic events that either result in physical elimination of autoreactive lymphocytes through apoptotic cell death (clonal deletion) or induce functional unresponsiveness (clonal anergy or exhaustion) of antigen-reactive immune cells [24]. Self-tolerance refers to the immune system's competence to recognize and protect cells expressing self-MHC/*self* antigenic peptide complexes while at the same time retaining its ability to propel immune responses against MHC/*foreign* peptide-bearing cells [24]. Thus, self-tolerance represents a crucial regulatory mechanism underlying immune homeostasis. In the cancer context, however, immune tolerance toward TAAs could facilitate tumor development and metastatic progression by impeding immunologic recognition and clearance of malignant cells [18]. Indeed, cancer takes advantage of various immunoevasive and tolerogenic processes to escape immune-mediated destruction [18]. In the following sections, we review the multifaceted immunoregulatory mechanisms underlying melanoma immune evasion, with a focus on TILs and their immunobiology.

3 Mechanisms of Melanoma Immune Evasion

3.1 Melanoma Differentiation Antigen Loss

Melanomas employ several complimentary strategies to evade or actively thwart antitumor immune responses. One mechanism by which melanoma cells can escape immune recognition is by suppressing their expression of MDAs. MDA loss has been demonstrated in several human melanoma cell lines [25]. Moreover, tumorigenic melanoma subpopulations isolated from patient biopsies demonstrated low to absent expression of several MAAs, including MART-1, gp100, NY-ESO-1, and MAGE-A [26, 27]. Mechanistically, inhibition of MDA promoter activity through a paracrine factor was found to partially account for diminished MDA expression by melanoma cells [28]. MDA downregulation has also been described in melanoma patients with metastatic [29] or lethal recurrent disease [30], potentially providing an explanation for the relative ineffectiveness of CTLs to fully eradicate melanomas. Together, these findings highlight that MDA loss represents an important mechanism of melanoma immune evasion (particularly from CTL recognition) that is associated with clinical virulence.

3.2 Reduced MHC Class I Expression

Another strategy through which melanomas escape immunologic clearance by CTLs is through decreased expression of MHC class I molecules. As outlined above, $CD8^+$ CTLs, and to a lesser degree, $CD4^+$ Th cells, rely on the surface expression of class I MHC antigens to recognize cancer cells as immunologic targets [20] (Fig. 1a). Partial or complete loss of MHC class I expression thus guards melanoma target cells from CTL-mediated lysis [29]. Notably, tumorigenic melanoma subpopulations express low to absent levels of MHC class I [26], a phenotype associated with disease progression and adverse clinical outcome in melanoma patients [31]. These insights have important implications for the relevant interpretation of TIL immunobiological features. Specifically, the influx of MDA-reactive TILs to the tumor site might not be indicative of an efficient antitumor immune response if the melanoma cells do not express sufficient levels of the respective MDA and/or MHC class I. TILs and their significance as biomarkers in melanoma prognosis and progression can thus only be properly evaluated in the context of the tumor environment and its immunologic properties.

3.3 Evading NK Cell-Mediated Destruction

Most investigations in the melanoma immunity field, including research analyzing TILs, have focused on T cells as immune effector populations. However, additional lymphocyte subsets, such as NK cells, are also capable of generating antimelanoma immune responses [32]. While low expression of MHC class I shields melanoma target cells from CTL attack, it simultaneously increases their susceptibility to NK-mediated lysis [32]. NK cytolytic activity is tightly regulated by a group of distinct immune receptors and their ligands [32]. Natural-killer group 2 member D (NKG2D) is one such receptor that delivers either activating or inhibitory signals to NK cells upon engagement to its ligands expressed by target cells [33]. Upregulation of inhibitory NKG2D ligands by melanoma target cells represents one immune escape mechanism from NK-specific destruction [34]. Melanomas have also been found to express low levels of activating NKG2D ligands, such as UL16-binding proteins (ULBP) [34], further suggesting melanoma escape from NK-mediated clearance.

3.4 Tumor-Mediated Deletion of Immune Effector Populations

In addition to evading CTL- and/or NK-mediated killing, melanomas also engage in active tolerance induction to dampen antitumor immunity [18]. As outlined above, clonal deletion of antigen-reactive T cells through apoptotic cell death is one process sustaining immunologic tolerance [24]. For example, the Fas (also known as CD95 and Apo-1) apoptotic pathway is a key mediator of T cell deletion [35]. Tumors use Fas/Fas ligand (Fas-L) signaling to evade immunologic destruction by CTLs [35]. For instance, Fas-L expression by melanoma cells triggered apoptosis of Fas-expressing CTLs and Fas inhibition on immune effector cells fueled experimental melanoma growth [36]. Notably, in metastatic tumors, TILs are often found in near proximity to Fas-L$^+$ tumor cells [36], further indicating a critical role of Fas-L signaling in melanoma immune evasion and neoplastic progression. In support of this notion, loss of Fas-L expression in metastatic lesions was associated with significantly prolonged median survival in melanoma patients [37]. Additional immunomodulatory molecules through which melanoma cells may induce apoptotic deletion of tumor-reactive T cell clones include programmed death 1 (PD-1) and its ligands [38, 39] (discussed in more detail below).

3.5 Clonal Anergy-Induced Tolerance

Tolerance can also be achieved through nondeletional immunologic processes that induce functional inactivation (clonal anergy) of antigen-reactive leukocytes [24]. Direct tolerization of diverse immune effector populations, such as CTLs, NK cells, or DCs, can be achieved via the secretion of immunosuppressive factors, such as transforming growth factor beta (TGF-β) or prostaglandin E2 (PGE2) [18]. Melanomas and other tumors produce high levels of soluble immunoregulatory mediators, including TGF-β and PGE2, to avoid immune-mediated clearance [40, 41]. Consequently, blockade of TGF-β signaling in immune effector populations generated antitumor immune responses capable of eradicating tumors in mice challenged with live tumor cells [40]. The presence or absence of immunomodulatory factors in the tumor environment is also crucial for distinguishing anergic from activated TILs.

Induction of clonal anergy can further result from impaired stimulation of antigen-reactive immune effector cells. Antigen-dependent T cell priming requires two distinct but complimentary signals [42]. On antigen encounter, naïve T-cells receive signal 1 through T-cell receptor (TCR/CD3) engagement with the MHC/antigenic peptide complex (Fig. 1b). Signal 2 is an antigen-independent stimulus provided through so-called costimulatory molecules [42] (Fig. 1b). Full T-cell activation requires positive costimulatory signaling interactions. In the absence of positive

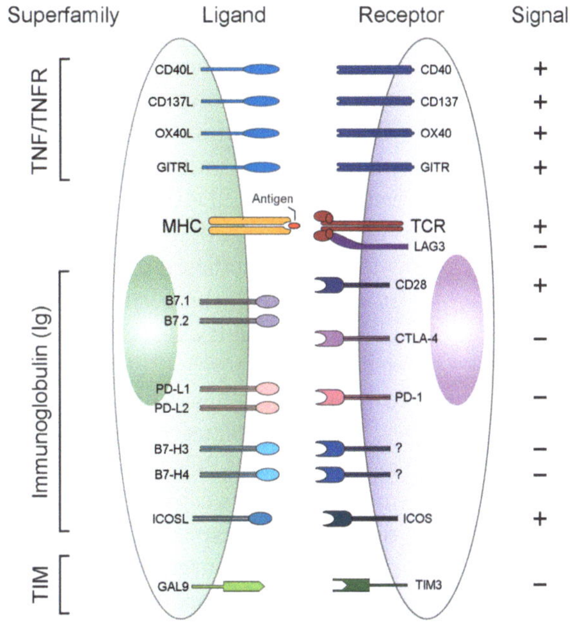

Fig. 2 Schematic overview of costimulatory and coinhibitory receptors and their ligands. Illustrated are select costimulatory and coinhibitory receptors and their respective ligands. Costimulatory molecules function to activate (+) immune effector responses, whereas coinhibitory signaling interactions downregulate (–) immunity upon T cell receptor (TCR) engagement with the major histocompatibility (MHC)/antigenic peptide complex. Costimulatory and coinhibitory molecules can be broadly grouped into three distinct superfamilies based on structural homology: (1) the tumor necrosis factor (TNF)/TNF receptor (TNFR) superfamily, (2) the immunoglobulin (Ig) superfamily, and (3) the emerging T cell Ig and mucin domain (TIM) superfamily. Costimulatory and coinhibitory ligands were originally described in antigen presenting cells (APCs) and their respective receptors in T cells. However, it is increasingly recognized that alternative immune cell compartments and nonlymphoid cells, including cancer cells, can also express costimulatory and coinhibitory ligands and receptors

costimulation, TCR binding leads to clonal anergy [24]. Similarly, so-called coinhibitory molecules (also known as immunologic checkpoints) function to downmodulate immune responses [43] (Fig. 1c). Based on structural homology, costimulatory and coinhibitory molecules can be assigned to three distinct superfamilies (Fig. 2), namely (a) the immunoglobulin (Ig) superfamily, which includes CD28, cytotoxic T lymphocyte antigen-4 (CTLA-4), and PD-1, (b) the tumor necrosis factor (TNF)/TNF receptor (TNFR) superfamily, in which the CD40 pathway is preeminent, and (c) the emerging T cell Ig and mucin domain (TIM) superfamily. Under physiologic conditions, the intricate balance between costimulatory and coinhibitory signals is crucial for the maintenance of self-tolerance [42].

3.6 Tumor-Induced Immune Tolerance

Melanomas, amongst other cancers, exploit costimulatory signaling interactions to modulate the immune response in favor of inexorable tumor growth [44]. For example, tolerance to a particular TAA can be induced via cross-presentation of the antigen by APCs unable to transmit positive costimulation [45]. Importantly, activation of the CD40 costimulatory pathway on such dysfunctional APCs was found to reverse immunologic tolerance concomitant with T cell-mediated experimental tumor regression [46]. In addition to CD40, the costimulatory ligands CD80 (B7.1) and CD86 (B7.2) and high expression of MHC class II are indicative of APC activation, whereas PD-L1 and PD-L2 are considered markers of tolerogenic APCs [43].

It is also plausible that melanoma cells themselves might serve as functional APCs. Findings of MHC class II-expressing human melanoma cells capable of stimulating autologous T cell proliferation [47] lend experimental support to this hypothesis. Maintenance of T cell anergy requires continues exposure to a particular antigen, which is accomplished by APCs in the lymph node [48]. Presentation of an MDA by MHC class II$^+$ melanoma cells in the absence of positive costimulation could thus foster functional unresponsiveness of MDA-reactive CTLs. In support of this possibility, MHC class II$^+$ melanoma cells rendered MHC class-II-restricted T cell clones anergic [49] and MHC class II immunoreactivity coincides with tumorigenic melanoma subsets [26] and correlates with disease progression and adverse clinical outcome in melanoma patients [50].

Melanomas can also directly deliver coinhibitory signals to immune effector populations to disrupt the antitumor immune response [44] (Fig. 1c). For example, expression of PD-L1 by melanoma cells conferred resistance to CTL-mediated target cell lysis [51] and blockade of this coinhibitory ligand on melanoma cells activated tumor-specific CTL responses in experimental animal models [38, 51] and melanoma patients [52]. Similarly, tumorigenic melanoma subpopulations demonstrate preferential expression of the immunologic checkpoint, PD-1 [26]. Because PD-1 receptor ligation not only confers changes to the receptor-expressing cell but may also deliver inhibitory signals into PD-1 ligand-positive immune subsets [43], PD-1 expression by melanoma cells might constitute a previously unrecognized mechanism of tumor immune evasion. Additional coinhibitory molecules expressed by tumor cells and also implicated in immunologic tolerance, include CD200 [53] and CD47 [54]. Of note, expression of coinhibitory molecules shields tumors not only from CTL responses, but also from additional immune effector populations, such as macrophages [54] and other mediators of both innate and adaptive immunity [44].

3.7 T Cell Exhaustion

Peripheral T cell tolerance can also be achieved via an immunologic phenomenon referred to as T cell exhaustion [55]. Whereas anergic T cells are insufficiently primed (e.g. in the absence of adequate costimulation) and thus do not develop into functional effector cells, exhausted T cells are adequately primed by a particular antigen and requisite costimulatory signals and therefore initially acquire immune effector functions. However, prolonged antigenic stimulation leads to progressive loss of T effector function and ultimately T cell exhaustion or unresponsiveness [55]. Melanomas induce T cell exhaustion to escape immunologic tumor control [55]. For instance, MDA-specific TILs isolated from metastatic tissues of melanoma patients demonstrated functional T cell impairment [56]. Strikingly, tumor-reactive CTLs isolated from the circulation of the same melanoma patients demonstrated immunoreactivity to MART-1 [56], indicating an inherent competence of the metastatic environment to shield the tumor from immune attack by locally inducing T cell exhaustion. In a separate study, upregulation of the immunoregulatory molecules PD-1 and TIM3 was associated with functional exhaustion of NY-ESO-1-specific T effector cells in patients with advanced melanoma [57]. The inhibitory receptors CD160 (also known as BY55), CTLA-4, and lymphocyte-activated gene 3 (LAG3) are additional markers of T cell exhaustion [55]. Importantly, in recent clinical trials, antibody-mediated blockade of CTLA-4 and PD-1 reactivated exhausted melanoma-specific T cells [58, 59] and improved overall survival in patients with advanced disease [59].

3.8 Treg Cell-Mediated Immune Evasion

Another mechanism underlying melanoma immune evasion is the induction, activation, and/or intratumoral recruitment of Treg cells [60]. Treg cells potently suppress activation and function of immune effector populations and are thus essential for maintaining self-tolerance. Phenotypically, Treg cells are generally defined by a $CD4^{+}CD25^{hi}$ phenotype and concurrent expression of the transcription factor, forkhead box P3 (Foxp3). Yet, alternative phenotypes, such as $CD8^{+}$ Treg cells, have also been described [60]. The intricate balance between costimulatory (e.g. CD28, 4-1BB) and coinhibitory (e.g. PD-L1, CTLA-4) signals and the presence of immunoregulatory cytokines (e.g. IL-2, TGF-β) govern Treg cell activation and function [60, 61]. In melanoma patients, Treg cells accumulate to high levels in tumors [62] and have been reported to exert inhibitory effects on immune effector cells, including tumor-reactive TILs [63]. Given their dominant role in tolerance induction, Treg cells are considered a major impediment for successful melanoma immunotherapy [60].

In summary, melanomas employ a plethora of immunoregulatory mechanisms to thwart endogenous antitumor immunity, including passive immune evasion via reduced expression of immunogenic MDAs, induction of clonal anergy and/or exhaustion of immune effector populations, and activation of tolerogenic immune cells. Furthermore, melanoma immunomodulatory functions have been implicated in disease progression and adverse clinical outcome in melanoma patients. Importantly, mechanistic insights into melanoma immune escape are pivotal for accurately interpreting immunophenotypic analyses of TILs. In our opinion, meaningful correlations between TIL immunophenotype and melanoma prognosis will further require detailed characterization of TIL immunobiological functions in the context of the immunoregulatory repertoire of a given tumor environment.

4 Tumor-Infiltrating Lymphocytes

4.1 History and Evolution of the Concept of TILs in Melanoma

As described in detail above, a complex host immunologic response may be directed against a melanoma. This phenomenon, which may result in elimination of part or all of the tumor, is termed regression and can be categorized into three temporal stages: early, intermediate, and late. Early regression is signified by the presence of TILs, i.e., lymphocytes in intimate association with tumor cells. It is generally agreed that to be regarded as TILs, lymphocytes must infiltrate and disrupt tumor nests and/or must be in direct contact with tumor cells (Fig. 3a). Intermediate and late regression result in partial or complete loss of the melanoma and are characterized by immature (intermediate) and mature (late) dermal fibrosis, often accompanied by the presence of melanophages and flattening of the epidermis (with loss of rete ridges).

It has long been recognized that lymphocytes may be observed in intimate association with tumor cells. Initially it was debated whether their presence enhanced the growth of the tumor by providing a fertile microenvironment or whether it represented the manifestation of a host immune response against the tumor [1]. Subsequently, it was reported that the presence of TILs was associated with a more favorable prognosis in patients with breast cancer [2]. More than 40 years ago Clark, Mihm and colleagues noted that early phase melanomas often elicit a significant superficial dermal lymphocyte reaction and that the presence of such a reaction associated with melanoma in situ may indicate the onset of early dermal invasive melanoma [3]. The importance of the immune system in modifying the natural history of melanoma was also highlighted by the recognition that occasionally, following the development of locoregional and/or distant metastases, the primary melanoma may undergo complete spontaneous regression [13]. The latter represents immune-mediated elimination of melanoma cells at the primary tumor site and can usually be recognized by the replacement of the tumor by fibrosis and pigment-laden

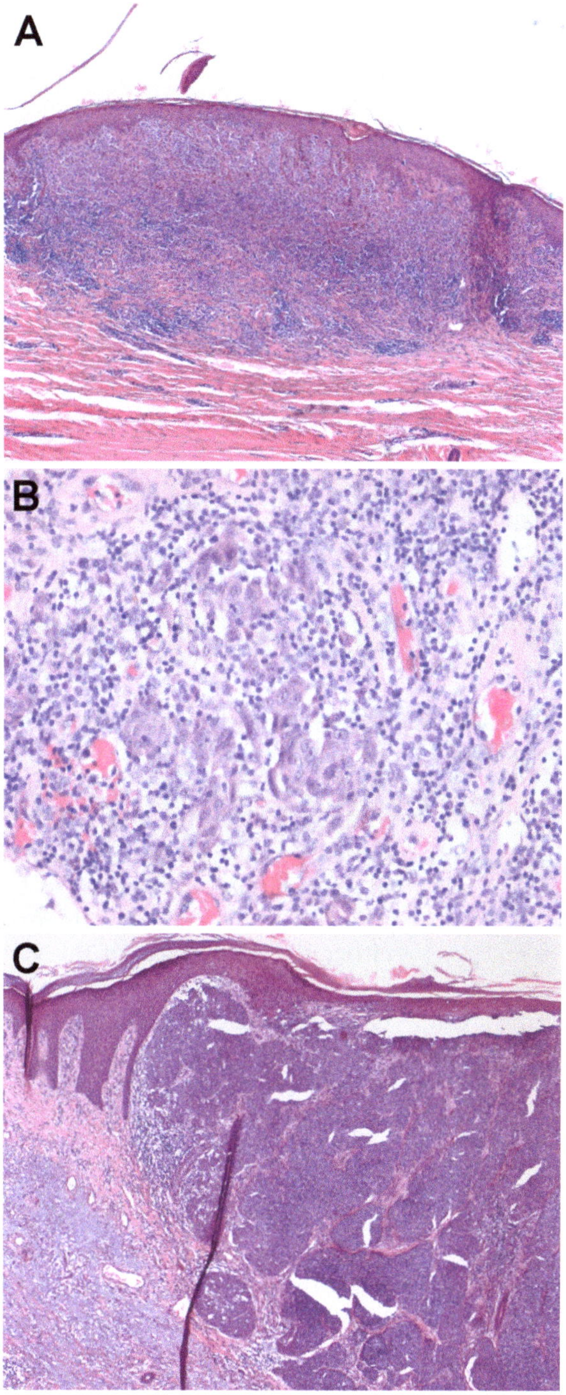

Fig. 3 Histologic examples of clinical melanomas with different types of TIL infiltrates. (**a**) Primary melanoma with a brisk TIL infiltrate characterized by a diffuse lymphoid infiltrate involving the lower one half of the vertical growth phase. (**b**) TIL infiltrate showing apposition of lymphocytes and tumor cells with disruption of tumor nests. (**c**) Nonbrisk TIL infiltrate in a primary melanoma

macrophages (the presence of which provides evidentiary support that this was, in fact, the primary tumor site).

In 1978, Larsen and Grude [64] reported that melanoma patients with a more prominent TIL response in their primary tumor had improved survival compared with those with a less prominent TIL infiltrate. In 1981, Day et al. [65] reported that patients with a moderate to marked infiltrate of lymphocytes within a primary cutaneous melanoma had a significantly better prognosis than those with sparse or absent TILs. Clark et al. [4], aided by careful morphologic analysis, later defined and classified the lymphocytic infiltrate into absent, "brisk," and "nonbrisk" categories according to their distribution and intensity (Fig. 4). They showed that TILs were prognostically significant in the vertical growth phase but not in the radial growth phase of melanomas and that dense intratumoral (but not peritumoral) lymphocytes were strongly associated with improved disease-free and overall survival. In 1996, utilizing the same histologic criteria for quantitating TILs in vertical growth phase primary melanomas, Mihm et al. showed that TILs in lymph node metastases were also associated with improved disease-free survival [6].

4.2 Schema for the Quantification of TILs

The most widely used grading scheme for quantifying the presence of TILs was originally described in detail by Clark et al. [4]. It divides the TIL infiltrate into three groups: absent, nonbrisk and brisk [4] (Table 1). "Absent" was defined as absence of lymphocytes or, if present, they were not directly apposed to tumor cells. A "nonbrisk" infiltrate was defined as a focal TIL infiltrate in the tumor. The TIL infiltrate was categorized as "brisk" if TILs involved either the entire base of the vertical growth phase of the tumor ("peripheral") or showed diffuse permeation of the vertical growth phase ("diffuse"). Clemente et al. [5] subsequently described and illustrated in great detail the different patterns of TILs in vertical growth phase melanomas and suggested that, for ease of understanding and communication, the two main patterns of "brisk" infiltrates (which have the same prognostic significance) be termed "diffuse" (Fig. 4a) and "peripheral" (Fig. 4b), respectively. They noted that in most brisk cases, the lymphocytes predominantly infiltrate the lower portion of the vertical growth phase along virtually the entire base of the tumor although they may occasionally involve the entire vertical growth phase (Fig. 4a). However, in some "brisk" cases, the infiltrate may only involve the lower one-half or lower one-third of the tumor (Fig. 4b). They emphasized that to qualify as "brisk," the lymphocytes must be diffusely interposed between tumor cells, surrounding and disrupting them, with evidence of scattered individual tumor cell necrosis (Fig. 3b). Clemente et al. [5] also stated that "nonbrisk" infiltrates were composed of one or more foci of infiltrating lymphocytes that may

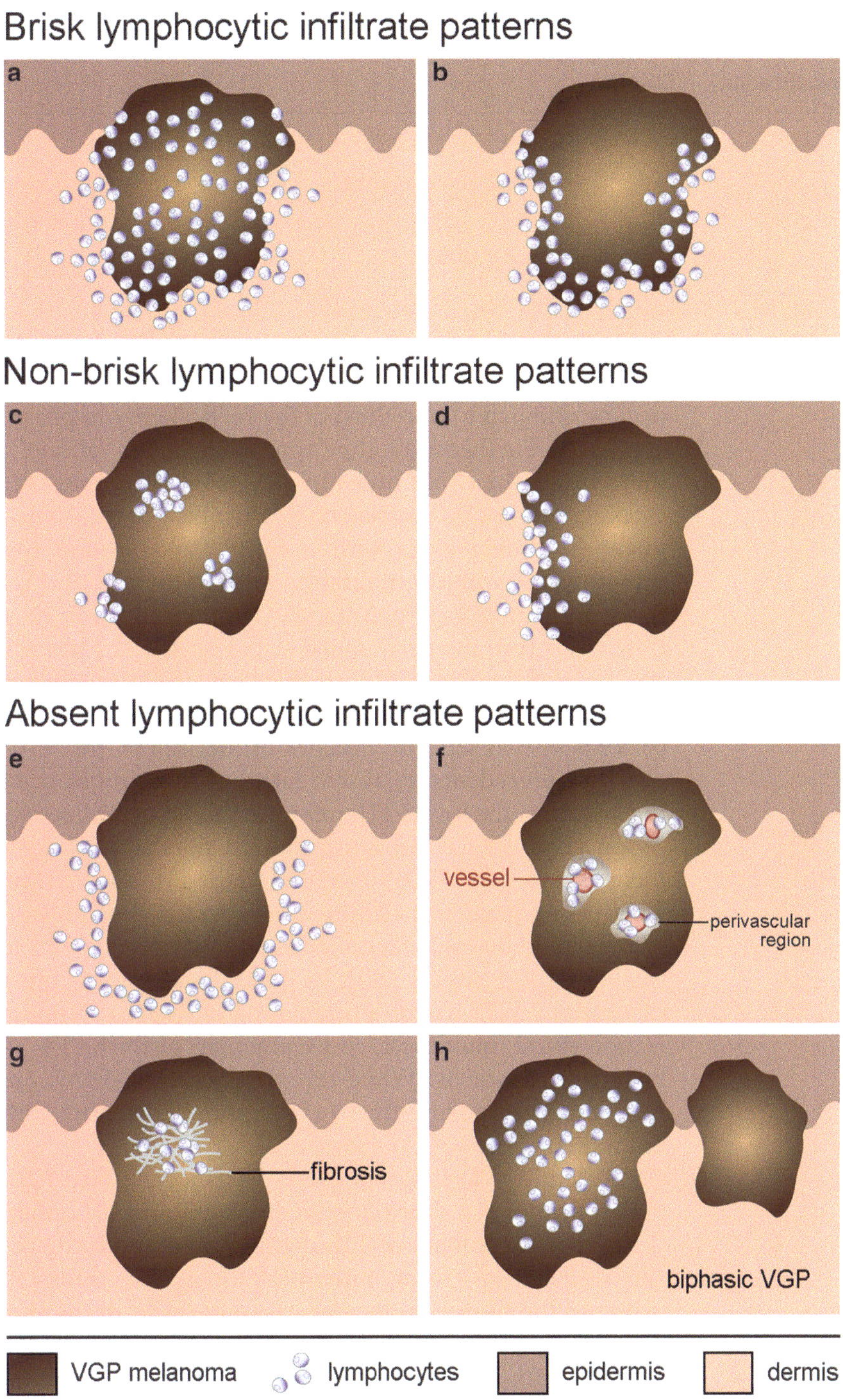

Fig. 4 Schematic figure illustrating the different types of TIL infiltrates in vertical growth phase (VGP) melanomas. (**a**, **b**) Brisk lymphocytic infiltrate patterns. (**c**, **d**) Nonbrisk lymphocytic infiltrate patterns. (**e**–**h**) Absent lymphocytic infiltrate patterns

Table 1
The "brisk"/"nonbrisk" system for quantitating TILs developed by Clark et al. [4]

TIL subclassification	Criteria
Absent	No lymphocytes directly apposed to tumor cells
Nonbrisk	Isolated, multifocal and segmental TIL infiltrate in the tumor
Brisk	Entire base of the tumor infiltrated by TILs ("peripheral") or TILs diffusely meeting tumor ("diffuse")

occupy one-half to one-third of the vertical growth phase (Figs. 3c and 4c, d). Furthermore, they noted that for the "absent" category there should be either no lymphocytes or, if present, the lymphocytes should not be associated with any part of the vertical growth phase (including cases with a dense band around the vertical growth phase without infiltration of the tumor itself (Fig. 4e)), or those with multifocal perivascular lymphocytes that do not infiltrate away from the perivascular site (Fig. 4f), or cases where TILs are confined to sites of fibrosis (Fig. 4g). Clemente and colleagues [5] also recommended that in cases where there are different TIL patterns in two separate nodules of melanoma, the TIL designation give precedence to absent rather than nonbrisk or brisk (i.e., the area with the lower TIL infiltrate should be utilized for classification (Fig. 4h)). One study showed good interobserver agreement (kappa score > 0.6) using the Clark TIL classification scheme when some prior instruction was provided, suggesting that this system could be easily taught and adopted to achieve an acceptable level of reproducibility [66]. In 2010, Rao et al. [67] further subcategorized TILs based upon their density (grades 1–3) and localization (focal, multifocal, and segmental) in thick (T4, >4.0 mm) primary melanomas. While the presence of TILs was associated with improved relapse-free survival, the TIL density and location did not correlate with outcome.

Recently, investigators from Melanoma Institute Australia (MIA) proposed a four-tier system for grading TIL infiltrates that is based on assessment of TIL density (mild, moderate or marked) and distribution (focal, multifocal, or diffuse across the entire extent of the tumor) in the dermal component of the tumor [68]. The TIL grades were defined as follows: grade 0—TILs absent; grade 1—either a mild or moderate focal or a mild multifocal TIL infiltrate; grade 2—either a marked focal, a moderate or marked multifocal, or a mild diffuse TIL infiltrate; grade 3—a moderate or marked diffuse TIL infiltrate (Table 2). Whilst the reported results suggest that it provides accurate prognostic information, further studies by independent observers utilizing independent datasets

Table 2
TIL grading system recently proposed by Melanoma Institute Australia investigators

	TIL density[a]		
TIL distribution	**Mild**	**Moderate**	**Marked**
Focal	1	1	2
Multifocal	1	2	2
Diffuse	2	3	3

[a]Absent TILs = TIL grade 0

Table 3
Comparison of the MIA TIL grading system and the schema of Clark et al. [4]

TIL involvement	TIL grade	Clark et al. [4]
TILs absent	0	Absent
Focal areas of infiltration in the tumor (isolated, multifocal, or segmental)	1 (or 2 if focal marked or multifocal moderate or marked infiltrate)	Nonbrisk
Entire base of the tumor	1–3 (depending on the distribution and density of the TILs)	Brisk
Diffuse permeation of the VGP	2–3 (depending on the density of TIL infiltrate)	Brisk

are required to validate the utility and reproducibility of this 4-tier TIL grading system (*see* Table 3 for a comparison of the MIA TIL grading system and the schema of Clark et al. [4]).

5 Role of TILs in Melanoma Prognosis

Accurate prediction of prognosis in melanoma patients is important to determine the need for further investigations, to guide appropriate management (particularly the appropriateness of postoperative adjuvant therapy), and for assignment of risk status in groups of patients entering clinical trials. Numerous studies have shown that the prognosis for patients who present with clinically localized primary cutaneous melanoma is most strongly associated with its tumor thickness but is also associated with other features of the primary tumor such as mitotic rate, ulcerative state, TILs and anatomic site, as well as patient characteristics, such as age and gender [69, 70]. Recent studies have suggested that the mitotic rate of the dermal component of a primary melanoma is a strong independent indicator of its metastatic potential, is a more powerful prognosticator than ulceration, and can provide more precise stratification of recurrence risk [71, 72]. In view of these findings, the presence or absence of mitoses has now been incorporated as a staging criterion for T1 tumors (≤1.0 mm in thickness) in the 7th edition of the American Joint Committee on Cancer (AJCC) staging system [73]. Furthermore, the AJCC Staging Committee recommends that mitotic rate be recorded using a standardized method in all melanoma pathology reports [73]. In recent times, additional prognostic information has been obtained by sentinel lymph node (SLN) biopsy, a minimally invasive procedure, which determines regional node field status with great accuracy [74]. Whilst it has long been known that TILs influence prognosis in melanoma patients, recent studies utilizing refined statistical techniques have highlighted the independent statistical significance of TILs both as a prognostic factor and as a predictor of SLN metastasis in melanoma patients [68]. These studies, utilizing patient cohorts derived from the modern era in which SLN biopsy is routinely performed as a staging procedure for patients with clinically localized primary cutaneous melanoma, have not only reaffirmed the prognostic value of TILs but have also confirmed its importance in patients undergoing SLN biopsy.

5.1 TILs as a Prognostic Factor in Cutaneous Melanoma

In primary melanomas, most studies point to a favorable prognostic effect of TILs. As described above, the first large study leading to this conclusion was reported by Larsen and Grude in 1978 [64]. In 1981, Day et al. [65] reported that patients with a moderate to marked infiltrate of lymphocytes within a primary cutaneous melanoma had a significantly better prognosis than those with sparse or absent TILs. Soon afterwards, Clark et al. [4] utilized careful morphologic analysis to more precisely define and quantify TIL infiltrates, allowing them to assess the prognostic significance of TILs in more detail. In their analysis of 264 patients, they showed that a dense intratumoral ("brisk") lymphocyte infiltrate in the vertical (but not radial) growth phase of melanoma was strongly and independently associated with improved disease-free and overall survival. A brisk TIL infiltrate was associated with 88 % 8 year survival compared with 75 and 59 % for patients with nonbrisk and absent TILs, respectively. In contrast, lymphocytes associated with the radial growth phase of melanomas or the presence of an abundance of peritumoral lymphocytes did not have prognostic significance.

The prognostic importance of TILs utilizing the classification scheme of Clark et al. [4] was subsequently confirmed by results from other studies [5, 6, 31, 75]. In 1996, a study by Clemente et al. [5] comprising of 285 patients with vertical growth phase primary cutaneous melanomas showed that the 5 year survival for patients with a brisk TIL infiltrate was 77 % compared with 53 and 37 % for those with nonbrisk and absent TIL infiltrates, respectively. In this study, both tumor thickness and TILs were independent predictors of outcome. Subsequently, Tuthill et al. [75] reported that a brisk TIL infiltrate was associated with 100 % 5 year survival in a study of 259 melanoma patients. However, some authors have reported prognostic value of TILs on univariate but not on multivariate analyses [76], while others have demonstrated no correlation between TILs and prognosis [15, 16, 64, 77]. In a population-based study of 548 melanoma patients, Barnhill et al. [77] found no significant association between TILs (classified as per Clark et al. [4]) and survival. Because TILs appear to be more prognostically important in vertical growth phase and thicker tumors in some studies [5], it has been suggested that possible reasons for the apparently discordant results in the latter studies may be related to the inclusion of a predominance of thin and radial growth phase melanomas, lack of adherence to the definition of TILs or failure to differentiate infiltrative and noninfiltrative lymphoid cells [5, 15, 77]. However, a number of studies have also suggested that TILs may have prognostic significance in the vertical growth phase of thin (<1.0 mm) melanomas [78, 79].

The studies cited above mostly preceded the current era of routine assessment of the tumor-harboring status of regional lymph nodes by SLN biopsy in patients with clinically localized primary cutaneous melanomas. However, a number of recently published larger studies have provided additional supportive evidence of the prognostic importance of TILs in melanoma patients in whom SLN biopsy was performed [15, 80–82]. Kruper et al. [80] showed that tumor thickness, mitotic rate and absent TILs were independent predictors of SLN metastasis in 327 patients with primary melanomas >1.0 mm in thickness. In a study of 887 patients published in 2007, Taylor and colleagues [15] reported that absent TILs (OR 0.48; 95 % CI 0.32–0.71; $p=0.0003$), as well as tumor thickness (OR 1.18; 95 % CI 1.11–1.26; $p<0.0001$), ulceration (OR 2.04; 95 % CI 1.38–3.03; $p=0.0004$) and male sex (OR 1.53; 95 % CI 1.03–2.26; $p=0.03$) predicted SLN positivity on multivariate analysis but the presence of TILs was not an independent predictor for survival [15]. In their study, 3.9 % of patients with a brisk TIL response had a positive SLN compared with 26.2 % of those with a nonbrisk TIL response [15]. Other authors have reported similar findings [81, 82]. Potentially, TIL data may be utilized to identify a subset of melanoma patients in whom the risk of SLN metastasis is so low that it may not be worthwhile performing this procedure. However, other studies have shown no correlation between TILs and SLN status [83, 84]. In another study, TILs and a dominant nodule within thick (>4.0 mm) primary melanomas were independent predictors of relapse-free survival in a study of 293 patients with long term follow up [67]. Furthermore, in an analysis of patients from the Sunbelt Melanoma Trial, reported in 2011, Burton et al. [82] found that 5 year overall

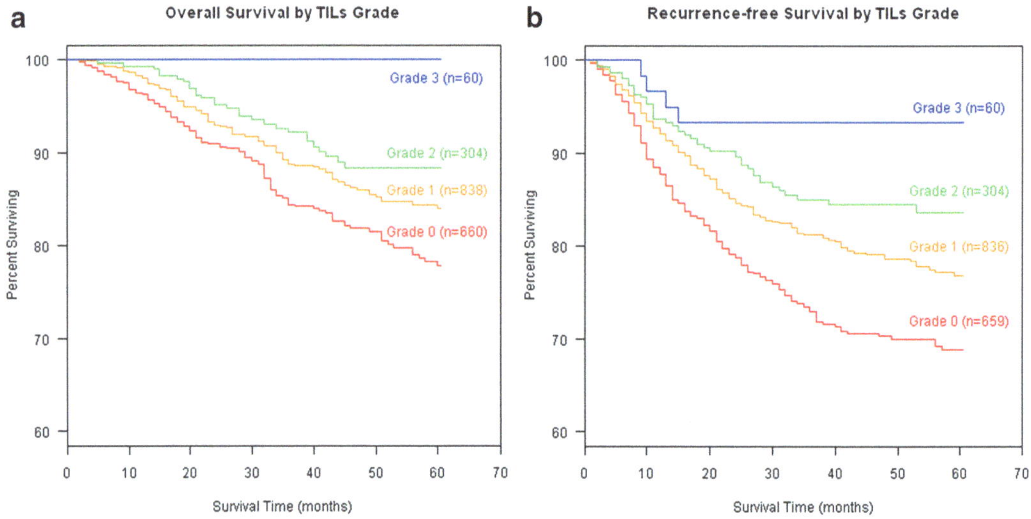

Fig. 5 Correlation of TIL grade with melanoma patient survival. (**a**) Overall survival in 1,865 melanoma patients stratified by TIL grade from a recent study by Melanoma Institute Australia investigators [68]. (**b**) Recurrence-free survival in 1,865 melanoma patients stratified by TIL grade from a recent study by Melanoma Institute Australia investigators [68]

survival in patients with a brisk TIL infiltrate was 95 % compared with 84 % in those with nonbrisk infiltrates ($p = 0.0083$).

In 2012, a study of 1,865 melanoma patients diagnosed and treated at MIA was reported [68]. This defined a novel four tiered grading system for TIL quantitation (Table 2) and represents the largest study reported to date assessing the prognostic significance of TILs in primary cutaneous melanomas as far as we are aware. The study showed that TIL grade is a powerful independent predictor of SLN status, melanoma-specific survival (Fig. 5a) and recurrence-free survival (Fig. 5b) in patients with clinically localized primary cutaneous melanoma ≥0.75 mm in thickness. There was a significant inverse association between SLN status and TIL grade (SLN positivity rates for each TIL grade: 0 = 27.8 %, 1 = 20.1 %, 2 = 18.3 %, 3 = 5.6 %; $p < 0.0001$). Predictors of SLN positivity were decreasing age ($p < 0.0001$), decreasing TIL grade ($p < 0.0001$), ulceration ($p = 0.003$), increasing tumor thickness ($p = 0.01$), satellitosis ($p = 0.03$) and increasing mitotic rate ($p = 0.03$). Tumor thickness ($p < 0.0001$), ulceration ($p < 0.0001$), satellitosis ($p < 0.0001$), mitotic rate ($p = 0.003$), TIL grade ($p < 0.0001$) and gender ($p = 0.01$) were independent predictors of melanoma-specific survival. In patients who underwent SLN biopsy, as expected, the tumor harboring status of the SLN was the strongest predictor of outcome. However TIL grade remained an independent predictor of outcome even when SLN status and other prognostic factors were taken into account. Patients with TIL grade 3 tumors had 100 % survival (Fig. 5a).

Whilst some previous studies have reported associations between TILs and some of these endpoints, this study is the first to find independent associations of TIL grade with all three outcomes (SLN status, disease-free and melanoma-specific survival). The findings have important implications for melanoma patient management and highlight the important role of the immune system in determining the clinical behavior of melanomas.

In recent studies, it has been demonstrated that the use of a structured or synoptic pathology report format for melanoma ensures completeness and validity of pathology reporting [85]. It also improves consistency of pathology reporting and presents information in a predictable and easy-to-read format that facilitates efficient extraction of information by clinicians and for registries, data collection and research purposes. In view of the prognostic importance of TILs (either as per the classification scheme of Clark et al. [4] or using the MIA TIL grade [68]), TIL status should be a component of synoptic reports for melanoma.

There are a number of limitations of current methods for staging and determining prognosis for melanoma patients. Firstly, there is a wide variation in clinical outcomes in the various AJCC stage categories, limiting the prognostic reliability of the stage groupings for individual patients. Secondly, the staging system does not account for change (improvement) in prognosis that occurs with time in surviving patients. Finally, most staging systems and other prognostic calculators do not take into account all of the known prognostic factors (including TILs) in melanoma patients. It is hoped that in the future, web-based prognostic calculators based on data derived from large cohorts of carefully annotated melanoma patients will be developed that take into account these issues and will be able to determine a more accurate prognostic estimate for individual patients.

In summary, most studies support the prognostic significance of "brisk"/prominent TILs in melanoma including a recent large study which confirmed that TILs were an independent predictor of both disease-free and melanoma-specific survival. In addition, in most studies where SLN biopsy was performed, absence of TILs predicted SLN positivity, which itself is the strongest predictor of shorter survival in patients with clinically localized primary cutaneous melanomas (*see* Table 4 for an overview of studies analyzing the association of TILs in primary melanomas with SLN status and/or overall survival).

5.2 TILs in Lymph Nodes and Effect on Prognosis

Malignant melanoma can metastasize by two principal routes other than by direct extension. These pathways include hematogenous as well as lymphatic spread. It appears that the most common route is by the lymphatic system [86]. The chosen lymphatic site is a regional lymph node basin that drains the area of the primary tumor. This route has been considered so important that for a long

Table 4
Studies analyzing the association of TILs in primary melanomas with sentinel lymph node status and/or overall survival

				Association with			
First author of study	Year of publication	No. of patients	TIL sub-groupings	SLN positivity	*P* value for SLN status	MSS (5 years)	*P* value for OS
Larsen	1978	361	+ +++	NP		78 % 91 %	Significant
Johnson	1985	262	+ +++	NP		48 % 60 %	<0.05
Clark	1989	264	Absent Nonbrisk Brisk	NP		59 %[a] 75 %[a] 88 %[a]	0.0015
Thorn	1994	498	None/slight Moderate Abundant	NP		56 % 76 % 94 %	Significant
Mansson-Brahme	1994	585	Grade of inflammatory response	NP			Significant
Clemente	1996	285	Absent Nonbrisk Brisk	NP		37 % 53 % 77 %	0.0003
Barnhill	1996	548	Absent Nonbrisk and Brisk	NP			NS
Mraz-Gernhard	1998	585	Absent Nonbrisk and brisk	UK	NS	NP	NP
Tuthill	2002	259	Absent Nonbrisk Brisk	NP		71 % 71 % 100 %	0.005
Taylor	2007	887	Absent Nonbrisk Brisk	26 % 16 % 4 %	0.0003	75 % 76 % (Nonbrisk and brisk combined)	NS
Mandala	2009	1,251	Absent Nonbrisk Brisk	22 % 12 % 18 %	0.02	90 % 95 %	NS
Rao	2010	293	Absent Nonbrisk Brisk	NP		54 % 54 % 72 %	NS

(continued)

Table 4 (continued)

First author of study	Year of publication	No. of patients	TIL sub-groupings	Association with SLN positivity	Association with P value for SLN status	Association with MSS (5 years)	P value for OS
Burton	2011	515	Nonbrisk	17.6 %	0.0087	84 %	0.0083
			Brisk	7 %		95 %	
Azimi	2012	1,865	TIL grade 0	28 %	<0.001	78 %	<0.001
			TIL grade 1	20 %		84 %	
			TIL grade 2	18 %		88 %	
			TIL grade 3	5 %		100 %	

[a]8 year survival
SLN sentinel lymph node, *MSS* melanoma-specific survival, *OS* overall survival, *NP* not performed, *NS* not significant, *UK* unknown

period of time complete excision plus a complete regional lymph node dissection were the treatment of choice in the management of a primary melanoma. More recently, attention has been drawn to the importance of the SLN, which is the first node in a lymph node chain to receive lymphatic drainage. In light of the work of Morton and his associates [74], the SLN biopsy and exhaustive histologic evaluation of the same have become the standard of care and are considered the optimal staging technique now available in the management of primary melanoma patients. With renewed interest in the biology of the host response, there have been extensive efforts to understand the immunological status of the SLNs [86]. This section will be devoted to the review of the various aspects of the biology of the SLN with emphasis on the humoral and cellular responses.

An early randomized control trial of stage II melanoma patients on IFN therapy with lymph node dissections showed that survival was most common in patients who had dense intra-tumoral lymphocytic infiltrates, both in the primary tumor and in all positive lymph node deposits [6]. In striking contrast, patients without infiltrates in the metastatic deposits had a much worse survival [6]. A subsequent study of several of these patients used identification of TCR beta variables, and demonstrated clonality of the lymphocytes both in the primary tumor and in the lymph nodes [87]. This finding implied a specific T cell antigen response in those patients. Together, these studies engendered further interest in understanding the biologic nature of the host response in metastatic nodes.

One of the most important functions of the lymph nodes is to handle antigen-primed DCs that come from the periphery via afferent lymphatics in the form of the "veiled cell" [88].

These veiled cells derive their name from the lack of the very prominent dendritic processes observed in the skin that are associated with antigen exposure [88]. Upon entering the lymph node, veiled cells reassume their dendritic profile and present antigens to naïve T cells [86]. This activity takes place in the paracortical region, where numerous T cells reside, and results in the formation of effector T cells, including cytotoxic (CD8+) and T helper (CD4+) cells with their various subtypes as well as tolerogenic immune cells, such as Tregs [86]. The cortex (also known as B cell zone) of the lymph node has a paracortical area overlying a follicular center. In the follicular center, antigens are presented to B cells that transform into plasma cells with the capacity to produce antibodies [86]. The deeper cortex mainly consists of T cells, including CD4(+) and CD8(+) populations. There are also alternative cell types in the lymph node, including fibrocytes that produce matrix proteins, such as collagens I and III. These collagens crosslink to form a meshwork of reticulin that provides structure and stability to the lymph node's overall architecture. The diverse cell types in the lymph node function both independently and interdependently.

Variations in the number of CD4(+) and CD8(+) T cells, and the production of tolerogenic cells have been demonstrated in SLNs that are positive for tumor and other adjacent nodes close to the SLN, in contrast to those at a distance from the positive node [89]. The remainder of this section will address these immunologic changes in SLNs and how they are considered to affect the host's response to the tumor. The secretagogues from the tumor itself are believed to be the predominant source of the manifold changes in the microenvironment of the SLN [86]. Tumor cell-derived soluble mediators include GMCSF, VEGF, IL-1, IL-6, IL-10, TGF-β, and prostaglandins (Fig. 6a, b). Under their influence, T cell numbers decrease while B cells concurrently increase in frequency in positive SLNs as compared to negative nodes. Of note, among the diminished T cells, a relative increase in highly immunosuppressive CD4(+)CD25(+)Foxp3(+) Tregs can be observed in positive versus negative SLNs [86].

Monocytes and DCs represent additional cell populations, apparently recruited to the lymph node by the aforementioned secretagogues. These immune cell subsets can be of either myeloid or lymphocytic origin. Myeloid-derived DCs are considered a classic, immunogenic APC. Plasmacytoid DCs of lymphocytic origin (also known as myeloid-derived suppressor cells (MDSCs)), on the other hand, are tolerogenic (Fig. 6a), and can be distinguished from their immunogenic counterparts based on their expression of the CD123 marker [86]. Monocytes are myeloid-derived cells that, like DCs, exhibit highly complex cytoplasmic processes when they are in an antigen-presenting phase [90]. They are markedly present in negative but greatly diminished in positive SLNs [89]. In the latter state, they have a round or "veiled" appearance,

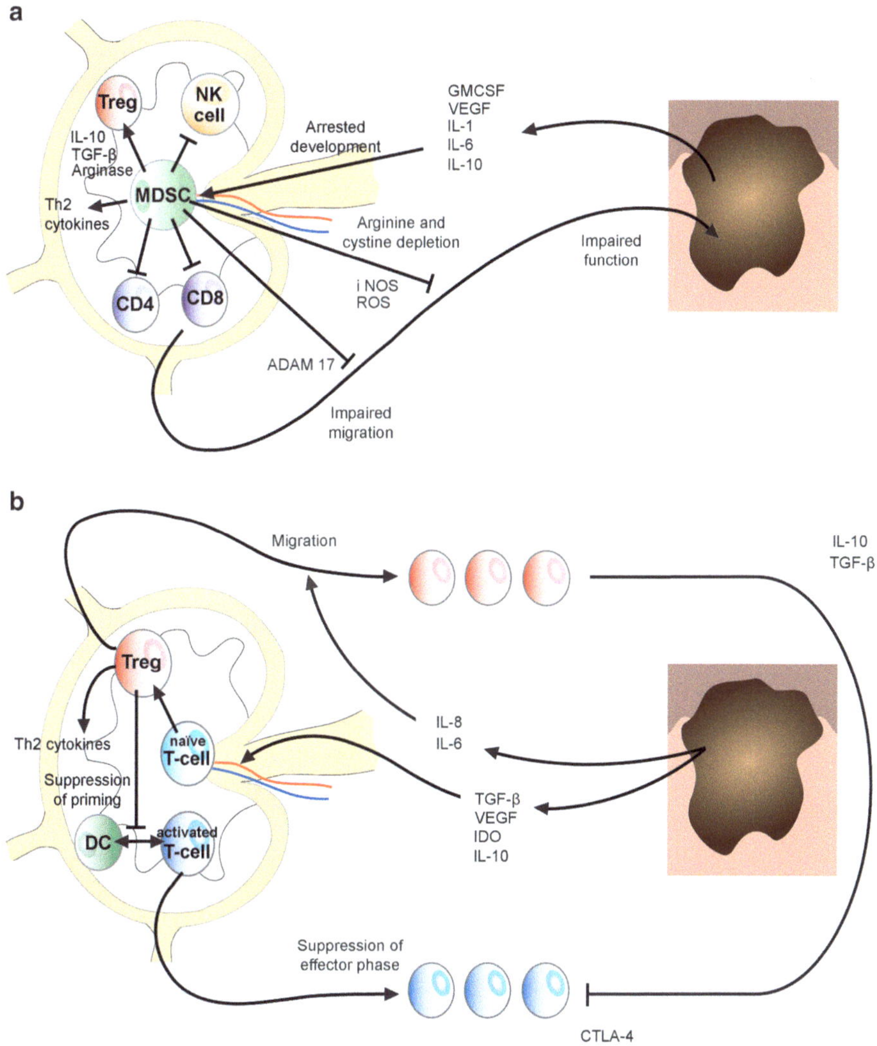

Fig. 6 Mechanisms of immunosuppression within the melanoma-draining lymph node. (**a**) Various mechanisms of myeloid-derived suppressor cell (MDSC)-mediated immunosuppression in the melanoma-draining lymph node. IL-10: interleukin-10; TGF-β: transforming growth factor-beta; Th2: T helper cell 2; GMCSF: granulocyte-macrophage colony-stimulating factor; VEGF: vascular endothelial growth factor; iNOS: inducible nitric oxide synthase; ROS: reactive oxygen species; ADAM 17: A disintegrin and metalloproteinase 17. (**b**) Various mechanisms of regulatory T cell (Treg)-mediated immunosuppression in the melanoma-draining lymph node. DC: dendritic cell; IDO: indoleamine 2,3-dioxigenase; CTLA-4: cytotoxic T-lymphocyte antigen 4. Adapted from [89] with permission

induced by tumor secretagogues or other cytokines of local origin [89]. Conversely, the plasmacytoid DCs of lymphocyte origin do not exhibit these remarkable dendritic processes, and many of them may appear to be veiled cells. However, they should not be confused with myeloid-derived, "veiled" cells, as they perform different functions [91]. In addition to myeloid DCs that are recruited to become immunogenic cells, there are alternative mononuclear cells in the peripheral blood that can give rise to immunosuppressive cells. Their mechanisms of suppression include increase in inducible nitric oxide synthase (iNOS), IL-1, IL-10 and ADAM 17 (Fig. 6a). These factors directly inhibit activation and migration of both CD4(+) and CD8(+) T cell populations [89] (Fig. 6a).

In addition to the various cytokines and chemokines produced by the tumor, Tregs also produce IL-10, as do tolerogenic DCs [92] (Fig. 6a, b). Importantly, tolerogenic DCs are also a major source of indoleamine-2,3-dioxigenase (IDO) [91]. The production of IDO inhibits T cell activity by catabolizing tryptophan to kynurenine [91]. Tryptophan is required for successful antigen presentation and sensitization of T cells [91]. IDO expression can be inhibited by IFN-γ [92]. However, in the presence of IL-10, plasmocytoid DCs maintain their IDO enzymatic activity, irrespective of exogenous IFN-γ [92]. This observation highlights the importance of IL-10 as a dominant immunosuppressive factor in the SLN. An additional mediator of both Treg and plasmocytoid DC maintenance and melanoma progression is VEGF. VEGF interactions with its receptor, neuropilin 1, expressed by Tregs and plasmocytoid DCs, were found to promote metastatic dissemination to the draining lymph node in tumor patients [93].

Finally, granulocyte macrophage colony stimulating factor (GMCSF) represents an additional key soluble mediator of the lymph node environment, with well-established roles in the recruitment of activated DCs [94]. In a phase I study, 11 of 21 evaluable stage IV melanoma patients vaccinated with autologous, irradiated melanoma cells engineered to produce GMCSF demonstrated prolonged survival [95]. The average survival time was approximately 3.5 years, with one patient surviving over 10 years [95]. Notably, metastatic lesions resected after vaccination demonstrated brisk or focal lymphocytic infiltrates with tumor necrosis as compared to pretreatment biopsies [95]. A subsequent vaccination study employing GMCSF-transduced melanoma cells yielded similar results in patients with metastatic melanoma [95]. Moreover, intradermal administration of GMCSF around the excision site of stage I primary melanoma tumors was found to increase the number and activation state of DCs in the paracortical areas of patient SLNs and enhanced their binding to T cells [96]. Together, these findings highlight that lymphocytes and tumor cells within positive SLNs are critically intertwined. However, the significance of this observation in the biology and progression of melanoma remains to be elucidated.

In summary, multiple immunologic factors support an immunosuppressive environment in positive SLNs (Fig. 6). These factors are produced initially by the tumor and then, under the influence of the tumor, also by other cellular components of the lymph node. Importantly, soluble mediators of the SLN environment serve as possible targets for specific agents such as small molecules or blocking antibodies that might counteract their effects. Release from the immunosuppressive mechanisms of the lymph node may further lead to better tumor control at the primary site.

6 Harnessing TILs to Improve Melanoma Immunotherapy

In addition to their potential significance as biomarkers of melanoma prognosis, TILs may also be predictive of therapeutic outcome in melanoma patients. TIL immunobiology might be particularly relevant for predicting and optimizing response to melanoma immunotherapy, which has evolved as a promising treatment option for patients with advanced disease [44]. Unfortunately, the immune distortions achieved by immunotherapeutic interventions might further complicate the analysis of TIL immunophenotype and function. Given its remarkable immunogenicity (discussed above), melanoma has been a major focus for the clinical advancement of cancer immunotherapies. However, a major obstacle for the development of efficient immunotherapeutic protocols has been the difficulty to successfully antagonize the numerous mechanisms of melanoma immune escape [44]. Melanoma immunotherapy can be broadly grouped into (a) immunomodulatory strategies aimed at reinforcing endogenous anti-melanoma immunity, (b) vaccination protocols involving whole cells, immunogenic peptides, or immunizing vectors to sensitize the immune system against the autologous tumor, and (c) adoptive cell transfer (ACT) of ex vivo expanded immune effector populations with melanoma target specificity [97]. This section will review examples of immunotherapeutic strategies aimed at activating melanoma-specific immunity and their potential effects on TILs, with a special emphasis on novel immune checkpoint inhibitors.

Therapeutic attempts to boost melanoma-specific immunity have included the administration of various nonspecific enhancers of immune effector responses. The proproliferative cytokine IL-2 is perhaps the best-studied nonspecific immune activator in the therapy of melanoma [14, 22, 23]. Expansion of MDA-specific T cell clones and increased CTL-mediated cytotoxicity have been proposed as mechanisms of action for IL-2 immunotherapy [98]. Numerous prospective clinical trials have demonstrated some utility of either IL-2 monotherapy or combinatorial approaches involving the cytokine for the treatment of metastatic melanoma [14, 22, 23]. Accordingly, the U.S. Food and Drug Administration (FDA) has approved IL-2 therapy for patients with advanced disease. However, most melanoma patients do not benefit from IL-2 immunotherapy as evident by complete response rates of only about 5–20 % [22, 23]. Immunohistochemical analysis of metastatic biopsies of IL-2-treated patients revealed that regressing melanomas harbored high levels of TILs, including both $CD4^+$ and $CD8^+$ T cells as well as macrophages [99]. Furthermore, MHC class II expression by melanoma cells appeared to be associated with therapeutic response [99]. However, neither these nor other immunohistochemical correlates were predictive of therapeutic response when evaluating pretreatment specimens [99]. A possible explanation for the refractoriness of melanoma to IL-2 therapy is suggested by the essential role of the cytokine not only for the activation for T effector responses [98] but also for the induction of Treg cells [60]. Indeed, IL-2 treatment was found to increase Treg TILs in melanoma patients [100].

Accordingly, Treg cell depleting strategies have been investigated in combination with IL-2 treatment or other immunotherapeutic approaches [101–103]. Treg cell-depleting agents include anti-CD25 (also known as IL-2 receptor (IL-2R)) antibodies or cytotoxic proteins conjugated to recombinant IL-2 [101–103], all of which induce cell death of CD25-expressing cells. However, current Treg cell depletion regimens have been less efficacious than anticipated, despite the constitutive expression of CD25 by Treg cells and the demonstrated effectiveness of CD25-directed therapies in successfully reducing Treg numbers [101]. Because CD25 is also a prominent regulator of T effector cell activation, one possible explanation for the inability of CD25-targeted regimens to sustain tumor regression could be the unwanted depletion of T effector populations.

Immunotherapy with IFN-α has also demonstrated reproducible activity in melanoma patients with advanced disease, as evident by objective response rates of approximately 15 % [104, 105]. Not unlike trials utilizing IL-2 [99], responders to IFN-α adjuvant therapy demonstrated significantly denser TIL infiltrates [105]. However, therapeutic outcome cannot be predicted based on current immunopathological analyses and the mechanisms underlying melanoma responsiveness to this proproliferative cytokine are not fully understood. IL-21 represents an additional nonspecific immune activator currently undergoing clinical testing in patients with metastatic melanoma [106].

More recently, additional therapeutics have been developed that target defined regulatory elements of patient immune cells to augment melanoma-specific immunity [44]. Among the most promising approaches in this regard is the inhibition of immunologic checkpoints [44]. As outlined in more detail above, immune checkpoints are negative regulators of the immune system that maintain immune homeostasis by modulating the amplitude and quality of numerous adaptive and innate effector mechanisms in favor of immunogenic tolerance. Tumors, including melanoma, exploit immune checkpoint signaling interactions as a major mechanism of both immune escape and immunotherapeutic resistance [44]. Mechanistically, immunologic checkpoint interference is thought to amplify melanoma-specific immunity (e.g. by reactivating exhausted or anergic T effector populations) while concurrently antagonizing mechanisms of tumor immune evasion (e.g. inhibition of Treg cell development and function) [44]. Therefore, therapeutic blockade of immunologic checkpoints could prove more efficient in inducing durable responses in melanoma patients than treatment with nonspecific immune activators.

CTLA-4 antibodies were the first of this class of immunotherapeutics to receive FDA approval for the treatment of metastatic melanoma [59]. CTLA-4 is predominantly expressed on T cells, where it dampens the amplitude of activation during early stages of T cell priming by counteracting CD28-mediated positive costimulatory signaling events [43]. CTLA-4 and CD28 share the same ligands, namely CD80 (also known as B7.1) and CD86 (also known as B7.2) (Fig. 1c), which are expressed by professional APCs, among other cell types [43]. CTLA-4 is believed to antagonize CD28-specific T cell activation because of its 100-to-2,000-fold greater affinity for CD80 and CD86 relative to that of CD28 and because CTLA-4 activation potently suppresses essential mediators of TCR signaling required for T cell survival [43]. Lethal lymphoproliferative disorders observed in CTLA-4 knockout mice further support a central role of CTLA-4 for sustaining T cell homeostasis [43]. In addition to downmodulating T effector responses, CTLA-4 enhances Treg cell immunosuppressive activity [61]. Antibodies that block CTLA-4 signaling would thus be predicted to potently augment antimelanoma immunity. Indeed, CTLA-4 inhibition was found to eliminate tumors concomitant with enhanced melanoma-specific CTL function in animal models of the disease [107]. In clinical trials, CTLA-4 inhibition demonstrated overall response rates of 8–18 % in patients with metastatic melanoma [59]. In a recent phase III study, treatment of patients with therapy-resistant, unresectable stage III or IV melanoma with the anti-CTLA-4 antibody "ipilimumab" resulted in improved overall survival compared to patients treated with a gp100 peptide vaccine [59]. Combination therapy of "tremelimumab," an alternative anti-CTLA-4 antibody, with IFN-α2b also showed promising durable antitumor efficacy in stage IV melanoma patients [104], warranting further testing in a randomized trial. Not surprisingly, given the prominent role of CTLA-4 in immune homeostasis, response to CTLA-4 immunotherapy often coincides with clinically significant inflammatory or autoimmune effects [59]. Studies of CTLA-4 blockade have also yielded insights into TIL behavior in the context of immune checkpoint interference [108]. For instance, while markedly increased numbers of TILs were detected as a result of CTLA-4 administration [108], the presence of Treg cells in metastatic melanoma appeared to inversely correlate with T effector TIL numbers and the extent of tumor necrosis [108], suggesting that Treg infiltrates may limit immune-mediated melanoma destruction in response to this form of immunotherapy.

More recently, additional inhibitors of immunologic checkpoint pathways have entered clinical trials for the treatment of advanced cancer, including monoclonal antibodies to PD-1 [58], PD-L1 [52], and LAG3 [44]. In contrast to the CTLA-4 receptor, which attenuates T cell stimulation during early phases of T cell priming, PD-1 signaling limits T cell activation at the time of an ongoing T effector response [43]. PD-1 has two known ligands, PD-L1 (also known as B7-H1) and PD-L2 (also known as B7-DC) (Fig. 1c). While PD-L1 is expressed by a wide range of both immune and nonimmune cells, including melanoma cells, PD-L2 expression is thought to be restricted to distinct APC subpopulations [43]. Together, the specific inhibition of immune evasion pathways that are directly delivered by the tumor and the predominant involvement of PD-1 in the effector phase of T cell immunity, suggest fewer autoimmune complications and greater antimelanoma activity of PD-1 pathway interference compared to CTLA-4 blockade [109]. Indeed, clinical trials of anti-PD-1 [58] and anti-PD-L1 antibody treatment [52] yielded objective response rates beyond 30 % [44] in patients with refractory solid tumors. Moreover, immune-related adverse events were significantly lower in both PD-1- and PD-L1-compared to CTLA-4 antibody-treated cancer patients, respectively [44]. These initial observations have sparked tremendous interest in the medical community, because they suggest that PD-1 pathway inhibition is likely to represent a new benchmark for antimelanoma immunotherapy [109].

Despite these seminal advances, a majority of melanoma patients still do not respond to these novel forms of immunotherapy and because the mechanisms underlying PD-1/PD-L1-driven tumor immune evasion are not fully understood, clinical response to PD-1 pathway interference is difficult to predict. Histologic and molecular characterization of pre- and post-immunotherapy specimens in general and TILs in particular could provide key insights for predicting patient response based on distinct immunoregulatory phenotypes. Central to this approach is the study of PD-1 and PD-1-ligand expression in the tumor environment [109]. In fact, PD-L1 immunoreactivity in metastatic melanoma tended to correlate with clinical response in PD-1-antibody treated patients [58]. However, neither the PD-L1 expression status of tumor cells nor that of TILs was found to correlate with better prognosis [39] or decreased overall survival of cancer patients [44], highlighting the requirement to further our understanding of the diverse cell types and signaling events involved in PD-1-driven melanoma immune escape and tumor progression.

An additional therapeutic avenue for potentiating the antitumor immune response is via active immunization protocols involving peptides, whole inactivated tumor cells, or antigen-pulsed DCs [97].

These active immunization approaches are often directed at MDAs or CTAs, including gp100, MART-1, or MAGE. Despite the frequently observed induction of tumor-specific immunity, including increased numbers of MDA-reactive TILs [19], in response to such vaccination regimens, only rare and highly sporadic regressions have been achieved in melanoma patients [97]. The common inefficacy of active immunization strategies in controlling melanoma progression could result from diminished expression of MDAs by melanoma target cells (discussed above) [28–30], among other tumor-mediated immune escape mechanisms [18].

Similar considerations may apply to ACT approaches involving infusion of cancer patients with ex vivo expanded immune effector populations with melanoma target specificity [97]. Comparable to cancer vaccines, ACT is often directed at well-established MDAs that are frequently downregulated in melanomas [97]. Additionally, ACT therapeutic outcomes may be profoundly limited by restricted in vivo homing properties or short life spans of ex vivo expanded tumor-specific immune effector cells [97]. Strategies aimed at improving ACT treatment efficacy include concurrent inhibition of coinhibitory receptors on tumor-reactive CTLs, transduction of melanoma-specific T cell clones with costimulatory molecules and/or growth factors, and prior depletion of host Treg cells [97].

The next frontier in melanoma therapy is to achieve high response rates and long-lasting remissions through the use of selectable biomarkers to provide a rationalized basis for personalized therapy [109]. The characterization of TILs and their immunobiology in the context of current therapeutic trials could provide invaluable insights in this regard. In addition to their tremendous potential for optimizing immunotherapeutic regimens, TILs could also help predict and monitor alternative treatment options. This possibility is supported by findings of elevated TIL frequencies in response to melanoma chemotherapy [110]. An increased understanding of TIL immunobiology and the improved characterization of distinct TIL immunophenotypes in the context of known immunomodulatory mechanisms of the tumor environment hold great promise for optimizing future therapy. However, much work is still needed before definitive conclusions about the significance of TILs as biomarkers in treatment selection can be drawn.

7 Conclusions

In this chapter the divergent roles of TILs in the dynamics of malignant melanoma progression and their significance for melanoma prognosis have been outlined and discussed. We have provided a detailed review of the immunology and histopathology of melanoma cell interactions with the inflammatory response, with emphasis on prediction of survival and SLN positivity. The impact of melanoma immunotherapy on TIL biology has also been reviewed. Overall, an increasing number of studies support the prognostic significance of distinct TIL infiltrates in melanoma and highlight their importance for evaluating response to melanoma immunotherapy. The sometimes contradictory findings of earlier studies likely reflect the great immunophenotypic and functional heterogeneity of TILs. By applying refined methodologies and immunobiological insight to future trials, TILs will increasingly serve as effective biomarkers, further improving prognosis and clinical management of melanoma.

Acknowledgments

We apologize to those colleagues whose work could not be cited due to space limitations. T. Schatton is the recipient of a Research Career Development Award from the Dermatology Foundation, an Innovative Research Grant from the Melanoma International Foundation, and a SPORE in Skin Cancer Developmental Project Grant (NIH/NCI).

References

1. Mantovani A, Allavena P, Sica A, Balkwill F (2008) Cancer-related inflammation. Nature 454:436–444
2. Moore OS Jr, Foote FW Jr (1949) The relatively favorable prognosis of medullary carcinoma of the breast. Cancer 2:635–642
3. Clark WH Jr, From L, Bernardino EA, Mihm MC (1969) The histogenesis and biologic behavior of primary human malignant melanomas of the skin. Cancer Res 29:705–727
4. Clark WH Jr, Elder DE, Guerry DT, Braitman LE, Trock BJ, Schultz D, Synnestvedt M, Halpern AC (1989) Model predicting survival in stage I melanoma based on tumor progression. J Natl Cancer Inst 81:1893–1904
5. Clemente CG, Mihm MC Jr, Bufalino R, Zurrida S, Collini P, Cascinelli N (1996) Prognostic value of tumor infiltrating lymphocytes in the vertical growth phase of primary cutaneous melanoma. Cancer 77: 1303–1310
6. Mihm MC Jr, Clemente CG, Cascinelli N (1996) Tumor infiltrating lymphocytes in lymph node melanoma metastases: a histopathologic prognostic indicator and an expression of local immune response. Lab Invest 74:43–47
7. Zhang L, Conejo-Garcia JR, Katsaros D, Gimotty PA, Massobrio M, Regnani G, Makrigiannakis A, Gray H, Schlienger K, Liebman MN, Rubin SC, Coukos G (2003) Intratumoral T cells, recurrence, and survival in epithelial ovarian cancer. N Engl J Med 348:203–213
8. Pages F, Berger A, Camus M, Sanchez-Cabo F, Costes A, Molidor R, Mlecnik B, Kirilovsky A, Nilsson M, Damotte D, Meatchi T, Bruneval P, Cugnenc PH, Trajanoski Z, Fridman WH, Galon J (2005) Effector memory T cells, early metastasis, and survival in colorectal cancer. N Engl J Med 353: 2654–2666
9. Hersey P, Bindon C, Edwards A, Murray E, Phillips G, McCarthy WH (1981) Induction of cytotoxic activity in human lymphocytes against autologous and allogeneic melanoma cells in vitro by culture with interleukin 2. Int J Cancer 28:695–703
10. Grimm EA, Mazumder A, Zhang HZ, Rosenberg SA (1982) Lymphokine-activated killer cell phenomenon. Lysis of natural killer-resistant fresh solid tumor cells by interleukin 2-activated autologous human peripheral blood lymphocytes. J Exp Med 155: 1823–1841
11. Muul LM, Spiess PJ, Director EP, Rosenberg SA (1987) Identification of specific cytolytic immune responses against autologous tumor

in humans bearing malignant melanoma. J Immunol 138:989–995

12. Ferradini L, Mackensen A, Genevee C, Bosq J, Duvillard P, Avril MF, Hercend T (1993) Analysis of T cell receptor variability in tumor-infiltrating lymphocytes from a human regressive melanoma. Evidence for in situ T cell clonal expansion. J Clin Invest 91:1183–1190
13. Bulkley GB, Cohen MH, Banks PM, Char DH, Ketcham AS (1975) Long-term spontaneous regression of malignant melanoma with visceral metastases. Report of a case with immunologic profile. Cancer 36:485–494
14. Rosenberg SA, Packard BS, Aebersold PM, Solomon D, Topalian SL, Toy ST, Simon P, Lotze MT, Yang JC, Seipp CA et al (1988) Use of tumor-infiltrating lymphocytes and interleukin-2 in the immunotherapy of patients with metastatic melanoma. A preliminary report. N Engl J Med 319:1676–1680
15. Taylor RC, Patel A, Panageas KS, Busam KJ, Brady MS (2007) Tumor-infiltrating lymphocytes predict sentinel lymph node positivity in patients with cutaneous melanoma. J Clin Oncol 25:869–875
16. Thorn M, Ponten F, Bergstrom R, Sparen P, Adami HO (1994) Clinical and histopathologic predictors of survival in patients with malignant melanoma: a population-based study in Sweden. J Natl Cancer Inst 86:761–769
17. Burnet M (1957) Cancer; a biological approach. I. The processes of control. Br Med J 1:779–786
18. Mapara MY, Sykes M (2004) Tolerance and cancer: mechanisms of tumor evasion and strategies for breaking tolerance. J Clin Oncol 22:1136–1151
19. Rosenberg SA (1999) A new era for cancer immunotherapy based on the genes that encode cancer antigens. Immunity 10: 281–287
20. Pandolfi F, Boyle LA, Trentin L, Kurnick JT, Isselbacher KJ, Gattoni-Celli S (1991) Expression of HLA-A2 antigen in human melanoma cell lines and its role in T-cell recognition. Cancer Res 51:3164–3170
21. Kalialis LV, Drzewiecki KT, Klyver H (2009) Spontaneous regression of metastases from melanoma: review of the literature. Melanoma Res 19:275–282
22. Atkins MB, Lotze MT, Dutcher JP, Fisher RI, Weiss G, Margolin K, Abrams J, Sznol M, Parkinson D, Hawkins M, Paradise C, Kunkel L, Rosenberg SA (1999) High-dose recombinant interleukin 2 therapy for patients with metastatic melanoma: analysis of 270 patients treated between 1985 and 1993. J Clin Oncol 17:2105–2116
23. Schwartzentruber DJ, Lawson DH, Richards JM, Conry RM, Miller DM, Treisman J, Gailani F, Riley L, Conlon K, Pockaj B, Kendra KL, White RL, Gonzalez R, Kuzel TM, Curti B, Leming PD, Whitman ED, Balkissoon J, Reintgen DS, Kaufman H, Marincola FM, Merino MJ, Rosenberg SA, Choyke P, Vena D, Hwu P (2011) gp100 peptide vaccine and interleukin-2 in patients with advanced melanoma. N Engl J Med 364:2119–2127
24. Hogquist KA, Baldwin TA, Jameson SC (2005) Central tolerance: learning self-control in the thymus. Nat Rev Immunol 5:772–782
25. Wang Z, Seliger B, Mike N, Momburg F, Knuth A, Ferrone S (1998) Molecular analysis of the HLA-A2 antigen loss by melanoma cells SK-MEL-29.1.22 and SK-MEL-29.1.29. Cancer Res 58:2149–2157
26. Schatton T, Schutte U, Frank NY, Zhan Q, Hoerning A, Robles SC, Zhou J, Hodi FS, Spagnoli GC, Murphy GF, Frank MH (2010) Modulation of T-cell activation by malignant melanoma initiating cells. Cancer Res 70: 697–708
27. Boiko AD, Razorenova OV, van de Rijn M, Swetter SM, Johnson DL, Ly DP, Butler PD, Yang GP, Joshua B, Kaplan MJ, Longaker MT, Weissman IL (2010) Human melanoma-initiating cells express neural crest nerve growth factor receptor CD271. Nature 466:133–137
28. Kurnick JT, Ramirez-Montagut T, Boyle LA, Andrews DM, Pandolfi F, Durda PJ, Butera D, Dunn IS, Benson EM, Gobin SJ, van den Elsen PJ (2001) A novel autocrine pathway of tumor escape from immune recognition: melanoma cell lines produce a soluble protein that diminishes expression of the gene encoding the melanocyte lineage melan-A/MART-1 antigen through down-modulation of its promoter. J Immunol 167:1204–1211
29. Khong HT, Wang QJ, Rosenberg SA (2004) Identification of multiple antigens recognized by tumor-infiltrating lymphocytes from a single patient: tumor escape by antigen loss and loss of MHC expression. J Immunother 27:184–190
30. Maeurer MJ, Gollin SM, Martin D, Swaney W, Bryant J, Castelli C, Robbins P, Parmiani G, Storkus WJ, Lotze MT (1996) Tumor escape from immune recognition: lethal recurrent melanoma in a patient associated with downregulation of the peptide transporter protein TAP-1 and loss of expression of the immunodominant MART-1/Melan-A antigen. J Clin Invest 98:1633–1641
31. van Houdt IS, Sluijter BJ, Moesbergen LM, Vos WM, de Gruijl TD, Molenkamp BG, van

den Eertwegh AJ, Hooijberg E, van Leeuwen PA, Meijer CJ, Oudejans JJ (2008) Favorable outcome in clinically stage II melanoma patients is associated with the presence of activated tumor infiltrating T-lymphocytes and preserved MHC class I antigen expression. Int J Cancer 123:609–615
32. Moretta A (2002) Natural killer cells and dendritic cells: rendezvous in abused tissues. Nat Rev Immunol 2:957–964
33. Bauer S, Groh V, Wu J, Steinle A, Phillips JH, Lanier LL, Spies T (1999) Activation of NK cells and T cells by NKG2D, a receptor for stress-inducible MICA. Science 285: 727–729
34. Solana R, Casado JG, Delgado E, DelaRosa O, Marin J, Duran E, Pawelec G, Tarazona R (2007) Lymphocyte activation in response to melanoma: interaction of NK-associated receptors and their ligands. Cancer Immunol Immunother 56:101–109
35. Strand S, Hofmann WJ, Hug H, Muller M, Otto G, Strand D, Mariani SM, Stremmel W, Krammer PH, Galle PR (1996) Lymphocyte apoptosis induced by CD95 (APO-1/Fas) ligand-expressing tumor cells–a mechanism of immune evasion? Nat Med 2:1361–1366
36. Hahne M, Rimoldi D, Schroter M, Romero P, Schreier M, French LE, Schneider P, Bornand T, Fontana A, Lienard D, Cerottini J, Tschopp J (1996) Melanoma cell expression of Fas(Apo-1/CD95) ligand: implications for tumor immune escape. Science 274: 1363–1366
37. Neuber K, Eidam B (2006) Expression of Fas ligand (CD95L) in primary malignant melanoma and melanoma metastases is associated with overall survival. Onkologie 29:361–365
38. Dong H, Strome SE, Salomao DR, Tamura H, Hirano F, Flies DB, Roche PC, Lu J, Zhu G, Tamada K, Lennon VA, Celis E, Chen L (2002) Tumor-associated B7-H1 promotes T-cell apoptosis: a potential mechanism of immune evasion. Nat Med 8:793–800
39. Taube JM, Anders RA, Young GD, Xu H, Sharma R, McMiller TL, Chen S, Klein AP, Pardoll DM, Topalian SL, Chen L (2012) Colocalization of inflammatory response with B7-h1 expression in human melanocytic lesions supports an adaptive resistance mechanism of immune escape. Sci Transl Med 4:127ra137
40. Gorelik L, Flavell RA (2001) Immune-mediated eradication of tumors through the blockade of transforming growth factor-beta signaling in T cells. Nat Med 7:1118–1122
41. Nicolaou A, Estdale SE, Tsatmali M, Herrero DP, Thody AJ (2004) Prostaglandin production by melanocytic cells and the effect of alpha-melanocyte stimulating hormone. FEBS Lett 570:223–226
42. Frauwirth KA, Thompson CB (2002) Activation and inhibition of lymphocytes by costimulation. J Clin Invest 109:295–299
43. Greenwald RJ, Freeman GJ, Sharpe AH (2005) The B7 family revisited. Annu Rev Immunol 23:515–548
44. Pardoll DM (2012) The blockade of immune checkpoints in cancer immunotherapy. Nat Rev Cancer 12:252–264
45. Sotomayor EM, Borrello I, Rattis FM, Cuenca AG, Abrams J, Staveley-O'Carroll K, Levitsky HI (2001) Cross-presentation of tumor antigens by bone marrow-derived antigen-presenting cells is the dominant mechanism in the induction of T-cell tolerance during B-cell lymphoma progression. Blood 98:1070–1077
46. Sotomayor EM, Borrello I, Tubb E, Rattis FM, Bien H, Lu Z, Fein S, Schoenberger S, Levitsky HI (1999) Conversion of tumor-specific CD4+ T-cell tolerance to T-cell priming through in vivo ligation of CD40. Nat Med 5:780–787
47. Guerry DT, Alexander MA, Herlyn MF, Zehngebot LM, Mitchell KF, Zmijewski CM, Lusk EJ (1984) HLA-DR histocompatibility leukocyte antigens permit cultured human melanoma cells from early but not advanced disease to stimulate autologous lymphocytes. J Clin Invest 73:267–271
48. Bai Y, Liu J, Wang Y, Honig S, Qin L, Boros P, Bromberg JS (2002) L-selectin-dependent lymphoid occupancy is required to induce alloantigen-specific tolerance. J Immunol 168:1579–1589
49. Becker JC, Brabletz T, Czerny C, Termeer C, Brocker EB (1993) Tumor escape mechanisms from immunosurveillance: induction of unresponsiveness in a specific MHC-restricted CD4+ human T cell clone by the autologous MHC class II+ melanoma. Int Immunol 5:1501–1508
50. Brocker EB, Suter L, Sorg C (1984) HLA-DR antigen expression in primary melanomas of the skin. J Invest Dermatol 82:244–247
51. Hirano F, Kaneko K, Tamura H, Dong H, Wang S, Ichikawa M, Rietz C, Flies DB, Lau JS, Zhu G, Tamada K, Chen L (2005) Blockade of B7-H1 and PD-1 by monoclonal antibodies potentiates cancer therapeutic immunity. Cancer Res 65:1089–1096
52. Brahmer JR, Tykodi SS, Chow LQ, Hwu WJ, Topalian SL, Hwu P, Drake CG, Camacho LH, Kauh J, Odunsi K, Pitot HC, Hamid O, Bhatia S, Martins R, Eaton K, Chen S, Salay

TM, Alaparthy S, Grosso JF, Korman AJ, Parker SM, Agrawal S, Goldberg SM, Pardoll DM, Gupta A, Wigginton JM (2012) Safety and activity of anti-PD-L1 antibody in patients with advanced cancer. N Engl J Med 366:2455–2465

53. Rygiel TP, Meyaard L (2012) CD200R signaling in tumor tolerance and inflammation: a tricky balance. Curr Opin Immunol 24:233–238
54. Jaiswal S, Chao MP, Majeti R, Weissman IL (2010) Macrophages as mediators of tumor immunosurveillance. Trends Immunol 31:212–219
55. Wherry EJ (2011) T cell exhaustion. Nat Immunol 12:492–499
56. Baitsch L, Baumgaertner P, Devevre E, Raghav SK, Legat A, Barba L, Wieckowski S, Bouzourene H, Deplancke B, Romero P, Rufer N, Speiser DE (2011) Exhaustion of tumor-specific CD8(+) T cells in metastases from melanoma patients. J Clin Invest 121:2350–2360
57. Fourcade J, Sun Z, Benallaoua M, Guillaume P, Luescher IF, Sander C, Kirkwood JM, Kuchroo V, Zarour HM (2010) Upregulation of Tim-3 and PD-1 expression is associated with tumor antigen-specific CD8+ T cell dysfunction in melanoma patients. J Exp Med 207:2175–2186
58. Topalian SL, Hodi FS, Brahmer JR, Gettinger SN, Smith DC, McDermott DF, Powderly JD, Carvajal RD, Sosman JA, Atkins MB, Leming PD, Spigel DR, Antonia SJ, Horn L, Drake CG, Pardoll DM, Chen L, Sharfman WH, Anders RA, Taube JM, McMiller TL, Xu H, Korman AJ, Jure-Kunkel M, Agrawal S, McDonald D, Kollia GD, Gupta A, Wigginton JM, Sznol M (2012) Safety, activity, and immune correlates of anti-PD-1 antibody in cancer. N Engl J Med 366:2443–2454
59. Hodi FS, O'Day SJ, McDermott DF, Weber RW, Sosman JA, Haanen JB, Gonzalez R, Robert C, Schadendorf D, Hassel JC, Akerley W, van den Eertwegh AJ, Lutzky J, Lorigan P, Vaubel JM, Linette GP, Hogg D, Ottensmeier CH, Lebbe C, Peschel C, Quirt I, Clark JI, Wolchok JD, Weber JS, Tian J, Yellin MJ, Nichol GM, Hoos A, Urba WJ (2010) Improved survival with ipilimumab in patients with metastatic melanoma. N Engl J Med 363:711–723
60. Jacobs JF, Nierkens S, Figdor CG, de Vries IJ, Adema GJ (2012) Regulatory T cells in melanoma: the final hurdle towards effective immunotherapy? Lancet Oncol 13:e32–e42
61. Wing K, Onishi Y, Prieto-Martin P, Yamaguchi T, Miyara M, Fehervari Z, Nomura T, Sakaguchi S (2008) CTLA-4 control over Foxp3+ regulatory T cell function. Science 322:271–275
62. Jandus C, Bioley G, Speiser DE, Romero P (2008) Selective accumulation of differentiated FOXP3(+) CD4 (+) T cells in metastatic tumor lesions from melanoma patients compared to peripheral blood. Cancer Immunol Immunother 57:1795–1805
63. Vence L, Palucka AK, Fay JW, Ito T, Liu YJ, Banchereau J, Ueno H (2007) Circulating tumor antigen-specific regulatory T cells in patients with metastatic melanoma. Proc Natl Acad Sci U S A 104:20884–20889
64. Larsen TE, Grude TH (1978) A retrospective histological study of 669 cases of primary cutaneous malignant melanoma in clinical stage I. 3. The relation between the tumour-associated lymphocyte infiltration and age and sex, tumour cell type, pigmentation, cellular atypia, mitotic count, depth of invasion, ulceration, tumour type and prognosis. Acta Pathol Microbiol Scand A 86A:523–530
65. Day CL Jr, Sober AJ, Kopf AW, Lew RA, Mihm MC Jr, Hennessey P, Golomb FM, Harris MN, Gumport SL, Raker JW, Malt RA, Cosimi AB, Wood WC, Roses DF, Gorstein F, Postel A, Grier WR, Mintzis MN, Fitzpatrick TB (1981) A prognostic model for clinical stage I melanoma of the upper extremity. The importance of anatomic subsites in predicting recurrent disease. Ann Surg 193:436–440
66. Busam KJ, Antonescu CR, Marghoob AA, Nehal KS, Sachs DL, Shia J, Berwick M (2001) Histologic classification of tumor-infiltrating lymphocytes in primary cutaneous malignant melanoma. A study of interobserver agreement. Am J Clin Pathol 115: 856–860
67. Rao UN, Lee SJ, Luo W, Mihm MC Jr, Kirkwood JM (2010) Presence of tumor-infiltrating lymphocytes and a dominant nodule within primary melanoma are prognostic factors for relapse-free survival of patients with thick (t4) primary melanoma: pathologic analysis of the e1690 and e1694 intergroup trials. Am J Clin Pathol 133:646–653
68. Azimi F, Scolyer RA, Rumcheva P, Moncrieff M, Murali R, McCarthy SW, Saw RP, Thompson JF (2012) Tumor-infiltrating lymphocyte grade is an independent predictor of sentinel lymph node status and survival in patients with cutaneous melanoma. J Clin Oncol 30:2678–2683
69. Balch CM, Soong SJ, Gershenwald JE, Thompson JF, Reintgen DS, Cascinelli N, Urist M, McMasters KM, Ross MI, Kirkwood

JM, Atkins MB, Thompson JA, Coit DG, Byrd D, Desmond R, Zhang Y, Liu PY, Lyman GH, Morabito A (2001) Prognostic factors analysis of 17,600 melanoma patients: validation of the American Joint Committee on Cancer melanoma staging system. J Clin Oncol 19:3622–3634

70. Balch CM, Soong SJ, Smith T, Ross MI, Urist MM, Karakousis CP, Temple WJ, Mihm MC, Barnhill RL, Jewell WR, Wanebo HJ, Desmond R (2001) Long-term results of a prospective surgical trial comparing 2 cm vs. 4 cm excision margins for 740 patients with 1–4 mm melanomas. Ann Surg Oncol 8:101–108
71. Azzola MF, Shaw HM, Thompson JF, Soong SJ, Scolyer RA, Watson GF, Colman MH, Zhang Y (2003) Tumor mitotic rate is a more powerful prognostic indicator than ulceration in patients with primary cutaneous melanoma: an analysis of 3661 patients from a single center. Cancer 97:1488–1498
72. Francken AB, Shaw HM, Thompson JF, Soong SJ, Accortt NA, Azzola MF, Scolyer RA, Milton GW, McCarthy WH, Colman MH, McGovern VJ (2004) The prognostic importance of tumor mitotic rate confirmed in 1317 patients with primary cutaneous melanoma and long follow-up. Ann Surg Oncol 11:426–433
73. Balch CM, Gershenwald JE, Soong SJ, Thompson JF, Atkins MB, Byrd DR, Buzaid AC, Cochran AJ, Coit DG, Ding S, Eggermont AM, Flaherty KT, Gimotty PA, Kirkwood JM, McMasters KM, Mihm MC Jr, Morton DL, Ross MI, Sober AJ, Sondak VK (2009) Final version of 2009 AJCC melanoma staging and classification. J Clin Oncol 27:6199–6206
74. Morton DL, Thompson JF, Cochran AJ, Mozzillo N, Elashoff R, Essner R, Nieweg OE, Roses DF, Hoekstra HJ, Karakousis CP, Reintgen DS, Coventry BJ, Glass EC, Wang HJ (2006) Sentinel-node biopsy or nodal observation in melanoma. N Engl J Med 355:1307–1317
75. Tuthill RJ, Unger JM, Liu PY, Flaherty LE, Sondak VK (2002) Risk assessment in localized primary cutaneous melanoma: a Southwest Oncology Group study evaluating nine factors and a test of the Clark logistic regression prediction model. Am J Clin Pathol 118:504–511
76. Gimotty PA, Van Belle P, Elder DE, Murry T, Montone KT, Xu X, Hotz S, Raines S, Ming ME, Wahl P, Guerry D (2005) Biologic and prognostic significance of dermal Ki67 expression, mitoses, and tumorigenicity in thin invasive cutaneous melanoma. J Clin Oncol 23:8048–8056
77. Barnhill RL, Fine JA, Roush GC, Berwick M (1996) Predicting five-year outcome for patients with cutaneous melanoma in a population-based study. Cancer 78:427–432
78. Gimotty PA, Guerry D, Ming ME, Elenitsas R, Xu X, Czerniecki B, Spitz F, Schuchter L, Elder D (2004) Thin primary cutaneous malignant melanoma: a prognostic tree for 10-year metastasis is more accurate than American Joint Committee on Cancer staging. J Clin Oncol 22:3668–3676
79. Mansson-Brahme E, Carstensen J, Erhardt K, Lagerlof B, Ringborg U, Rutqvist LE (1994) Prognostic factors in thin cutaneous malignant melanoma. Cancer 73:2324–2332
80. Kruper LL, Spitz FR, Czerniecki BJ, Fraker DL, Blackwood-Chirchir A, Ming ME, Elder DE, Elenitsas R, Guerry D, Gimotty PA (2006) Predicting sentinel node status in AJCC stage I/II primary cutaneous melanoma. Cancer 107:2436–2445
81. Mandala M, Imberti GL, Piazzalunga D, Belfiglio M, Labianca R, Barberis M, Marchesi L, Poletti P, Bonomi L, Novellino L, Di Biagio K, Milesi A, Guerra U, Tondini C (2009) Clinical and histopathological risk factors to predict sentinel lymph node positivity, disease-free and overall survival in clinical stages I-II AJCC skin melanoma: outcome analysis from a single-institution prospectively collected database. Eur J Cancer 45:2537–2545
82. Burton AL, Roach BA, Mays MP, Chen AF, Ginter BA, Vierling AM, Scoggins CR, Martin RC, Stromberg AJ, Hagendoorn L, McMasters KM (2011) Prognostic significance of tumor infiltrating lymphocytes in melanoma. Am Surg 77:188–192
83. Mraz-Gernhard S, Sagebiel RW, Kashani-Sabet M, Miller JR 3rd, Leong SP (1998) Prediction of sentinel lymph node micrometastasis by histological features in primary cutaneous malignant melanoma. Arch Dermatol 134:983–987
84. Wong SL, Brady MS, Busam KJ, Coit DG (2006) Results of sentinel lymph node biopsy in patients with thin melanoma. Ann Surg Oncol 13:302–309
85. Karim RZ, van den Berg KS, Colman MH, McCarthy SW, Thompson JF, Scolyer RA (2008) The advantage of using a synoptic pathology report format for cutaneous melanoma. Histopathology 52:130–138
86. Cochran AJ, Huang RR, Lee J, Itakura E, Leong SP, Essner R (2006) Tumour-induced immune modulation of sentinel lymph nodes. Nat Rev Immunol 6:659–670

87. Clemente C, Rao S, Lupetti R, Tragni G, Pisarra P, Bersani I, Parmiani G, Mihm MC Jr, Sensi M (1998) Immunohistochemical analysis of the T-cell receptor beta-chain variable regions expressed by T lymphocytes infiltrating primary human melanoma. Lab Invest 78:619–627
88. Howard CJ, Hope JC (2000) Dendritic cells, implications on function from studies of the afferent lymph veiled cell. Vet Immunol Immunopathol 77:1–13
89. Grotz TE, Mansfield AS, Jakub JW, Markovic SN (2012) Regional lymphatic immunity in melanoma. Melanoma Res 22:9–18
90. Shi C, Pamer EG (2011) Monocyte recruitment during infection and inflammation. Nat Rev Immunol 11:762–774
91. Munn DH, Mellor AL (2007) Indoleamine 2,3-dioxygenase and tumor-induced tolerance. J Clin Invest 117:1147–1154
92. Lee JH, Torisu-Itakara H, Cochran AJ, Kadison A, Huynh Y, Morton DL, Essner R (2005) Quantitative analysis of melanoma-induced cytokine-mediated immunosuppression in melanoma sentinel nodes. Clin Cancer Res 11:107–112
93. Battaglia A, Buzzonetti A, Baranello C, Ferrandina G, Martinelli E, Fanfani F, Scambia G, Fattorossi A (2009) Metastatic tumour cells favour the generation of a tolerogenic milieu in tumour draining lymph node in patients with early cervical cancer. Cancer Immunol Immunother 58:1363–1373
94. Dranoff G, Soiffer R, Lynch T, Mihm M, Jung K, Kolesar K, Liebster L, Lam P, Duda R, Mentzer S, Singer S, Tanabe K, Johnson R, Sober A, Bhan A, Clift S, Cohen L, Parry G, Rokovich J, Richards L, Drayer J, Berns A, Mulligan RC (1997) A phase I study of vaccination with autologous, irradiated melanoma cells engineered to secrete human granulocyte-macrophage colony stimulating factor. Hum Gene Ther 8:111–123
95. Soiffer R, Lynch T, Mihm M, Jung K, Rhuda C, Schmollinger JC, Hodi FS, Liebster L, Lam P, Mentzer S, Singer S, Tanabe KK, Cosimi AB, Duda R, Sober A, Bhan A, Daley J, Neuberg D, Parry G, Rokovich J, Richards L, Drayer J, Berns A, Clift S, Cohen LK, Mulligan RC, Dranoff G (1998) Vaccination with irradiated autologous melanoma cells engineered to secrete human granulocyte-macrophage colony-stimulating factor generates potent antitumor immunity in patients with metastatic melanoma. Proc Natl Acad Sci U S A 95:13141–13146
96. Vuylsteke RJ, Molenkamp BG, Gietema HA, van Leeuwen PA, Wijnands PG, Vos W, van Diest PJ, Scheper RJ, Meijer S, de Gruijl TD (2004) Local administration of granulocyte/macrophage colony-stimulating factor increases the number and activation state of dendritic cells in the sentinel lymph node of early-stage melanoma. Cancer Res 64:8456–8460
97. Restifo NP, Dudley ME, Rosenberg SA (2012) Adoptive immunotherapy for cancer: harnessing the T cell response. Nat Rev Immunol 12:269–281
98. Itoh K, Tilden AB, Balch CM (1986) Interleukin 2 activation of cytotoxic T-lymphocytes infiltrating into human metastatic melanomas. Cancer Res 46:3011–3017
99. Rubin JT, Elwood LJ, Rosenberg SA, Lotze MT (1989) Immunohistochemical correlates of response to recombinant interleukin-2-based immunotherapy in humans. Cancer Res 49:7086–7092
100. Ahmadzadeh M, Rosenberg SA (2006) IL-2 administration increases CD4+ CD25(hi) Foxp3+ regulatory T cells in cancer patients. Blood 107:2409–2414
101. Dannull J, Su Z, Rizzieri D, Yang BK, Coleman D, Yancey D, Zhang A, Dahm P, Chao N, Gilboa E, Vieweg J (2005) Enhancement of vaccine-mediated antitumor immunity in cancer patients after depletion of regulatory T cells. J Clin Invest 115:3623–3633
102. Attia P, Maker AV, Haworth LR, Rogers-Freezer L, Rosenberg SA (2005) Inability of a fusion protein of IL-2 and diphtheria toxin (Denileukin Diftitox, DAB389IL-2, ONTAK) to eliminate regulatory T lymphocytes in patients with melanoma. J Immunother 28:582–592
103. Powell DJ Jr, de Vries CR, Allen T, Ahmadzadeh M, Rosenberg SA (2007) Inability to mediate prolonged reduction of regulatory T cells after transfer of autologous CD25-depleted PBMC and interleukin-2 after lymphodepleting chemotherapy. J Immunother 30:438–447
104. Tarhini AA, Cherian J, Moschos SJ, Tawbi HA, Shuai Y, Gooding WE, Sander C, Kirkwood JM (2012) Safety and efficacy of combination immunotherapy with interferon alfa-2b and tremelimumab in patients with stage IV melanoma. J Clin Oncol 30:322–328
105. Moschos SJ, Edington HD, Land SR, Rao UN, Jukic D, Shipe-Spotloe J, Kirkwood JM (2006) Neoadjuvant treatment of regional stage IIIB melanoma with high-dose interferon alfa-2b induces objective tumor regression in association with modulation of tumor infiltrating host cellular immune responses. J Clin Oncol 24:3164–3171

106. Petrella TM, Tozer R, Belanger K, Savage J, Wong R, Smylie M, Kamel-Reid S, Tron V, Chen BE, Hunder NN, Hagerman L, Walsh W, Eisenhauer EA (2012) Interleukin-21 has activity in patients with metastatic melanoma: a phase II study. J Clin Oncol 30: 3396–3401
107. Leach DR, Krummel MF, Allison JP (1996) Enhancement of antitumor immunity by CTLA-4 blockade. Science 271:1734–1736
108. Hodi FS, Butler M, Oble DA, Seiden MV, Haluska FG, Kruse A, Macrae S, Nelson M, Canning C, Lowy I, Korman A, Lautz D, Russell S, Jaklitsch MT, Ramaiya N, Chen TC, Neuberg D, Allison JP, Mihm MC, Dranoff G (2008) Immunologic and clinical effects of antibody blockade of cytotoxic T lymphocyte-associated antigen 4 in previously vaccinated cancer patients. Proc Natl Acad Sci U S A 105:3005–3010
109. Ribas A (2012) Tumor immunotherapy directed at PD-1. N Engl J Med 366: 2517–2519
110. Hong M, Puaux AL, Huang C, Loumagne L, Tow C, Mackay C, Kato M, Prevost-Blondel A, Avril MF, Nardin A, Abastado JP (2011) Chemotherapy induces intratumoral expression of chemokines in cutaneous melanoma, favoring T-cell infiltration and tumor control. Cancer Res 71:6997–7009

Chapter 17

Pathological Staging of Melanoma

David E. Elder

Abstract

Staging of cancer is a shorthand system of describing the extent of disease. Pathological staging, often called microstaging, uses the methods of histopathology to achieve this goal. Microstaging for melanoma utilizes attributes that are associated with outcome, generally in association with prognostic models that allow for estimation of survival rates, based on large groups of patients with similar tumors. Microstaging can be performed on primary tumors and to a lesser extent on metastases. Attributes that are important in microstaging in primary tumors include, in particular, those that are utilized in the AJCC/UICC staging system. These are, more or less in order of importance, Breslow's thickness, ulceration, and mitogenicity (the presence or absence of mitoses). Other attributes that have relevance to prognosis at least in some well-conducted studies include tumor-infiltrating lymphocytes, lymphovascular invasion, perineural invasion, Clark's level of invasion, the presence or absence of vertical growth phase and of regression, and other attributes. The pathologic interpretation and significance of these "prognostic variables" are discussed in this chapter. In addition, prognostic models including the AJCC staging system are presented in some detail.

Key words Melanoma, Staging, Microstaging, AJCC, Prognosis

1 Introduction

Staging of cancer typically includes three major categories of disease: (a) tumor localized to the primary site (T), (b) having regional lymph node metastasis (N), and (c) with distant metastasis (M). Staging systems categorize patients into groups whose prognosis differs significantly from one another, and are of clinical value when treatment also differs among the groups. Staging systems empirically test the hypothesis that the selected staging categories define populations of patients that differ with respect to survival. The American Joint Commission on Cancer and the Union Internationale Contra Cancer (AJCC/UICC) TNM system for melanoma prognosis and staging is presented later in this review and represents the standard of care for melanoma management [1]. The system includes pathologic staging utilizing microscopic attributes of primary tumors, which may be termed "microstaging," and also clinical staging, for example, by palpation of lymph nodes,

Magdalena Thurin and Francesco M. Marincola (eds.), *Molecular Diagnostics for Melanoma: Methods and Protocols*, Methods in Molecular Biology, vol. 1102, DOI 10.1007/978-1-62703-727-3_17,

as well as imaging and laboratory studies. Other prognostic models are available in the literature and may be useful for decision making in particular situations. This review is based extensively on a summary of staging attributes published recently in the Armed Forces Institute of Pathology Fascicle on Melanocytic Tumors of the Skin [2].

Prognostic models may be rather accurately predictive when applied to large groups of cases, but should be used with caution in prognosticating for individual patients. Microstaging of primary tumors by standard techniques may retain some predictive power when applied to patients with regional nodal metastases. However, microstaging is most effective when applied to patients with localized tumors in whom the clinically apparent disease is confined to the local site. A proportion of these cases will have occult nodal metastases. Indeed, an important current use of microstaging is to predict the likelihood that nodal metastases are present, information which is used in planning for regional lymphadenectomy and adjuvant therapy [3, 4].

Staging and microstaging predict survival through the use of clinical and histologic "prognostic variables" (or "prognostic attributes"). A prognostic variable is an attribute of a primary melanoma that has been statistically associated with survival. Most of the known survival associations have been determined empirically, and the discovery of such associations can suggest relationships of biological interest. For example, the favorable survival association of an attribute such as an infiltrative lymphocytic response at the base of the vertical growth phase [5] suggests that there is an effective host resistance to the tumor.

The variables that are of prognostic value are determined histologically or clinically and are entered in a database for correlation with survival. The precision of microstaging depends on the number and power of variables that are considered simultaneously, though a few of these, such as tumor thickness, are sufficiently powerful predictors of survival that it may be sufficient to consider them as single variables for some routine clinical purposes. The application of multivariate analysis to melanoma databases was an important advance in the development of a sophisticated microstaging process [6]. Multivariate analysis considers a given putative prognostic variable in relation to other variables to determine whether its relationship with survival is "independent." An independent prognostic variable adds explanatory power to the survival function in the presence of other known independent variables. Variables found in a multivariate analysis to be "dependent" may derive their association with survival from correlations with other variables, and in part for this reason, the exact variables that enter any given prognostic model differ slightly from one database to another. For example, levels of invasion, ulceration, the location of the lesion, and the sex of the patient are all predictive of survival as single variables, but each of these factors has been found to be dependent in some but not all of the published prognostic models. This fact should not, however, lead to the conclusion that any of these properties is necessarily irrelevant to survival. Because the results of analyses in different databases often differ appreciably, putative prognostic associations should ideally be confirmed by another analytic method, and in another database. Several models have been described for melanoma that meet at least some of these requirements, and these models are tools for categorizing patients according to expected survival. This categorization has value in clinical decision-making, and is of particular importance in the stratification of clinical trials.

Issues relating to melanoma staging and microstaging have been reviewed by Gershenwald et al. [7]. A protocol for the examination of specimens from patients with melanoma of the skin has been developed by the College of American Pathologists, and includes detailed definitions of terms and a template for structured reporting [8]. Some of the areas that have been or continue to be at issue include the relevance of level of invasion versus tumor thickness, optimal cutoffs for tumor thickness, importance of ulceration, the grouping of satellites with in-transit metastases, the inclusion of microsatellites and local recurrences as a separate staging criterion, the replacement of size of nodal mass with number of positive nodes, the importance of nodal metastases in more than one nodal basin, the significance of minimal nodal disease, and the prognostic significance of categories of distant metastases. Issues relating to staging of primary tumors and their locoregional metastases are discussed in sections following.

The current global standard for staging of melanoma, as other cancers, is the AJCC/UICC system, which is based on the TNM methodology of assessing the primary Tumor, the regional lymph Nodes, and regional and distant Metastases. The latest (2009) edition of this staging system will be discussed in detail at the end of this essay [9]. First, attributes of potential use in staging and microstaging will be discussed, in some cases for their historical and explanatory value.

2 Microstaging Attributes (Pathologic and Clinical)

2.1 Phase of Tumor Progression

Melanomas have been categorized into two "phases" of progression, namely the vertical growth phase or tumorigenic melanoma, in which a mass lesion is formed, and the radial growth phase, in which these is a patch or a plaque, but no mass. As discussed above, metastasis is very rare in melanomas that are confined to the radial growth phase, i.e., nontumorigenic melanomas, implying that tumorigenicity is important in the development of clinically evident metastases. In two studies from the prospectively accrued database of the University of Pennsylvania's Pigmented Lesion Clinic, there were no deaths from melanoma in these nontumorigenic melanomas, in which the survival was estimated at 100 ± 1 % [10, 11]. However, our extended experience and that of others has demonstrated a low but definite mortality rate in these cases of the order of 1–2 %. In a population-based study, the survival of patients with vertical growth phase was 84 %, compared to 98.2 % when vertical growth phase was absent (nontumorigenic or microinvasive melanomas) [12]. The rare examples of metastasizing nontumorigenic cases may reflect sampling error of small primaries, where a small vertical growth phase could be missed even after multiple sectioning. It is also theoretically possible that a small group of cells, or even a single cell, might in rare instances have metastasized without leaving a residual trace at the primary site. However, most of these lesions in our experience have either had mitotic activity in the dermis (nontumorigenic but mitogenic melanomas), or have been cases of largely or completely regressed melanomas. Some of these lesions have been found in the region of lymph nodes containing metastatic tumor or have been associated with distant metastases, suggesting that the primary tumor may have regressed after the metastatic event. All of these occurrences are rare indeed. When mitogenicity is included, tumorigenicity loses its independent prognostic significance in most but not all datasets.

2.2 Clark's Levels of Invasion

Described by Clark in 1967, the characterization of melanomas into five levels of invasion was the first widely accepted microstaging method for malignant melanoma [13]. The levels of invasion define a stepwise progression of biological properties that are associated with increasingly aggressive behavior of melanoma cells. An understanding of levels of invasion is of descriptive value in the concept of tumor progression in melanomas. The levels of invasion were defined as follows: Level I: melanoma cells are confined to the epidermis (in situ melanoma). The major acquired property that distinguishes level I cells from normal melanocytes is their propensity for apparently inexorable growth, but these cells lack the ability to traverse the basement membrane and are therefore limited to the normal micro-environment of melanocytes, the epidermis, albeit often with "pagetoid" escape upward from the dermal-epidermal junction. In level II invasion, melanoma cells extend from the epidermis into the papillary dermis, but the papillary dermis is not filled or expanded. The biologic property that distinguishes most level II melanomas from level I is their ability to traverse the basement membrane and invade the dermis. However, the cells are nontumorigenic in most cases, suggesting that they have the capacity to invade and survive in the papillary dermis, but not to proliferate there. Level III invasion, in contrast, represents a true tumor in the vast majority of cases, in the old sense of the term as a swelling or a mass. The lesional cells have the capacity to survive and also to proliferate in the papillary dermis, forming a vertical growth phase nodule that fills and expands the papillary dermis. This ability to form an expansile tumor nodule appears to represent a qualitatively new property acquired by the evolving neoplastic cells. Level IV invasion constitutes infiltration of tumor cells among reticular dermis collagen fibers. Since the papillary dermis represents a micro-environment that is specialized to support epithelium, i.e., the normal epidermis and adnexa), while the "leathery" reticular dermis is less hospitable, the progression to level IV invasion perhaps reflects properties of the melanoma cells that are of significance in terms of tissue infiltration and invasion, and thus of the potential for metastasis. For example, the cells might have acquired receptors or growth factors that alter their relationships with their stroma. Level V invasion represents infiltration of tumor cells from the reticular dermis into the subcutaneous fat. This may be the only stage in the hierarchy of levels that represents a quantitative rather than qualitative change in the properties of the tumor cells.

Level of invasion is highly associated with survival when considered as a single variable. In a population-based study, which may avoid referral and other biases that could be associated with findings from specialized clinic populations, the survival of patients with level II melanoma was 98.8 %, level III 92.5 %, level IV 76.7 %, and level V 75 % [12]. These 5-year survival figures are considerably better than the longer survival data from most specialized clinic databases. For example, in the Penn Pigmented Lesion Group, at about the same time, the 8-year survival for patients with level II melanomas was 96.3 %, compared with 76.1 %, 60.7 %, and 38.5 % for levels II, IV, and V, respectively [5]. In most but not all studies, including the recent very large AJCC model, levels of invasion lose prognostic significance when other factors such as thickness and mitogenicity are known [14].

2.3 Breslow's Tumor Thickness

First introduced as a means of microstaging melanomas by Breslow in 1970 [15], the evaluation of tumor thickness by micrometer measurement from the top of the granular layer to the deepest tumor cell soon came to be recognized as the single strongest prognostic variable for melanoma apparently confined to the primary site. Over the last few years, its use as a single variable has appropriately supplanted that of levels of invasion, as several studies have indicated that the levels add little information to thickness in large series of melanoma cases, especially when mitotic rate is known.

In his original publications, based on only 98 cases, Breslow identified a group of melanomas thinner than 0.76 mm which rarely metastasized, and the good prognosis of this group of cases has been repeatedly confirmed since. In the Connecticut Tumor Registry population-based study of Barnhill et al., the 5-year survival of patients with melanomas <0.76 mm in thickness was 97.9 %, while survival for 0.76–1.69 mm was 91.7 %, for

1.7–3.6 mm was 72.8 %, and for >3.6 mm was 57.5 % [12]. In the Penn Pigmented Lesion Group, the corresponding 10-year survival rates were 96 %, 83 %, 59 %, and 29 %, respectively [16].

Breslow also identified a group of tumors in the range 0.76–1.5 mm that appeared to benefit from elective lymph node dissection, but he later attributed this apparent benefit to surgical selection bias [17]. However, the thickness ranges mentioned above remained for many years in common use as "break-points" delineating categories of patients at increasing risk. In such a scheme, "low-risk" patients are those with tumors less than 0.76 mm in greatest thickness. Patients with tumors 0.76–1.50 mm in greatest thickness have been designated "low-intermediate risk," while those with tumors 1.5–3.99 mm are at "high-intermediate risk," and those with tumors thicker than 4.0 mm are at very high risk for recurrence.

More recently, the break-points of 1, 2, and 4 mm have been selected by the American Joint Committee on Cancer Staging for use in the TNM classification [18]. There has been controversy as to the most appropriate "break-points," and as to whether risk in fact increases in the stepwise fashion implied by these intervals [19, 20]. With regard to decisions about sentinel node staging, breakpoints of 0.75 and 0.50 mm have been considered. Although fairly good evidence in favor of a linear progression has been presented [21], the categorization of cases into thickness intervals of the sort mentioned above is in general more convenient than the use of a linear function.

While the pathologic evaluation of thickness may seem straightforward, there are some potential difficulties. By definition, thickness is measured from the top of the granular layer to the deepest invasive tumor cell. This means that a tumor with marked epidermal hyperplasia could be measured as quite "thick" when the invasive tumor, in fact, consists only of a few cells in the dermis. In this circumstance it is appropriate to add a note to the pathology report, giving an estimate of the thickness of the dermal component, and mentioning that the prognosis may be better than that which would have been expected by thickness alone. The presence of ulceration also creates some difficulties in determining thickness. By convention in an ulcerated neoplasm, the thickness should be measured from the ulcer bed (the surface of the ulcer) to the deepest invasive tumor cell. It is possible that the significance of ulceration as a prognostic variable in some databases results from "down staging" of the tumor in terms of its thickness, since such tumors presumably were thicker prior to the occurrence of the ulceration. The phenomenon of tumor spread downwards in the basal epithelium of skin appendages, a common feature in melanomas, also creates difficulties in choosing the deepest tumor cell for evaluation of thickness. When cells are in the epithelium of skin appendages they are not invasive and thus can be ignored because thickness measurements by definition are based on invasive tumor. When tumor cells invade outward from a skin appendage into the adventitial dermis which surrounds the appendage and is a continuation of the papillary dermis, they may represent the equivalent of Level II or Level III invasion, depending upon whether or not the adventitial dermis is filled and expanded. We do not measure the depth of the melanoma from the surface to these invasive tumor cells in the adventitial dermis, preferring to choose an area of the neoplasm where invasive cells extend directly from the surface epidermis. Rarely, melanoma cells will invade the reticular dermis directly from a site of periadnexal adventitial spread, resulting in a focus of reticular dermal invasion that is deeper than where the lesion more conventionally invades directly from the overlying epidermis. While measurement of this deeper focus may be provided as a worst-case scenario, in addition to the more conventional measurement, it should be emphasized that the biological and prognostic significance of such foci has not as yet been fully determined. Microscopic satellites in the reticular dermis have been used as the point of thickness measurement by some observers [22], but we prefer to measure the deepest invasive contiguous tumor cell, while commenting on the presence of microscopic satellites in the reticular dermis, or fat as the case may be. Finally, the thickness cannot be determined in tangentially sectioned or curetted melanomas.

In a theoretical model of tumor growth, it has been demonstrated that time was the most important factor contributing to tumor thickness. Other important factors included tumor cell motility, particularly when stimulated by stromal elements, a lower rate of tumor cell loss, and pronounced proliferation associated with high numbers of cell cycle generations in the tumor cells. These findings were in agreement with experimental data indicating that metastatic capacity may depend on increased motility, stroma-induced motility stimulation, evasion from the host immune system, and genetic instability made manifest during cell cycling [23].

2.4 Dermal Mitotic Rate

The analysis of mitotic rate, like that of thickness, is a relatively simple quantitative determination that can be done by any pathologist using simple equipment. The prognostic significance of mitotic rate was recognized by Cochran in an early (1968) prognostic model [24]. Schmoeckel and his colleagues also used mitotic rate to generate a prognostic index based on the product of mitotic rate and thickness [25]. While some substantial studies have failed to establish an independent relationship between mitotic rate and survival [26, 27], there is now consensus that the dermal mitotic rate is among the strongest of predictive variables [9]. Mitoses in the epidermal component of the radial growth phase are irrelevant to prognosis (though they are of diagnostic value), and it is possible that a failure to make this distinction could have accounted for discrepancies in reported results. Mitotic rate is recorded in a "hot spot" as the maximal number of mitoses per square millimeter of vertical growth phase tumor. The most mitotically active area of the tumor is identified, and then mitoses are counted over at least 1 mm^2, which represents about 3–4 high-power fields in most modern wide-field 40× objectives. In a small dermal component with one or a few mitoses, it is no longer considered appropriate to extrapolate with a correction factor, and the number of mitoses present is reported as the rate per sq mm, and as a whole number. The exact area of a high-power field should be determined for each microscope using a millimeter scale on the stage to determine the diameter of the field, and the standard formula to determine the area of the circle. If there are no mitoses, the rate should be reported as zero (0), and if there is only a single mitosis, the rate should be reported as one (1) per mm^2, irrespective of the surface area of the lesion that may be available for observation (i.e., whether this is smaller than 1 mm^2 or larger) [28].

Mitotic rate is found in most studies to be highly predictive of survival [5, 12, 24, 29]. In a population-based study, mitotic rate was the only independent predictive attribute in addition to thickness. The survival was 98.7 % for patients with a mitotic rate of zero, 85.1 % when the mitotic rate was 0.1–6.0, and 68.2 % when the rate was over 6 mitoses/mm^2 [12]. In a recent large scale analysis of 13,296 patients from the multi-institutional AJCC database, 10-year survival ranged from 93 % for patients whose tumors had 0 mitosis/mm^2 to 48 % for those with >20/mm^2 ($p<0.001$). In a multivariate analysis of 10,233 patients from this database, the independent predictive factors for survival in order of significance were: tumor thickness, mitotic rate, patient age, ulceration, anatomic site, and patient sex (all $p<0.001$). Clark's level of invasion was not an independent predictor of survival in this database [29].

Mitotic rate in the Clark prognostic model used (as an adjunct to standard AJCC staging) in our practice is determined in the vertical growth phase, and is categorized as "absent," "low" (fewer than 6/mm^2), or "high" (6 or greater). As is also the case with thickness measurements, there is a strong dose–response relationship between mitotic rate and survival, in that the survival becomes progressively worse as the mitotic rate increases [5]. Biologically, it is certainly reasonable to suppose that tumors with a higher proliferative fraction as judged by the presence of more numerous mitoses might be more aggressive neoplasms.

For AJCC staging, "present" or "absent" are the two categories that should be used. The term "<1/mm^2" should not be used to indicate a low but nonzero MR, despite the fact that this term was used in the 2009 publication of the new system [9]. The following statement was developed by a group of pathologists and clinicians, and presented by Gershenwald et al. on behalf of the AJCC Staging Committee [28]: "As detailed in the seventh edition of the AJCC Cancer Staging Manual, the recommended approach to enumerating mitoses is to first find the areas in the dermis containing the most mitotic figures, the so-called hot spot. After counting the mitoses in the hot spot, the count is extended to adjacent fields until an area corresponding to 1 mm^2 is assessed. If no hot spot can be found and mitoses are sparse and randomly scattered throughout the lesion, then a representative mitosis is chosen, and beginning with that field, the count is then extended to adjacent fields until an area corresponding to 1 mm^2 is assessed. The count is then expressed as the number of mitoses/mm^2. To accurately record mitoses, calibration of individual microscopes is recommended; as a guide, 1 mm^2 corresponds to an area corresponding to approximately four high-power fields at 40× in most, but not all, microscopes. For classifying T1 (i.e., up to and including 1 mm) melanomas, the threshold for a nonulcerated melanoma to be defined as T1b is ≥1mitoses/mm^2. When the invasive component of tumor is <1 mm^2 (in area), the number of mitoses present in 1 mm^2 of dermal tissue that includes the tumor should be enumerated and recorded as a number per square millimeter. Alternatively, in tumors whose invasive component comprises an area of >1 mm^2, the simple presence or absence of a mitosis can be designated as at least 1/mm^2 (i.e., "mitogenic") or 0/mm^2 (i.e., "nonmitogenic"), respectively. At some institutions, when mitotic figures are not found after examining numerous fields, the mitotic count has been described as <1/mm^2. For most tumor registries, the designation "< 1/mm^2" is synonymous with zero, as has been customarily used in the past. Although this practice may be continued for historical data, the AJCC Melanoma Staging Committee urges pathologists to use the approach outlined above beginning in 2010."

2.5 Tumor-Infiltrating Lymphocytes and Other Immunocompetent Cells in the Vertical Growth Phase

The host inflammatory response to melanoma is a diagnostically important microscopic feature, but the interpretation of its relationship to survival poses considerable complexities. To understand the relationship, it is important to consider the radial and vertical growth phases separately. In the radial growth phase, a brisk host response is commonly present, and this may result in the appearance of areas of partial regression, that may correlate at the clinical level with the impression of the patient that the melanoma is "breaking up" and "going away," a belief that may in some cases delay presentation to a physician. This phenomenon of regression is discussed in the next section.

A host response also exists to the vertical growth phase, though it is generally less than that to the radial growth phase. In the development of the 1989 Clark prognostic model [5], we characterized the host response to the vertical growth phase as either infiltrative (tumor infiltrating lymphocytes, TIL), or noninfiltrative. In the infiltrative pattern, lymphocytes extend among tumor cells, often rosetting around individual cells and sometimes associated with observable degeneration of the tumor cells so surrounded, while in the noninfiltrative pattern, lymphocytes do not extend among individual tumor cells, but rather infiltrate the dermis that abuts the tumor. We and others have found infiltrating, but not noninfiltrating, lymphocytes in the vertical growth phase to be significantly associated with survival. Indeed, this "TIL" response was second only to mitotic rate in predictive power as judged by the survival odds ratio in the Clark model. In addition, in multiple studies since the first by Kruper et al. in 2006, it has been found that the TIL response in the primary tumor, along with Breslow thickness and other attributes, was predictive of the presence of a positive sentinel node [30–35]. The TIL response is characterized as "brisk" (a dense continuous band of lymphocytes among tumor cells across the entire base or throughout the tumor), "nonbrisk" (a discontinuous band or focal collection of lymphocytes among tumor cells at the base or within the tumor), or "absent" [8]. There is a strong dose–response relationship between the TIL grade and survival and/or sentinel node status, as reviewed elsewhere in this volume. In a formal study, it has been demonstrated that the reproducible categorization of TIL can be easily taught, and can be applied with an acceptable level of reproducibility in routine diagnostic practice [36].

Some of the antigens that are recognized by TIL have been identified in ex vivo studies, but most of these have not been studied for their correlation with the host response in situ. One study addressed this question for the melanoma-associated antigen (MAGE) family, which consists of a number of antigens recognized by cytotoxic T lymphocytes. Positive immunostaining for MAGE was associated with a brisk TIL response involving the vertical growth phase. Because, as discussed above, tumor-infiltrating lymphocytes in melanoma are associated with longer survival, these findings suggest a potential prognostic role for MAGE [37].

2.6 Radial Growth Phase Regression

Probably as a consequence of lesional cell destruction by cytotoxic T cells, it is common for localized areas of partial disappearance to occur in melanoma lesions, almost always confined to the radial growth phase compartment, though a similar phenomenon may rarely be apparent in the vertical growth phase, and even in metastases. This may be noticed by patients who may feel that the melanoma is "breaking up" and "going away." Unfortunately, the disappearance is often not complete. Paradoxically, the presence of partial regression has been found in some but not all studies to correlate with metastasis of thin melanomas [38–41], or with worsened prognosis in tumorigenic melanomas [5]. In our experience, regression has been present in about a third of the metastasizing thin melanomas we have seen, but vertical growth phase is usually also present (with only rare exceptions). It is possible that a small tumorigenic and/or mitogenic component might have present in the area of regression before it regressed. In any case, in our experience, regression is the only attribute of the radial growth phase that has a significant (negative) correlation with survival [5].

Regression in the radial growth phase is defined by us as a local area within a melanoma where there is diffuse fibroplasia in the papillary dermis and usually a lymphocytic infiltrate, often with melanophages and prominent vessels, with absence of melanoma in both the epidermis and the dermis. Adjacent to this area of "regressive fibroplasia" (on one side or the other, or on both sides), there is usually melanoma present in either the epidermis or dermis, or both. This phenomenon may be termed "locally complete" regression. Frequently, diffuse fibroplasia otherwise indistinguishable from "regressive fibroplasia" is observed in the presence of melanoma cells in the overlying epidermis. This finding, which we interpret as a stromal response to the tumor, is not considered by us to represent "locally complete regression." Conversely, occasional examples of putative complete disappearance of a melanoma ("globally complete regression") are observed. In these cases, there is no residual diagnostic melanoma and the diagnosis is necessarily inferential, but may be supported by a convincing clinical history of an evolving and then regressing lesion consistent with a primary melanoma. Unfortunately, a few of these "globally" or "completely" regressed melanomas have been found, concurrently or in follow-up, to have been associated with regional lymph node or distant metastases, which presumably occurred before the complete regression of the primary lesion.

Kang et al. have provided a detailed description and definition of three phases of regression as follows: "Early" regression: "Zone of papillary dermis and epidermis within a recognizable melanoma, characterized by dense infiltrates of lymphocytes disrupting/replacing nests of melanoma cells within the papillary dermis and possibly the epidermis as compared to adjoining zones of tumors; degenerating melanoma cells may or may not be recognizable. There is no recognizable fibrosis." Intermediate regression in addition to the above was characterized by: "reduction (loss) in the amount of tumor (a disruption in the continuity of the tumor) or absence of tumor in the papillary dermis and possibly the epidermis, and replacement by varying admixtures of lymphoid cells and increased fibrous tissue (as compared to normal papillary dermis) in this zone. Variable telangiectasia and melanophages may be present." In late regression in addition to the above there was "marked reduction" or "loss" of tumor in the zone of regression, and there was "replacement and expansion of the papillary dermis by extensive fibrosis (usually dense and horizontally disposed)" as well as variable telangiectasia, lymphocytes, melanophages, and effacement of the epidermis [42]. Our own definition more or less corresponds to that of "late" regression when there is loss of tumor in the area of regression ("locally complete" regression).

Using the definitions of Kang et al., interobserver reproducibility was good (90 % or better) between two observers for presence or absence of regression, but agreement rates fell and the patterns were often mixed for the subdivision described above.

2.7 Ulceration

The association of ulceration of a primary melanoma with unfavorable survival has been reviewed in several large databases. Ulcer width but not depth correlated with survival in an early study [43], but width is not considered in the recent AJCC staging system [9]. As noted above, it is possible that an ulcer might serve to "down-stage" a melanoma by resulting in a spuriously low thickness measurement. In the Connecticut Tumor Registry population-based study, the survivals were 91.6 % and 66.2 % for patients without and with ulceration, respectively [12]. A working group recently defined an ulcer as a local full-thickness loss of continuity of the epithelium, with evidence of a host response such as fibrin, inflammation, granulation tissue, or fibrosis, and with thinning, effacement or reactive hyperplasia of the adjacent epithelium at the periphery of the ulcer, and demonstrated that diagnosis using these criteria was reproducible [44]. Erosions that lack evidence of a response may represent a biopsy artifact. A prior shave biopsy may exactly resemble an ulcer as defined above, but should not be so classified in prognostic models.

2.8 Microscopic Satellites

In some analyses, the presence of microscopic satellites is an independent adverse prognostic variable. Satellites are discrete foci of tumor in the connective tissue discontinuous from the main tumor, and are considered to most likely represent locoregional metastases [45]. In older and some current literature, satellites were distinguished from "in-transit metastases" by an arbitrary cutoff limit of 5 cm from the primary tumor. However, the latest AJCC staging scheme merges satellite metastases around a primary melanoma and in-transit metastases into a single staging entity that is grouped into stage III disease [18]. Most of these lesions represent macroscopically visible lesions. A category of "microscopic satellites" has also been described and has been defined as the presence of deposits of tumor >0.05 mm in size and >0.3 mm from the deepest tumor cells [46]. These were associated with diminished survival in a multivariable analysis. While satellites are not independent variables in some studies [5], this may have been because they are relatively uncommon, so that the studies lack power to observe a survival effect. In a matched pair study designed to focus on this question, satellites were significantly associated with a worse outcome [47]. In a population-based study, the survivals were 90 % and 66.7 % for patients without ($n = 512$) and with ($n = 18$) satellites, respectively [12]. Anecdotally, satellites appear to be associated with increased risk for local recurrence even after a formal wide excision has been done. It must be emphasized, however, that microscopic satellites are relatively rare events, and their hypothetical presence does not justify arbitrary wide excisions designed to "capture" melanoma cells in the process of spreading from their primary site. Accordingly, metastases that develop after complete excision of a primary melanoma that does not recur locally must be the consequence of spread from the primary site prior to the excision.

2.9 Lymphovascular Invasion

This phenomenon may be considered as closely related to satellites, as most satellites presumably occur as a result of angiolymphatic invasion. A similar phenomenon has been described as "extravascular migratory metastasis" by Barnhill [48]. It is generally not possible to distinguish between vascular (VI) and lymphatic invasion (LI), except with special stains. The latter demonstrate that most of the involved vessels are lymphatics. Definite angiolymphatic invasion is uncommonly observed with routine stains, which may at least in part explain its failure to find independent significance in most of the early multivariable studies. In a population-based study, the survivals were 89.1 % and 42.9 % for patients without (n=533) and with (n=7) angiolymphatic invasion, respectively [12]. It seems likely that angiolymphatic invasion, when present, is likely to be associated with a poor prognosis. In most studies that have been adequately powered and have used sensitive techniques, Lymphovascular invasion (LVI) has been associated with survival and/or sentinel node status, as reviewed elsewhere in this volume. Xu et al., using double staining immunohistochemistry recently found invasion of lymphatic spaces (LI) to be independently prognostic for metastasis in primary melanoma. A multivariate model for ten-year metastasis identified tumor thickness, mitotic rate (MR), LI, and anatomic site as independent prognostic factors. A prognostic tree identified patients with stage IB melanomas and LI as a group with thin melanomas and poor prognosis. Survival curves for time to first metastasis demonstrated significantly poorer prognosis for patients with LI compared to those without it for both stages IB and IIA. The recognition of LI is increased by the double staining method, however its detection is insufficiently predictive of sentinel node involvement to permit it to serve as a surrogate for the procedure [49].

2.10 Morphometric Attributes

Nuclear morphometry has been used in an effort to correlate nuclear parameters with survival. In one study of thick primary melanomas, area, perimeter, roundness and aspect ratio of 200 nuclei (100 in the superficial areas and 100 in the lower area) were considered to represent an additional prognostic tool with statistical significance [50]. In a case–control study, 24 thin metastasizing melanomas were compared with 48 matched nonmetastasizing cases by morphometric assessment of nuclear area, shape and density, nucleolar area, analysis of DNA content and expression of proliferating cell nuclear antigen (PCNA). Multivariable analysis showed significant differences between metastasizing and nonmetastasizing melanomas with regard to the nuclear correlation coefficient ($p=0.005$), standard deviation of nuclear shape NCI ($p=0.017$), and nuclear density ($p=0.030$), indicating that thin melanomas with pleomorphic and possibly densely packed nuclei are associated with recurrence. The other attributes studied were not significant [51]. In general, these studies have been disappointing in terms of their lack of ability to provide automated analysis of prognostic attributes, of sufficient clinical utility for inclusion in working models.

2.11 Age, Sex, and Anatomic Location

Demographic or clinical factors that have been associated with survival in melanoma patients have included age, anatomic site, sex, and stage. The effect of age is the least consistent, but some studies have found better prognosis for younger patients [16, 27]. This may be particularly true for melanomas that develop in infancy and childhood, although larger studies are needed before definitive statements can be made. In addition, it is of interest that, despite a higher rate of sentinel node metastasis, patients under 30 years of age do not have a worse survival, due to their having a more favorable clinicopathologic profile [52]. The superior survival of female patients, and of patients whose melanomas are on the limbs compared to the trunk, has been demonstrated in most multivariable studies [16, 53, 54], but interactions among these variables often complicate interpretation of the findings.

2.12 Lymph Node Metastases

Stage is the most important single factor in melanoma, and the prognostic models discussed above and below have demonstrated most of their predictive capacities in patients with clinically localized tumors (AJCC stages I and II). Beyond these localized stages, stage III, defined as regional lymph node metastasis, is associated with a dramatic deterioration of prognosis, which has been estimated overall as a 40 % reduction in the 5-year survival [55]. Regional lymph node metastases can be discovered at the time of primary tumor diagnosis (usually as a sentinel node procedure as discussed elsewhere in this book), or at a later time, or they may occur without an identifiable primary lesion. According to one study, the prognosis for each group was about the same, if measured from the time of discovery of the metastasis [56]. The characteristics of the primary retain some reduced significance in some subsets of patients with regional lymph node metastases, particularly when the extent of nodal disease is limited. In a recent analysis of the AJCC database, the number of involved nodes was the most significant prognostic factor. Five-year survival correlated inversely with number of involved nodes regardless of micrometastatic (i.e., nonpalpable and discovered at sentinel node biopsy) or macrometastatic (palpable) status. When stratified by number of tumor-positive nodes and tumor burden, 5-year survival rates for patients with one, two, or three tumor-positive nodes (microscopic *v* macroscopic) were 71 % versus 50 % ($p < 0.001$), 65 % and 43 % ($p < 0.001$), and 61 % and 40 % ($p = 0.004$), respectively. In contrast, 5-year survival was identical in both groups (36 %) when four or more nodes contained tumor. When primary ulceration was included in the stratification, there was great variation in 5-year survival, ranging from 29 to 82 % [57]. In another recent study of the effect of tumor load, patients with a category of "submicrometastases" that were <0.1 mm in diameter, and present in the subcapsular area of the node only, had an nonsentinel node positivity rate of 2 % and an estimated 5- and 10-year melanoma-specific survival (MSS) of

95 %. It was concluded that these patients may be over treated by a routine completion node dissection and have a survival indistinguishable from that of sentinel node negative patients [58].

3 Survival Models for Melanoma Patients

Many groups have developed prognostic models for melanoma in an effort to provide accurate predictions of survival probability and thus to assist in formulating a basis for clinical decision making. Because the models are derived from the study of populations of cases, they necessarily have limited accuracy when applied to the individual patient, especially when applied outside the group originally used for model-building. Nevertheless, the models provide information of value when considering the extent of primary therapy, the use of adjuvant therapy with differing degrees of toxicity, and the frequency and extent of follow-up, as well as in patient's personal planning. As discussed above, Clark and Breslow introduced very powerful single variables, namely levels of invasion [13, 59] and tumor thickness [15, 60], that successively revolutionized the field of prognostication for melanoma. A few years later, the introduction of extensive multivariable modeling of a large clinicopathologic database by Day, Lew, and colleagues allowed for the effect of these attributes to be considered in relation to each other and to other clinical and statistical attributes [6]. These seminal studies are of interest to this day and have provided a basis for additional modeling efforts that aim to address a range of issues from individualized prognosis to stratification for clinical trials.

Among the many available prognostic models, the best developed, which we consider to have potential value in clinical practice and research, include those of Clark et al. [5], Soong et al. [61], and Cochran et al. [27]. Differences in study design, as well as other variables peculiar to the databases, no doubt explain variation in the attributes that have been considered to be independently associated with survival in these and other similar studies. Soong, for example, found thickness, ulceration, surgical treatment (elective node dissection), anatomic site, and pathologic stage to be independently associated with survival in a Cox model, while Clark et al. found ulceration, treatment, and pathologic stage to be dependent while mitotic rate, tumor-infiltrating lymphocytes, and the gender of the patient were independent variables [5]. In the study of Cochran et al., five variables were linked to survival: gender, site of primary, age relative to 60 years, Breslow thickness, and presence and width of ulceration [27]. Mitotic rate and "intratumoral inflammation" were not independently significant in this study. Some of these differences, perhaps, may be explained by the fact that most studies have not distinguished radial growth phase, with their near perfect freedom from metastasis, from the vertical growth phase cases among which there is considerable survival variation. In addition, these earlier models in general did not have prognostic information from sentinel node staging. Although other differences in study design could be invoked to explain some of the variance, differences in referral pattern of cases and random variation in outcome among the databases must also exist, suggesting that no one of the models that have been presented to date can be considered to be definitive. It is also worth noting again that survival rates in the one available detailed population-based study appear to be superior to those in most referral center-based studies, again suggesting the possibility of referral or other local bias [12].

It is worth mentioning in considering prognostic models that prognostication for individual melanoma patients is still highly imperfect in a "n of 1" setting. Even for patients who may have an excellent predicted probability of survival, a small percentage will in fact develop metastatic disease and may die from their melanoma. Conversely, patients with the most high-risk tumors as judged by prognostic modeling still may survive their disease. As the "low-risk" AJCC stage I cases with Breslow thickness of 1 mm or less account for an increasing proportion of new melanoma cases, a correspondingly high proportion of deaths that will occur for melanoma in the future will derive from cases judged to be "low risk" by current "state-of-the-art" prognostic modeling. This consideration provides an impetus, and an opportunity, to refine these prognostic models so as to recognize subsets of cases at different levels of risk.

The AJCC Staging system, which is currently standard of care, will be discussed in more detail at the end of this chapter. Here, we consider a prognostic model that was developed and is still in use at the Hospital of the University of Pennsylvania, and that provides interesting insights as to interactions among the prognostic attributes discussed above.

3.1 Clark Progression-Based Survival Model

In developing a model for predicting survival in stage I melanoma, Clark et al. considered that survival is 100 % in radial growth phase melanomas irrespective of thickness or any other risk factor [5]. Therefore an optimum model for prediction of survival should be based first on the phase of tumor progression, followed by further characterization of the factors associated with survival in vertical growth phase (tumorigenic) cases, i.e., those melanomas that have potential competence for metastasis but that exhibit substantial variance in the probability of metastasis. Vertical growth phase cases include some where the probability of metastasis is almost zero, while other cases are at extremely high risk. Thickness explains some but not all of this variance. This group studied 484 patients, all of whom had been followed for 8 years or until death, by the Pigmented Lesion Group at the University of Pennsylvania. The model was developed in a test group of 386 patients, and

Table 1
Odds ratios for independent predictors of survival (Clark et al. 1989 [5])

Prognostic variable	Categories	Adjusted odds ratio
Mitotic rate	0/mm^2	11.69
	0.1–6.0/mm^2	3.49
	>6.0/mm^2	1.00
TIL	Brisk	11.31
	Nonbrisk	3.51
	Absent	1.00
Thickness	<1.70 mm	4.04
	>1.70 mm	1.00
Anatomic site	Extremities	3.80
	Axial/volar	1.00
Sex	Female	2.92
	Male	1.00
Regression	Absent	2.79
	Present	1.00

The adjusted odds ratio expresses the likelihood of death, compared to a patient whose tumor lacks the attribute under consideration, all other attributes being held constant. For example, a patient whose melanoma has a mitotic rate higher than 6 is almost 12 times as likely to die as a patient whose tumor has no mitoses, all other variables being equal

validated in a group of 98 patients whose cases had not been used for building the model.

The survival for 122 patients with no vertical growth phase (radial growth phase only) was 100 ± 1 %. A logistic regression model for 8-year survival of the 264 patients with vertical growth phase melanomas in clinical stage I characterized six variables as independent predictors of survival. In order of relative predictive weight for favorable survival, the six independent variables were: relatively low mitotic rate (0 or <6/mm^2); presence of brisk or moderate tumor-infiltrating lymphocytes (TILs); thickness <1.70 mm; location on extremity skin excluding volar/subungual skin; female sex, and; absence of regression in the radial growth phase. Odds ratios for the predictors of survival, indicative of the relative risk associated with each factor, are shown in Table 1. The relatively small survival odds effect for thickness compared to other series is likely explained by the fact that much of the predictive power of thickness in early studies derives from the excellent survival of "thin" melanomas. The good survival of these thin melanomas, however, is likely due to more than 90 % of them being in the nontumorigenic radial growth phase, and thus almost incapable of metastasis. This model differs from models like that of Soong [61], and of Cochran et al. [27], in that it was developed only on cases with vertical growth phase tumors. The output from the logistic regression analysis provides an estimate of survival probabilities, presented in a simple tabular format (Table 1).

Table 2
Probabilities of 8-year survival for vertical growth phase (AJCC 1 or 2)

			Female				Male			
Mitoses	**TIL**	**Regression**	**Arm, leg**		**Axial, subvol**		**Arm, leg**		**Axial, subvol**	
Thickness (mm)			<1.7	>1.7	<1.7	>1.7	<1.7	>1.7	<1.7	>1.7
0.0/mm^2	Brisk	Absent	1.0	0.99	1.0	0.98	1.0	0.98	0.99	0.95
		Present	1.0	0.99	0.99	0.95	0.99	0.96	0.96	0.86
	Nonbrisk	Absent	1.0	0.98	0.98	0.94	0.99	0.95	0.96	0.84
		Present	0.99	0.95	0.96	0.85	0.97	0.88	0.89	0.66
	Absent	Absent	0.99	0.94	0.95	0.82	0.96	0.85	0.86	0.60
		Present	0.96	0.86	0.87	0.61	0.89	0.67	0.69	0.35
0.1–6.0/mm^2	Brisk	Absent	1.0	0.98	0.98	0.94	0.99	0.95	0.95	0.84
		Present	0.99	0.95	0.96	0.84	0.97	0.87	0.88	0.65
	Nonbrisk	Absent	0.99	0.95	0.95	0.82	0.96	0.86	0.87	0.61
		Present	0.96	0.86	0.87	0.62	0.90	0.68	0.70	0.36
	Absent	Absent	0.95	0.83	0.84	0.57	0.87	0.63	0.65	0.31
		Present	0.88	0.64	0.66	0.32	0.71	0.38	0.40	0.14
>6.0/mm^2	Brisk	Absent	0.99	0.94	0.95	0.81	0.96	0.85	0.86	0.60
		Present	0.96	0.85	0.86	0.61	0.89	0.67	0.68	0.35
	Nonbrisk	Absent	0.95	0.84	0.84	0.57	0.88	0.63	0.65	0.31
		Present	0.88	0.64	0.66	0.32	0.72	0.38	0.40	0.14
	Absent	Absent	0.85	0.59	0.61	0.28	0.67	0.33	0.34	0.12
		Present	0.68	0.34	0.35	0.12	0.42	0.15	0.16	0.04

Data from [5]

Application of the Clark survival model: The model is applied as a two-step procedure by first identifying cases of pure radial growth phase melanoma. For these cases, the predicted survival is 100 ± 1 %. Then, the prognosis for tumorigenic cases is obtained from the probability formula, expressed in tabular form. The model generates a survival probability at 8 years with confidence intervals (Table 2). For example, a 52 year old man with a nodular melanoma of the thigh that was 3.99 mm thick, having a mitotic rate of 3.6, nonbrisk TIL and no regression, had a survival probability of 0.86 (range 0.69–0.94), and was in fact alive at 13.2 years after therapy. A 47 year old man had a superficial spreading melanoma of the abdomen that was 0.76 mm thick, with a mitotic rate of 13.6, absent TIL, and regression in the radial phase. His predicted survival probability was 0.16 (range 0.06–0.37), and he died 18.8 months after therapy. The predicted survivals of the two patients illustrated above in a model based on thickness alone were 0.32 and 0.88, respectively. When the model was applied to the validation sample of 98 cases, 89 % of the outcomes were correctly predicted.

In an evaluation of the model in a different dataset, Tuthill et al. found in 259 patients that tumor-infiltrating lymphocytes, primary site, and thickness had independent predictive value. Using the Clark logistic regression prediction model, 8-year survival was predicted in 72.9 % of 166 patients and melanoma-specific mortality in 43 % of 74 patients. The combined or overall accuracy of the model was only 64 % [62]. This dataset was a group of patients who were to be randomized into a clinical trial and did not include patients with melanomas of Breslow thickness <0.76, and therefore is not directly comparable. Nevertheless, these data indicate the need for independent confirmation, and also illustrate the fact that the accuracy of any model will be best in the dataset in which it was developed, or a very similar dataset [63]. Gimotty et al. pointed out that the percent of patients correctly predicted by a model will depend on the "case-mix" of a cohort. To demonstrate this interrelationship, these authors identified a new validation cohort from their database based on the original eligibility criteria for the Clark model. This new cohort included 691 patients with primary melanoma who also had complete data on all variables in the model (approximately 46 % of those seen between 1980 and 1990). In this validation cohort, 40 % of these patients had thin lesions, less than 0.75 mm. For the 511 of these lesions with vertical growth phase, predicted probabilities were computed using the original Clark model. It was found that 84 % of the patients were correctly classified, exactly as found with the original model. When the Tuthill et al. thickness eligibility criterion was then applied removing all patients in the new validation cohort whose lesion thickness was less than or equal to 0.75 mm (322 vertical growth phase lesions), the proportion of patients correctly predicted decreased to 76 % [63].

3.2 Model for Survival Prediction in "thin" (AJCC Stage 1) Melanoma

Recognizing that tumor mitotic rate is not universally available in pathology reports, Gimotty et al. recently used data from 26,291 patients with thin melanomas from the US population-based Surveillance, Epidemiology, and End Results (SEER) cancer registry, to develop a model which was then validated using 2,389 patients seen by the University of Pennsylvania's Pigmented Lesion Group (PLG). In the SEER-based classification tree, which included thickness, anatomic level, ulceration, site, sex, and age, 10-year survival rates ranged from 89.1 to 99 %. Prognostication and related clinical decision making in the majority of patients with melanoma can be improved now using this validated, SEER-based classification.

The survival rates for the validated model are shown in Table 3. This model is evidence based and peer reviewed and can be used now for purposes of prognostication and therapy. It should be noted that the survival rates, in general, are considerably better than those in the AJCC prognostic table for stage IA. This difference is likely to be due to selection bias in the latter series, compared to the population-based SEER data.

Table 3

Expanded AJCC classification for thin melanomas (<1 mm)

Category	Number of cases	Survival
	(SEER database, 10-year survival rate)	
Not ulcerated		
Level II, thickness < 0.78 mm, age < 60	10,648	99.0
Level II, thickness < 0.78 mm, age > 60	5,258	97.5
Level III, thickness < 0.78 mm, other sites	4,169	96.8
Level III, thickness < 0.78 mm, head and neck	664	92.1
Level II/III, thickness > 0.78 mm, women	1,397	95.6
Level II/III, thickness > 0.78 mm, men	1,608	90.6
Level IV/V	2,213	91.4
Ulcerated		
Level II/III	215	88.9
Level IV/V	119	69.8

Data from [14]

A new PLG-based tree was also developed which identified groups using level, tumor cell mitotic rate, and sex, and had better discrimination, with survival rates ranging from 83.4 to 100 %; however, this new model would require validation in another data set before it could be used in practice [14], and has now been supplanted by the current AJCC staging system (Table 4).

3.3 TNM Staging System for Melanoma (AJCC/UICC)

The tumor-node-metastasis (TNM) system of tumor staging considers factors related to the primary tumor, to regional lymph nodes (and other regional soft tissues), and to distant metastases to result in a classification that is associated with the probability of survival. The system is evidence based and can be used as a guide to treatment. The factors considered in the primary tumor (T) category include some of the microstaging attributes discussed above. Thus, the TNM classification combines staging and microstaging information in a single format. In the current and recent prior systems, the T attributes are classified pathologically after excision of the melanoma (pT), as described below [9]. The TNM model therefore considers pathologic attributes of the primaries, but staging for metastases is defined in part clinically, for example, lymph node metastases are defined in terms of the number of lymph nodes involved as well as volume, coded as "micrometastasis" if lymph node metastasis has been diagnosed at sentinel node biopsy or at elective lymphadenectomy, or as "macrometastasis" if clinically positive and pathologically confirmed by therapeutic lymphadenectomy. Among macrometastases, the size of nodes is no longer used in staging, based on evidence that the number of nodes but not their size is significant prognostically. In other prognostic models, it has been demonstrated that microstaging of the primary tumor retains

Table 4
Melanoma TNM classification (adapted from [9])

T classification

	Thickness	Ulceration status
T1	≤ 1.0 mm	a: without ulceration and mitosis $<1/\text{mm}^2$ b: with ulceration or mitosis $\geq 1/\text{mm}^2$
T2	1.01–2.0 mm	a: without ulceration b: with ulceration
T3	2.01–4.0 mm	a: without ulceration b: with ulceration
T4	>4.0 mm	a: without ulceration b: with ulceration

N classification

	No. of metastatic nodes	Nodal metastatic mass
N0	0	Not applicable
N1	1 node	a: micrometastasis[a] b: macrometastasis[b]
N2	2–3 nodes	a: micrometastasis[a] b: macrometastasis[b] c: in-transit met(s)/satellite(s) Without metastatic nodes
N3	4 or more metastatic nodes, or matted nodes, or in-transit metastases/satellites with metastatic nodes	

M classification

M1b	Site	Serum lactate dehydrogenase
M1a	Distant skin, subcutaneous, or nodal metastases	Normal
M1b	Lung metastases	Normal
M1c	All other visceral metastases	Normal
	Any distant metastasis	Elevated

[a]Micrometastases are diagnosed after sentinel or elective lymphadenectomy
[b]Macrometastases are defined as clinically detectable nodal metastases confirmed pathologically

prognostic significance in melanoma patients who are clinically negative but pathologically positive for metastases to regional nodes, and this is also reflected in the new AJCC staging system, where ulceration of the primary tumor retains significance in some patients with nodal metastases [9].

3.4 AJCC Staging System

7th Edition, 2009

The latest AJCC staging system was presented in 2009 by Balch et al. [9]. The major change recommended for TNM and stage grouping criteria was the addition of mitogenicity as a stage modifier for AJCC stage I primary melanomas. In studies of more than 59,000 melanoma cases from 16 international groups, the mitotic rate of the primary melanoma was identified as an independent factor and a mitotic rate >1 was been incorporated into the staging system as a T1b stage modifier, replacing Clark level IV. In addition, it was stated that immunohistochemical detection of nodal metastases is acceptable, with no lower limit of size to designate N+ disease. The possible existence of a lower limit of size (such as submicroscopic micrometastases <0.1 mm) is the subject of ongoing clinical trials and recent reports [58]. In addition, in our opinion, the pathologist should be convinced that the immunohistochemically positive cells are melanoma cells and not nevus cells, Schwann cells, or some artifact.

The latest revision (2009) of the TNM categories is presented in Table 4 and the final stage groupings are in Table 5. Clinical staging includes microstaging of the primary melanoma and clinical/radiologic evaluation for metastases. By convention, clinical staging should be used after complete excision of the primary melanoma, with clinical assessment for regional and distant metastases. Pathologic staging includes microstaging of the primary melanoma and pathologic information about the regional lymph nodes after partial or complete lymphadenectomy. Pathologic stage 0 or stage 1A patients do not require pathologic evaluation of their lymph nodes. There are no stage III subgroups for clinical staging. The definitions have been recommended by the AJCC Melanoma Staging Committee and approved by both the AJCC Executive Committee and the TNM Committee of the International Union Against Cancer (Union Internationale Contra Cancer, UICC). These new definitions incorporate substantial revisions from previous (1983, 1997, and 2001) versions of the melanoma staging categories and classifications [64–66].

The TNM staging system differs from previously used, simple primarily clinical staging systems (localized, regional, and metastatic disease) in that pathological attributes of the primary neoplasm ("microstaging attributes") are considered in the definition of the first three stages of the "Stage Groups." Tumors in Stage Groups I and II are nonmetastatic (Table 5). Stage IV is always metastatic beyond the region.

The AJCC Melanoma Staging Committee has listed the following guidelines that it has used to determine the criteria for the TNM classification and the stage groupings. First, the staging system should be practical, reproducible, and applicable to the diverse needs of all medical disciplines. Second, the criteria should accurately reflect the biology of melanoma based on consistent

Table 5
Stage groupings for cutaneous melanoma (adapted from [9])

Clinical staging				Pathologic staging			
0	T	N	M		T	N	M
0	Tis	N0	M0	0	Tis	N0	M0
IA	T1a	N0	M0	IA	T1a	N0	M0
IB	T1b	N0	M0	IB	T1b	N0	M0
	T2a	N0	M0		T2a	N0	M0
IIA	T2b	N0	M0	IIA	T2b	N0	M0
	T3a	N0	M0		T3a	N0	M0
IIB	T3b	N0	M0	IIB	T3b	N0	M0
	T4a	N0	M0		T4a	N0	M0
IIC	T4b	N0	M0	IIC	T4b	N0	M0
III	Any T	N>N0	M0	IIIA	T1-4a	N1a	M0
					T1-4a	N2a	M0
				IIIB	T1-4b	N1a	M0
					T1-4b	N2a	M0
					T1-4a	N1b	M0
					T1-4a	N2b	M0
				IIIC	T1-4b	N1b	M0
					T1-4b	N2b	M0
					T1-4b	N2c	M0
					Any T	N3	M0
IV	Any T	Any N	Any M1	IV	Any T	Any N	Any M1

outcome results of patients treated at multiple institutions from multiple countries. Third, the criteria used should be evidence-based and reflect the dominant prognostic factors consistently identified in Cox multivariate regression analyses. Fourth, the criteria should be relevant to current clinical practice and regularly incorporated in clinical trials. Fifth, the required data should be sufficiently easy for tumor registrars to identify in medical records to code staging information [66].

Given the complexity of current staging systems, which may be expected to increase in the future, the AJCC has created a preliminary computerized model for survival prediction, which can be accessed at www.melanomaprognosis.org [67]. This model was developed in a database of 25,734 patients with localized melanoma from the 2008 American Joint Committee on Cancer (AJCC) Melanoma Database. The predictive model was developed in a development data set ($n = 14{,}760$) contributed by nine major groups and was validated on an independent validation data set ($n = 10{,}974$) consisting of patients from a separate melanoma center. Another similar model has recently been developed that provides superior survival estimates compared with the AJCC model for patients undergoing SLN biopsy [68]. This online tool is available at www.melanomacalculator.com and will likely provide information that can be used to guide adjuvant therapy decisions and stratification in future clinical trials.

3.4.1 Survival in Patients with Lymph Node Metastatic Melanoma

The survival for patients with lymph node metastatic melanoma is somewhat variable, but generally poor. For some patients with limited nodal disease (stage IIIA), the 10-year survival is above 50 % [66]. As previously noted, it is of interest that, despite a higher rate of sentinel node metastasis, patients under 30 years of age do not have a worse survival, due to their having a more favorable clinicopathologic profile [52]. Therefore, the discovery of lymph node metastases, especially when confined to a single node, should not be regarded as a death sentence. In addition, as previously discussed, the survival of patients with "submicroscopic" nodal involvement is very good and may be indistinguishable from that of patients with negative nodes [58].

3.4.2 Survival in Patients with Distant Metastatic Melanoma

Barth et al. undertook a retrospective analysis of data for 1,521 patients with AJCC stage IV melanoma treated by the staff of the John Wayne Cancer Institute. The median survival time of the 1,521 patients was 7.5 months; the estimated 5-year survival rate was 6 %. Three independent variables significantly predicted survival: initial site of metastases; disease-free interval before distant metastases; and stage of disease preceding distant metastases. Patients could be divided into three distinct prognostic groups based on the initial site of metastases: cutaneous, nodal, or gastrointestinal metastases (median survival of 12.5 months; estimated 5-year survival rate 14 %); pulmonary metastases (8.3 months, 4 %); and metastases to the liver, brain, or bone (4.4 months, 3 %). There was no significant change in the survival rate of patients with AJCC stage IV melanoma during the 22-year review period [69]. The development of targeted therapy and immunotherapy for melanoma will hopefully result in improvement of these grim statistics in the near future.

References

1. Edge SB, Byrd DR, Compton C, Fritz AG (2009) AJCC cancer staging manual, 7th edn. Springer, New York
2. Elder DE, Murphy GF (2011) American registry of pathology, in collaboration with the Armed Forces Institute of Pathology. Melanocytic tumors of the skin, vol 12, Washington, DC
3. Karakousis GC, Gimotty PA, Botbyl JD et al (2006) Predictors of regional nodal disease in patients with thin melanomas. Ann Surg Oncol 13:1–9
4. Kesmodel SB, Karakousis GC, Botbyl JD et al (2005) Mitotic rate as a predictor of sentinel lymph nodepositivity in patients with thin melanomas. Ann Surg Oncol 12: 449–458
5. Clark WH Jr, Elder DE, Guerry DIV et al (1989) Model predicting survival in stage I

melanoma based on tumor progression. J Natl Cancer Inst 81:1893–1904
6. Lew RA, Day CL Jr, Harrist TJ, Wood WC, Mihm MC Jr (1983) Multivariate analysis. Some guidelines for physicians. JAMA 249:641–643
7. Gershenwald JE, Buzaid AC, Ross MI (2000) Classification and staging of melanoma. Clin Lab Med 20:785–815
8. Frishberg DP, Balch C, Balzer BL et al (2009) Protocol for the examination of specimens from patients with melanoma of the skin. Arch Pathol Lab Med 133:1560–1567
9. Balch CM, Gershenwald JE, Soong SJ et al (2009) Final version of 2009 AJCC melanoma staging and classification. J Clin Oncol 27:6199–6206
10. Guerry DIV, Synnestvedt M, Elder DE, Schultz D (1993) Lessons from tumor progression: the invasive radial growth phase of melanoma is common, incapable of metastasis, and indolent. J Invest Dermatol 100:342S–345S
11. Elder DE, Guerry DIV, Epstein MN et al (1984) Invasive malignant melanomas lacking competence for metastasis. Am J Dermatopathol 6:55–62
12. Barnhill RL, Fine JA, Roush GC, Berwick M (1996) Predicting five-year outcome for patients with cutaneous melanoma in a population-based study. Cancer 78:427–432
13. Clark WH Jr (1967) A classification of malignant melanoma in man correlated with histogenesis and biologic behavior. In: Montagna W, Hu F (eds) Advances in the biology of the skin, vol VIII. Pergamon, New York, pp 621–647
14. Gimotty PA, Elder DE, Fraker DL et al (2007) Identification of high-risk patients among those diagnosed with thin cutaneous melanomas. J Clin Oncol 25:1129–1134
15. Breslow A (1970) Thickness, cross-sectional areas and depth of invasion in the prognosis of cutaneous melanoma. Ann Surg 172:902–908
16. Schuchter L, Schultz DJ, Synnestvedt M et al (1996) A prognostic model for predicting 10-year survival in patients with primary melanoma. Ann Intern Med 125:369–375
17. Breslow A (1975) Tumor thickness, level of invasion and node dissection in stage I cutaneous melanoma. Ann Surg 182:572–575
18. Balch CM, Buzaid AC, Atkins MB et al (2000) A new American Joint Committee on cancer staging system for cutaneous melanoma. Cancer 88:1484–1491
19. Day CL Jr, Lew RA, Mihm MC Jr et al (1981) The natural break points for primary-tumor thickness in clinical stage I melanoma. N Engl J Med 305:1155 [letter]
20. Balch CM, Soong S-J, Shaw HM, Milton GW (1985) An analysis of prognostic factors in 4000 patients with cutaneous melanoma. In: Balch CM, Milton GW, Shaw HM, Soong S-J (eds) Cutaneous melanoma. Clinical management and treatment results worldwide, 1st edn. Lippincott, Philadelphia, pp 321–352
21. Vollmer RT, Seigler HF (2001) Using a continuous transformation of the Breslow thickness for prognosis in cutaneous melanoma. Am J Clin Pathol 115:205–212
22. Cochran AJ, Bailly C, Cook M et al (1997) Recommendations for the reporting of tissues removed as part of the surgical treatment of cutaneous melanoma. Hum Pathol 28: 1123–1125
23. Smolle J (1995) Biological significance of tumor thickness. Theoretical considerations based on computer simulation. Am J Dermatopathol 17: 281–286
24. Cochran AJ (1968) Method of assessing prognosis in patients with malignant melanoma. Lancet 2:1062–1064
25. Schmoeckel C, Braun-Falco O (1978) Prognostic index in maligant melanoma. Arch Dermatol 114:871–873
26. Attis MG, Vollmer RT (2007) Mitotic rate in melanoma: a reexamination. Am J Clin Pathol 127:380–384
27. Cochran AJ, Elashoff D, Morton DL, Elashoff R (2000) Individualized prognosis for melanoma patients. Hum Pathol 31:327–331
28. Gershenwald JE, Soong SJ, Balch CM (2010) 2010 TNM staging system for cutaneous melanoma...and beyond. Ann Surg Oncol 17: 1475–1477
29. Thompson JF, Soong SJ, Balch CM et al (2011) Prognostic significance of mitotic rate in localized primary cutaneous melanoma: an analysis of patients in the multi-institutional American Joint Committee on cancer melanoma staging database. J Clin Oncol 29:2199–2205
30. Kruper LL, Spitz FR, Czerniecki BJ et al (2006) Predicting sentinel node status in AJCC stage I/II primary cutaneous melanoma. Cancer 107:2436–2445
31. Taylor RC, Patel A, Panageas KS, Busam KJ, Brady MS (2007) Tumor-infiltrating lymphocytes predict sentinel lymph node positivity in patients with cutaneous melanoma. J Clin Oncol 25:869–875
32. Mandala M, Imberti GL, Piazzalunga D et al (2009) Clinical and histopathological risk factors to predict sentinel lymph node positivity, disease-free and overall survival in clinical stages I-II AJCC skin melanoma: outcome analysis from a single-institution prospectively

collected database. Eur J Cancer 45: 2537–2545
33. van Houdt IS, Sluijter BJ, van Leeuwen PA et al (2009) Absence of Granzyme B positive tumour-infiltrating lymphocytes in primary melanoma excisional biopsies is strongly associated with the presence of sentinel lymph node metastasis. Cell Oncol 31:407–413
34. Burton AL, Roach BA, Mays MP et al (2011) Prognostic significance of tumor infiltrating lymphocytes in melanoma. Am Surg 77:188–192
35. Azimi F, Scolyer RA, Rumcheva P et al (2012) Tumor-infiltrating lymphocyte grade is an independent predictor of sentinel lymph node status and survival in patients with cutaneous melanoma. J Clin Oncol 30:2678–2683
36. Busam KJ, Antonescu CR, Marghoob AA et al (2001) Histologic classification of tumor-infiltrating lymphocytes in primary cutaneous malignant melanoma. A study of interobserver agreement. Am J Clin Pathol 115:856–860
37. Busam KJ, Iversen K, Berwick M, Spagnoli GC, Old LJ, Jungbluth AA (2000) Immunoreactivity with the anti-MAGE antibody 57B in malignant melanoma: frequency of expression and correlation with prognostic parameters. Mod Pathol 13:459–465
38. Massi D, Franchi A, Borgognoni L, Reali UM, Santucci M (1999) Thin cutaneous malignant melanomas (< or =1.5 mm): identification of risk factors indicative of progression. Cancer 85:1067–1076
39. Taran JM, Heenan PJ (2001) Clinical and histologic features of level 2 cutaneous malignant melanoma associated with metastasis. Cancer 91:1822–1825
40. Gromet MA, Epstein WL, Blois MS (1978) The regressing thin malignant melanoma: a distinctive lesion with metastatic potential. Cancer 42:2282–2292
41. Ronan SG, Eng AM, Briele HA, Shioura NN, Das Gupta TK (1987) Thin malignant melanomas with regression and metastases. Arch Dermatol 123:1326–1330
42. Kang S, Barnhill RL, Mihm MC Jr, Sober AJ (1993) Histologic regression in malignant melanoma: an interobserver concordance study. J Cutan Pathol 20:126–129
43. Balch CM, Wilkerson JA, Murad TM, Soong SJ, Ingalls AL, Maddox WA (1980) The prognostic significance of ulceration of cutaneous melanoma. Cancer 45:3012–3017
44. Spatz A, Cook MG, Elder DE, Piepkorn M, Ruiter DJ, Barnhill RL (2003) Interobserver reproducibility of ulceration assessment in primary cutaneous melanomas. Eur J Cancer 39:1861–1865
45. Day CL Jr, Harrist TJ, Gorstein F et al (1981) Malignant melanoma. Prognostic significance of "microscopic satellites" in the reticular dermis and subcutaneous fat. Ann Surg 194: 108–112
46. Harrist TJ, Rigel DS, Day CL Jr et al (1984) "Microscopic satellites" are more highly associated with regional lymph node metastases than is primary melanoma thickness. Cancer 53:2183–2187
47. León P, Daly JM, Synnestvedt M, Schultz DJ, Elder DE, Clark WH Jr (1991) The prognostic implications of microscopic satellites in patients with clinical stage I melanoma. Arch Surg 126:1461–1468
48. Barnhill RL, Lugassy C (2004) Angiotropic malignant melanoma and extravascular migratory metastasis: description of 36 cases with emphasis on a new mechanism of tumour spread. Pathology 36:485–490
49. Xu X, Chen L, Guerry D et al (2011) Lymphatic invasion is independently prognostic of metastasis in primary cutaneous melanoma. Clin Cancer Res 18:229–237
50. Mauri MF, Boi S, Micciolo R, Cristofolini M, Dalla Palma P (1997) Morphometric analysis in prognostic evaluation of stage I thick cutaneous melanomas. Anal Quant Cytol Histol 19:311–315
51. Bjornhagen V, Mansson-Brahme E, Lindholm J, Mattsson A, Auer G (1993) Morphometric, DNA and PCNA in thin malignant melanomas. Med Oncol Tumor Pharmacother 10:87–94
52. Chagpar RB, Ross MI, Reintgen DS et al (2007) Factors associated with improved survival among young adult melanoma patients despite a greater incidence of sentinel lymph node metastasis. J Surg Res 143:164–168
53. Clemente CG, Mihm MG, Bufalino R, Zurrida S, Collini P, Cascinelli N (1996) Prognostic value of tumor infiltrating lymphocytes in the vertical growth phase of primary cutaneous melanoma. Cancer 77:1303–1310
54. Aitchison TC, Sirel JM, Watt DC, MacKie RM (1995) Prognostic trees to aid prognosis in patients with cutaneous malignant melanoma. Scottish Melanoma Group. BMJ 311: 1536–1539
55. Reintgen DS, Albertini J, Miliotes G (2001) The accurate staging and modern day treatment of malignant melanoma. Cancer Res Ther Control 4:183
56. Stadelmann WK, Rapaport DP, Soong S-J, Reintgen DS, Buzaid AC, Balch CM (1998) Prognostic clinical and pathologic features. In: Balch CM, Houghton AN, Sober AJ, Soong S-J (eds) Cutaneous melanoma, 3rd edn.

Quality Medical Publishing, Inc., St Louis, MO, pp 11–36

57. Balch CM, Gershenwald JE, Soong SJ et al (2010) Multivariate analysis of prognostic factors among 2,313 patients with stage III melanoma: comparison of nodal micrometastases versus macrometastases. J Clin Oncol 28: 2452–2459
58. van der Ploeg AP, van Akkooi AC, Rutkowski P et al (2011) Prognosis in patients with sentinel node-positive melanoma is accurately defined by the combined Rotterdam tumor load and dewar topography criteria. J Clin Oncol 29:2206–2214
59. Clark WH Jr, From L, Bernardino EA, Mihm MC Jr (1969) The histogenesis and biologic behavior of primary human malignant melanomas of the skin. Cancer Res 29:705–727
60. Breslow A (1980) Prognosis in cutaneous melanoma: tumor thickness as a guide to treatment. Pathol Annu 15:1–22
61. Soong S-J (1985) A computerized mathematical model and scoring system for predicting outcome in melanoma patients. In: Balch CM, Milton GW, Shaw HM, Soong S-J (eds) Cutaneous melanoma. Clinical management and treatment results worldwide, 1st edn. J.B.Lippincott Company, Philadelphia, pp 353–370
62. Tuthill RJ, Unger JM, Liu PY, Flaherty LE, Sondak VK (2002) Risk assessment in localized primary cutaneous melanoma: a Southwest Oncology Group study evaluating nine factors and a test of the Clark logistic regression prediction model. Am J Clin Pathol 118: 504–511
63. Gimotty PA, Guerry D, Elder DE (2002) Validation of prognostic models for melanoma. Am J Clin Pathol 118:489–491
64. Beahrs OH, Myers MH (1983) Manual for staging of cancer. Lippincott, Philadelphia
65. Buzaid AC, Ross MI, Balch CM et al (1997) Critical analysis of the current American Joint Committee on cancer staging system for cutaneous melanoma and proposal of a new staging system. J Clin Oncol 15:1039–1051
66. Balch CM, Buzaid AC, Soong SJ et al (2001) Final version of the american joint committee on cancer staging system for cutaneous melanoma. J Clin Oncol 19:3635–3648
67. Soong SJ, Ding S, Coit D et al (2010) Predicting survival outcome of localized melanoma: an electronic prediction tool based on the AJCC melanoma database. Ann Surg Oncol 17:2006–2014
68. Callender GG, Gershenwald JE, Egger ME et al (2012) A novel and accurate computer model of melanoma prognosis for patients staged by sentinel lymph node biopsy: comparison with the American Joint Committee on cancer model. J Am Coll Surg 214:608–617
69. Barth A, Wanek LA, Morton DL (1995) Prognostic factors in 1,521 melanoma patients with distant metastases. J Am Coll Surg 181:A193–A201

Chapter 18

Genotyping of Human Leukocyte Antigen (HLA) Ancestral Haplotypes as Prognostic Marker in Cancer Using PCR Analysis

Lisa Villabona, Emilia Andersson, Maddalena Marchesi, and Giuseppe V. Masucci

Abstract

The major histocompatibility complex (MHC) comprises a set of genes that are essential to immunity and surveillance against neoplastic transformation. MHC antigens not only regulate antitumor immune responses in experimental animal models but also directly correlate with survival and prognosis of patients with various types of cancers. Effective recognition of tumor cells by effector T cells may be affected by the genotype and the extent of expression of human leukocyte antigen (HLA)-peptide complexes. Therefore, MHC antigens may serve as potential biomarkers for prognosis and allow selection of cancer patients for specific therapy. We describe PCR-based method to determine the HLA genotype in healthy individuals and patients using blood and tumor tissue as DNA source.

Key words HLA genotyping, Ancestral haplotype 62.1, Malignant melanoma, Survival, HLA-A typing from formalin-fixed paraffin embedded tissue DNA

Abbreviations

HLA	Human leucocyte antigen
MHC	Major histocompatibility complex
APM	Antigen presenting machinery
AHH	Ancestral HLA haplotype
PCR	Polymerase chain reaction
MM	Malignant melanoma
EOC	Epithelial ovarian cancer
OS	Overall survival
TTM1	Time from diagnosis to first metastasis
SFM1	Survival time from metastasis
FFPE	Formalin fixed paraffin embedded
PBL	Peripheral blood lymphocytes

Magdalena Thurin and Francesco M. Marincola (eds.), *Molecular Diagnostics for Melanoma: Methods and Protocols*, Methods in Molecular Biology, vol. 1102, DOI 10.1007/978-1-62703-727-3_18, © Springer Science+Business Media New York 2014

1 Introduction

The immune system has an important function for controlling tumor growth and eliminating metastasizing tumor cells. A prerequisite for T cell recognition of tumor cells is a functioning antigen presentation of the tumor-associated antigens on the cell surface by the human leukocyte antigen (HLA) class I and II on the tumor cells, which is needed for an effective T cell immune response [1]. Several investigators have pointed out different possible roles played by HLA class I and II antigens in the immune surveillance against tumors. In melanoma, renal cell carcinoma, and chronic myeloid leukemia the expression of certain HLA alleles can predict the response to immunological treatments such as vaccine or cytokine therapy [2–6]. As a prognostic factor, HLA has been studied in association with lung [7] and head and neck tumors [8].

Antigenic peptide recognition by $CD8^+$ and $CD4^+$ T lymphocytes through MHC class I and class II molecules, respectively on the surface of antigen-presenting cells initiate a priming of the adaptive immune system for destruction of tumor cells as well as to eliminate invading pathogens. The major histocompatibility complex (MHC) class I molecules are therefore vital components of the adaptive immune system [9] and critical to the immunological recognition of tumor cells. As a result defects in the expression and/or function of MHC antigens provide tumor cells with an escape mechanism from recognition and destruction by the host's immune system [10–14].

1.1 The Major Histocompatibility Complex

MHC, located on the short arm of chromosome 6 (6p21.3), is one of the most intensively studied chromosomal regions in humans. Recently, the human genome has been depicted in block-like structures characterized by areas of high linkage disequilibrium (LD) creating the so-called haplotype blocks of variable length, separated by regions of low LD, that correspond to recombination hot spots [15–18]. This arrangement facilitates the discovery of genes that predispose individuals to diseases through "haplotype-tagging" single-nucleotides polymorphism, reducing the number of markers needed in the mapping process [19]. Haplotype blocks are an algorithmic definition of a region in the human genome characterized by reduced haplotype diversity or strong LD, rather than a biological phenomenon.

"Ancestral haplotype" is a term used to describe conserved haplotypes that appear to be identical among individuals who are not known to be directly related. These ancestral haplotypes have a specific content of alleles at all MHC loci and have a particular genomic length. In the Caucasoid population, approximately 30 ancestral haplotypes and recombinants among them, account for almost 90 % of the haplotypes found during genetic family studies [20].

The HLA loci typically span 3.6 Mb [21] and extend to 7.6 Mb with the telomeric repeats. The adjacent sequences within the super locus contain several genes regulating immune function and demonstrate synteny to the mouse MHC [21, 22]. About 28 % of the expressed transcripts from the genes, within the super locus, are potentially implicated in the immune response. For this reason, it is not unexpected that this genetic region is linked to a large number of autoimmune and immune-mediated diseases [23].

1.2 HLA-A2 and Ancestral Haplotypes as Prognostic Factors

We have been studying the correlation of ancestral HLA haplotypes (AHH) as a prognostic factor in several different malignancies. HLA-A2 represents an independent negative clinical prognostic factor in patients with advanced ovarian cancer [24]. The higher frequency of this allele found in Scandinavian countries significantly decreases moving further south in Europe. In parallel, ovarian and prostate cancer mortality rates decrease with latitude and correlates with the demographic changes in HLA-A2 expression. Moreover, an overrepresentation of the HLA-A2 phenotype was observed in both ovarian and prostate cancer in Swedish patients compared to the normal population [25].

We have published data describing the analysis of 162 paraffin-embedded epithelial ovarian cancer specimens, stained with antibodies against the HLA class I and II antigens, β_2-microglobulin, and components of the antigen presenting machinery (APM). Immunohistochemical analysis demonstrated a high frequency of aberrant expression of MHC class I and II antigens and APM components. HLA-A2 expression, stage III–IV disease, and serous adenocarcinoma histology were independently predictive of poor survival. Down regulation of HLA class I and II antigens was significantly more frequent in tumor tissues from HLA-A02* positive patients with serous adenocarcinoma surgical stage III–IV [26].

The relationship of HLA and cancer further extend the correlation of single alleles with cancer survival and prognosis. Ancestral HLA Haplotypes (AHH) represent clusters of alleles that occur at a higher frequency in certain populations than predicted. These ancestral haplotypes correlate with survival and prognosis in diverse malignancies.

For example, the AHH 8.1 (A*01-B*08-TNF-308A) is predictive for a shorter progression free and overall survival in non-Hodgkin's lymphoma [27] and, as our group has shown, malignant melanoma [28]. We studied the 62.1 AHH [(A2) B15 Cw3 DRB1*04] allele in patients with advanced metastatic melanoma and ovarian cancer (Figs. 1 and 2). The effect of HLA genotypes on prognosis defined by Kaplan-Meier and Cox-Mantel methods were analyzed in these patients. AHH 62.1 in clinical stage IV patients was significantly and independently associated with the decreased survival rate from the time of appearance of metastasis, although the period from the primary diagnosis to metastasis was

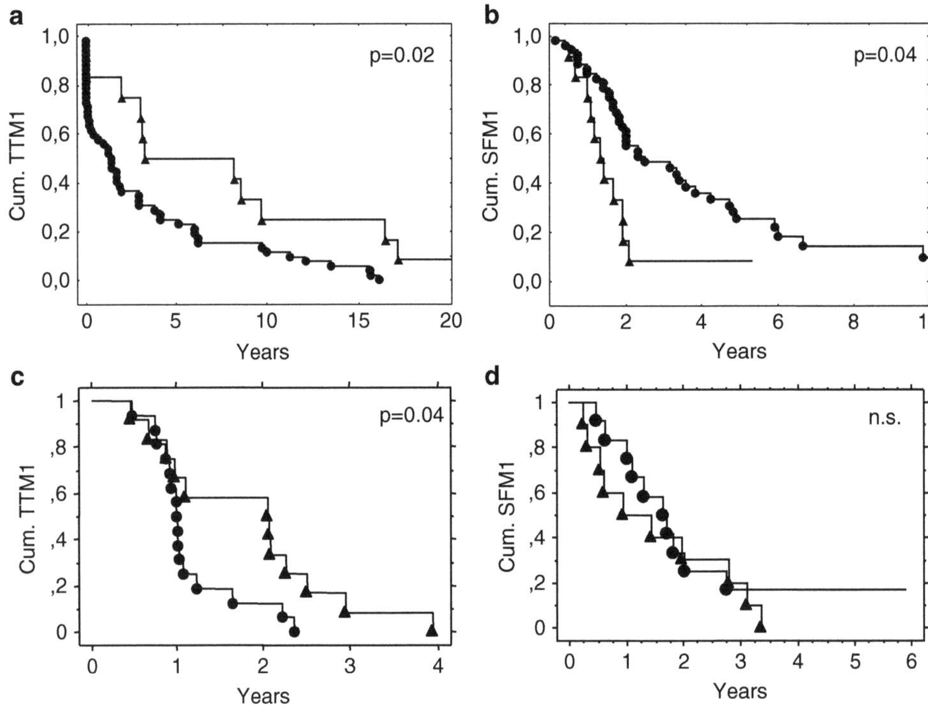

Fig. 1 Kaplan-Meier analysis of time from primary diagnosis to first metastasis (TTM1) and survival from first metastasis (SFM1), with log-rank mantel-Cox test Malignant Melanoma patients. (**a**) TTM1, stage IV patients, AHH 62.1 (B15 Cw3 DRB1*04) positive (*filled triangle*) and negative (*filled circle*); (**b**) SFM1, stage IV patients, AHH 62.1 positive (*filled triangle*) and negative (*filled circle*). Ovarian Cancer Stage III–IV (**c**) TTM1 patients, AHH 62.1 (B15 Cw3 DRB1*04) positive (*filled triangle*) and negative (*filled circle*); (**d**) SFM1, stage III–IV patients, AHH 62.1 positive (*filled triangle*) and negative (*filled circle*)

the longest in patients with this haplotype. Thus, AHH 62.1, known to be associated with autoimmune diseases, in these cohorts of melanoma and ovarian cancer patients correlates with an initial strong anti-tumor capacity with longer metastasis-free period but deteriorate rapidly when the disease advances (Fig. 1a–d).

One of the possible mechanisms underlying this aggressive tumor progression is escape from immune surveillance [29–31]. We might consider the possibility that a haplotype, such as AHH 62.1, may efficiently control the presence of possible residual tumor cells after surgery as long as they are discernible by the immune system (Fig. 2). Paradoxically the presence of altered haplotypes might induce a selection and overgrowth of tumor cells that become "invisible" due to the loss of HLA expression which is often associated with deficient expression of components of antigen processing and presentation machinery [32]. In this escape scenario, in patients with AHH 62.1 tumor cells are selected by genomic loss of part or the entire HLA loci, rearrangement of the HLA allele or failure to express certain HLA alleles on the cell surface [33, 34]. These immune escape variants may also bear mutated

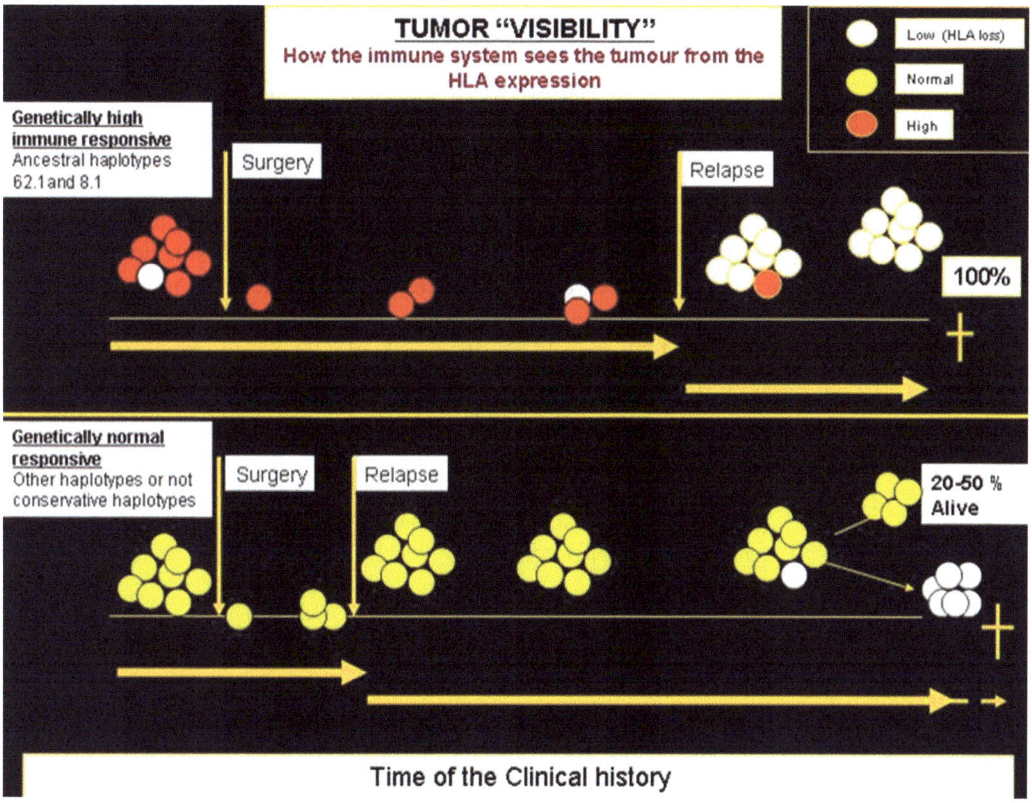

Fig. 2 The highly immune-responsive haplotypes initially promote a strong immune response and can therefore have a long initial relapse-free period. The strong immunologic response unfortunately provokes a high pressure for HLA loss and immune escape, which leads to rapid progression and death. Less-responsive HLA types have a shorter time to initial relapse but less pressure to create clones that are invisible for the immune system and hence longer survival after relapse

oncogenes, which contribute to the more aggressive nature of the tumor manifested by rapidly disseminating disease [33]. Haplotypes other than the ones described above may stimulate a lower level of antitumor effector T cells activity ensuing in a shorter time to relapse. However, the lower selection pressure exerted on the tumor cells by this immune haplotype sustains the immune recognition of the tumor cells.

1.3 Remarks

One of the challenges in the management of cancer patients is the limited knowledge of prognostic factors for those with metastatic disease that foresee their outcome following conventional therapy (surgery, radiation, and chemotherapy). Our investigations validate the hypothesis that HLA typing of patients may provide an additional prognostic factor or predict treatment outcome in patients with advanced ovarian, prostate cancers and malignant melanoma at the diagnosis. In fact, our finding suggests that the HLA-A2 genotype and ancestral haplotypes 62.1 and 8.1 are highly associated with poor prognosis and inadequate response to treatment. The implications are that these patients can be identified at earlier stages before the development of metastatic disease and thereby provide a larger window of opportunity for intensive follow up, early intervention, and aggressive treatment.

HLA typing might be a valuable tool to identify patients who would benefit the greatest from aggressive therapies from those who will not receive additional benefit and should be spared adverse effects of more aggressive regimens. Furthermore, the underlying molecular mechanisms utilized by tumor cells to deregulate HLA expression, may provide novel opportunities for targeted therapy or especially for immunotherapies that really not solely on HLA type I or II restricted T cells. Additional therapeutic modalities that impede immune escape by tumors through down regulation of HLA expression may also increase the survival and prognosis of advance cancer patients when utilized in combinatorial therapy approaches.

2 Materials

2.1 Blood and Tissue Sample Collection

1. Blood samples were collected from patients with confirmed malignant melanoma and epithelial ovarian cancer.
2. Formalin fixed paraffin embedded (FFPE) tumor tissue blocks from consented patients available for the pathology departments (*see* **Note 1**).
3. Lymphoprep for peripheral blood lymphocytes (PBL) isolation (Axis-Shield PoC AS, Oslo, Norway).
4. Citrate tubes for collecting blood samples (10 ml).

2.2 DNA Extraction

1. Roche High-Pure DNA extraction kit for blood and FFPE tissue samples (Roche, Molecular Biochemicals). The kit contains: Lysis, Elution, Binding, and Washing buffers and Proteinase K).
2. Xylene.
3. 100 % ethanol.

2.3 HLA Typing of Blood-Derived DNA for Complete Allele Genotyping

1. Olerup sequence-specific primer (SSP) HLA Typing Kit for complete allele HLA genotype containing: Olerup SSP primer trays, PCR Master Mix, and Adhesive PCR seals (Olerup SSP AB, Stockholm, Sweden).
2. PCR Master Mix contains: 2 U of Taq polymerase, 200 μM of each dNTP, 50 mM KCl, 1.5 mM $MgCl_2$, 10 mM Tris–HCl pH 8.3, 0.001 % w/v gelatine, 5 % glycerol and 100 μg/ml Cresol Red.

Table 1
Primer sequences

Primers	Name	Sequence	Comments
HLA-A2 forward	A*577LL	5′GGA GCC CCG CTT CAT CGC A3′	Do not include alleles:
HLA-A2 reverse	A*503invLL	5′CTC CCC GTC CCA ATA CTC CGG A3′	A*020109, 0248, 0250, 0255
S14 forward	S14sense	5′TCA AAA GGG GAA GGA AAA GA3′	
S14 reverse	S14antisense	5′CAG TGA CAT GGA CAA AAG TG3′	

2.4 HLA-A2 Locus-Specific Determination in FFPE-Derived DNA

1. HLA-A2 primers (for HLA-A2 only) (Table 1) and S14 primers (human ribosomal gene S14 primers) (CybereGene AB; Stckholm, Sweden).
2. PCR MasterMix from Olerup SSP HLA Typing Kit (Olerup SSP AB).
3. Taq polymerase (Applied Biosystems).

2.5 SDS Polyacrylamide Gel Electrophoresis

1. Electrophoresis-grade agarose (Seakem LE; Lonza Rockland, Inc).
2. Tris buffered saline buffer for electrophoresis (TBE, 0.5×), TBE buffer (1×): 89 mM Tris–borate, 2 mM disodium EDTA, pH 8.0.
3. DNA size marker to cover range of 50–1,000 bp (e.g., GeneRuler™ 1 kb Plus DNA ladder, Fermentas).
4. Ethidium bromide dropper bottle.
5. Gel-loading pipetting device.
6. Electrophoresis apparatus/power supply.
7. UV transilluminator.
8. Photographic or image documentation system.

2.6 Other Equipment

1. Vortex mixer.
2. Microcentrifuge.
3. Thermocycler with heated lid, we use thermocycler from GeneAmp PCR system 9700 (Applied Biosystems).
4. Microwave oven or hot plate for heating agarose solutions.
5. NanoDrop technology device for determining the yield and quantity of purified DNA (GE Lifesciences, Uppsala, Sweden).

3 Methods

3.1 DNA Extraction from PBL

1. Blood samples were drawn from patients and collected in 10 ml citrate tubes. PBL were isolated from collected blood samples by addition of Lymphoprep according to manufacturer's

instruction. The lymphocyte suspension is adjusted to 2–3 × 10^6 cells/ml.

2. PBL containing samples of 200 μl were treated with 1 ml Lysis Buffer. Samples are mixed by vortexing, incubated at 80 °C for 30 min and then centrifuged at 12,000 × *g* for 10 min.
3. Collect supernatant into a new reaction tube with 400 μl Binding Buffer (to inactivate nucleases) and 80 μl Proteinase K. Incubate at 72 °C for 10 min and add 200 μl Isopropanol.
4. Load sample onto a filter cartridge placed on a collection tube and centrifuge at 5,000 × g for 1 min.
5. Wash twice with 450 μl Wash Buffer by centrifugation at 5,000 × *g* for 2 min.
6. After final washing step, dry samples by a centrifugation at maximum speed for 10 min.
7. DNA in the filter is then eluted with 50 μl Elution Buffer into a new reaction tube by centrifugation at 5,000 × *g* for 1 min.
8. Finally, the DNA amount and purity were measured by NanoDrop technology (*see* **Note 2**).

3.2 DNA Extraction from FFPE Tissue Samples

1. Day one—Deparaffinization. 4 μm of tissue was sliced from the FFPE blocks and transferred to 2 ml microcentrifuge tubes.
2. Remove the paraffin by adding 800 μl xylene and 500 μl 100 % ethanol, centrifuge at 8,000 × *g*, discard supernatant. Repeat this step twice.
3. Clean from xylene by adding 1 ml 100 % ethanol, centrifuge at max speed and discard supernatant. Dry away all traces of ethanol on heating plate at 97 °C.
4. Add 100 μl Lysis Buffer, 40 μl Proteinase K and 16 μl 10 % SDS to disrupt tissue pellet. Incubate overnight at 55 °C on shaker.
5. Day two—DNA isolation. Mix the sample with 325 μl of Binding Buffer and transfer the mixture onto the Filter Cartridge. Centrifuge at 8,000 × *g*, discard flow through, and dry the filter by centrifugation at max speed.
6. Wash with 800 μl Washing Buffer I, centrifuge at 8,000 × *g* and discard flow through. Wash with 800 μl Washing Buffer II, centrifuge at 8,000 × *g* and discard flow through. Finally, wash with 400 μl Washing Buffer II, centrifuge at 8,000 × *g* and discard flow through. Repeat wash steps twice and then dry by centrifuging at max speed.
7. Elute DNA by adding 90 μl Eluting Buffer to the membrane. Change collection tubes into microcentrifuge tubes and centrifuge at max speed.
8. Remove trace proteins by adding 10 μl Lysis Buffer, 40 μl Proteinase K, and 18 μl 10 % SDS and incubate at 55 °C for 1 h.

9. Bind DNA again to membrane in fresh collection tubes by mixing sample with 325 μl of Binding Buffer and loading it onto the membrane. Centrifuge at 8,000 × *g*, discard flow through, and centrifuge to dry the filter at max speed.
10. Elute DNA by adding 50 μl Elution Buffer to the membrane; incubate in room temperature for 1 min. Change collection tubes to microcentrifuge tubes. Centrifuge at max speed.
11. Amount and purity can then be measured by NanoDrop technology.

3.3 HLA Genotyping in Patients from Blood-Derived DNA

1. HLA-typing was performed according to the protocol used by the laboratory for routine HLA testing at Karolinska University Hospital Huddinge using the tray Olerup SSP HLA Typing Kit.
2. Add Master Mix and distilled water into a 1.5 ml tube, amount according to the table provided in kit. Vortex to mix and pulse-spin to bring all liquid down.
3. Add 8 μl of Master Mix-water mix and 2 μl water into the indicated negative control well on the primer tray.
4. Add the amount of DNA indicated in the provided table into the remaining Master Mix. Vortex and pulse spin.
5. Aliquot 10 μl of reaction mixture into each well except the negative control on the primer tray.
6. Cover the tray with provided seals. Check that all wells are completely covered to prevent evaporative loss.
7. Run amplification consisting of an initial denaturation of 2 min at 94 °C followed by 10 cycles of 94 °C for 10 s and 65 °C for 60 s, then 20 cycles of 94 °C for 10 s, 61 °C for 50 s and finally 72 °C for 30 s.
8. Run the PCR product loading the content of each well on gel electrophoresis at 120 V for 20 min on a 2 % agarose gel, stain with ethidium bromide, and visualize under UV light (Fig. 3).
9. Interpret the typing results with the lot-specific interpretation and specificity tables or worksheet provided with the Olerup SSP HLA Typing kit (*see* **Note 3**).

3.4 HLA-A2 Allele-Specific Determination in FFPE-Derived DNA

1. Dilute DNA to a concentration of 30 ng/μl (*see* **Note 2**).
2. Add 4 μl (120 ng) sample DNA into an amplification mixture containing 2.0 pmol of each primer (Table 1) and 6 μl Master Mix.
3. Use water as negative control and DNA extracted from patient with known HLA-A2 positivity as positive control.
4. Run an amplification consisting of an initial denaturation of 2 min at 94 °C followed by 10 cycles of 94 °C for 10 s and

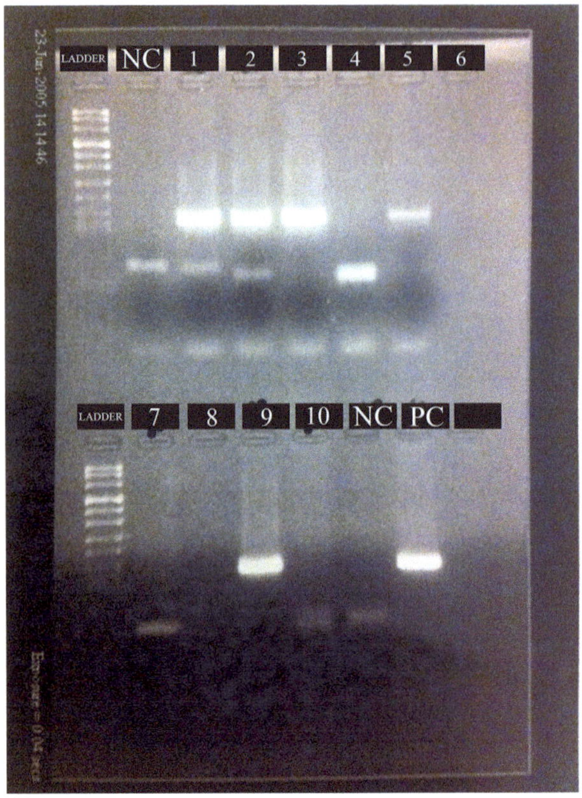

Fig. 3 Nine samples tested for HLA-A2 positivity. NCs are negative controls. PC is a positive control. Samples 1–3, 5, and 9 are samples from HLA A2 positive patients. Samples 4, 6, 7–8 are samples from HLA-A2 negative patients or samples, which are unamplifiable

65 °C for 60 s, then 20 cycles of 94 °C for 10 s, 61 °C for 50 s and finally 72 °C for 30 s.

5. Run gel electrophoresis at 120 V for 20 min using 2 % agarose gel and ethidium bromide staining and visualize in UV light (Fig. 4). Samples from HLA-A2 positive patients give rise to an amplicon of 124 bp, HLA-A2 negative patients give rise to no amplicon (*see* **Notes 3–6**).

3.5 Verification of Amplifiable DNA by S14 PCR (See Note 7*)*

1. Add 4 μl (120 ng) of sample DNA into an amplification mixture containing 5 μl 10× PCR buffer, 200 μM of each dNTP, 1.5 mM $MgCl_2$, 4 μg/μl BSA, 15 pmol of each S14 primer and 10 U Taq polymerase.
2. Use water as negative control and previously tested positive sample as positive control.
3. Run amplification in automated thermocycler initiated by a denaturation step at 94 °C for 1 min, followed by 40 amplification cycles consisting of denaturation at 94 °C for 30 s, annealing at 50 °C for 30 s and elongation at 72 °C for 5 min.

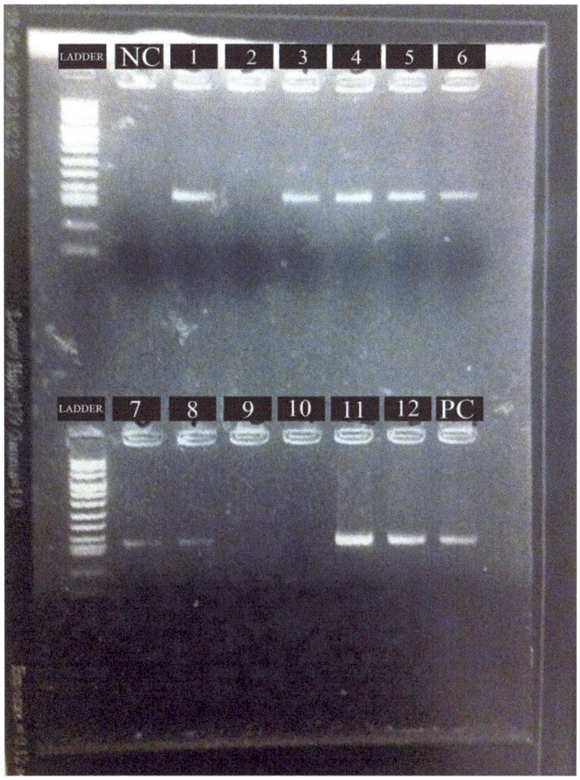

Fig. 4 Twelve samples (different cohort from figure 3) tested for S14. NC is a negative control. PC is a positive control. Samples 1, 3–8, 11–12 are amplifiable samples. Samples 2, 9, and 10 are unamplifiable and can thus not be determined if they are amplifiable for HLA-A2

4. Run gel electrophoresis on 3 % agarose gel and ethidium bromide staining and visualize in UV light. Samples from HLA-A2 positive patients give rise to an amplicon of 124 bp; S14 PCR give 150 bp amplions and nonamplifiable DNA gives no amplicon (*see* **Notes 5** and **6**).

3.6 Statistics for Calculating Clinical Correlations

1. HLA gene and haplotype frequency calculation: HLA class I and II phenotype frequency were calculated by dividing the number of alleles present for each HLA type by the total number of patients.
2. Homozygotes were tallied once. Haplotype frequency was determined using the maximum likelihood method [35, 36]. The statistical significance of the frequencies of individual HLA alleles or haplotypes with the cohort of patients compared to Healthy Swedish Donors (HSD) was calculated using Fisher's exact test. Two-tailed p-values were utilized to detect positive and negative associations. Results with a P value of <0.05, adjusted for Bonferroni correction [37], were regarded to be significant.

3. Survival analysis: The χ^2 trend test was used to examine patients' characteristics for discrete categorical variables or factors.

4 Notes

1. HLA typing is performed routinely for organ transplantation queries. The methods used are mostly DNA based, but require a DNA of good quality, which usually can be extracted from fresh blood samples. When performing retrospective studies of correlation with cancer patients disease progression in many cases blood samples are no longer available. In that case FFPE blocks with cancer tissue are used as a source of genomic DNA.
2. DNA samples to be used for HLA-A2 PCR should be resuspended in dH_2O. The purified DNA should have an A260/A280 ratio between 1.6 and 2.0 to obtain optimal band visualization by electrophoresis. DNA concentrations exceedingg 50 ng/μl will increase the risk for nonspecific amplifications and weak extra bands.
3. The above described method descriminates HLA-A2 positive and HLA-A2 negative samples by a PCR amplification. After the PCR process, the amplified DNA fragments are size-separated, e.g., by agarose gel electrophoresis, visualized by staining with ethidium bromide and exposure to ultraviolet light, documented by photography and interpreted. Positive PCR product indicates HLA-A2 positive patient. It does not however indicate if the patient is homo- or heterozygous for HLA-A2.
4. Examine the gel photo carefully and determine the positive lanes. A faster-migrating, shorter band will be seen in a gel lane if specific HLA allele(s) was amplified. This indicates a positive test result. The relative lengths of the specific PCR products as given in the lot-specific product inserts when interpreting the gel results.
5. The positive control used may be DNA from a person with known HLA-A2 positivity. It is run in a separate gel lane. The absence of positive control band with no specific PCR product indicates failed PCR reaction.
6. The presence of PCR product in negative control lane(s) indicates contamination with PCR product(s) and voids all test results. Primer oligomers ranging from 40 to 60 base pairs in size might be observed in the negative control late(s). This does not represent contamination.
7. The verification of amplifiable DNA is important when working with FFPE material, because of its poor quality. We have used PCR for S14 which is a house keeping gene and present in all cells. Other genes like β2 microglobulin are also available for use.

Acknowledgments

These studies were mainly supported by grants from the Cancer Society in Stockholm and the King Gustaf V Jubilee Fund and the Swedish Cancer Society, the Karolinska Institute/Stockholm County ALF grant. Sequences for HLA-A2 primers were kindly provided by Dr. Olle Olerup at Olerup SSP AB.

References

1. Wallich R, Bulbuc N, Hammerling GJ, Katzav S, Segal S, Feldman M (1985) Abrogation of metastatic properties of tumour cells by de novo expression of H-2K antigens following H-2 gene transfection. Nature 315(6017): 301–305
2. Hoon DS, Okamoto T, Wang HJ, Elashoff R, Nizze AJ, Foshag LJ, Gammon G, Morton DL (1998) Is the survival of melanoma patients receiving polyvalent melanoma cell vaccine linked to the human leukocyte antigen phenotype of patients? J Clin Oncol 16(4):1430–1437
3. Lee JE, Abdalla J, Porter GA, Bradford L, Grimm EA, Reveille JD, Mansfield PF, Gershenwald JE, Ross MI (2002) Presence of the human leukocyte antigen class II gene DRB1*1101 predicts interferon gamma levels and disease recurrence in melanoma patients. Ann Surg Oncol 9(6):587–593
4. Onishi T, Ohishi Y, Iizuka N, Imagawa K (1996) Phenotype frequency of human leukocyte antigens in Japanese patients with renal cell carcinoma who responded to interferon-alpha treatment. Int J Urol 3(6):435–440
5. Franzke A, Buer J, Probst-Kepper M, Lindig C, Framzle M, Schrader AJ, Ganser A, Atzpodien J (2001) HLA phenotype and cytokine-induced tumor control in advanced renal cell cancer. Cancer Biother Radiopharm 16(5):401–409
6. Bain C, Merrouche Y, Puisieux I, Blay JY, Negrier S, Bonadona V, Lasset C, Lanier F, Duc A, Gebuhrer L, Philip T, Favrot MC (1997) Correlation between clinical response to interleukin 2 and HLA phenotypes in patients with metastatic renal cell carcinoma. Br J Cancer 75(2):283–286
7. So T, Takenoyama M, Sugaya M, Yasuda M, Eifuku R, Yoshimatsu T, Osaki T, Yasumoto K (2001) Unfavorable prognosis of patients with non-small cell lung carcinoma associated with HLA-A2. Lung Cancer 32(1):39–46
8. Tisch M, Kyrberg H, Weidauer H, Mytilineos J, Conradt C, Opelz G, Maier H (2002) Human leukocyte antigens and prognosis in patients with head and neck cancer: results of a prospective follow-up study. Laryngoscope 112(4):651–657
9. Townsend ARM, Gotch FM, Davey J (1985) Cytotoxic T cells recognize fragments of the influenza nucleoprotein. Cell 42(2):457
10. Sioud M (2009) Does our current understanding of immune tolerance, autoimmunity, and immunosuppressive mechanisms facilitate the design of efficient cancer vaccines? Scand J Immunol 70(6):516–525
11. Campoli M, Ferrone S (2008) Tumor escape mechanisms: potential role of soluble HLA antigens and NK cells activating ligands. Tissue Antigens 72(4):321–334
12. Algarra I, Collado A, Garrido F (1997) Protein bound polysaccharide PSK abrogates more efficiently experimental metastases derived from H-2 negative than from H-2 positive fibrosarcoma tumor clones. J Exp Clin Cancer Res 16(4):373–380
13. Andersson E, Villabona L, Bergfeldt K, Carlson JW, Ferrone S, Kiessling R, Seliger B, Masucci GV (2012) Correlation of HLA-A02* genotype and HLA class I antigen down-regulation with the prognosis of epithelial ovarian cancer. Cancer Immunol Immunother 61:1243–1253
14. Browning M, Dunnion D (1997) HLA and cancer: implications for cancer immunotherapy and vaccination. Eur J Immunogenet 24(4): 293–312
15. Blomhoff A, Olsson M, Johansson S, Akselsen HE, Pociot F, Nerup J, Kockum I, Cambon-Thomsen A, Thorsby E, Undlien DE, Lie BA (2006) Linkage disequilibrium and haplotype blocks in the MHC vary in an HLA haplotype specific manner assessed mainly by DRB1*03 and DRB1*04 haplotypes. Genes Immun 7(2):130–140
16. Reich DE, Cargill M, Bolk S, Ireland J, Sabeti PC, Richter DJ, Lavery T, Kouyoumjian R, Farhadian SF, Ward R, Lander ES (2001) Linkage disequilibrium in the human genome. Nature 411(6834):199–204

17. Gabriel SB, Schaffner SF, Nguyen H, Moore JM, Roy J, Blumenstiel B, Higgins J, DeFelice M, Lochner A, Faggart M, Liu-Cordero SN, Rotimi C, Adeyemo A, Cooper R, Ward R, Lander ES, Daly MJ, Altshuler D (2002) The structure of haplotype blocks in the human genome. Science 296(5576):2225–2229
18. Alper CA, Larsen CE, Dubey DP, Awdeh ZL, Fici DA, Yunis EJ (2006) The haplotype structure of the human major histocompatibility complex. Hum Immunol 67(1–2):73
19. Johnson GC, Esposito L, Barratt BJ, Smith AN, Heward J, Di Genova G, Ueda H, Cordell HJ, Eaves IA, Dudbridge F, Twells RC, Payne F, Hughes W, Nutland S, Stevens H, Carr P, Tuomilehto-Wolf E, Tuomilehto J, Gough SC, Clayton DG, Todd JA (2001) Haplotype tagging for the identification of common disease genes. Nat Genet 29(2):233–237
20. Degli-Esposti MA, Leaver AL, Christiansen FT, Witt CS, Abraham LJ, Dawkins RL (1992) Ancestral haplotypes: conserved population MHC haplotypes. Hum Immunol 34(4):242
21. The MHC sequencing consortium (1999) Complete sequence and gene map of a human major histocompatibility complex. Nature 401(6756):921–923
22. Horton R, Wilming L, Rand V, Lovering RC, Bruford EA, Khodiyar VK, Lush MJ, Povey S, Talbot CC Jr, Wright MW, Wain HM, Trowsdale J, Ziegler A, Beck S (2004) Gene map of the extended human MHC. Nat Rev Genet 5(12):889–899
23. Thorsby E (1997) Invited anniversary review: HLA associated diseases. Hum Immunol 53(1): 1–11
24. Gamzatova Z, Villabona L, Dahlgren L, Dalianis T, Nillson B, Bergfeldt K, Masucci GV (2006) Human leucocyte antigen (HLA) A2 as a negative clinical prognostic factor in patients with advanced ovarian cancer. Gynecol Oncol 103(1):145–150
25. De Petris L, Bergfeldt K, Hising C, Lundqvist A, Tholander B, Pisa P, Van Der Zanden HG, Masucci G (2004) Correlation between HLA-A2 Gene Frequency, Latitude, Ovarian and Prostate Cancer Mortality Rates. Med Oncol 21(1):49–52
26. Andersson E, Villabona L, Bergfeldt K, Carlson JW, Ferrone S, Kiessling R, Seliger B, Masucci GV (2012) Correlation of HLA-A02* genotype and HLA class I antigen down-regulation with the prognosis of epithelial ovarian cancer. (2012). Cancer Immunol Immunother 61(8):1243–1253
27. Nowak J, Kalinka-Warzocha E, Juszczynski P, Bilinski P, Mika-Witkowska R, Zajko M, Bienvenu J, Coiffier B, Salles G, Warzocha K (2007) Association of human leukocyte antigen ancestral haplotype 8.1 with adverse outcome of non-Hodgkin's lymphoma. Genes Chromosomes Cancer 46(5):500–507
28. Helgadottir H, Andersson E, Villabona L, Kanter L, van der Zanden H, Haasnoot GW, Seliger B, Bergfeldt K, Hansson J, Ragnarsson-Olding B, Kiessling R, Masucci GV (2009) The common Scandinavian human leucocyte antigen ancestral haplotype 62.1 as prognostic factor in patients with advanced malignant melanoma. Cancer Immunol Immunother 58(10):1599–1608
29. Khong HT, Restifo NP (2002) Natural selection of tumor variants in the generation of "tumor escape" phenotypes. Nat Immunol 3(11):999–1005
30. Dunn GP, Bruce AT, Ikeda H, Old LJ, Schreiber RD (2002) Cancer immunoediting: from immunosurveillance to tumor escape. Nat Immunol 3(11):991–998
31. Kim R, Emi M, Tanabe K (2007) Cancer immunoediting from immune surveillance to immune escape. Immunology 121(1):1–14
32. Cabrera T, Lara E, Romero JM, Maleno I, Real LM, Ruiz-Cabello F, Valero P, Camacho FM, Garrido F (2007) HLA class I expression in metastatic melanoma correlates with tumor development during autologous vaccination. Cancer Immunol Immunother 56(5): 709–717
33. Anichini A, Mortarini R, Nonaka D, Molla A, Vegetti C, Montaldi E, Wang X, Ferrone S (2006) Association of antigen-processing machinery and HLA antigen phenotype of melanoma cells with survival in American Joint Committee on Cancer stage III and IV melanoma patients. Cancer Res 66(12):6405–6411
34. Maeurer MJ, Gollin SM, Storkus WJ, Swaney W, Karbach J, Martin D, Castelli C, Salter R, Knuth A, Lotze MT (1996) Tumor escape from immune recognition: loss of HLA-A2 melanoma cell surface expression is associated with a complex rearrangement of the short arm of chromosome 6. Clin Cancer Res 2(4):641–652
35. Schipper RF, D'Amaro J, Bakker JT, Bakker J, van Rood JJ, Oudshoorn M (1997) HLA gene haplotype frequencies in bone marrow donors worldwide registries. Hum Immunol 52(1): 54–71
36. Schipper RF, D'Amaro J, de Lange P, Schreuder GM, van Rood JJ, Oudshoorn M (1998) Validation of haplotype frequency estimation methods. Hum Immunol 59(8):518–523
37. Svejgaard A, Ryder LP (1994) HLA and disease associations: detecting the strongest association. Tissue Antigens 43(1):18–27

Chapter 19

B7-H Abnormalities in Melanoma and Clinical Relevance

Barbara Seliger

Abstract

Melanoma have been shown to escape immune surveillance by different mechanisms such as loss of HLA class I antigens, upregulation of nonclassical HLA-G antigen and Fas, increased secretion of immune suppressive cytokines and metabolites as well as altered expression of co-stimulatory and coinhibitory signals. Recently, an important role of B7-H1 and B7-H4 in the immune escape of melanoma has been described. High mRNA and/or protein expression levels of these coinhibitory molecules were detected in both melanoma cell lines and melanoma lesions when compared to melanocytes. However, their clinical relevance is currently controversially discussed regarding a correlation of B7-H family members with tumor grading and staging as well as survival of patients in melanoma.

Key words MHC antigens, Coinhibitory molecules, Immune escape, Melanoma

Abbreviations

APC	Antigen presenting cell
BTLA	B- and T-lymphocyte attenuator
CTL	Cytotoxic T lymphocyte
CTLA4	Cytotoxic T-lymphocyte antigen 4
HLA	Human leukocyte antigen
IFN	Interferon
mAb	Monoclonal antibody
MFI	Mean specific fluorescence intensity
PBS	Phosphate buffered saline
PD1	Programmed cell death
TCR	T cell receptor
TIL	Tumor-infiltrating lymphocyte
β_2-m	β_2-Microglobulin

Magdalena Thurin and Francesco M. Marincola (eds.), *Molecular Diagnostics for Melanoma: Methods and Protocols*, Methods in Molecular Biology, vol. 1102, DOI 10.1007/978-1-62703-727-3_19, © Springer Science+Business Media New York 2014

1 Introduction

The activation of T lymphocytes is tuned by a combination of two signals delivered through the T cell receptor (TCR)-CD3 and accessory signals, which could be either stimulatory or inhibitory. The first signal is mediated through the interaction of the MHC/peptide complex on professional antigen presenting cells (APC), which is not sufficient to induce the full activation of naïve T cells. Therefore, it requires a second antigen-independent signal, which is provided by classical members of the B7 family, B7-1 (CD80) and B7-2 (CD86), which interact with the costimulatory (CD28) or coinhibitory (CTLA-4) receptors [1, 2]. During the last decade, a number of ligands/counter receptors have been identified with homology to the prototypes. These so called B7 homologues (B7-H) are often expressed in tumors of distinct histology including melanoma as well as in cells of the tumor microenvironment [3–5] and play a critical role in the maintenance of self-tolerance, in the initiation and progression of tumors as well as in the regulation of the innate and adaptive anti-tumor immunity. Currently, some of the B7-H family members are investigated as therapeutic targets, since they have been shown to negatively interfere with anti-tumoral immune responses in tumor-bearing hosts [6–8]. Thus the expression analysis of B7 family members is also important for the monitoring of (immuno) therapy response and as a prognostic marker of patients.

1.1 Characteristics of Costimulatory and Coinhibitory Pathways

The prototype of costimulatory signals is provided by the interaction between B7-1 (CD80) and B7-2 (CD86) ligands on antigen-presenting cells (APC) and CD28 and CTLA4 expressed on T cells [9]. After receiving the second signal from the APC, the T cell will only require the first signal for future activation and effector function against nonself antigens. In humans, both B7-1 and B7-2 are needed for complete activation of naïve T cells and are involved on the balance of activating and inhibitory signals. Both ligands exert distinct expression patterns: While B7-1 is inducible; B7-2 is constitutively expressed on APCs, but further upregulated upon their activation. The ligation of B7-1 and B7-2 with the receptor CD28 caused a costimulatory signal, while ligation of B7-1 and B7-2 with CTLA-4, which is transiently expressed in T cells, caused an inhibitory effect on T cell activation thereby blocking T cell responses and maintaining peripheral tolerance [2, 10].

The B7-H family has rapidly expanded during the last years (Table 1; [9]). These B7-H molecules share structural similarities with the classical B7 molecules and some also bind to members of the CD28 family thereby exerting costimulatory and coinhibitory functions. These include B7-H1 (PDL-1, CD274) and B7-DC (PDL-2, CD273), which bind to the programmed cell death

Table 1
The characteristics of the B7 superfamily members

B7 molecule	Alternate names	Receptor	Function
B7-1	CD80	CD28, CTLA4	Stimulatory
B7-2	CD86	CD28, CTLA4	Stimulatory
B7-H2	ICOS-L	ICOS, CD28, CTLA4	Stimulatory
B7-H1	PDL1, CD274	PD1 (CD279)	Inhibitory
B7-DC	PDL2, CD273	PD1, unknown	Inhibitory
B7-H3	CD276	TLT2?	Inhibitory (stimulatory)
B7-H4	B7-x, B7-S1	Unknown	Inhibitory
B7-H6		NKp30	Stimulatory
BTLN2		Unknown	Inhibitory

(PD-1) receptor and B7-H2 (ICOS-L, CD275), which is the ligand for the inducible costimulator ICOS. B7-H1 is constitutively expressed on multiple cell types including activated B and T cells, myeloid and dendritic cells (DC) as well as endothelial cells, B7-DC expression is restricted to DC and macrophages. Their expression and function could be modulated by cytokines, such as IL-4, IL-13 and interferon (IFN)-γ. Both B7-H1 and B7-DC molecules mediate negative costimulatory signals through its PD-1 receptor, block T cell effector functions and promote T cell apoptosis [7, 11]. In contrast to B7-H1 and B7-DC, B7-H2 delivers positive costimulatory signals through its engagement with ICOS or CD28. B7-H2 is constitutively expressed on B cells, macrophages, DC and some T cell subpopulations as well as on lung, kidney, liver, and testicular tissues. Furthermore, it is induced on $CD4^{+}$ and $CD8^{+}$ T cells during T cell activation. Therefore, the B7-H2 pathway is critical for the delivery of T cell helper function, thereby promoting the immunity ([9]. B7-H3 (CD276), which is involved in the fine-tuning of the immune response [12], is constitutively expressed on T cells, B cells, macrophages and DC as well as on many nonimmune tissues and could be upregulated by IFN-γ or downregulated by IL-4. The functional properties of the B7-H3 receptor appear to be rather complex and the evidence available suggest both a costimulatory and coinhibitory activity of this molecule. Thus the triggering of B7-H3 via the TLT-2 receptor is controversial discussed [13, 14]. The B7-H4 (B7S1, B7×) mRNA is widely expressed in many human lymphoid and nonlymphoid tissues, but its protein expression is limited. B7-H4 is not constitutively expressed in naïve T and B cells as well as a dendritic cells (DC) macrophages and monocytes, but is inducible after stimulation with cytokines. Until now the receptor for B7-H4 has not yet been identified. Although the B and T cell attenuator (BTLA) has been suggested as receptor for B7-H4, it does not directly bind to B7-H4. Furthermore, B7-H4 has been demonstrated to negatively interfere with T cell responses by inhibition of T cell proliferation, cytokine secretion and cytotoxicity [12, 15–17]. Based on this function the B7 family members are engaged in distinct stimulatory and inhibitory pathways and therefore differentially affect immune responses.

1.2 Heterogeneous Expression and Function of B7-H Molecules on Melanoma Cells

The PD-1/PDL1 pathway is critical for the peripheral tolerance and plays an essential role in chronic viral infections as well as in anti-tumor immune responses [6, 18]. The delivery of an inhibitory signal through B7-H1 and B7-DC has been demonstrated to mediate peripheral tolerance and inhibit T cell growth and cytokine production [7, 19]. Many tumors such as renal cell carcinoma (RCC), non-small cell lung cancer, gastric, breast, ovarian, pancreatic, cervical and bladder carcinoma as well as melanoma express B7-H1, which downregulates specific T cell responses [3, 20, 21]. However, there exist controversial data on the expression pattern of B7-H1 in primary and metastatic melanoma lesions: While B7-H1 expression was only observed in a minority of primary tumors and was increased in primary tumors of stage III and IV as well as in metastasis [22–25], others showed high levels of B7-H1 expression in melanoma lesions independent of the tumor grading and staging ([26]. Interestingly, B7-H1 expression was mainly found at the invasion front of melanoma, which appears to correlate with the IFN-γ production of the tumor microenvironment [24]. Indeed, the tumor microenvironment plays an important role in inducing PD1 expression on T cells that infiltrate or surround melanoma cells. The increased frequencies of PD1+, melanoma antigen specific T cells in the blood of advanced melanoma patients suggest an enhanced immune dysfunction [24].

Furthermore, it has been demonstrated that B7-H2 is expressed in a high frequency of melanoma [25, 27], while melanocytes express B7-H2 mRNA, but no protein. In addition, B7-H3 and B7-H4 are highly expressed in most melanoma cells. In addition B7-H4 expression was found on many human tumor tissues and cell lines, such as colon, prostate and lung carcinoma, while it is rarely expressed on normal tissues [28]. Upon its binding to an unknown receptor on T cells, it is inhibiting the tumor-specific T cell activation and proliferation [29]. Studies of different laboratories detected B7-H4 mRNA and/or protein expression at a high frequency in melanoma cell lines and melanoma tissues when compared to melanocytes. B7-H4 expression directly promotes the malignant transformation of melanoma cells [25] and the levels of B7-H4 expression is correlated with tumor TNM staging and/or patients' survival. Furthermore, soluble B7-H4 was often found in blood samples of tumor patients and might represent a diagnostic

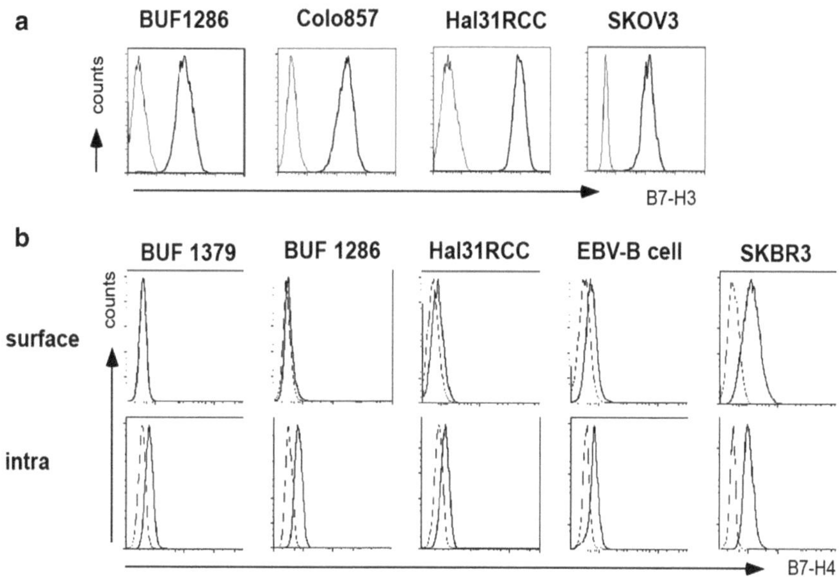

Fig. 1 Flow cytometric analysis of B7-H3 and B7-H4 of two representative melanoma cell lines (BUF1286 and Colo857), as described in Subheading 4. (**a**) Surface B7-H3 expression (*bold lines*) on melanoma cell lines and *thin lines* represent an isotype-matched IgG that served as a control. (**b**) Surface and intracellular B7-H4 (*bold lines*) expression on melanoma cell lines. *Thin line* represents a respective isotype control. The results are presented in histograms of a representative staining of at least three independent experiments. Tumor cells with known B7-H3 and B7-H4 expression served as positive controls

marker for some tumor patients [28]. Thus, both coinhibitory molecules provide a potential therapeutic target to inhibit the progression of this disease.

Despite B7-H4 mRNA expression was detected in almost all melanoma cells, in particular the frequency of B7-H4 surface expression, is lower, suggesting a posttranscriptional regulation of these molecules. However, melanoma lacking B7-H4 surface expression often express high levels of intracellular B7-H4 protein, which was determined by flow cytometry using an anti-B7-H4 monoclonal antibody. A representative constitutive intracellular and surface expression of B7-H4 of the cell lines Bufl286 and Bufl379 is shown (*see* Fig. 1). EBV-transformed B cells, the B7-H4-expressing mammary carcinoma cell line SKBR3 and the colorectal carcinoma cell line served as a positive or negative control, respectively. So far, the additive and competitive effects of the expression of B7-H family members, their mode of regulation and their role in the T cell/tumor interaction have not yet been analyzed in detail. This might lead to a better tuning of the T cell immune response.

1.3 Clinical Relevance of Altered B7-H Expression in Melanoma

In the last decade, an adverse clinical association with the expression of B7-H family members was found in tumors of distinct origin [5] suggesting that these molecules might be used as molecular biomarkers associated with disease progression and survival of tumor patients. Although B7-H1 is expressed in many human

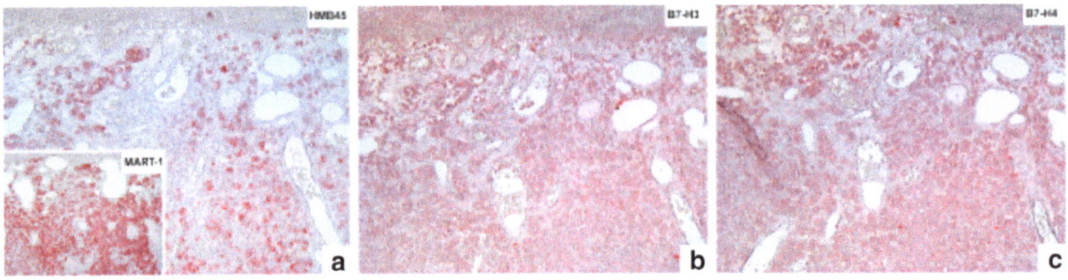

Fig. 2 Immunohistochemical analysis of B7-H expression on melanoma lesions and normal skin surrounding the tumor. Immunohistochemical staining of paraffin-embedded tissues from patients with primary melanoma for B7-H3 and B7-H4 expression using anti-B7-H3 (**b**) and anti-B7-H4 (**c**) antibodies as described [25]. Staining with a MART1 and gp100 melanoma markers specific antibodies served as a control (**a**)

tumors its prognostic relevance is controversially discussed: An increased B7-H1 expression on e.g. RCC is significantly correlated with a bad prognosis [30–32], while in other malignancies opposite results have been described [22]. In melanoma B7-H1 expression was increased during tumor progression with lower levels in primary melanoma lesions when compared to metastases [23]. Upon analysis of the prognostic value of B7-H1 expression on melanoma [26] demonstrated a positive association with a reduced patient's survival suggesting the use of B7-H1 expression as an independent poor prognostic factor in melanoma, while other authors showed no negative association of B7-H1 expression with the patients' survival in this disease [23, 24]. The reason for this discrepancy might explained by the use of different antibodies and material (paraffin-embedded vs. fresh frozen tissues), the small number of melanoma tissues analyzed, the cohort of patients (female vs. male, molecular characteristics) and a different read out for immunohistochemistry [26, 33]. Indeed a recent study performing comparative immunohistochemical analysis of paraffin-embedded and frozen melanoma lesions with 11 distinct mAbs demonstrated that the frequency of B7-H1^{+} melanoma lesions was much higher using frozen tissues when compared to paraffin-embedded tissues. In addition, the quality of staining was significantly dependent on the antibody used for immunohistochemistry [23].

Next to B7-H1, immunohistochemical analyses of B7-H3 and B7-H4 revealed a positive staining pattern for B7-H3 and B7-H4 in most primary melanoma lesions and corresponding metastasis (*see* Fig. 2), but not in healthy skin. Furthermore, a significant positive correlation between the expression of B7-H4 in lymph node metastasis when compared to primary melanoma lesions was observed [25].

1.4 The Role of B7 Costimulatory/Coinhibitory Molecules in the Tumor Microenvironment

A strong association between B7-H1 expression on melanoma and the presence of PD1 positive tumor-infiltrating lymphocytes (TIL) has been reported [34]. PD1 expression is upregulated in CD8^{+} T cells from melanoma patients during progression and metastasis formation [24], which is accompanied by T cell dysfunction [35].

B7-H1 expressing melanoma cells were almost colocalized to adjacent uvant to TIL. This colocalization was also detected in inflamed benign nevi suggesting that B7-H1 expression might represent a host response to inflammation [36]. This is further supported by the presence of IFN-γ at the interface between B7-H1+ tumors and TIL [36]. However, the B7-H1/PD1 signal pathway might still be of prognostic relevance since other immune cell interactions such as T cell/APC might be also involved in this process. Therefore, it has been suggested that B7-H2 expression is a potential source of costimulation of tumor-infiltrating T cells leading to CD4+ T cell activation and cytokine production. Recently, Tregs present in melanoma and metastatic melanoma lymph nodes have been shown to express ICOS on the cell surface [37, 38], which interacts with B7-H2 on the melanoma. This leads to costimulation of Tregs associated with high expression levels of CD25, FoxP3 and ICOS thereby driving Treg activation and their expansion in the tumor microenvironment, which might represent an novel immune escape mechanism [39]. This is in line with reduced number of Tregs in the tumor microenvironment by blockade of B7-H2 in vivo [27]. However, the role of ICOS stimulation on Treg and effector T cells requires to be addressed.

In addition to B7-H1, there exist evidence that the tumor microenvironment is instrumental for the expression of B7-H3 and B7-H4 [40, 41]. Factors released by tumors such as IFN-γ and IL-10 can stimulate B7-H expression in tumor-infiltrating immune cells, including myeloid DC, T cells, NK cells, macrophages, but also in MDSC [42]. Furthermore, B7-H4 expression is commonly detected on antigen presenting cells due to high levels of IL-6 rand IL-10, but lack of IL-4 and GM-CSF in the microenvironment of human cancers [5, 29]. Furthermore, the number of infiltrating T cells in tumor tissues that express B7-H4 was much lower than those lacking B7-H4 expression. These data suggest that B7-H4 over expressing melanoma cells may reflect a more aggressive biologic potential and therefore may play a role in the tumor immune surveillance of this disease. The correlation of clinical data demonstrated that the B7-H4 expression in primary tumor significantly correlated with the survival of patients [25]. In contrast, there exists no correlation of clinical data and immune cell infiltrates with the expression of B7-H3 in melanoma. Similar holds for the expression of B7-H1 expression.

1.5 Impaired Antitumor Immunity of B7-H1 and B7-H4, but not of B7-H3 Molecules in Melanoma

Among distinct mechanisms of tumor-induced immune suppression resulting in resistance to CTL-mediated lysis, both experimental animal studies and in vitro experiments suggested that the coinhibitory molecules B7-H1 and B7-H4 play an important role negatively interfering with CD8+ T cell effector functions [43, 44]. This is in line with a report from [38] demonstrating that a combined induction of TIM-3 and B7-H1 in advanced melanoma is associated with a dysfunction of tumor antigen-specific CTL.

Furthermore, PD1 expression is often upregulated in these antigen-specific T cells as well as ex vivo, $CD8^+$ T cells of melanoma patients' thereby impairing immune response [35]. The impact of the expression of B7 family members on the immune responses was monitored in two experimental settings. The first employed primary and established melanoma cell lines constitutively expressing the B7-H molecules, while the second approach used melanoma cells, in which B7-H molecules were overexpressed or inhibited by shRNA or monoclonal antibodies (mAb). High levels of B7-H1 expression have been shown to block T cell responses directed against melanoma. This was mediated by the inhibition of the activation, proliferation as well as clonal expansion of $CD4^+$ and $CD8^+$ T cells, which was accompanied by a suppressed production of IL-2 and IFN-γ and inhibition of alloreactive CTL by cell cycle arrest In vivo and in vitro blockade of endogeneous B7-H1 as well as PD1 expression by specific mAb promoted T cell responses. These results suggest that the interaction of B7-H4 with its receptor plays an inhibitory role in T cell activation. For analyzing the effect of B7-H3 and B7-H4 molecules on immune cell responses model systems lacking or over expressing B7-H3 or B7-H4 were generated and employed for in vitro cocultivation experiments of T cells with tumor cells in the presence or absence of B7-H molecules. The $CD8^+$ effector T cell function was determined regarding the cytotoxic activity and cytokine expression [25]. Using this approach it could be demonstrated that the cytotoxicity and cytokine production of $CD8^+$ T cells as determined by chromium release assay, CD107 degranulation assay, ELISA or intracellular flow cytometric staining is independent of the B7-H3 expression. In contrast, B7-H4 expression on melanoma cells inhibits the antigen-specific $CD8^+$ T cell response, in particular the IFN-γ, IL-2 and TNF-α production. This was demonstrated with a MART1-specific T cell clone as well as $CD8^+$ T cells obtained from a healthy HLA-$A2^+$ volunteer. However, the cytotoxic activity of the antigen-specific T cells is independent of B7-H4 expression.

It is noteworthy that in addition to the regulation of T cell immunity, B7-H family members, such as B7-H2 and B7-H6 have been shown to also influence the innate immune response [45].

2 Conclusions

Melanoma cell lines could exert immune escape mechanisms by over expressing the B7-H family members B7-H1 and B7-H4, while the role of B7-H2 and B7-H3 in immune evasion of melanoma still requires further investigations. These abnormalities lead to a reduced T cell response, which is associated with a reduced patients' survival. However, the determination of the expression pattern of B7-H molecules and the elucidation of the molecular mechanisms of their altered expression pattern should be performed carefully since it could occur at different levels. Furthermore, it might be mediated also by indirect processes such as signal transduction pathways or transcription factors. Targeting these immune checkpoints by inhibiting the B7-H expression might enhance the antitumor immunity of melanoma patients.

3 Materials

3.1 Immunoreagents

1. The primary B7-H-specific fluorochrome (PE) conjugated antibodies for direct immunofluorescence and immunoglobulin (Ig) (APC and Alexa647) conjugated control antibodies for fluorescence-activated cell sorting (FACS) are listed in Table 2.
2. For staining experiments anti-B7-H specific antibodies were used at 1–20 mg/ml. Mouse IgG mAb was used as an isotype control at the same concentrations.

3.2 Chemicals

1. Phosphate buffered saline (PBS. pH 7.2–7.4, PAA Laboratories, Pasching, Austria).
2. Fetal calf serum (FCS), (Life Technologies).
3. RPMI medium (PAA Laboratories, Pasching Austria).
4. L-alanine and L-glutamine (Biochrome AG).
5. Interferon (IFN)-γ) (R & D Systems).
6. Trypsin Solution, 1× (Sigma).

Table 2
B7-H antibodies used in the study

Antibodies	Isotype	Clones	Company
IgG1-PE		679.1Mc7	Beckman Coulter
B7-H1-PE	mouse IgG1	MIH1	eBioscience
B7-H2-PE	mouse IgG2b	2D3	Biolegend
B7-H3-PE	mouse IgG1	185504	R&D Systems
IgG1-APC		MOPC-21	BD Biosystems
IgG2b-APC		133303	R&D Systems
B7-H1-APC	mouse IgG1	MIH1	eBioscience
B7-H2-APC	mouse IgG2b	136726	R&D Systems
B7-H3-APC	mouse IgG1	185504	R&D Systems
IgG1-Alexa647		MOPC-21	BD Biosystems
B7-H4-Alexa 647	mouse IgG1	MIH43	Serotec

7. 2 % Paraformaldehyde (Merck).
8. Cytofix/cytoperm reagent kit (BD Biosciences).
9. Saponin (Sigma).

3.3 Materials

1. T25 flasks (Sarstedt).
2. FACS tubes (Sarstedt).
3. Allegra x15R Benchtop Centrifuge (Beckman Coulter).
4. IKA MS 2 MiniShaker Vortex Mixer (Gemini BV).

3.4 Flow Cytometers

1. FACScan instrument (BD Biosciences).
2. FACS-Calibur flow cytometer (BD Biosciences).
3. FACS-Canto II Flow Cytometer (BD Biosciences).
4. BD FACS DIVA SoftwareCanto or CellQuest Pro FACSsoftware.

4 Methods

4.1 Cell Culture and Treatment Modalities

1. Different melanoma cell lines were cultured in standard RPMI medium containing 10 % FCS, 2 mM L-glutamine and respective antibiotics.
2. Cells were treated for 48 h with IFN-γ (20 U/ml) to determine B7-H protein expression.

4.2 Fluorescence-Activated Cell Sorting (FACS) Analysis Using Antibodies Directed Against B7-H Molecules

4.2.1 Preparation of Cells for Flow Cytometry

1. For determination of B7-H surface expression untreated and IFN-γ treated melanoma cells were subjected to flow cytometric analysis using the respective anti-B7-H antibodies. Appropriate isotype matching IgG antibodies served as a control (Table 2).
2. Subconfluent melanoma cells cultured in T25 flasks were left untreated or treated with IFN-γ (20 U/ml) for 48 h.
3. Cells were washed twice with PBS, than briefly trypsinized for 5 min.
4. Trypsinization was stopped by adding PBS with 1 % FCS.
5. Cells were washed twice in PBS/1 % FCS and counted.
6. Cells were suspended in PBS/1 % FCS and cell number was adjusted to a concentration of 1×10^6 cells/ml.

4.2.2 Membrane Staining

1. Incubation of fluorescent B7-H specific mAb (5 μl) with 100 μl of cell suspension in each tube.
2. Incubation of fluorescent IgG control mAb (5 μl) with 100 μl of cell suspension.
3. After vortexing cells were incubated at room temperature for 20 min.

4. Cells were washed twice with 2 ml PBS/1 % FCS followed by centrifugation at 400 × *g* at room temperature for 5 min.
5. Aspirate the supernatant and fix the cells with 0.5 ml of 2 % paraformaldehyde/PBS.
6. Quick vortexing of cells.
7. Incubation of cell mixture at room temperature for 10 min in the dark.
8. Washing twice with 2 ml PBS.
9. Removal of the supernatant and addition of 100 μl PBS.
10. Storage of fixed and stained cells at +4 °C for maximum 24 h.
11. Determination of fluorescence on a BD flow cytometer. The results were expressed as mean fluorescence intensity (MFI) ±SD of three independent experiments using DIVA Software Canto.
12. Representative histograms demonstrating surface expression of B7-H3 on melanoma cells and control cells of known B7-H3 expression are shown on Fig. 1a. FACS analysis using B7-H4 specific antibody did not reveal B7-H4 positivity of surface staining in melanoma cells (*see* Fig. 1b).

4.2.3 Intracellular Staining of Selected B7-H Proteins

1. For detection of selected B7-H intracellular proteins (B7-H1, B7-H2, B7-H3 and B7-H4) untreated or IFN-γ-treated melanoma cells were fixed and permeabilized in Cytofix/cytoperm according to the manufacturer's instructions (*see* **Note 1**).
2. Cells were washed twice with saponin (1 % in PBS) (*see* **Notes 2** and **3**).
3. Perform intracellular staining by resuspending the cells in 50 μl of the predetermined optimal concentration of a fluorochrome-conjugated anti- B7-H antibody or appropriate negative control antibody dilution in 1× Perm Wash buffer. Incubate 20–30 min on ice in the dark (*see* **Note 4**).
4. Wash cells with 1 ml of 1× Perm Wash Buffer per sample. Collect cells by centrifugation at 400 × *g* at 5oC for 5 min.
5. Aspirate supernatant, resuspend stained cells and fix with 2 % paraformaldehyde at room temperature for 10 min.
6. Cells were washed twice with PBS before flow cytometric analysis (*see* **Note 5**).
7. Fluorescence intensity was determined on a flow cytometer using the CellQuest software.
8. Representative results are presented as histograms (*see* Fig. 1b). FACS analysis using B7-H4 specific antibody revealed B7-H4 positivity of intracellular staining in melanoma cells (*see* Fig. 1b).

5 Notes

1. The permeabilization buffer creates holes in the membrane thereby allowing the intracellular staining antibodies to enter the cell effectively. Subsequent washing steps, antibody additions, and incubations after cell permeabilization should be performed using the Permeabilization Solution to keep cells permeabilized.
2. The permeabilization substance as well as time of permeabilization could differ and depend on the cell line analyzed. Therefore this step has to be optimized for each cell line and antibody used.
3. Often high intracellular levels were found in particular for B7-H3 and B7-H4 molecules (*see* Fig. 1).
4. The optimal antibody concentrations for intracellular stains tend to be lower than for the same antibody used for extracellular stains. Optimal antibody concentration for specific application should be predetermined by running a titration series.
5. For most antibodies stained cells can be left in Stain Buffer and analyzed the next day. Extended incubation prior to analysis may result in reduced fluorescent signals.

Acknowledgements

This work was supported from grants of the Mildred Scheel Cancer Foundation, the Wilhelm Sander Foundation and the intramural Wilhelm Roux Program.

References

1. Harding FA et al (1992) CD28-mediated signalling co-stimulates murine T cells and prevents induction of anergy in T-cell clones. Nature 356(6370):607–609
2. Sharpe AH, Freeman GJ (2002) The B7-CD28 superfamily. Nat Rev Immunol 2(2):116–126
3. Driessens G, Kline J, Gajewski TF (2009) Costimulatory and coinhibitory receptors in anti-tumor immunity. Immunol Rev 229(1): 126–144
4. Seliger B, Quandt D (2012) The expression, function, and clinical relevance of B7 family members in cancer. Cancer Immunol Immunother 61(8):1327–1341
5. Zou W, Chen L (2008) Inhibitory B7-family molecules in the tumour microenvironment. Nat Rev Immunol 8(6):467–477
6. Flies DB, Chen L (2007) The new B7s: playing a pivotal role in tumor immunity. J Immunother 30(3):251–260
7. Keir ME et al (2008) PD-1 and its ligands in tolerance and immunity. Annu Rev Immunol 26:677–704
8. Postow MA, Harding J, Wolchok JD (2012) Targeting immune checkpoints: releasing the restraints on anti-tumor immunity for patients with melanoma. Cancer J 18(2): 153–159
9. Greenwald RJ, Freeman GJ, Sharpe AH (2005) The B7 family revisited. Annu Rev Immunol 23:515–548
10. Seliger B et al (2008) The complex role of B7 molecules in tumor immunology. Trends Mol Med 14(12):550–559

11. Dong H et al (2002) Tumor-associated B7-H1 promotes T-cell apoptosis: a potential mechanism of immune evasion. Nat Med 8(8): 793–800
12. Yi KH, Chen L (2009) Fine tuning the immune response through B7-H3 and B7-H4. Immunol Rev 229(1):145–151
13. Chapoval AI et al (2001) B7-H3: a costimulatory molecule for T cell activation and IFN-gamma production. Nat Immunol 2(3): 269–274
14. Leitner J et al (2009) B7-H3 is a potent inhibitor of human T-cell activation: No evidence for B7-H3 and TREML2 interaction. Eur J Immunol 39(7):1754–1764
15. Prasad DV et al (2003) B7S1, a novel B7 family member that negatively regulates T cell activation. Immunity 18(6):863–873
16. Sica GL et al (2003) B7-H4, a molecule of the B7 family, negatively regulates T cell immunity. Immunity 18(6):849–861
17. Zang X et al (2003) B7×: a widely expressed B7 family member that inhibits T cell activation. Proc Natl Acad Sci U S A 100(18): 10388–10392
18. Wilcox RA et al (2012) The B7 homologues and their receptors in hematologic malignancies. Eur J Haematol 88(6):465–475
19. Nishimura H, Honjo T (2001) PD-1: an inhibitory immunoreceptor involved in peripheral tolerance. Trends Immunol 22(5):265–268
20. Arigami T et al (2011) Clinical significance of the B7-H4 coregulatory molecule as a novel prognostic marker in gastric cancer. World J Surg 35(9):2051–2057
21. Iwai Y et al (2002) Involvement of PD-L1 on tumor cells in the escape from host immune system and tumor immunotherapy by PD-L1 blockade. Proc Natl Acad Sci U S A 99(19): 12293–12297
22. Blank C et al (2006) Blockade of PD-L1 (B7-H1) augments human tumor-specific T cell responses in vitro. Int J Cancer 119(2): 317–327
23. Gadiot J et al (2011) Overall survival and PD-L1 expression in metastasized malignant melanoma. Cancer 117(10):2192–2201
24. Kronig H et al (2012) PD-1 expression on Melan-A-reactive T cells increases during progression to metastatic disease. Int J Cancer 130(10):2327–2336
25. Quandt D et al (2011) B7-h4 expression in human melanoma: its association with patients' survival and antitumor immune response. Clin Cancer Res 17(10):3100–3111
26. Hino R et al (2010) Tumor cell expression of programmed cell death-1 ligand 1 is a prognostic factor for malignant melanoma. Cancer 116(7):1757–1766
27. Martin-Orozco N et al (2010) Melanoma cells express ICOS ligand to promote the activation and expansion of T-regulatory cells. Cancer Res 70(23):9581–9590
28. He C et al (2011) The inhibitory role of b7-h4 in antitumor immunity: association with cancer progression and survival. Clin Dev Immunol 2011:695834
29. Zheng X et al (2012) Expression of costimulatory molecule B7-H4 in human malignant tumors. Onkologie 35(11):700–705
30. Mumprecht S et al (2009) Programmed death 1 signaling on chronic myeloid leukemia-specific T cells results in T-cell exhaustion and disease progression. Blood 114(8):1528–1536
31. Thompson RH et al (2005) Costimulatory molecule B7-H1 in primary and metastatic clear cell renal cell carcinoma. Cancer 104(10): 2084–2091
32. Thompson RH et al (2004) Costimulatory B7-H1 in renal cell carcinoma patients: Indicator of tumor aggressiveness and potential therapeutic target. Proc Natl Acad Sci U S A 101(49):17174–17179
33. Curtin JA et al (2005) Distinct sets of genetic alterations in melanoma. N Engl J Med 353(20):2135–2147
34. Tjin EP et al (2011) T-cell immune function in tumor, skin, and peripheral blood of advanced stage melanoma patients: implications for immunotherapy. Clin Cancer Res 17(17): 5736–5747
35. Fourcade J et al (2010) Upregulation of Tim-3 and PD-1 expression is associated with tumor antigen-specific CD8+ T cell dysfunction in melanoma patients. J Exp Med 207(10): 2175–2178
36. Taube JM et al (2012) Colocalization of inflammatory response with B7-h1 expression in human melanocytic lesions supports an adaptive resistance mechanism of immune escape. Sci Transl Med 4(127):127–137
37. Strauss L et al (2008) Expression of ICOS on human melanoma-infiltrating CD4+CD25high Foxp3+ T regulatory cells: implications and impact on tumor-mediated immune suppression. J Immunol 180(5):2967–2980
38. Viguier M et al (2004) Foxp3 expressing CD4+CD25(high) regulatory T cells are overrepresented in human metastatic melanoma lymph nodes and inhibit the function of infiltrating T cells. J Immunol 173(2): 1444–1453
39. Fu T, HE Q, Sharma P (2011) The ICOS/ICOSL pathway is required for optimal antitumor

responses mediated by anti-CTLA-4 therapy. Cancer Res 71(16):5445–5454
40. Zang X et al (2010) Tumor associated endothelial expression of B7-H3 predicts survival in ovarian carcinomas. Mod Pathol 23(8): 1104–1112
41. Fujimura T et al (2012) Regulatory T cells stimulate B7-H1 expression in myeloid-derived suppressor cells in ret melanomas. J Invest Dermatol 132(4):1239–1246
42. Blank C, Gajewski TF, Mackensen A (2005) Interaction of PD-L1 on tumor cells with PD-1 on tumor-specific T cells as a mechanism of immune evasion: implications for tumor immunotherapy. Cancer Immunol Immunother 54(4):307–314
43. Fourcade J et al (2009) PD-1 is a regulator of NY-ESO-1-specific CD8+ T cell expansion in melanoma patients. J Immunol 182(9): 5240–5249
44. Brandt CS et al (2009) The B7 family member B7-H6 is a tumor cell ligand for the activating natural killer cell receptor NKp30 in humans. J Exp Med 206(7):1495–1503
45. Li Y, Wang Q, Mariuzza RA (2011) Structure of the human activating natural cytotoxicity receptor NKp30 bound to its tumor cell ligand B7-H6. J Exp Med 208(4):703–714

Chapter 20

Melanoma Susceptibility Genes and Risk Assessment

Alexander Marzuka-Alcalá, Michele Jacobs Gabree, and Hensin Tsao

Abstract

Familial melanoma accounts for approximately a tenth of all melanoma cases. The most commonly known melanoma susceptibility gene is the highly penetrant *CDKN2A* (p16INK4a) locus, which is transmitted in an autosomal dominant fashion and accounts for approximately 20–50 % of familial melanoma cases. Mutated p16INK4a shows impaired capacity to inhibit the cyclin D1-CDK4 complex, allowing for unchecked cell cycle progression. Mutations in the second protein coded by *CDKN2A*, p14ARF, are much less common and result in proteasomal degradation of p53 with subsequent accumulation of DNA damage as the cell progresses through the cell cycle without a functional p53-mediated DNA damage response. Mutations in *CDK4* that impair the inhibitory interaction with p16INK4a also increase melanoma risk but these mutations are extremely rare. Genes of the melanin biosynthetic pathway, including *MC1R* and *MITF*, have also been implicated in melanomagenesis. *MC1R* variants were traditionally thought to increase risk for melanoma secondary to intensified UV-mediated DNA damage in the setting of absent photoprotective eumelanin. Accumulation of pheomelanin, which appears to have a carcinogenic effect regardless of UV exposure, may be a more likely mechanism. Impaired SUMOylation of the E318K variant of MITF results in increased transcription of genes that confer melanocytes with a pro-malignant phenotype. Mutations in the tumor suppressor *BAP1* enhance the metastatic potential of uveal melanoma and predispose to cutaneous/ocular melanoma, atypical melanocytic tumors, and other internal malignancies (COMMON syndrome). Genome-wide association studies have identified numerous low-risk alleles. Although several melanoma susceptibility genes have been identified, risk assessment tools have been developed only for the most common gene implicated with hereditary melanoma, *CDKN2A*. MelaPRO, a validated model that relies on Mendelian inheritance and Bayesian probability theories, estimates carrier probability for *CDKN2A* and future risk of melanoma taking into account a patient's family and past medical history of melanoma. Genetic testing for *CDKN2A* mutations is currently available but the Melanoma Genetics Consortium recommends offering such testing to patients only in the context of research protocols because clinical utility is uncertain.

Key words Familial melanoma, Hereditary melanoma, CDKN2A, p16INK4a, P14ARF, MC1R, MITF, BAP1, Genome-wide association studies, Cancer risk assessment, MelaPRO, COMMON syndrome

Magdalena Thurin and Francesco M. Marincola (eds.), *Molecular Diagnostics for Melanoma: Methods and Protocols*, Methods in Molecular Biology, vol. 1102, DOI 10.1007/978-1-62703-727-3_20, © Springer Science+Business Media New York 2014

1 Introduction

Mutations in a number of genes involved in cell proliferation and melanin biosynthesis increase the risk of melanoma development. Inheritance of these genes may manifest as hereditary melanoma, which tends to occur in multiple members of the same family (also known as familial melanoma); as multiple primary melanomas in a given individual; or as a primary melanoma with onset at an early age.

The percentage of melanomas arising in individuals who have one or more first-degree relatives with melanoma is approximately 5–12 % [1]. The identification of individuals at risk of developing hereditary melanoma is important in order to implement strategies for reducing the burden of early disease. The purpose of this chapter is to provide an overview of genes that increase susceptibility to melanoma, to present tools for risk assessment, and to discuss current management strategies for families with increased melanoma risk.

2 Melanoma Susceptibility Genes

2.1 High-Risk Loci and Pathways

The *CDKN2A/CDK4/Rb* pathway. The most commonly involved melanoma susceptibility locus is the tumor suppressor *CDKN2A* located on chromosome 9p21. This genetic unit encodes for two distinct proteins: p16INK4a, a cell cycle inhibitory protein, and p14ARF, an inducer of cell cycle arrest and apoptosis (Fig. 1) [2–4]. These proteins are derived from exons 1a, 2, and 3 (p16INK4a) and exons 1b, 2, and 3 (p14ARF); thus, these functionally distinct proteins capitalize on differential splicing and alternative reading frame use. The mutations are inherited in an autosomal dominant fashion with variable penetrance and their frequency in families with at least three patients with melanoma varies across continents, from 20 % in Australia to 45 % in North America to 57 % in Europe [5]. Furthermore, approximately 10–15 % of individuals with multiple primary melanomas who lack a family history of melanoma also carry germline *CDKN2A* mutations [6, 7].

Of the two proteins coded by *CDKN2A*, exons 1a (p16INK4a specific) and 2 (p16INK4a and p14ARF) appear to harbor most of the mutations arguing that p16INK4a may be the preferential target. The p16INK4a protein inhibits cyclinD1/CDK4, which in turn limits the phosphorylation of RB. Hypophosphorylated RB inhibits the transcription factor E2F thereby reducing S phase genes and arresting the cell in the G1 phase. Cells lacking a functional RB, and therefore incapable of inhibiting E2F, show a lack of cell cycle arrest in the setting of p16INK4a activation, indicating that loss of p16INK4a, activation of Cdk4, or loss of RB have similar effects on G1 progression. Loss of p16INK4a results in progression of the cell cycle through the G1 phase and a resumption of cell cycling [8].

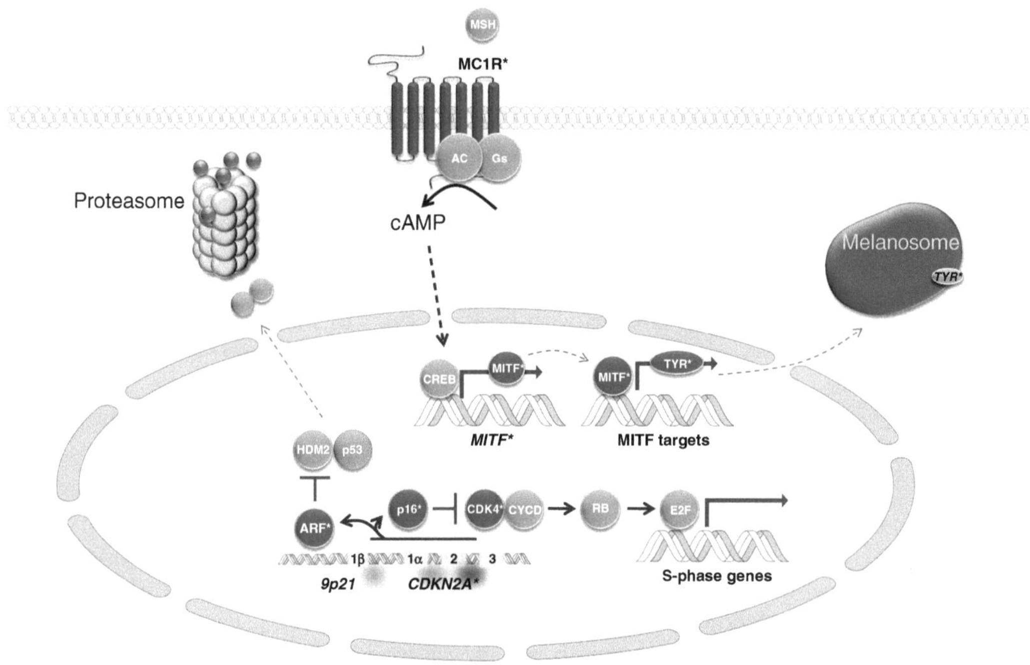

Fig. 1 Melanoma susceptibility genes. Mutations in the *CDKN2A/CDK4/Rb* and the *MC1R/MITF* pathways predispose to melanoma. The tumor suppressor locus *CDKN2A* codes for two proteins: p16INK4a and p14ARF. Deficiency of p16INK4a permits formation of a complex between CDK4 and cyclin D1, which results in hyperphosphorylation of Rb, consequent release of the E2F transcription factor and induction of S-phase genes by E2F. Absence of p14ARF increases MDM2-mediated ubiquitination of p53, which condemns p53 to degradation in the proteasome. As the cell cycle progresses, DNA damage accumulates in the setting of deficient p53. MC1R variants appear to predispose to melanoma by two separate mechanisms, nonpigmentary and pigmentary, as some variants have been associated with melanoma only while others have been associated with both melanoma and red hair/fair skin phenotype. The canonical red hair variants appear to compromise the ability of MC1R to respond to MSH. The mutant E318K MITF shows impaired posttranslational modification, resulting in increased expression of genes associated with malignant potential

Increased G1-S progression thus represents a common pathway for increased risk of hereditary melanoma [9].

On the other hand, p14ARF inhibits MDM2, an E3 ubiquitin ligase that condemns the p53 tumor suppressor for destruction. The net effect of p14ARF loss is decreased p53 transcriptional activity due to heightened MDM2. Although germline exon 1b mutations (i.e., p14ARF-specific) have been described, these are relatively less common than those in exon 1a and exon 2 [10–14].

The risk of developing melanoma has been estimated in both the familial and population-wide settings. The penetrance of *CDKN2A* mutations among familial melanoma has been examined in European, Australian, and American families with multiple cases of melanoma [15]. Overall, penetrance estimates reached 0.30 by age 50 and 0.67 by age 80 years. Penetrance varied among the three geographical regions based on melanoma population incidence rates with the United States showing the highest penetrance of 0.50 by age 50 and Australia showing the highest penetrance of 0.91 by age 80. These variations suggest that ambient sunlight and other familial modulating loci may influence penetrance. In a population-based analysis, the lifetime risk of melanoma in individuals harboring a *CDKN2A* mutation appeared to be much lower: 14 % by age 50, 24 % by age 70, and 28 % by age 80 [16]. These findings suggest that *CDKN2A* mutation carriers in the general population are at lower risk of developing melanoma than those in families with multiple cases of melanoma perhaps because of other risk modifying loci that are co-inherited with *CDKN2A* in the familial context.

A GenoMEL (Melanoma Genetics Consortium) study showed that several factors should raise suspicion that underlying *CDKN2A* mutations are present in a family with melanoma. In the context of a positive family history of melanoma, high number of individuals with melanoma, early age of onset of melanoma, multiple primary melanomas, and cases of pancreatic cancer have been shown to be predictors of *CDKN2A* mutation status [5]. Families with at least three patients with melanoma from North America, Australia, and Europe were used in the GenoMEL study. In North America, the risk of *CDKN2A* mutations was 44 % in families with 5 relatives diagnosed with melanoma and 80 % in those with 6 or more relatives with melanoma. A median age of melanoma diagnosis of less than 34 years in families with at least three patients with melanoma was associated with much greater frequency of mutations, at approximately 65 %, than a median age of melanoma diagnosis of greater than 50 years, at approximately 10 %. The presence of at least one relative with multiple primary melanomas accounted for a mutation frequency of 74 % compared to 10 % in similar families without patients with multiple primary melanomas. More than 75 % of families with at least three patients with melanoma and one relative with pancreatic cancer had mutations detected in *CDKN2A*. In the absence of a family history of melanoma, multiple primary melanomas, or pancreatic cancer; early age of melanoma onset alone is not a strong predictor of a germline *CDKN2A* mutation [17, 18].

Germline mutations in *CDKN2A* have been observed in a subset of patients with familial atypical multiple mole and melanoma (FAMMM) syndrome, an autosomal dominant cancer syndrome characterized by numerous clinically and histologically atypical melanocytic nevi (i.e., dyplastic nevi) and cutaneous melanoma [19]. Though the presence of multiple dysplastic nevi is a known risk factor for melanoma [20], the dysplastic nevus phenotype alone, in the absence of melanoma, does not appear to predict *CDKN2A* mutational status [3, 21]. Another cancer that has been linked to germline *CDKN2A* mutagenesis is pancreatic cancer. It has been observed that mutations that impair the function of the p16INK4a protein may increase the risk of developing pancreatic cancer. In contrast, wild-type alleles and mutations that result in a functionally intact protein do not exhibit this increased risk [22].

A review of the literature determined that families that meet certain criteria should be referred for genetic evaluation and consideration of *CDKN2A* testing because of high likelihood of underlying *CDKN2A* mutations [23]. In moderate to high melanoma incidence areas, such as Australia and certain regions of the United States, these criteria include: (1) individuals with three or more primary invasive melanomas; or (2) families with at least one invasive melanoma and two or more cases of melanoma and/or pancreatic cancer among first- or second-degree relatives on the same side of the family. In contrast, the threshold for referral is lower in patients from low melanoma incidence areas and includes the following criteria: (1) Two or more primary invasive melanomas; or (2) individuals with melanoma and one or more first- or second-degree relatives on the same side of the family with melanoma and/or pancreatic cancer. The frequency of *CDKN2A* mutations increases with greater number of primary melanomas and in the presence of a family history of melanoma. Patients from low incidence areas having at least four melanomas have been shown to carry *CDKN2A* mutations in 29–100 % of cases [23]. A BayesMendel model has been recently developed to more accurately predict *CDKN2A* carrier probability [24]. MelaPRO is comparable to BRCAPRO though MelaPRO incorporates ambient melanoma incidence into the calculation function while BRCAPRO does not. MelaPRO is free and available online (http://bcb.dfci.harvard.edu/bayesmendel/melapro.php).

CDK4 is another melanoma susceptibility gene transmitted in an autosomal dominant manner. To date, all germline mutations have been reported in the p16INK4a-binding region and specifically at Arg24. When altered, CDK4 resists p16INK4a inhibition and promotes progression through the cell cycle when complexed with cyclin D1. Germline *CDK4* mutations appear to be extremely rare [25–28]. Consistent with the common signaling pathway to which p16INK4a and CDK4 belong, the few families with *CDK4* mutations exhibit essentially the same phenotype as those with germline *p16* mutations.

The BAP1 locus. BAP1 (BRCA1-associated protein-1/ubiquitin carboxy-terminal hydrolase) is a tumor suppressor gene that has been implicated with metastatic phenotype in uveal melanomas, where 84 % of metastasizing tumors have been found to have inactivating somatic mutations [29]. Inactivating germline mutations of *BAP1* (Fig. 2) have also been linked to a new autosomal dominant syndrome consisting of multiple, pink, melanocytic neoplasms and cutaneous melanoma and with a cancer syndrome characterized by mesothelioma and uveal melanoma [30, 31]. Given the range of findings, Njauw et al. suggested that the BAP1

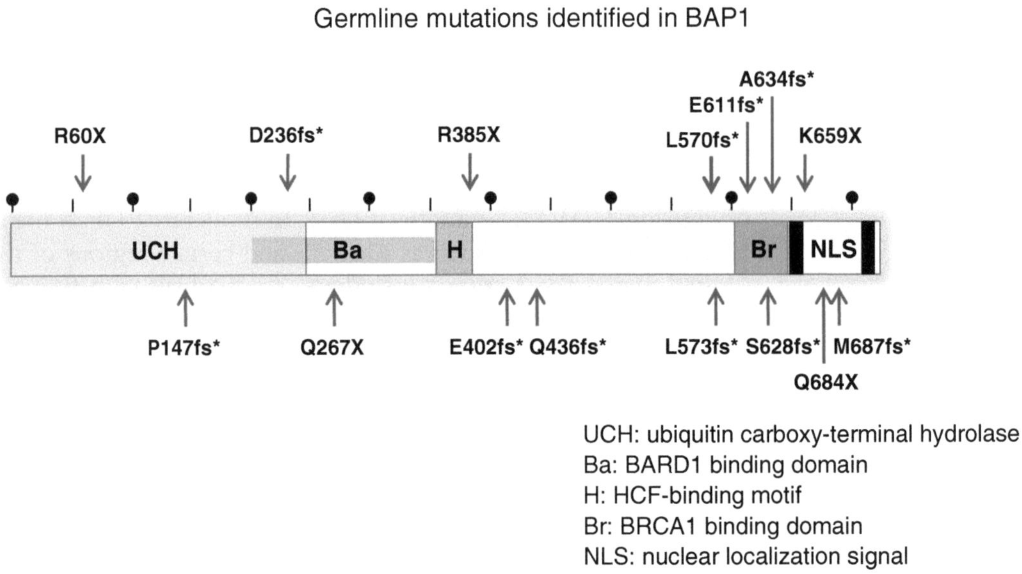

Fig. 2 Germline mutations identified in *BAP1*. BAP1 is a tumor suppressor gene with a ubiquitin carboxy-terminal hydrolase (UCH) domain. This gene has been recently associated with a cancer syndrome consisting of cutaneous/ocular melanoma, atypical melanocytic proliferations, and other internal malignancies (COMMON complex). Numerous mutations in various domains of the protein have been found to date. There appears to be a cluster of mutations in the C-terminus

phenotypic complex be termed *c*utaneous/*o*cular *m*elanoma, atypical *m*elanocytic proliferations, and *o*ther internal *n*eoplasms, such as mesothelioma (COMMON) syndrome [32, 33].

The contribution of germline *BAP1* mutations to cutaneous melanoma risk was evaluated in 200 individuals with hereditary cutaneous melanoma, 7 of which also had a family history of ocular melanoma (CM-OM families) [32]. Two out of seven (29 %) probands from the CM-OM families and 1/193 (0.52 %) probands from the CM-non-OM families showed *BAP1* mutations ($p = 0.003$). A germline *BAP1* mutation, specifically the splice variant c.1709C>G (p.Leu570fs*40), has been associated with paragangliomas in a Danish family with uveal melanoma and a variety of other tumors [34].

2.2 Low-to-Moderate-Risk Loci and Pathways

Pigmentation traits are linked to development of melanoma: fair skin, red hair, inability to tan, and tendency to freckle are phenotypic risk factors for melanoma [35, 36]. Melanin is a pigment that protects the skin from the damaging effects of ultraviolet radiation. Two types of melanin exist: eumelanin and pheomelanin. Eumelanin is responsible for constitutive pigmentation among darker skin tones. Binding of MSH ligand to the melanocytic 7-pass transmembrane receptor MC1R (Fig. 1), activates cytoplasmic adenylate cyclase, which in turn increases intracellular cyclic AMP levels [10, 37]. The increase in cAMP triggers a downstream signaling pathway that involves phosphorylation of the cAMP response element-binding protein (CREB) through protein kinase A and expression of microphthalmia transcription factor (*MITF*). MITF then drives expression of genes involved in melanin biosynthesis.

Activation of wild-type MC1R increases the proportion of eumelanin relative to pheomelanin. Individuals with germline *MC1R* variants show diminished eumelanization and increased sun sensitivity. In fact, more than 80 % of individuals with red hair or fair skin that tans poorly harbor *MC1R* variants compared to 20 % of individuals with brown or black hair [38]. The percentage is even lower, at 4 %, for individuals who show a good tanning response. These observations indicate MC1R is a regulatory checkpoint of pigmentation phenotype and an important player in the tanning response.

Certain *MC1R* variants have been associated with melanoma only (p.I155T, p.R163Q), while others have been associated with melanoma and red hair phenotype (p.D84E, p.R142H, p.R151C, p.R160W, and p.D294H), suggesting that nonpigmentary and pigmentary pathways for the increased risk of melanoma associated with *MC1R* variants exist [39, 40]. The mechanism behind the increased melanoma risk has been traditionally thought to be increased UV damage to melanocytes from low levels of photoprotective eumelanin. Although UV attenuation is clearly an important component, DNA repair is also critical as patients with xeroderma pigmentosum, a rare genodermatosis caused by enzymatic defects in the nucleotide excision repair pathway, exhibit a >1,000-fold greater risk of skin cancer, including melanoma, than the general population [41]. Although the UV-dependent mechanism of increased melanoma susceptibility is logical, recent studies indicate that pheomelanin, which accumulates in the setting of certain *MC1R* gene variants and causes the red hair/fair skin phenotype, increases the risk of melanoma in a UV-independent fashion [42].

Microphthalmia-associated transcription factor (MITF) is a crucial regulatory protein of melanocytes. It modulates a variety of genes involved in differentiation and pigmentation and it has also been found to play a role in melanoma [43]. In addition, a novel germline variant of *MITF* that predisposes to melanoma has been identified through whole-genome sequencing of probands from several families with hereditary melanoma [44]. The E318K variant showed an altered small-ubiquitin-like modifier (SUMO) motif and impaired SUMOylation at that site. Impaired SUMOylation increased the transcriptional activity of MITF, enhancing melanocyte clonogenicity, migration, and invasion; all properties associated with a malignant phenotype [45]. The mutation was also associated with multiple primary melanomas, increased nevus count, and nonblue eye color.

Table 1
SNPs associated with melanoma identified through genome-wide association studies [46]

GWAS, SNPs, and melanoma				
Chromosomal region	**Candidate gene**	**SNP**	**Minor allele frequency**	**Per-allele odds ratio (95 % CI) for risk of melanoma**
2q33-q34	*CASP8*	rs13016963	0.33	1.25 (1.07, 1.46)
5p15.33	*TERT-CLPTM1L*	rs401681	0.46	1.08 (0.93, 1.25)
5p13.2	*SLC45A2*	rs16891982	0.03	0.72 (0.44, 1.18)
6p25-p23	*IRF4*	rs12203592	0.24	0.80 (0.67, 0.95)
9p21	*CDKN2A/MTAP*	rs7023329	0.49	0.86 (0.73, 1.00)
11q14-q21	*TYR*	rs1393350	0.27	1.34 (1.14, 1.58)
11q22-q23	*ATM*	rs1801516	0.14	0.88 (0.71, 1.09)
16q24.3	*MC1R*	rs258322	0.10	1.83 (1.44, 2.32)
20q11.2-q12	*ASIP*	rs4911442	0.13	1.35 (1.08, 1.68)
21q22.3	*MX2*	rs45430	0.38	0.90 (0.77, 1.05)
22q13.1	*PLA2G6*	rs6001027	0.37	0.78 (0.66, 0.91)

2.3 Additional Loci from Genome-Wide Association Studies (GWAS)

A number of genome-wide association studies have identified new, low-risk, melanoma susceptibility loci (Table 1). These include single nucleotide polymorphisms (SNPs) at *ATM*, *MX2*, and *CASP8* [46]; variants at the 1q21.3 locus (possible candidates in this region include *ARNT* and *SETDB1*) [47, 48]; SNPs at *MTAP* (a gene adjacent to *CDKN2A* on 9p21) and *PLA2G6* on 22q13.1 [49]; and SNPs at *TYR* [50].

3 Risk Assessment and Management

3.1 Risk Assessment

Families suggestive of a hereditary melanoma syndrome should be referred for genetic counseling and risk assessment. The risk assessment process should include at minimum a 3-generation pedigree, recording each individual's age or age at death and information regarding cancer diagnoses, including the type of cancer and age at diagnosis. Whenever possible, medical records should be obtained to confirm cancer diagnoses. The pedigree should be comprised of affected and unaffected relatives. In addition, ethnicity should be recorded as well as any other pertinent factors, such as sun exposure or smoking history.

3.2 Risk Assessment Tools

As germline *CDKN2A* mutations are the most commonly known, high penetrance mutations associated with hereditary melanoma; efforts to estimate hereditary melanoma risk have focused on the development of tools to assess the probability that an individual carries germline *CDKN2A* mutations. Two models currently exist: MELPREDICT, which relies on a logistic regression model, and MelaPRO, which integrates Mendelian inheritance and Bayesian probability theories [24, 51]. MelaPRO outperforms MELPREDICT in estimating carrier probability. Furthermore, it also estimates the future risk of melanoma in unaffected individuals. To use MelaPRO, the individual's detailed family and past medical history of melanoma is entered into the program. MelaPRO then provides a carrier probability and an estimate of the future risk of developing melanoma if the proband is free of the disease at the time of genetic counseling. MelaPRO's flexible platform allows for assimilation of future biological information to achieve improved risk assessment. However, it is important to note that this model does not incorporate pancreatic cancer as a risk factor for *CDKN2A* mutations. While MelaPRO is a useful program for assessing *CDKN2A* mutation probability in families with melanoma, it is important to note that other hereditary syndromes also contain melanoma as a component feature. Therefore, when reviewing a family history it is important to consider all cancer diagnoses in the assessment. MelaPRO can be accessed online (http://www4.utsouthwestern.edu/breasthealth/cagene/).

3.3 Management of Familial Melanoma

The American Society of Clinical Oncology (ASCO) provides guidelines to cancer specialists regarding the use of genetic testing for cancer susceptibility [52]. Genetic testing should be considered when a patient has a personal or family history of cancer suggestive of an underlying hereditary component, the test can be adequately interpreted, and the results will guide diagnosis and management. Furthermore, prior to testing, the patient should be provided with genetic counseling, which should also include pre- and posttest counseling and risk assessment, with discussion of risks and benefits of genetic testing, including the likelihood of detecting a cancer susceptibility mutation, the potential impact on medical management, the psychological implications of testing, possible effects on family members and relationships, and concerns regarding confidentiality and insurance coverage.

The advantage of genetic testing and risk assessment is tangible in the setting of high-penetrance mutations for which tests provide clinical utility. In other words, a genetic test is advantageous if it accurately identifies mutations that increase the risk of cancer development to such an extent as to warrant the implementation of validated strategies, which can be in the form of preventive medical or surgical interventions, behavioral changes, or heightened screening, to reduce that risk. Tests for mutations of low or uncertain risk and tests that will not guide management of a genetic condition lack sufficient benefit to be endorsed. The disadvantages of clinically ambiguous test results include unjustified alarm, unnecessary screening and preventive care, and false reassurance.

No widely accepted guidelines for the management of families with hereditary risk of melanoma exist. The Melanoma Genetics Consortium, however, concluded that under most circumstances clinical genetic testing for *CDKN2A* mutations in families at risk of hereditary melanoma or in individuals with multiple primary melanomas should be considered with caution in part because of its uncertain clinical utility [53, 54]. Even so, some clinicians advocate management schemes for families with confirmed or high suspicion for *CDKN2A*-mutated hereditary melanoma under special circumstances [55]. In moderate to high melanoma incidence regions, families with at least three relatives afflicted with melanoma on the same side of the family, multiple primary melanomas, or a family history that includes both melanoma and pancreatic cancer should be offered formal genetic counseling and the opportunity to participate in research protocols. Through the genetic counseling process, they should also be informed of all aspects of *CDKN2A* genetic testing, including the risks, benefits, and limitations, such as uncertain clinical utility of the test. Individuals with a known *CDKN2A* mutation should be referred for heightened screening in the form of skin examinations every 3–6 months with a health professional trained to recognize the features of early melanoma. Referral to a gastroenterologist for pancreatic cancer screening under certain circumstances, such as known *CDKN2A* mutation and a family history of pancreatic cancer, should be discussed with the patient. It is important to note, however, that the effectiveness of pancreatic surveillance for individuals at increased risk of pancreatic cancer remains under investigation. Individuals who have not pursued genetic testing or are negative for a *CDKN2A* mutation may still be at increased risk of melanoma due to other cryptic high-risk alleles and should be monitored accordingly based on personal and/or family history. Finally, individuals who are found to have a variant of uncertain significance in the *CDKN2A* gene should also be monitored for cancer as dictated by personal and family history [56]. *BAP1* testing constitutes an area of future investigation as its benefits are currently unknown.

4 Conclusions

An understanding of the genetic basis for melanoma will allow for earlier identification of high-risk individuals and, over time, a potentially useful means of stratifying preventive strategies. Familial melanoma accounts for approximately a tenth of all melanoma cases. Traditional positional and candidate approaches have been useful in uncovering high-risk susceptibility genes including *CDKN2A*, *CDK4*, and *BAP1*. A recent explosion in genome-wide approaches has added insight into the heritable factors that contribute to sporadic melanoma. Genetic loci involved in the regulation of pigmentation appear to be front-and-center to melanoma risk at the individual level.

Although multiple melanoma susceptibility genes have been identified, risk assessment tools have been developed only for the most common gene, *CDKN2A*. MelaPRO, a validated model that relies on Mendelian inheritance and Bayesian probability theories, estimates carrier probability for *CDKN2A* and future risk of melanoma taking into account a patient's family and past medical history of melanoma. Genetic testing for *CDKN2A* mutations is currently available but the Melanoma Genetics Consortium recommends offering such testing to patients only in the context of research protocols in part due to the uncertain clinical utility.

Acknowledgements

Supervision of this scholarly activity was made possible by a grant from NIH to H.T. (K24 CA149202).

References

1. Goldstein AM, Tucker MA (2004) Familial melanoma and its management. In: Eeles R, Easton D, Eng C, Ponder B (eds) Genetic predisposition to cancer, 2nd edn. Arnold Publishers Ltd, London
2. Kamb A, Shattuck-Eidens D, Eeles R et al (1994) Analysis of the p16 gene (CDKN2A) as a candidate for the chromosome 9p melanoma susceptibility locus. Nat Genet 8:23–26
3. Hussussian CJ, Struewing JP, Goldstein AM et al (1994) Germline p16 mutations in familial melanoma. Nat Genet 8:15–21
4. Goldstein AM, Tucker MA (2001) Genetic epidemiology of cutaneous melanoma: a global perspective. Arch Dermatol 137:1493–1496
5. Goldstein AM, Chan M, Harland M et al (2007) Features associated with germline CDKN2A mutations: a GenoMEL study of melanoma-prone families from three continents. J Med Genet 44:99–106
6. Hashemi J, Platz A, Ueno T et al (2000) CDKN2A germ-line mutations in individuals with multiple cutaneous melanomas. Cancer Res 60:6864–6867
7. Monzon J, Liu L, Brill H et al (1998) CDKN2A mutations in multiple primary melanomas. N Engl J Med 338:879–887
8. Koh J, Enders GH, Dynlacht BD et al (1995) Tumour-derived p16INK4a alleles encoding proteins defective in cell-cycle inhibition. Nature 375:506–510
9. Lukas J, Parry D, Aagaard L et al (1995) Retinoblastoma-protein-dependent cell-cycle inhibition by the tumour suppressor p16. Nature 375:503–506
10. Tsao H, Chin L, Garraway LA et al (2012) Melanoma: from mutations to medicine. Genes Dev 26(11):1131–1135
11. Udayakumar D, Mahato B, Gabree M et al (2010) Genetic determinants of cutaneous melanoma predisposition. Semin Cutan Med Surg 29(3):190–195
12. Pomerantz J, Schreiber-Agus N, Liegeois NJ et al (1998) The Ink4a tumor suppressor gene product, p19Arf, interacts with MDM2 and neutralizes MDM2's inhibition of p53. Cell 92:713–723
13. Stott FJ, Bates S, James MC et al (1998) The alternative product from the human CDKN2A locus, p14(ARF), participates in a regulatory feedback loop with p53 and MDM2. EMBO J 17:5001–5014
14. Zhang Y, Xiong Y, Yarbrough WG et al (1998) ARF promotes MDM2 degradation and stabilizes p53: ARF-INK4a locus deletion impairs both the Rb and p53 tumor suppression pathways. Cell 92:725–734
15. Bishop DT, Demenais F, Goldstein AM et al (2002) Geographical variation in the penetrance of CDKN2A mutations for melanoma. J Natl Cancer Inst 19:894–903
16. Begg CB, Orlow I, Hummer AJ et al (2005) Lifetime risk of melanoma in CDKN2A mutation

carriers in a population-based sample. J Natl Cancer Inst 97(20):1507–1515
17. Whiteman DC, Milligan A, Welch J et al (1997) Germline CDKN2A mutations in childhood melanoma. J Natl Cancer Inst 89:1460
18. Tsao H, Zhang X, Kwitkiwski K et al (2000) Low prevalence of germline CDKN2A and CDK4 mutations in patients with early-onset melanoma. Arch Dermatol 136:1118–1122
19. Foulkes WD, Flanders TY, Pollock PM et al (1997) The CDKN2A (p16) gene and human cancer. Mol Med 3(1):5–20
20. Tucker MA, Halpern A, Holly EA et al (1997) Clinically recognized dysplastic nevi. A central risk factor for cutaneous melanoma. JAMA 277:1439–1444
21. Puig S, Ruiz A, Castel T et al (1997) Inherited susceptibility to several cancers but absence of linkage between dysplastic nevus syndrome and CDKN2A in a melanoma family with a mutation in the CDKN2A (P16INK4A) gene. Hum Genet 101:359–364
22. Goldstein AM, Fraser MC, Struewing JP et al (1995) Increased risk of pancreatic cancer in melanoma-prone kindreds with p16INK4 mutations. N Engl J Med 333:970–974
23. Leachman SA, Carucci J, Kohlman W et al (2009) Selection criteria for genetic assessment of patients with melanoma. J Am Acad Dermatol 61(4):677
24. Wang W, Niendorf KB, Patel D et al (2010) Estimating CDKN2A carrier probability and personalizing cancer risk assessments in hereditary melanoma using MelaPRO. Cancer Res 70(2):552–559
25. Nikolaou V, Kang X, Stratigos A et al (2011) Comprehensive mutational analysis of CDKN2A and CDK4 in Greek patients with cutaneous melanoma. Br J Dermatol 165(6): 1219–1222
26. Zuo L, Weger J, Yang Q et al (1996) Germline mutations in p16INK4a binding domain of *CDK4* in familial melanoma. Nat Genet 12:97–99
27. Fitzgerald MG, Harkin DP, Silva-Arrieta S et al (1996) Prevalence of germline mutations in p16, p19ARF, and CDK4 in familial melanoma: analysis of a clinic-based population. Proc Natl Acad Sci 93:8541–8545
28. Soufir N, Avril MF, Chompret A et al (1998) Prevalence of p16 and CDK4 germline mutations in 48 melanoma-prone families in France. The French Familial Melanoma Study Group. Hum Mol Genet 7:209–216
29. Harbour JW, Onken MD, Roberson ED et al (2010) Frequent mutation of BAP1 in metastasizing uveal melanomas. Science 330(6009):1410–1413
30. Wiesner T, Obenauf AC, Murali R et al (2011) Germline mutations in BAP1 predispose to melanocytic tumors. Nat Genet 43(10):1018–1021
31. Testa JR, Cheung M, Pei J et al (2011) Germline BAP1 mutations predispose to malignant mesothelioma. Nat Genet 43(10): 1022–1025
32. Njauw CN, Kim I, Piris A et al (2012) Germline BAP1 inactivation is preferentially associated with metastatic ocular melanoma and cutaneous-ocular melanoma families. PLoS One 7(4):e35295
33. Carbone M, Korb FL, Baumann F et al (2012) BAP1 cancer syndrome: malignant mesothelioma, uveal and cutaneous melanoma, and MBAITs. J Transl Med 10(1):179
34. Wadt K, Choi J, Chung JY et al (2012) A cryptic BAP1 splice mutation in a family with uveal and cutaneous melanoma, and paraganglioma. Pigment Cell Melanoma Res. doi:10.1111/pcmr.12006
35. Gandini S, Sera F, Cattaruzza MS et al (2005) Meta-analysis of risk factors for cutaneous melanoma. I. Common and atypical naevi. Eur J Cancer 41:28–44
36. Gandini S, Sera F, Cattaruzza MS et al (2005) Meta-analysis of risk factors for cutaneous melanoma. III. Family history, actinic damage, and phenotypic factors. Eur J Cancer 41:2040–2059
37. Miller AJ, Tsao H (2010) New insights into pigmentary pathways and skin cancer. Br J Dermatol 162(1):22–28
38. Valverde F, Healy E, Jackson I et al (1995) Variants of the melanocyte-stimulating hormone receptor gene are associated with red hair and fair skin in humans. Nat Genet 11:328–330
39. Kennedy C, ter Huurne J, Berkhout M et al (2001) Melanocortin 1 receptor (*MC1R*) gene variants are associated with an increased risk of cutaneous melanoma which is largely independent of skin type and hair color. J Invest Dermatol 117:294–300
40. Raimondi S, Sera F, Gandini S et al (2008) MC1R variants, melanoma, and red hair color phenotype: a meta-analysis. Int J Cancer 122: 2753–2760
41. Kraemer KH, Lee MM, Andrews AD et al (1994) The role of sunlight and DNA repair in melanoma and nonmelanoma skin cancer. The xeroderma pigmentosum paradigm. Arch Dermatol 130(8):1018–1021
42. Mitra D, Luo X, Wargo J et al (2011) Why redheads are at increased risk of melanoma: a novel BRAF mutant mouse model. Pigm Cell Melanoma R 24:1016

43. Levy C, Khaled M, Fisher DE et al (2006) MITF: master regulator of melanocyte development and melanoma oncogene. Trends Mol Med 12(9):406–413
44. Yokoyama S, Woods S, Boyle GM et al (2011) A novel recurrent mutation in *MITF* predisposes to familial and sporadic melanoma. Nature 480:99–103
45. Bertolotto C, Lesueur F, Giuliano S et al (2011) A SUMOylation-defective MITF germline mutation predisposes to melanoma and renal carcinoma. Nature 480:94–98
46. Barrett JH, Iles MM, Harland M et al (2011) Genome-wide association study identifies three new melanoma susceptibility loci. Nat Genet 43(11):1108–1113
47. Amos CI, Wang LE, Lee JE et al (2011) Genome-wide association study identifies novel loci predisposing to cutaneous melanoma. Hum Mol Genet 20(24):5012–5023
48. Macgregor S, Montgomery GW, Liu JZ et al (2011) Genome-wide association study identifies a new melanoma susceptibility locus at 1q21.3. Nat Genet 43(11):1114–1118
49. Falchi M, Bataille V, Hayward NK et al (2009) Genome-wide association study identifies variants at 9p21 and 22q13 associated with development of cutaneous nevi. Nat Genet 41(8):915–919
50. Bishop DT, Demenais F, Iles MM et al (2009) Genome-wide association study identifies three loci associated with melanoma risk. Nat Genet 41(8):920–925
51. Niendorf KB, Goggins W, Yang G et al (2006) MELPREDICT: a logistic regression model to estimate CDKN2A carrier probability. J Med Genet 43:501–506
52. Robson ME, Storm CD, Weitzel J et al (2010) Policy statement update: genetic and genomic testing for cancer susceptibility. J Clin Oncol 28:893–901
53. Kefford R, Bishop JN, Tucker M et al (2002) Genetic testing for melanoma. Lancet Oncol 3:653–654
54. Kefford RF, Newton Bishop JA, Bergman W et al (1999) Counseling and DNA testing for individuals perceived to be genetically predisposed to melanoma: a consensus statement of the Melanoma Genetics Consortium. J Clin Oncol 17:3245–3251
55. Niendorf KB, Tsao H (2006) Cutaneous melanoma: family screening and genetic testing. Dermatol Ther 19:1–8
56. Rulyak SJ, Kimmey MB, Veenstra DL et al (2003) Cost-effectiveness of pancreatic cancer screening in familial pancreatic cancer kindreds. Gastrointest Endosc 57:23–29

Part IV

Uveal Melanoma

Chapter 21

Clinical, Pathologic, and Imaging Features and Biological Markers of Uveal Melanoma

Alia B. Rashid and Hans E. Grossniklaus

Abstract

Uveal melanoma has unique clinical and pathologic features including virtually exclusive metastasis to the liver in high-risk cases. In this chapter, the clinical findings in uveal melanoma and diagnostic methods including imaging tests and serum markers are described. Additionally, the histopathologic features including the modified Callender classification and immunohistochemical findings of uveal melanoma are described.

Key words Uveal melanoma, Clinical features, Histopathology, Biological markers, Imaging, Prognosis

1 Introduction

Uveal melanoma affects the uveal tissues of the eye—namely, the iris, ciliary body, and choroid. Over 90 % of all uveal melanomas (UM) involve the choroid [1]. A recent study of 8,033 cases of uveal melanoma revealed that based on age (young, mid adults, and older adults) at presentation, the tumor center was located in iris (21, 4, 2 %; $P<0.0001$), ciliary body (8, 5, and 7 %; $P=0.0225$), or choroid (7, 91, and 90 %; $P<0.0001$) [2]. UM is the most common primary intraocular malignancy in adults [3]. Approximately 1,200–1,500 new cases are diagnosed each year in the United States, and UM accounts for about 5 % of all melanomas [3]. The mean age-adjusted incidence of uveal melanoma in the United States was 5.1 per million (95 % CI, 4.8–5.3) [4]. The incidence in light-skinned (non-Hispanic) Caucasians has been reported as between 8 and 196 times greater than that in African races [3, 5–7]. Known risk factors for UM include light skin color, cutaneous freckles and nevi, red or blonde hair, and light-colored irides [8–10]. Unlike in cutaneous melanoma, the link between UM and increased sun exposure or UV light is not clear cut. An association between sunlight or UV light exposure and UM has been made by some studies [9, 11], while more recently it was shown that the rates of

Magdalena Thurin and Francesco M. Marincola (eds.), *Molecular Diagnostics for Melanoma: Methods and Protocols*, Methods in Molecular Biology, vol. 1102, DOI 10.1007/978-1-62703-727-3_21, © Springer Science+Business Media New York 2014

UM have not increased over the past several decades, unlike the rates of cutaneous melanoma, in response to increased UV light exposure [12]. Males seem to be affected slightly more than females [4, 7], and a study by Bergman et al. [13] showed that the peak incidence for females occurs almost a decade earlier than in males. Older patients have a significantly worse survival rate [14]. Approximately 50 % of patients diagnosed with uveal melanoma will die as a result of hematogenous spread of metastases, most commonly to the liver [15, 16]. The tumor burden from metastases to the liver is typically high by the time of detection through abnormal liver function tests (LFTs) or imaging studies [17]. The median survival time following the detection of metastatic disease is extremely poor, ranging from 2 months to about 1 year, despite improvements in treatment for local uveal melanoma [18–20]. At this time there are no effective treatments for metastatic uveal melanoma; however several therapies are clinically in use or under investigation in multicenter clinical trials, so the importance of accurate prognostication in order to give patients the best chance of survival has never been higher. Early diagnosis of UM is important not only because it may improve the chance of survival through prevention of metastasis by appropriate intervention or therapy, but also because it will allow patients more time to arrange their medical care or make important life decisions.

2 Clinical and Histologic Features

There are several well-established guidelines for the staging of histopathology specimens from eyes with suspected uveal melanoma. These include the system used by the Collaborative Ocular Melanoma Study (COMS) group and the American Joint Committee on Cancer (AJCC) TNM staging system (Table 1).

The first histological classification system for uveal melanomas was devised by Callender in 1931, and this was then further modified in 1983 by McLean et al. to improve prognostic classification [22]. The AJCC has utilized the modified Callender system and adapted this to define the TNM staging system for uveal melanoma [23]. The College of American Pathologists has taken this classification system a step further, to incorporate all clinical and histopathological data, in order to provide the most accurate prognostic classification system to date [24]. There are several key clinical and histopathological observations that are most useful in determining the outcome of a diagnosis of uveal melanoma. The features that correlate with a poor prognosis include a larger tumor basal diameter, ciliary involvement, extrascleral extension, an epithelioid cell type, mean diameter of the ten largest nucleoli (MLN), presence of mitotic figures, presence of lymphocytic infiltrates, and architecture of the microcirculation [25–28].

Table 1

Summary of high-risk clinical and histologic features for uveal melanoma metastasis and disease-related mortality [21]

Clinical features	Histologic features
Older age	Epithelioid cell type
Large tumor basal diameter	High mitotic rate
Tumor thickness	Closed PAS-positive loops
Ciliary body involvement	Mean diameter of ten largest nucleoli
Extraocular extension	Degree of pigmentation
Diffuse growth pattern	Inflammation
Ring melanoma	Vascular invasion
Optic nerve involvement	Tumor necrosis

2.1 Clinical High-Risk Features

2.1.1 Older Age

Age is a factor that has been presented as both a valuable and significant high-risk prognosticator for death as well as being purported to be of no significance in outcome from diagnosis of UM [14, 16, 25, 29]. The English literature reports the median age at diagnosis of UM to range between 57 and 64 years of age [16]. An explanation for this controversy may lie in the mistaken reporting of the cause of death in patients diagnosed with UM when considering that older patients may have other comorbidities which may contribute to or mask the actual cause of death. It is also important to consider the potential for a lead-time bias, whereby older patients may have had a UM present in the eye for longer, giving a greater chance for greater LTD, extraocular extension (EOE), or metastasis [30].

2.1.2 Largest Tumor Diameter

Numerous studies cite the largest basal tumor diameter (LTD) as the best predictor of metastatic disease [15, 20, 31–33]. It is the most widely used clinical factor used for prognostication, partly because it has been shown to correlate with extraocular spread and the likelihood of recurrence in the eye [34, 35]. A 2009 study by Damato et al. investigated the significance of LTD in posterior uveal melanoma in correlation with histologic and cytogenetic predictors and mortality [30]. This study involved a large cohort of 1,776 patients with posterior UM and found that metastatic death correlated with LTD ($P<0.001$). Using multivariate Cox analysis, they found a significant correlation between metastatic death and several histopathologic and cytogenetic factors: largest basal tumor diameter ($P<0.001$), epithelioid cells ($P=0.009$), high mitotic rate ($P<0.001$), closed connective tissue loops ($P<0.001$), and chromosome 3 loss ($P<0.001$). The prevalence of these risk factors was stratified according to the largest basal tumor diameter and found that predictors of metastatic death were more prevalent in tumors with a greater LTD and subsequently that there was an inverse correlation between LTD size and survival time. They postulated that this inverse relationship may be because tumors with greater LTD had been present for longer, thus introducing a lead-time bias, or that due to a high mitotic rate in more aggressive tumors the doubling time may have been shorter. This study supports the hypothesis that uveal melanomas are larger at the time of diagnosis because of their aggressiveness and not vice versa. The same study found that LTD also correlated with reduced survival times in patients reported to have died from other conditions ($P = 0.01$), possibly through mistaken reporting of the cause of death, or that older patients tended to have tumors with greater LTD (t-test, $P < 0.001$).

2.1.3 Tumor Thickness

The majority of studies looking at prognostic factors for UM have used either tumor thickness or largest tumor basal diameter in their models for estimating prognosis [15, 36]. Despite using various measurements, all have shown that tumor size has a significant prognostic effect on morbidity and mortality. The COMS group found that echographic measurements of tumor thickness (apical height) were found to be concordant to within 2 mm of histopathological measurements, 90 % of the time [37]. A recent study to determine the rate of metastasis according to tumor thickness in 8,033 cases of uveal melanoma provides the most precise measurement correlations [38]. In order to avoid complications from the use of artificial size measurements, i.e., small, medium, and large, the tumor thickness was measured exactly in millimeters, using ultrasonographic calipers. Using multivariate analysis, tumor thickness was found to be a significant predictive factor of metastasis, with each millimeter increase in thickness imparting a 1.06 hazard ratio. The exception to this finding was for melanomas less than 1 mm in thickness in the iris or 2 mm in the ciliary body and choroid, which had a slightly higher risk of metastasis than those with a greater thickness, most likely due to the inclusion of diffuse melanoma within that bracket. The rate of metastasis at 10 years ranged from 6 % (0–1.0 mm thickness) to 51 % (>10 mm thickness).

2.1.4 Ciliary Body Involvement

Uveal melanomas that involve the ciliary body appear to have greater mortality rates than those that do not involve the ciliary body. There are several factors to consider in trying to explain this outcome. Firstly, the location of a uveal melanoma that involves the ciliary body—if it originates close to the ciliary body it is unlikely to cause visual symptoms until it is of considerable size, and if the tumor originates in the choroid it usually has to have grown to a large size in order to involve the ciliary body. Either way, tumors that involve the ciliary body tend to be larger when they are diagnosed, and this factor significantly affects mortality rates [32, 33]. Secondly, the route of extraocular spread of melanoma from the ciliary body is the aqueous channels, and a study by Coupland et al. found that spread of UM via aqueous channels occurred in 29.8 % of metastatic cases [35]. McLean et al. [39] performed a multivariate survival analysis for choroidal-ciliary body melanomas using both Kaplan–Meier and univariate Cox analyses and found that there was a significant association between involvement of the ciliary body and mortality rates. However, the use of multivariate Cox and Gamel–Boag models revealed that ciliary body involvement was no longer significant. Importantly, they found that UM with ciliary body involvement were significantly more likely to be of a mixed cell type, with larger nucleoli, and have a larger tumor base, all factors which are associated with higher mortality.

2.1.5 Extraocular Extension

In eyes that have been enucleated, EOE of UM is found in approximately 13 % of cases [16, 20, 40]. Several studies have shown a poorer prognosis for UM with EOE, attributing this outcome to increased malignancy of the tumor [16, 40] and specifically to an association with the presence of histopathologic features of malignancy [41]. The size of the extraocular tumor has been associated with increased mortality and orbital recurrence as its dimensions increase [40, 41]. There are several possible routes for EOE of UM, including the aqueous drainage channels of Schlemm's canal, the anterior and posterior ciliary arteries, the four vortex veins, the long and short ciliary nerves, the optic nerve, and finally, direct scleral perforation. A study by Zografos reported that spread of UM along vortex veins was the only route of EOE that predicted increased metastatic mortality. A 2008 study by Coupland investigated the routes of EOE in UM [35]. A review of the histopathological and cytogenetic analysis of 847 patients with UM who were treated by enucleation found that EOE was present in 124 (14.6 %) patients. Of those, spread of UM via aqueous channels occurred in 29.8 %, ciliary arteries in 27.4 %, vortex veins in 18.5 %, ciliary nerves in 8.8 %, optic nerve in 0.8 %, and a variety of combinations of these routes in 10.4 %. By taking histopathologic evaluation into account, it was found that EOE correlated strongly with large basal tumor diameter ($P<0.001$), anterior tumor extension/angle involvement ($P<0.001$), epithelioid cellularity ($P=0.002$), and closed connective tissue loops ($P=0.002$). Cytogenetics revealed a strong correlation with monosomy 3 ($P=0.001$). A log rank analysis showed that EOE correlated with metastatic death independently of the route of spread, and a multivariate Cox analysis revealed this correlation to be statistically significant ($P<0.001$) yet still weaker than those for metastatic death and epithelioid cells, mitotic rate, closed connective tissue loops, or largest basal tumor diameter. Importantly, the size of the extraocular tumor was not

Table 2
Significance of routes of EOE

Route of EOE	$N=124$ total (%)	Correlation with histopathologic findings	Correlation with clinical findings
Aqueous channels	37 (29.8 %)	Inverse correlation with largest basal tumor diameter ($P=0.005$) and tumor height ($P<0.001$)	Angle involvement ($P<0.001$)
Ciliary arteries	34 (27.4 %)	Posterior tumor extension to the disc ($P=0.008$)	Nasal tumor location ($P=0.002$)
Vortex veins	28 (18.5 %)	Large basal tumor diameter ($P<0.001$)	Ciliary body involvement ($P=0.001$) and weak correlation with sagittal tumor location ($P=0.03$)
Ciliary nerves	11 (8.9 %)	Large basal tumor diameter ($P=0.002$) and weak correlation with mitotic rate ($P=0.03$)	–
Optic nerve	1 (0.8 %)	Large basal tumor diameter ($P=0.002$) and weak correlation with mitotic rate ($P=0.03$)	–
Combination of routes	13 (10.4 %)	–	–

Adapted from a study by Coupland et al. [35]

found to be significant ($P=0.1$). These findings indicate that the route of EOE is dependent on the UM location, as previously suggested by other studies, and that extraocular spread is an indicator of greater malignancy and intraocular tumor size rather than being a cause of systemic metastasis (Table 2).

2.1.6 Diffuse Pattern

A diffuse pattern in uveal melanoma is rare and represents only about 5 % of posterior uveal melanomas [42, 43]. These lesions typically are minimally elevated, with a predominantly horizontal growth pattern and a large basal tumor diameter. The diffuse-type tumors have been associated with high-risk features such as epithelioid cell type and EOE, which inevitably leads to a poor prognosis [42, 43]. Another reason for the poorer prognosis of this type of UM is that it is difficult to diagnose clinically, resulting in frequent misdiagnosis and delayed diagnosis. A 1968 study by Font [42] found that the diagnosis of choroidal melanoma was not suspected at the time of enucleation in 40 % of cases with the most common misdiagnoses being glaucoma, retinal detachment, choroidal nevus, or chronic uveitis. It has also been misdiagnosed as many other lesions including serous retinal detachment, scleritis, and central serous chorioretinopathy [44, 45]. The earlier that a correct diagnosis can be made, the better the chances of survival for the patient.

Key clinical signs that can arouse suspicion for the diagnosis of a diffuse uveal melanoma are tumor thickness ≥2 mm, location near the optic disc, the presence of lipofuscin or subretinal fluid, or complaints of symptoms such as pain or blurring of vision [46]. A study by Shields et al. [47] of 111 cases of diffuse UM found that the clinical findings that could predict metastatic disease by both univariate and multivariate analysis were LTD ≥18 mm, optic nerve invasion, and poorly defined tumor margins. Univariate analysis also found transcleral extension to be a significant prognostic factor. Additionally, they found that the probability of metastatic disease developing was 16 % at 3 years, 24 % at 5 years, and 36 % at 10 years post diagnosis, using Kaplan–Meier survival estimates. LTD showed the most significant increase in the risk of metastatic disease development, with a 1 mm increase in basal diameter equating to a relative risk increase of 1.172.

2.1.7 Ring Melanoma

Ring melanoma is a very rare variant of UM where the tumor is often found to be a circumferential growth around the eye. It involves the ciliary body and is usually quite advanced at the time of diagnosis [48]. This is usually due to the fact that the patients have few symptoms, but when they do, most typically complain of blurred vision which is then improved by refractive lenses and dismissed. The blurring of vision is likely to be a result of the compressive effects of the ring of tumor subluxating the lens. Other symptoms of ring melanoma, such as increased or decreased intraocular pressure, retinal or choroidal detachments and choroidal effusions, episcleral sentinel vessels, shallowing of the anterior chamber, and lens changes, can often confuse the clinical picture, leading to delayed or misdiagnosis [49–51]. A study by Demirci [52] of 8,800 patients with UM found only 0.3 % to have a diagnosis of ring melanoma of the ciliary body, and of these 42 % were missed at initial presentation. The main visual symptom was blurred vision, found in three-quarters of the patients with ring melanoma, with the rest being asymptomatic. Transillumination was blocked, ultrasound examination revealed hollowness with intrinsic pulsations in all cases, multilobulated masses were found in 83 %, and episcleral sentinel vessels were found in 74 %; these findings can be crucial in differentiating ring melanoma from simulating conditions. Only 30 % of cases had complete circumferential invasion of the ciliary body. Mixed-cell type predominated (74 %).

2.1.8 Optic Nerve Involvement

The rate of infiltration of the optic nerve by UM has been quoted as between 0.6 and 5 % of cases of UM [53–55]. There is an association with juxtapapillary location, non-spindle cell type, high intraocular pressure, and blindness [53–55]. Recently, large basal tumor diameter was found to be a highly statistically significant risk factor for optic nerve spread, and a weaker correlation was found with mitotic rate [35]. The study by Lindegaard et al. [54] reviewed

2,758 cases of UM and found optic nerve involvement in 5.7 %, of which just over half were confined to the prelaminar or laminar part of the optic nerve, the rest invading to postlaminar locations. Interestingly, they found that the mean age of patients with postlaminar invasion was significantly older than those with prelaminar or laminar invasion (70 years vs. 63 years). They also noted that postlaminar patients had significantly lower visual acuities (light perception or no light perception), higher intraocular pressures (>24 mmHg), larger tumor basal diameters (>15 mm), and an increased chance of EOE and recurrence when compared to cases with prelaminar and laminar optic nerve invasion. Juxtapapillary location was significantly associated with prelaminar or laminar location. In addition, it was found that all patients in the study who had optic nerve invasion also had CNS metastases, possibly due to seeding through the cerebrospinal fluid following postlaminar invasion by the tumor. When looking at mortality (all cause vs. melanoma related) in a univariate model, a significant difference was found between patients with postlaminar invasion and prelaminar/laminar invasion or controls. This may be because the patients with postlaminar invasion were older than patients in the other groups, with larger tumors and an increased frequency of recurrence. Prelaminar/laminar invasion-related mortality did not show any significant differences when compared to controls. However optic nerve invasion was not found to be a significant factor in survival when it was included in a multivariate analysis [32].

2.2 Histological High-Risk Features

2.2.1 Cell Type

McLean et al. developed the modified Callender system to categorize cell types in uveal melanoma [22]. They differentiated four cell types—spindle cell nevus, spindle cell melanoma (consisting of either spindle A or B cells), epithelioid cell melanoma, and mixed-cell melanoma.

Spindle cells are typically well-differentiated melanocytes, most often seen in small tumors in the early stages of disease. These cells have long, oval-shaped nuclei, which may contain nucleoli, and are highly cohesive and fusiform in shape. Epithelioid cells on the other hand are generally poorly differentiated melanocytes. They appear as large, polyhedral cells, with abundant cytoplasm and large round-to-oval nuclei with prominent nucleoli and can occasionally appear as multinucleated cells. They lack cohesion and are typically spaced far apart in the tumor architecture. They have a more pleomorphic appearance than spindle cells do and are seen more frequently in large tumors, indicating the more aggressive nature of the tumor. Mixed-cell melanomas are composed of both spindle and epithelioid cell types. According to COMS if less than one-half of the tumor is composed of epithelioid cells, then it is considered a mixed-cell tumor. The importance of cell type in a melanoma has been strongly linked to tumor growth and mortality rates. McLean et al. found that independent of tumor size, cell type was a significant prognostic indicator for mortality. The mortality rates for spindle cell type vs. epithelioid cell type in small tumors (<10 mm) were 6.5 and 47 %, respectively, and for larger tumors, the mortality rates were 18 and 64 %, respectively [56]. Epithelioid cell type has also been found to be a predictor for recurrence following local transcleral resection of UM [57].

2.2.2 Mean Diameter of the Ten Largest Nucleoli (MLN)

The Callender classification includes the MLN in its assessment of prognostic outcome from UM. Some studies have postulated that MLN can be replicated more consistently than the assignment of tumor cell type from the modified Callender classification [58].

The mean diameter of the ten largest nucleoli (MLN) is a value derived by measuring the largest diameter of the nucleoli of tumor cells on cross section cut from an FFPE tumor tissue sample. The method used has varied from observation of the cells at 1,000× through to 3,000× in different studies and measuring the largest dimension either at the microscope or on a digitized image [58–61]. The method itself requires an experienced observer, but when considering the variability in the methods used to obtain this value it can be seen that there may be considerable inter-observer variability, and as a result, the MLN has been touted as both a significant factor associated with a poorer prognosis [58, 61] and in other studies as an insignificant prognostic indicator [59, 60].

Pe'er et al. [60] tested both the intra- and inter-observer reproducibility of this technique using two observers. They found a statistically significant difference between the inter-observer MLN values but noted a weakly statistically significant association between the measurement sets. Intra-observer values showed a high degree of agreement. When they attempted to draw correlations between MLN and other variables (LTD, mitotic figures, age), no significant correlations were found. Similarly, analysis using both univariate and multivariate analysis of MLN in Cox models found that MLN had no significant prognostic predictive value on time to death or outcome after enucleation. Coleman et al. [59] tried to determine the most significant and reproducible cytomorphometric nuclear variables and similarly concluded that MLN was not significant in either univariate or multivariate Cox analyses, although the univariate analysis did show a trend toward significance. They did however find a strong correlation for MLN with Callender cell type ($p < 0.0007$).

In contrast to these findings, Gamel et al. [62] had compared the relative value of MLN with other covariable factors in assessing prognostic outcome, finding that with a univariate analysis Cox proportional hazards model, MLN correlated equally with LTD, cell type, and standard deviation of nucleolar area, with death from metastatic UM. Multivariate analysis found that combining MLN with LTD yielded a substantial increase in prognostic value. They concluded that the relatively easy measurement and reproducibility

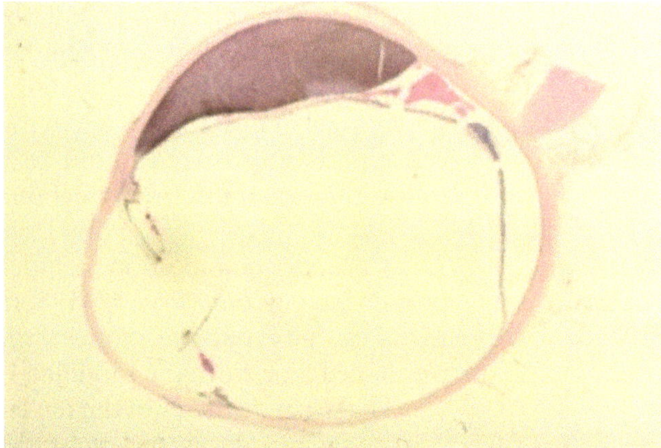

Fig. 1 Image showing an H&E-stained slide of a choroidal melanoma. Prognostic factors such as basal diameter and tumor thickness as well as intra- and extra-ocular extension can be identified histopathologically

of MLN could make it a useful cytologic index in determining the malignant potential of uveal melanomas.

Following this disconcordance in the evaluation of MLN from different studies, Seregard et al. [61] aimed to specifically determine the prognostic accuracy of MLN along with vascular patterns with a PC-10 immunostain in uveal melanoma. With the aid of the immunostain MLN, along with other variables, was found to have prognostic significance in both univariate and multivariate Cox analyses, although in the multivariate model, MLN had the lowest degree of significance amongst the covariables. A correlation matrix drawn from this data found that tumors with a high MLN value were more often of mixed or epithelioid cellularity.

In summary, studies have produced discordant results with respect to the significance of MLN on prognostic determination, which may be due to deviations in the protocols used to elucidate the MLN value in each study. It seems that with the assistance of immunostaining the accuracy of MLN determination has improved its significance in Cox analyses and hence its prognostic potential (Fig. 1).

2.2.3 High Mitotic Rate

The presence of mitotic figures indicates proliferative activity in a tissue. The conventional way to establish the degree of proliferative activity is to calculate the mitotic count. This is achieved by counting the number of mitotic figures seen per 40 high-power fields (HPF) using the 40× objective in H&E-stained sections of the tissue [56]. This method can produce inconsistent results due to inter-observer variability, and the technique itself requires experienced pathologists in order to perform it well. Van Diest et al. [63] established the criteria required to assess mitotic figures as follows: (1) the absence of the nuclear membrane, signifying the end of prophase; (2) the presence of condensed chromosomes, clotted (early metaphase), arranged in a plane (metaphase/anaphase), or in separate clots (telophase) with the clots counted as one mitotic figure; and (3) ignoring the hyperchromatic and apoptotic nuclei. Problems with this technique include difficulty in identifying mitotic figures in the presence of apoptotic cells or karyorrhexis as well as the potential for obscuration of mitotic figures by crush artifact or overstaining by the hematoxylin stain. A recent study by Angi et al. [64] tried a new technique for staining the tissue sections for analysis of mitotic figure counts. They compared the traditional method using H&E staining with a newer method—the use of phospho-histone H3 (PHH3), an antibody marker used for mitotic counting in other types of tumor [65]. In addition to the features described by van Diest et al, the mitotic figures in the PHH3-stained sections had to show positive staining to be counted. Angi et al. found that PHH3-stained mitotic figures could be easily identified in highly pigmented tumors, near necrotic areas, tumors with dense cellularity, or where the nuclei were distorted or few in number and at low magnifications. In nearly all the cases, the PHH3 counts were the same or greater than the H&E-stained counts. The greater counts found by using PHH3 staining aided in drawing a significant correlation between mitotic count and the presence of extracellular matrix loops. Both markers showed a similar correlation with metastatic death using a univariate Cox analysis ($p = 0.020$ H&E, $p = 0.029$ PHH3), concluding that a high mitotic count was associated with an increased risk of metastasis.

2.2.4 Microcirculation

Uveal melanomas disseminate hematogenously, and so angiogenesis plays a key role in the biology of UM and metastasis [66]. There are two aspects of angiogenesis in tumor biology which promote tumorigenicity—remodeling of the vascular bed and production of new blood vessels [67]. Initially, pathologists focused on the prognostic significance of new vessel location and density within a tumor, as a high vascular density had been found to correlate with poor prognosis in several other forms of cancer [68–74]. In uveal melanomas, remodeling of the microcirculation into regions of specific patterns was shown through analysis of histological sections [27]. The microcirculatory patterns were demonstrated on histological sections by use of a modified PAS stain, where hematoxylin counterstaining was not used. A green filter was used in the microscope to view the magenta patterns of the microcirculation in the tumor tissue as black patterns, which enabled the patterns to be imaged with a photomicroscope. This method was not affected by permanganate bleaching for highly pigmented melanomas. This work by Folberg described the microcirculation patterns found in UM tumors—closed vascular loops, incomplete vascular loops (arcs) with and without branching, microvascular networks composed of back-to-back loops, PAS-positive parallel vascular channels with and without cross-linking, incorporation of normal vessels into the tumor, and focal avascular zones [75].

In ciliary body and choroidal nevi, only four vascular patterns have been observed: normal vessels, straight vessels, parallel vessels without cross-linking, and avascular zones [76]. In this study Rummelt et al. looked at 234 cases of UM, of which 21 % contained a nevus-like circulation, and the rest contained the vascular patterns not found in nevi. Interestingly, the melanomas that had nevus-like vascular patterns had a tendency to be both smaller and located posterior to the equator than melanomas who exhibited vascular patterns not found in choroidal nevi. In addition, the mortality associated with melanomas that lacked a nevus-like microcirculation was more than double that for melanomas with a nevus-like vascular pattern (32.4 % vs. 14.3 %, $p = 0.012$). Similarly, the survival curves at 15-year follow-up were 84.8 and 60.4 %, respectively ($p = 0.0007$). The study concluded that it was likely that there are three types of melanocytic uveal lesion: benign nevi with no capacity for metastasis, melanomas with a nevus-like microcirculation that have a limited capacity for metastasis and better prognosis and survival times, and melanomas with aggressive vascular patterns that are strongly associated with metastasis and poorer prognosis. This suggestion was further strengthened by Folberg et al. [75] who used Kaplan–Meier survival curves based on deaths from metastatic UM to find that at 10 years post diagnosis, survival was significantly better in patients who did not have tumors with loops, networks, or parallel vessels with cross-linking patterns. When a Cox proportional hazards model was devised to include conventional prognostic factors, the most important variable was found to be the network pattern, which it must be remembered are compromised of back-to back microvascular loops. Cox proportional hazards have also been used to determine the importance of conventional prognostic variables such as cell type and mean of the ten largest nucleoli (MLN). Cell type has been found to be of little significance in prognostication or indeed not even entering the Cox models once microvascular patterns are included in the models [75]. Similarly, MLN do not enter the Cox models when microvascular patterns are included [60]. Although cell type does not appear in the Cox models if microcirculation patterns are entered, it still has relevance, as a study by Folberg showed that the presence of networks was associated with epithelioid cell type and the absence of this cell type was associated with avascular zones [27]. The association between loops and networks and death from metastatic disease has been confirmed by several studies [28, 33, 61].

2.2.5 Pigmentation

There is considerable variation in the color of uveal melanomas, ranging from an amelanotic yellow-white to dark brown, and approximately 25 % of all UM are amelanotic (Fig. 2). In addition

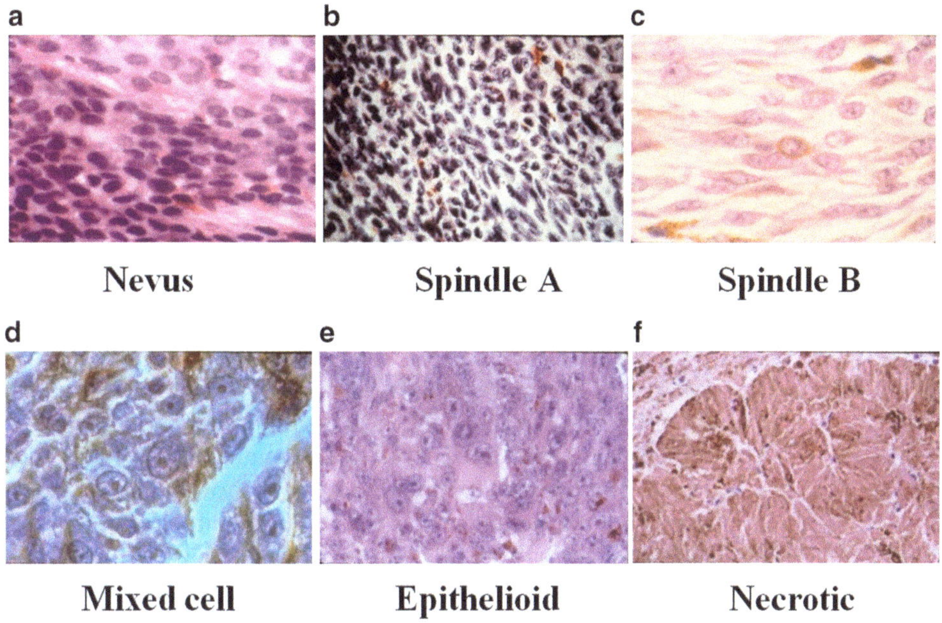

Fig. 2 The different cell types found in uveal melanomas

Table 3
COMS classification system for pigmentation of uveal melanomas

Category of pigmentation	Uniform pigmentation	Variable pigmentation
None	No pigmentation	No pigmentation
Minimal	Cytologic detail evident	One-third or less pigmented
Moderate	Cytologic detail partially obscured	One-third to two-thirds pigmented
Heavy	Cytologic detail obscured	Two-thirds to complete pigmentation

to the pigmentation provided by melanin in the cells, the color of the tumors can vary according to the presence of blood vessels, lipofuscin, and subretinal fluid on the surface of the tumor. Once the presence of a tumor begins to affect the overlying retinal pigment epithelium (RPE), the RPE can degenerate into orange lipofuscin granules or decompensate, causing a buildup of subretinal fluid and subsequently a serous retinal detachment, which can affect the perceived color of the tumor.

On histological examination, the true degree of pigmentation of a UM becomes apparent, and it is this factor which is used in prognostication. The COMS categorized uveal melanomas based on their degree of pigmentation (Table 3 and Fig. 3) [77].

The COMS found an association between tumor size, cell type, and degree of pigmentation: larger tumors and an epithelioid cell type were associated with heavy pigmentation. None of the amelanotic

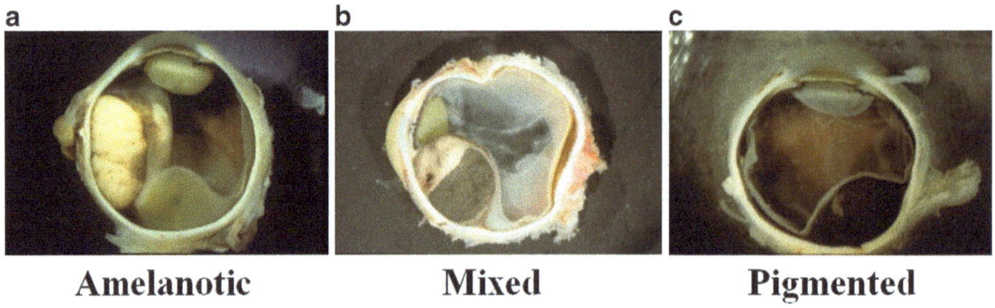

Fig. 3 Uveal melanomas in situ show the variability in pigmentation

melanomas were classified as epithelioid, even those in the large-size category. Interestingly, increasing pigmentation was correlated with necrosis with 66.2 % of heavily pigmented tumors and only 38.7 % of minimally pigmented tumors showing signs of necrosis. Increasing pigmentation, larger size, and epithelioid cell type were all associated with greater number of macrophages, which in turn was significantly associated with necrosis. Heavy pigmentation has been associated with a poor prognosis [20, 78]. Shammas et al. [79] found that the degree of pigmentation in large tumors had an effect on the prognostic outcome if the tumor ruptured through Bruch's membrane, and mortality increased from 19 % for amelanotic lesions to 65 % for heavily pigmented tumors.

2.2.6 Inflammation

An inflammatory phenotype is an indicator of poor prognosis in uveal melanoma. This is characterized by the presence of a lymphocytic infiltrate and increased expression of HLA antigens [80]. The lymphocytic infiltrate in UM consists predominantly of T-suppressor/cytotoxic lymphocytes, with B-lymphocytes present in insignificant quantities [81]. Approximately a quarter of cases of UM reveal an inflammatory infiltrate upon microscopic examination. A study by de La Cruz [26] looked at 1,193 cases of UM and found that an increase in the number of lymphocytes seen per 20 HPF was associated with reduced survival rates ($P<0.0001$) even when other risk factors were controlled. Although this finding seems contradictory, the explanation lies in the fact that the eye is an immune-privileged site, with no lymphatic drainage channels. As such, the only way an immune response can be induced is by extrascleral spread of the uveal melanoma through hematogenous routes. Hence, an immune response will only be found in uveal melanomas that have already metastasized.

3 Immunohistochemical Markers

Many different immunohistochemical stains have been tried in the prognostic testing of uveal melanoma, namely, HMB-45, Ki-67, S100, MART-1 (Melan-A), NKI-C3, NSE, and p53. The most commonly used stains are HMB-45, S100, Ki-67, and Melan-A.

3.1 HMB-45

HMB-45 is a monoclonal antibody that binds a cytoplasmic antigen produced by fetal melanocytes and melanoma cells [82, 83]. It had originally been found to be a highly specific and sensitive immunohistochemical marker for cutaneous malignant melanomas with >90 % of melanomas showing positive staining for HMB-45 [82, 84, 85]. In primary uveal melanomas, HMB-45 has been shown to detect 99 % of lesions, with the strongest expression of the marker at the invasive edge [83]. Burnier et al. [86] evaluated the expression of HMB-45 as well as S100 and neuron-specific enolase (NSE) in uveal melanocytic tumors. They found that all three markers showed a greater intensity of staining in uveal melanomas than nevi. HMB-45 showed strong staining in all the uveal melanomas tested, whereas the S100 and NSE showed positive staining in only 40 and 55 % of UM, respectively. Additionally HMB-45 positively stained UM that were necrotic, unlike the other two markers. Luyten et al. [87] also found HMB-45 to be superior to the other markers for staining UM (>93 %) and furthermore were able to determine that HMB-45 was significantly more sensitive than S100 in detecting metastatic lesions. Overall, HMB-45 was found to be more specific and sensitive than both S100 and NSE in detecting uveal melanocytic tumors [86, 87].

3.2 S100

S100 is a protein family that belongs to the EF hand proteins [88], and the isoform αβ is found in melanocytes [89]. This can be useful in distinguishing between metastatic carcinoma and a melanocytic tumor [90]. Although S100 is one of the most commonly used diagnostic markers used for uveal melanoma it has the problem of being expressed in many non-melanocytic tumors, giving it low specificity, and in addition, the expression of S100 can be affected by the use of routine FFPE tissue, giving false-negative results all too commonly [90]. Despite the lower specificity of S100 compared to other immunohistochemical markers used for UM, it has been found to be a sensitive marker, staining >90 % of primary uveal melanomas [86, 91].

3.3 Ki-67

Ki-67 is a nuclear protein expressed during the active phase of the cell cycle and is therefore used as a marker for cell proliferation [92]. Although it has been used to identify cell proliferation in uveal melanoma, its main use has been in detecting the differences in cell proliferation rates between UM that have been irradiated and those that have not had radiation treatment [93, 94]. As previously mentioned, a high proliferation rate of tumor cells is associated with metastasis and death, so it can be inferred that strong expression of Ki-67 in UM can be an indicator of a worse prognosis. The expression of Ki-67 has also been shown to be associated with the formation of microvascular networks [95]. One study by Al-Jamal et al. [96] looked at Ki-67 immunoreactivity with respect to other prognostic factors. They found that there was a trend toward high proportion of Ki-67 immunopositive cells (high proliferation rate) with the presence of non-spindle cell-type UM. No similar trends were found between Ki-67 immunoreactivity and other prognostic factors. Univariate analysis of survival found that UM-related mortality was significantly higher with the presence of Ki-67-positive cells. Multivariate analysis showed that the presence of Ki-67-positive cells was still useful as an independent predictor of prognosis, but the significance decreased as other variables were introduced into the model.

3.4 Melan-A

Melan-A is a product of the MART-1 gene and is a melanocytic differentiation antigen protein specific for melanocytic cells [97]. In cutaneous melanoma, Melan-A has been found to be more sensitive than HMB-45 and with a higher specificity for melanocytic lesions, making it useful in diagnostic antibody panels [98]. Heegaard et al. [99] compared Melan-A with HMB-45 and S100 in ocular melanomas and found that Melan-A had a higher sensitivity (100 %) than HMB-45 (55 %) in iris melanomas and a similar sensitivity to HMB-45 in choroidal melanomas. 100 % of epithelioid cell choroidal melanomas stained with the Melan-A and HMB-45, compared to 80 % with S100. Melan-A was also noted to stain in a similar pattern to S100, only it stained much more strongly than S100 in iris melanomas. Additionally, Melan-A stains only cytoplasm, whereas S100 stains both cytoplasm and nuclear components, making Melan-A more specific. Fernandes et al. [100] looked at the correlation of Melan-A staining with clinicopathological parameters as well as whether the influence of irradiation on UM would affect the expression of Melan-A staining in a diagnostic antibody panel. They did not find any significant association between the expression of Melan-A and radiotherapy, cell type, lymphocytic infiltration, presence of closed vascular loops, gender, age, or LTD.

4 Liver Function Tests

In North America, LFTs are used routinely in screening for metastatic disease from uveal melanoma, as the primary focus of metastasis by hematogenous spread is the liver in up to 95 % of cases [15, 31, 101]. The median survival time from diagnosis of metastasis ranges from 2 months to about 1 year, and among the patients who die from metastatic disease, the liver is nearly always involved [102, 103]. Although there are no current treatments available that are known to significantly prolong survival and quality of life, clinicians continue to try and identify liver metastases as early as possible in the hope that they can try adjuvant therapies to prolong survival or at the very least give their patients sufficient time to plan their medical care and futures. In the United States, biannual screening for UM metastasis is performed by doing LFTs followed by imaging of the liver if abnormalities are detected in the LFTs [104]. Although screening for UM metastases using LFTs remains popular in North America, its diagnostic value has been questioned recently, with several studies finding LFTs to have relatively low sensitivity [105–108]. In Europe, imaging of the liver using ultrasound seems to be the preferred method over monitoring of LFTs, for screening for metastatic disease [106].

The most commonly ordered tests in an LFT work-up include alkaline phosphatase (AP), lactate dehydrogenase (LDH), aspartame transferase (AST), alanine transferase (ALT), and occasionally gamma glutamyl transpeptidase (GGT).

4.1 Alkaline Phosphatase

AP is found in tissues throughout the body with highest concentrations in the liver, biliary ducts, kidneys, and bones. AP is an enzyme located in the cells that line the biliary ducts, and therefore levels will elevate in infiltrative diseases of the liver such as cancer. It is also elevated significantly in osteoblastic activity, which is important to note when considering a growing child with UM or older patients with bone disease. In addition it is important to note that AP levels can also be lowered by conditions such as various anemias, chronic myelogenous leukemia, use of estrogen therapy, e.g., in postmenopausal women, recent cardiac surgery, hypothyroidism, and malnutrition, all of which are very likely to affect the population that are most likely to develop a UM.

4.2 Lactate Dehydrogenase

LDH is an enzyme found not only in the hepatocytes of the liver but also in many other body tissues. LDH is released from cells when they are damaged and so is a direct marker of tissue damage. In cancer, where the cells have increased metabolic activity and a high turnover rate the LDH level can be markedly elevated.

4.3 Aspartate Transaminase and Alanine Transaminase

ALT is also known as serum glutamic pyruvate transaminase (SGPT), is an enzyme present in the liver parenchymal cells, and shows marked diurnal variation. AST is also known as serum glutamic oxaloacetic transaminase (SGOT) and is an enzyme found in liver parenchymal cells that is typically elevated in acute hepatocellular injury. AST is found more widely spread in the body, in tissues such as the heart, kidneys, and skeletal muscle, red bloods cells, and brain, and will be elevated in injury to these tissues. Although ALT is also found in cardiac muscle, kidneys, and skeletal muscle, it is found in clinically negligible quantities in those tissues and therefore serves as a much more accurate marker for liver injury than AST.

4.4 Gamma-Glutamyl Transferase

GGT is an enzyme found in the cell membranes of the biliary ducts and has a similar response to AP but seems to be a more sensitive marker for cholestatic injury than AP. In addition, it aids in the analysis of AP elevations, as it is not affected by bony injury or disease, unlike AP. This issue is very pertinent when dealing with the population of patients with UM where the mean age at diagnosis is around 60 years old and the likelihood of concomitant bone disease may be highly prevalent.

5 Comparison of LFTs

The problem with LFTs is that they are relatively insensitive markers when there is only mild liver dysfunction and so are unlikely to be very useful in catching very early metastatic disease, when chances of intervention are most likely to succeed [105, 107]. In the COMS reports, in an analysis of LFTs in patients who had received local treatment for UM, but before metastatic disease was found, the sensitivity, specificity, PPV, and NPV of having at least 1 abnormal LFT were 14.7, 92.3, 45.7, and 71.0 %, respectively [104]. A study by Eskelin [109] looking at the screening methods used for metastatic UM found that at least 1 LFT was abnormal (in a panel of AP, LDH, AST, and ALT) in 70 % of patients with metastatic disease, with the overall sensitivity of AST, ALT, and AP ranging from 0.27 to 0.43, but LDH was notably more sensitive at 0.67. The specificity of all the LFTs ranged from 0.90 to 0.96, again with LD coming out on top. Subsequently, LD was calculated to have the best likelihood ratio for both a positive and negative test, being the most sensitive with the highest PPV. Some studies found that elevations in LD and AP and GGT may have prognostic significance in metastatic disease as they may reflect the hepatic tumor burden [17, 110, 111]. A study by Kaiserman et al. [17] evaluated the trends in LFTs prior to detection of hepatic metastases in UM, looking at both the mean levels and the changes in LFT levels at various time points prior to detection of the metastases with imaging. They found that the mean levels of all the LFT in the panel did not reveal any abnormality more than 6 months before the metastases were detected by imaging. However in the 6-month period prior to detection of the metastases a rise in the LFTs was noted but with most values staying within normal limits. AP, GGT, and LDH seemed to peak around the time of diagnosis, whereas AST and ALT appeared to peak approximately 6 months after detection of metastases. The mean levels of LDH and GGT were seen to rise above the normal limit, and this finding was consistent with other studies which found these two markers to be the most sensitive of the LFT panel [17, 105, 107, 109]. Both of these enzymes are found in cells of the biliary ducts, and a rise in their levels would indicate cholestasis, which may be a result of the presence of micro-metastases in the liver. When likelihood ratios (LR) for predicting the presence of hepatic metastases were compared in Eskelin's study, AP and LDH had the best LR 6 months before and also at the time of detection of metastases, which would

Table 4
Rates for LFTs

LFT	Sensitivity (%)	Specificity (%)	PPV (%)	NPV (%)	Likelihood ratio +
ALT	17.0	96.2	11.6	97.5	4.4
AST	26.1	95.7	15.1	97.8	6.0
GGT	35.2	90.0	9.4	97.9	3.5
LDH	39.8	92.2	13.2	98.1	5.1
AP	23.9	95.3	13.1	97.7	5.1
LDH and AP	19.3	99.1	38.6	97.6	21.2

Adapted from Table 2 of Mouriaux et al. [108]

indicate that they are the best predictive LFTs. The study concluded that AP and GGT were predictive only above the upper normal limit, while LDH and AST could be considered predictive at rise of 80 % over the normal limit.

A very recent study by Mouriaux et al. [108] has taken the view that LFTs are not helpful in the early diagnosis of metastatic UM. Eighty-eight patients who developed metastases during annual screening with LFTs were compared to 174 patients who had UM but not metastatic disease. In addition to estimates for sensitivity, specificity, PPV, and NPV, a cost evaluation was undertaken (Table 4).

The highest PPV was found for a combination of LDH and AP, at 38.6 %. PPVs are clinically useful, as they indicate the probability of metastases with an abnormal LFT, but in this study low PPV values suggested that LFTs were not useful as prognostic tools. Mouriaux et al. found that metastases were detected after at least 1 abnormal LFT in 45 % of patients. They found that there was no significant difference between the proportions of false-positive results (abnormal LFTs without metastasis) between the two groups of patients; however this could be because true positives may not have actually been included in the control group. This is important to note as false positives may result in liver imaging which both is costly and in some cases could result in unnecessary exposure to radiation or contrast agents. In some cases repeat testing of an abnormal LFT may be justified if the clinician feels that the situation warrants it, e.g., recent use by a patient of alcohol or a course of medication, which may have affected the result. In the group with metastases, 51 patients (58 %) were found to have at least one abnormal LFT result. As hepatic metastases have been found in up to 90 % of UM patients with metastatic disease, it could be expected that abnormal LFTs would be detected in 90 % of patients with metastatic UM. The fact that this study, as well as others [17, 109], finds the rate of abnormal LFT results at the point of detection of hepatic metastases to be substantially lower than 90 % may be explained by the fact that the metastatic burden on liver function may not be high enough to increase the LFTs to abnormal levels in some patients. It could also point to the fact that the liver may not necessarily be the first site of extraocular spread. In this predominantly older population of patients, the very likely possibility of other comorbidities may skewer the LFT levels to higher or lower than would be expected from a measure of just the hepatic function due to the fact that many of the tests in the LFT panel are not specific to the liver.

Mouriaux also calculated the cost-effectiveness of screening and found that the mean cost of LFT screening, including cost of imaging where requested, was about $273/year per patient in the United States, of which $10.13 was the cost for the 5 LFTs.

6 Serum Markers

As UM tends to spread to the liver first [112] tests for liver function and anatomical imaging are crucial to detect the presence of metastases and predict prognosis. Despite improvements in treatment for the intraocular tumor, the survival rate has changed very little over the last few decades due to a high metastatic tumor burden once the metastases are finally detected. A recent development is the use of sensitive biomarkers to detect early metastases to the liver. For cutaneous malignant melanoma, there are several available diagnostic tests to detect associated molecules, such as S-100β [113] and melanoma-inhibitory activity (MIA) [114] as well as LASA-P (lipid-bound sialic acid), NSE, and LDH as established by the AJCC. Another serum marker, osteopontin (OPN), was noted to have elevated levels in the blood of patients with a variety of metastatic cancers [115]. S-100β serum levels had been shown to be a useful prognostic marker for cutaneous melanoma in stage II and III disease, with changes in the levels of serum S-100β reported to reflect the changes in tumor burden and hence providing the ability to predict a positive response to chemotherapy and immunotherapy [116, 117]. For uveal melanoma, the exact biomarkers most useful in prognostic evaluation are still being established; however the role of OPN, S-100β, and MIA as prognostic serum markers for predicting earlier hepatic metastasis appears promising [116, 118, 119].

7 Imaging

In the COMS trials, the mortality rate from metastatic melanoma at 5 years was found to be up to 30 % for large tumors, although at the time of diagnosis, metastatic disease was detected in fewer than 1 % of the cases of UM [104, 120]. This discrepancy may be explained by the presence of micro-metastases at the time of diagnosis that were not detectable by the methods used in the COMS trials. Hence earlier and more accurate detection of metastatic disease in UM may lead to improved prognosis through better directed treatment modalities. The COMS advocates the combination of liver function tests, chest radiographic imaging, and abdominal (hepatic) ultrasound screening preoperatively and then biannually [104].

7.1 Chest Radiography

Several studies, including the COMS, have recommended that a chest radiograph (CXR) be taken preoperatively to rule out any primary lung tumors or metastases [104, 107, 109]. Estimates of the frequency of metastases to the eye from lung primaries range from 17 to 39 % [121, 122]. However, cases of pulmonary metastases from UM are very rare [123, 124]. A recent review of patients with UM found that a large proportion were metastases from lung primaries; however CXR was not able to rule out the diagnosis of primary lung cancer, and further investigation was needed [121]. As such, although a CXR is considered crucial during the initial work-up of patients with UM to rule out the possibility of lung primaries, it holds little value as part of a follow-up screening program for extraocular metastasis due to its low yield and the risks imposed by repeated exposure to radiation from CXR [108, 109]. It may be prudent to continue using CXR in follow-up screening for those patients with a smoking history or that have complained of pulmonary symptoms.

7.2 Abdominal Ultrasound

At the time of diagnosis, hepatic metastases are noted in between 40 and 60 % of patients, and this number increases up to 95 % of patients with time [103, 104, 110, 125]. Screening for metastatic disease in the United States relies on clinical examination findings, LFTs and CXR, whereas in Europe abdominal ultrasound is the preferred screening method and has been recommended by several studies [103, 126, 127]. Abdominal ultrasound has the advantages of being both noninvasive and safe, eliminating the risk of radiation found with CT scans. It is more widely available than CT and MRI scanning and is relatively much cheaper to perform. The ability of liver US to detect all the existing hepatic metastases in a patient was reported to be 37 % [111]; however as there are often multiple metastatic foci, a study by Eskelin [109] looking at the use of abdominal ultrasound as a screening method for metastatic UM found that abdominal US revealed unequivocal hepatic metastases in 78 % of patients and lesions suggestive of metastases in a further 11 %, which were confirmed as metastatic lesions by FNA or CT. A comparison of abdominal US with CT found that both modalities independently detected 89 % of lesions. They concluded that semiannual screening using a combination of LFTs and abdominal US would detect >95 % of patients with metastatic disease.

7.3 Computed Tomography

Although UM metastasizes most frequently to the liver, half of UM patients will also develop extrahepatic metastases, most commonly to the brain, bone, lungs, or skin [19, 31, 41]. A retrospective analysis of 91 patients who had CT scanning within a month of their UM diagnosis found that CT had a 100 % sensitivity and negative-predictive value rate and specificity was 91 % [128]. The positive predictive value was only 27 % but can be attributed to the detection of benign hepatic lesions by the CT imaging modality. Another study analyzed the sensitivity of different imaging modalities for metastases in UM and found that US detected 37 %, MRI detected 67 %, and CT detected 77 % [111]. Additionally, combining CT with arterial portography was found to be the most sensitive method by far, which could be used for initial staging but not for follow-up screening. Although CT has been found to be highly sensitive to the presence of abnormal lesions, its low PPV, high cost, and risk from high radiation doses prevent it from being used widely as a follow-up screening tool. Use of CT in semiannual screening may be beneficial for patients with UM with high-risk clinical and histopathologic features, especially if more effective treatments become available in the future [109].

7.4 Positron Emission Tomography/Computed Tomography

Positron emission tomography/computed tomography (PET/CT) uses radioactive ^{18}F-fluorodeoxyglucose (FDG) to produce functional images from PET, which are then combined with high-resolution anatomical images from CT. Whole-body imaging using PET/CT for staging and screening purposes has been gaining acceptance for cutaneous melanoma, lymphoma, gastrointestinal malignancies, colorectal cancers, and non-small-cell cancers, to name a few [129]. PET/CT has been compared to PEt alone, revealing a significant improvement in lesion delineation with the dual-modality imaging resulting in the authors postulating it as a useful tool for determining the areas for biopsy [130]. Whole-body imaging using PET/CT compared to MRI for tumor staging showed that although the two modalities performed similarly in detecting metastases, PET/CT was shown to be superior for overall TNM staging purposes [131]. This is due to the propensity of the FDG-enhanced PET scan in revealing the functional activity around lesions, allowing delineation of active or quiescent/benign lesions. The use of FDG in PET/CT allows the differentiation of malignant from benign lesions by determining the variability in glucose uptake in the lesion compared to surrounding tissue and comparing the results to standardized uptake values (SUV). Recently, the use of PET/CT has been studied in more detail with respect to screening for metastatic UM. Both Freudenberg [132] and Finger [133] have advocated the use of PET/CT in staging for UM, guiding further imaging or biopsy investigations and hence directing treatment decisions.

A recent study by Orcurto [134] compared FDG-PET/CT and MRI in patients with hepatic metastases from uveal melanoma. They scanned 10 patients with biopsy-proven liver metastases from UM with both imaging techniques and found that of the 108 liver lesions that were detected, 31 % were seen by both modalities, 65 % by MRI alone, but only 4 % by PET/CT alone. Furthermore, they found that PET/CT only detected 11 % of the lesions seen on MRI that were less than 1.2 cm in size ($P < 0.0001$) and concluded that MRI was far superior to PET/CT in detection of small (<1.2 cm) liver metastases. They did note however that the PET/CT scan was able to detect changes in FDG uptake that were unrelated to change in size of the lesion, suggesting that this modality could be useful in determining the response to therapy. When compared to the other imaging modalities, PET/CT is very expensive and still faces the problem of false-positive findings which require further investigation [133]. Although PET/CT is an expensive option, the potential for discovering occult metastases and being able to initiate appropriate therapy in a timely manner, thus avoiding unnecessary and expensive procedures, can make it cost effective. Its potential role in assessing early response of metastases to therapy is the one to be considered most seriously in improving the management of metastatic UM.

7.5 Abdominal Magnetic Resonance Imaging

Although UM metastasizes most commonly to the liver, half of UM patients will also develop extrahepatic metastases. One study looking at the sensitivity of imaging techniques found that MRI detected lesions only 67 % of the time, compared to CT which detected lesions 77 % of the time [111]. MRI has the advantage of providing high-resolution images and not being a source of radiation exposure; however it is expensive and has an appreciable false-positive rate. A recent comparison of MRI with FDG-PET by Servois looked at the sensitivity of the two imaging modalities in the preoperative diagnosis of metastatic uveal melanoma [135]. They found that sensitivity and positive predictive value for MRI were 67 and 95 %, respectively, compared to 41 and 100 % for FDG-PET and that this difference was statistically significant using the McNemar test ($P < 0.01$), concluding that MRI was superior to FDG-PET for staging of liver metastases from UM.

7.6 Comparison of Prognostic Tests (Table 5)

From looking at the different modalities available for prognostic prediction, we can see that although LFTs have low sensitivity and positive predictive values for detecting metastatic disease to the liver, they have a comparable specificity and NPV (>90 %) to the far more costly imaging tests. The concern with false positives generated by liver function testing is that those results induce costly liver imaging which may unnecessarily expose the patient to harmful radiation or contrast agents.

Table 5

Comparison of the tests used in uveal melanoma for prognostic evaluation

Test	Study	Sensitivity (%)	Specificity (%)	Positive predictive value (%)	Negative predictive value (%)
Liver function test *At least 1 abnormal LFT	COMS [104]	14.7	92.3	45.7	71.0
Chest radiograph *Obtained ≤90 days from diagnosis	COMS [104]	35	98	65	93
Abdominal computed tomography *Within 1 month of diagnosis	Feinstein [128]	100	91	27	93
Positron emission tomography	Francken [140]	100	67	88	100

Adapted from Wyckoff et al. [136]

Recent studies comparing liver function tests with serum markers for uveal melanoma have found that both types of test have some predictive value in the early detection of metastatic uveal melanoma to the liver [137]. Missotten et al. [138] found that the best blood tests for identifying metastatic disease were LDH, GGT, S100β, and MIA. Hendler et al. [137] confirmed these findings and additionally noted that GGT was elevated at time = 0, showing that there was no lead-time for this test. They also found that OPN had a statistically significant lead-time of more than 6 months. In view of these findings, at a minimum, it is advisable to obtain a panel of LFTs every 6 months from the time of diagnosis and compare serial results in order to detect any elevations early, referring for further investigation as necessary. It is also advisable to request serum markers at the same time, as these tests have been shown to be more specific than the LFTs in predicting liver metastases.

The use of molecular cytogenetic testing to identify uveal melanomas at high risk of metastasis is an emerging field. The prognostic significance of monosomy 3 and loss on chromosomes 1p, 3, 6q, 8p, and 9p and gains on 1q, 6p, and 8q has been identified and continues to be explored [139]. This topic is explained in greater detail in two chapters in this volume.

8 Conclusion

At present the prognosis of uveal melanoma, once it has metastasized, is poor. Considerable improvements in the identification of histopathologic parameters with prognostic significance, combined with the use of multimodal imaging, as well as prognostic testing through serum biomarkers or molecular cytogenetics may in the future allow for more accurate prognostication. Identifying the high-risk clinicopathological and genetic features of tumors may contribute to improving life expectancy through appropriate and timely intervention.

References

1. Damato BE, Coupland SE (2012) Differences in uveal melanomas between men and women from the British Isles. Eye (Lond) 26(2): 292–299
2. Shields CL et al (2012) Clinical spectrum and prognosis of uveal melanoma based on Age at presentation in 8,033 cases. Retina 32(7): 1363–1372
3. Egan KM et al (1988) Epidemiologic aspects of uveal melanoma. Surv Ophthalmol 32(4):239–251
4. Singh AD, Bergman L, Seregard S (2005) Uveal melanoma: epidemiologic aspects. Ophthalmol Clin North Am 18(1):75–84, viii
5. Hu DN et al (2005) Population-based incidence of uveal melanoma in various races and ethnic groups. Am J Ophthalmol 140(4): 612–617
6. Margo CE, Mulla Z, Billiris K (1998) Incidence of surgically treated uveal melanoma by race and ethnicity. Ophthalmology 105(6):1087–1090
7. Singh AD, Topham A (2003) Incidence of uveal melanoma in the United States: 1973-1997. Ophthalmology 110(5):956–961
8. Gallagher RP et al (1985) Risk factors for ocular melanoma: Western Canada Melanoma Study. J Natl Cancer Inst 74(4):775–778
9. Seddon JM et al (1990) Host factors, UV radiation, and risk of uveal melanoma. A case-control study. Arch Ophthalmol 108(9): 1274–1280
10. van Hees CL et al (1994) Are atypical nevi a risk factor for uveal melanoma? A case-control study. J Invest Dermatol 103(2):202–205
11. Tucker MA et al (1985) Sunlight exposure as risk factor for intraocular malignant melanoma. N Engl J Med 313(13):789–792
12. Singh AD, Turell ME, Topham AK (2011) Uveal melanoma: trends in incidence, treatment, and survival. Ophthalmology 118(9):1881–1885
13. Bergman L et al (2002) Incidence of uveal melanoma in Sweden from 1960 to 1998. Invest Ophthalmol Vis Sci 43(8):2579–2583
14. Burr JM et al (2007) Survival from uveal melanoma in England and Wales 1986 to 2001. Ophthalmic Epidemiol 14(1):3–8
15. Kujala E, Makitie T, Kivela T (2003) Very long-term prognosis of patients with malignant uveal melanoma. Invest Ophthalmol Vis Sci 44(11):4651–4659
16. Seregard S, Kock E (1995) Prognostic indicators following enucleation for posterior uveal melanoma. A multivariate analysis of long-term survival with minimized loss to follow-up. Acta Ophthalmologica Scandinavica 73(4):340–344
17. Kaiserman I, Amer R, Pe'er J (2004) Liver function tests in metastatic uveal melanoma. Am J Ophthalmol 137(2):236–243
18. Bedikian AY (2006) Metastatic uveal melanoma therapy: current options. Int Ophthalmol Clin 46(1):151–166
19. Kath R et al (1993) Prognosis and treatment of disseminated uveal melanoma. Cancer 72(7):2219–2223
20. Seddon JM et al (1983) A prognostic factor study of disease-free interval and survival following enucleation for uveal melanoma. Arch Ophthalmol 101(12):1894–1899
21. Chowers I, Amer R, Pe'er J (2002) The correlation among different immunostaining evaluation methods for the assessment of proliferative activity in uveal melanoma. Curr Eye Res 25(6):369–372
22. McLean IW et al (1983) Modifications of Callender's classification of uveal melanoma at the armed forces institute of pathology. Am J Ophthalmol 96(4):502–509
23. Edge SD, BD Carducci MA, Compton CC. (2009) Chapter 43: Malignant melanoma of the uvea. In: AJCC cancer staging manual. Springer: New York, NY
24. Grossniklaus HE, Kivela T, Harbour JW, Finger P (2011) Protocol for the examination of specimens from patients with uveal melanoma. College of American Pathologists Cancer Protocols 2011 [cited 2011 November 2011]; Uveal Melanoma 3.1.0.1:[Available from: http://www.cap.org/apps/docs/committees/cancer/cancer_protocols/2012/UvealMelanom_12protocol.pdf
25. Augsburger JJ, Gamel JW (1990) Clinical prognostic factors in patients with posterior

uveal malignant melanoma. Cancer 66(7): 1596–1600
26. de la Cruz PO Jr, Specht CS, McLean IW (1990) Lymphocytic infiltration in uveal malignant melanoma. Cancer 65(1):112–115
27. Folberg R et al (1992) The morphologic characteristics of tumor blood vessels as a marker of tumor progression in primary human uveal melanoma: a matched case-control study. Hum Pathol 23(11):1298–1305
28. Makitie T et al (1999) Microvascular loops and networks as prognostic indicators in choroidal and ciliary body melanomas. J Natl Cancer Inst 91(4):359–367
29. Diener-West M et al (2001) The COMS randomized trial of iodine 125 brachytherapy for choroidal melanoma, II: characteristics of patients enrolled and not enrolled. COMS Report No. 17. Arch Ophthalmol 119(7): 951–965
30. Damato B, Coupland SE (2009) A reappraisal of the significance of largest basal diameter of posterior uveal melanoma. Eye (Lond) 23(12):2152–2160, quiz 2161-2
31. Diener-West M et al (2005) Development of metastatic disease after enrollment in the COMS trials for treatment of choroidal melanoma: Collaborative Ocular Melanoma Study Group Report No. 26. Arch Ophthalmol 123(12):1639–1643
32. Isager P, Ehlers N, Overgaard J (2004) Prognostic factors for survival after enucleation for choroidal and ciliary body melanomas. Acta Ophthalmol Scand 82(5):517–525
33. McLean IW, Keefe KS, Burnier MN (1997) Uveal melanoma. Comparison of the prognostic value of fibrovascular loops, mean of the ten largest nucleoli, cell type, and tumor size. Ophthalmology 104(5):777–780
34. Bellmann C et al (2010) Uveal melanoma: management and outcome of patients with extraocular spread. Br J Ophthalmol 94(5):569–574
35. Coupland SE, Campbell I, Damato B (2008) Routes of extraocular extension of uveal melanoma: risk factors and influence on survival probability. Ophthalmology 115(10):1778–1785
36. Diener-West M et al (1992) A review of mortality from choroidal melanoma. II. A meta-analysis of 5-year mortality rates following enucleation, through 1988. Arch Ophthalmol 110(2):245–250
37. Comparison of clinical, echographic, and histopathological measurements from eyes with medium-sized choroidal melanoma in the collaborative ocular melanoma study: COMS report no. 21. (2003) Arch Ophthalmol, 121(8): p. 1163–1171
38. Shields CL et al (2009) Metastasis of uveal melanoma millimeter-by-millimeter in 8033 consecutive eyes. Arch Ophthalmol 127(8):989–998
39. McLean IW et al (1995) Choroidal-ciliary body melanoma. A multivariate survival analysis of tumor location. Ophthalmology 102(7):1060–1064
40. Pach JM et al (1986) Prognostic factors in choroidal and ciliary body melanomas with extrascleral extension. Am J Ophthalmol 101(3):325–331
41. Affeldt JC et al (1980) Prognosis in uveal melanoma with extrascleral extension. Arch Ophthalmol 98(11):1975–1979
42. Font RL, Spaulding AG, Zimmerman LDM (1968) a clinicopathologic report of 54 cases. Transactions—American Academy of Ophthal ology and. Otolaryngology 72(6):877–895
43. Reese AB, Howard GM (1967) Flat uveal melanomas. Am J Ophthalmol 64(6): 1021–1028
44. Reichel E et al (1995) Occult choroidal melanoma presenting as a serous macular detachment. Retina 15(2):167–169
45. Yap EY, Robertson DM, Buettner H (1992) Scleritis as an initial manifestation of choroidal malignant melanoma. Ophthalmology 99(11):1693–1697
46. Shields CL et al (1995) Risk factors for growth and metastasis of small choroidal melanocytic lesions. Ophthalmology 102(9): 1351–1361
47. Shields CL et al (1996) Diffuse choroidal melanoma. Clinical features predictive of metastasis. Arch Ophthalmol 114(8):956–963
48. Shields JA, Shields CL (1999) Atlas of Intraocular Tumors. Lippincott Williams & Wilkins, Philadelphia, PA
49. Chaudhry IM, Moster MR, Augsburger JJ (1997) Iris ring melanoma masquerading as pigmentary glaucoma. Arch Ophthalmol 115(11):1480–1481
50. Diekstall F, Demeler U (1988) Therapy-resistant increase in ocular pressure–a rare differential diagnosis: ring melanoma. Fortschr Ophthalmol 85(1):98–100
51. Vasquez LM et al (2008) Ring melanoma of the ciliary body: clinical and ultrasound biomicroscopic characteristics. Can J Ophthalmol 43(2):229–233
52. Demirci H et al (2002) Ring melanoma of the ciliary body: report on twenty-three patients. Retina 22(6):698–706, quiz 852-3
53. Christmas NJ et al (1991) Secondary optic nerve tumors. Surv Ophthalmol 36(3): 196–206
54. Lindegaard J, Heegaard S, Prause JU (2002) Histopathologically verified non-vascular optic nerve lesions in Denmark 1940-99. Acta Ophthalmol Scand 80(1):32–37
55. Shammas HF, Blodi FC (1978) Peripapillary choroidal melanomas. Extension along the

optic nerve and its sheaths. Arch Ophthalmol 96(3):440–445
56. McLean MJ, Foster WD, Zimmerman LE (1977) Prognostic factors in small malignant melanomas of choroid and ciliary body. Arch Ophthalmol 95(1):48–58
57. Damato BE, Paul J, Foulds WS (1996) Risk factors for residual and recurrent uveal melanoma after trans-scleral local resection. Br J Ophthalmol 80(2):102–108
58. McCurdy J, Gamel J, McLean I (1991) A simple, efficient, and reproducible method for estimating the malignant potential of uveal melanoma from routine H & E slides. Pathol Res Pract 187(8):1025–1027
59. Coleman K et al (1996) Prognostic value of morphometric features and the callender classification in uveal melanomas. Ophthalmology 103(10):1634–1641
60. Pe'er J et al (1994) Mean of the ten largest nucleoli, microcirculation architecture, and prognosis of ciliochoroidal melanomas. Ophthalmology 101(7):1227–1235
61. Seregard S et al (1998) Prognostic accuracy of the mean of the largest nucleoli, vascular patterns, and PC-10 in posterior uveal melanoma. Ophthalmology 105(3):485–491
62. Gamel JW, McCurdy JB, McLean IW (1992) A comparison of prognostic covariates for uveal melanoma. Invest Ophthalmol Vis Sci 33(6):1919–1922
63. van Diest PJ et al (1992) Reproducibility of mitosis counting in 2,469 breast cancer specimens: results from the Multicenter Morphometric Mammary Carcinoma Project. Hum Pathol 23(6):603–607
64. Angi M et al (2011) Immunohistochemical assessment of mitotic count in uveal melanoma. Acta Ophthalmol 89(2):e155–e160
65. Tapia C et al (2006) Two mitosis-specific antibodies, MPM-2 and phospho-histone H3 (Ser28), allow rapid and precise determination of mitotic activity. Am J Surg Pathol 30(1):83–89
66. Folberg R et al (1997) The microcirculation of choroidal and ciliary body melanomas. Eye (Lond) 11(Pt 2):227–238
67. Vernon RB, Sage EH (1995) Between molecules and morphology. Extracellular matrix and creation of vascular form. Am J Pathol 147(4):873–883
68. Ajili F et al (2012) Prognostic impact of angiogenesis in nonmuscle invasive bladder cancer as defined by microvessel density after immunohistochemical staining for CD34. Ultrastruct Pathol 36(5):336–342
69. Benckert C et al (2012) Impact of microvessel density on lymph node metastasis and survival after curative resection of pancreatic cancer. Surg Today 42(2):169–176
70. Dutta S et al (2012) The relationship between tumour necrosis, tumour proliferation, local and systemic inflammation, microvessel density and survival in patients undergoing potentially curative resection of oesophageal adenocarcinoma. Br J Cancer 106(4):702–710
71. Iakovlev VV et al (2012) Microvascular density as an independent predictor of clinical outcome in renal cell carcinoma: an automated image analysis study. Lab Invest 92(1):46–56
72. Wang J et al (2012) Lymphatic microvessel density as a prognostic factor in non-small cell lung carcinoma: a meta-analysis of the literature. Mol Biol Rep 39(5):5331–5338
73. Folkman J (1985) Tumor angiogenesis. Adv Cancer Res 43:175–203
74. Weidner N et al (1991) Tumor angiogenesis and metastasis–correlation in invasive breast carcinoma. N Engl J Med 324(1):1–8
75. Folberg R et al (1993) The prognostic value of tumor blood vessel morphology in primary uveal melanoma. Ophthalmology 100(9):1389–1398
76. Rummelt V et al (1994) Microcirculation architecture of melanocytic nevi and malignant melanomas of the ciliary body and choroid. A comparative histopathologic and ultrastructural study. Ophthalmology 101(4):718–727
77. Histopathologic characteristics of uveal melanomas in eyes enucleated from the Collaborative Ocular Melanoma Study. (1998) COMS report no. 6. Am J Ophthalmol 125(6):745–766
78. McLean IW, Saraiva VS, Burnier MN (2004) Pathological and prognostic features of uveal melanomas. Can J Ophthalmol 39(4):343–350
79. Shammas HF, Blodi FC (1977) Prognostic factors in choroidal and ciliary body melanomas. Arch Ophthalmol 95(1):63–69
80. Ly LV et al (2010) Inflammatory cytokines in eyes with uveal melanoma and relation with macrophage infiltration. Invest Ophthalmol Vis Sci 51(11):5445–5451
81. Durie FH et al (1990) Analysis of lymphocytic infiltration in uveal melanoma. Invest Ophthalmol Vis Sci 31(10):2106–2110
82. Gown AM et al (1986) Monoclonal antibodies specific for melanocytic tumors distinguish subpopulations of melanocytes. Am J Pathol 123(2):195–203
83. Steuhl KP et al (1993) Significance, specificity, and ultrastructural localization of HMB-45 antigen in pigmented ocular tumors. Ophthalmology 100(2):208–215
84. Ordonez NG, Ji XL, Hickey RC (1988) Comparison of HMB-45 monoclonal antibody and S-100 protein in the immunohisto-

chemical diagnosis of melanoma. Am J Clin Pathol 90(4):385–390
85. Wick MR, Swanson PE, Rocamora A (1988) Recognition of malignant melanoma by monoclonal antibody HMB-45. An immunohistochemical study of 200 paraffin-embedded cutaneous tumors. J Cutan Pathol 15(4): 201–207
86. Burnier MN Jr, McLean IW, Gamel JW (1991) Immunohistochemical evaluation of uveal melanocytic tumors. Expression of HMB-45, S-100 protein, and neuron-specific enolase. Cancer 68(4):809–814
87. Luyten GP et al (1996) Metastatic uveal melanoma. A morphologic and immunohistochemical analysis. Cancer 78(9):1967–1971
88. Schafer BW, Heizmann CW (1996) The S100 family of EF-hand calcium-binding proteins: functions and pathology. Trends Biochem Sci 21(4):134–140
89. Baudier J, Glasser N, Gerard D (1986) Ions binding to S100 proteins. I. Calcium- and zinc-binding properties of bovine brain S100 alpha alpha, S100a (alpha beta), and S100b (beta beta) protein: Zn2+ regulates Ca2+ binding on S100b protein. J Biol Chem 261(18):8192–8203
90. Cochran AJ et al (1983) Detection of cytoplasmic S-100 protein in primary and metastatic intraocular melanomas. Invest Ophthalmol Vis Sci 24(8):1153–1155
91. Cochran AJ et al (1993) S-100 protein remains a practical marker for melanocytic and other tumours. Melanoma Res 3(5):325–330
92. Gerdes J et al (1984) Cell cycle analysis of a cell proliferation-associated human nuclear antigen defined by the monoclonal antibody Ki-67. J Immunol 133(4):1710–1715
93. Mooy CM et al (1990) Ki-67 immunostaining in uveal melanoma. The effect of pre-enucleation radiotherapy. Ophthalmology 97(10):1275–1280
94. Schilling H, Sehu KW, Lee WR (1997) A histologic study (including DNA quantification and Ki-67 labeling index) in uveal melanomas after brachytherapy with ruthenium plaques. Invest Ophthalmol Vis Sci 38(10): 2081–2092
95. Chowers I et al (2001) Comparison of microcirculation patterns and MIB-1 immunoreactivity in iris and posterior uveal melanoma. Ophthalmology 108(2):367–371
96. Al-Jamal RT, Kivela T (2006) KI-67 immunopositivity in choroidal and ciliary body melanoma with respect to nucleolar diameter and other prognostic factors. Curr Eye Res 31(1):57–67
97. Chen YT et al (1996) Serological analysis of Melan-A(MART-1), a melanocyte-specific protein homogeneously expressed in human melanomas. Proc Natl Acad Sci U S A 93(12):5915–5919
98. Blessing K, Sanders DS, Grant JJ (1998) Comparison of immunohistochemical staining of the novel antibody melan-A with S100 protein and HMB-45 in malignant melanoma and melanoma variants. Histopathology 32(2):139–146
99. Heegaard S, Jensen OA, Prause JU (2000) Immunohistochemical diagnosis of malignant melanoma of the conjunctiva and uvea: comparison of the novel antibody against melan-A with S100 protein and HMB-45. Melanoma Res 10(4):350–354
100. Fernandes BF et al (2007) Immunohistochemical expression of melan-A and tyrosinase in uveal melanoma. J Carcinog 6:6
101. Kivela T, Eskelin S, Kujala E (2006) Metastatic uveal melanoma. Int Ophthalmol Clin 46(1):133–149
102. Zakka KA et al (1980) Malignant melanoma. Analysis of an autopsy population. Ophthalmology 87(6):549–556
103. Gragoudas ES et al (1991) Survival of patients with metastases from uveal melanoma. Ophthalmology 98(3):383–389, discussion 390
104. Diener-West M et al (2004) Screening for metastasis from choroidal melanoma: the Collaborative Ocular Melanoma Study Group Report 23. J Clin Oncol 22(12):2438–2444
105. Donoso LA et al (1985) Metastatic uveal melanoma. Pretherapy serum liver enzyme and liver scan abnormalities. Arch Ophthalmol 103(6):796–798
106. Gombos DS et al (2004) Geographic disparities in diagnostic screening for metastatic uveal melanoma. Ophthalmology 111(12):2254–2258
107. Hicks C, Foss AJ, Hungerford JL (1998) Predictive power of screening tests for metastasis in uveal melanoma. Eye (Lond) 12(Pt 6):945–948
108. Mouriaux F et al (2012) Liver function testing is not helpful for early diagnosis of metastatic uveal melanoma. Ophthalmology 119(8):1590–1595
109. Eskelin S et al (1999) Screening for metastatic malignant melanoma of the uvea revisited. Cancer 85(5):1151–1159
110. Bedikian AY et al (1995) Treatment of uveal melanoma metastatic to the liver: a review of the M. D. Anderson Cancer Center experience and prognostic factors. Cancer 76(9):1665–1670
111. Leyvraz S et al (1997) Treatment of ocular melanoma metastatic to the liver by hepatic arterial chemotherapy. J Clin Oncol 15(7): 2589–2595

112. Mudhar HS et al (2004) A critical appraisal of the prognostic and predictive factors for uveal malignant melanoma. Histopathology 45(1):1–12
113. Bonfrer JM et al (1998) The luminescence immunoassay S-100: a sensitive test to measure circulating S-100B: its prognostic value in malignant melanoma. Br J Cancer 77(12):2210–2214
114. Bosserhoff AK et al (1999) MIA, a novel serum marker for progression of malignant melanoma. Anticancer Res 19(4A):2691–2693
115. Rittling SR, Chambers AF (2004) Role of osteopontin in tumour progression. Br J Cancer 90(10):1877–1881
116. Bonfrer JM, Korse CM, Israels SP (1997) Serum S-100 has prognostic significance in malignant melanoma. Anticancer Res 17(4B):2975–2977
117. Hauschild A et al (1999) S100B protein detection in serum is a significant prognostic factor in metastatic melanoma. Oncology 56(4):338–344
118. Kadkol SS et al (2006) Osteopontin expression and serum levels in metastatic uveal melanoma: a pilot study. Invest Ophthalmol Vis Sci 47(3):802–806
119. Reiniger IW et al (2005) "Melanoma inhibitory activity" (MIA): a promising serological tumour marker in metastatic uveal melanoma. Graefes Arch Clin Exp Ophthalmol 243(11):1161–1166
120. Hawkins BS (2004) The Collaborative Ocular Melanoma Study (COMS) randomized trial of pre-enucleation radiation of large choroidal melanoma: IV. Ten-year mortality findings and prognostic factors. COMS report number 24. Am J Ophthalmol 138(6):936–951
121. Meziani L et al (2012) Uveal metastasis revealing lung cancer. J Fr Ophtalmol 35(6):420–425
122. Shields CL et al (1997) Survey of 520 eyes with uveal metastases. Ophthalmology 104(8):1265–1276
123. Harada S et al (1983) Solitary pulmonary metastasis of choroidal malignant melanoma: report of an unusual case. Endoscopy 15(6):363–364
124. Tishler M, Greif J, Topilsky M (1986) Solitary pulmonary metastasis of choroidal malignant melanoma simulating primary lung cancer. Eur J Respir Dis 68(3):215–217
125. Frenkel S et al (2009) Long-term survival of uveal melanoma patients after surgery for liver metastases. Br J Ophthalmol 93(8):1042–1046
126. Sato T et al (1997) Time to systemic metastases in patients with posterior uveal melanoma. Cancer Invest 15(2):98–105
127. Summanen P et al (1993) Survival of patients and metastatic and local recurrent tumor growth in malignant melanoma of the uvea after ruthenium plaque radiotherapy. Ophthalmic Surg 24(2):82–90
128. Feinstein EG et al (2010) Hepatic abnormalities identified on abdominal computed tomography at diagnosis of uveal melanoma. Arch Ophthalmol 128(3):319–323
129. Schoder H, Larson SM, Yeung HW (2004) PET/CT in oncology: integration into clinical management of lymphoma, melanoma, and gastrointestinal malignancies. J Nucl Med 45(Suppl 1):72S–81S
130. Cohade C et al (2003) Direct comparison of (18)F-FDG PET and PET/CT in patients with colorectal carcinoma. J Nucl Med 44(11):1797–1803
131. Antoch G et al (2003) Whole-body dual-modality PET/CT and whole-body MRI for tumor staging in oncology. JAMA 290(24):3199–3206
132. Freudenberg LS et al (2004) Whole-body fluorine-18 fluordeoxyglucose positron emission tomography/computed tomography (FDG-PET/CT) in staging of advanced uveal melanoma. Surv Ophthalmol 49(5):537–540
133. Finger PT et al (2005) Whole body PET/CT for initial staging of choroidal melanoma. Br J Ophthalmol 89(10):1270–1274
134. Orcurto V et al (2012) (18) F-fluorodeoxyglucose positron emission tomography/computed tomography and magnetic resonance imaging in patients with liver metastases from uveal melanoma: results from a pilot study. Melanoma Res 22(1): 63–69
135. Servois V et al (2010) Preoperative staging of liver metastases from uveal melanoma by magnetic resonance imaging (MRI) and fluorodeoxyglucose-positron emission tomography (FDG-PET). Eur J Surg Oncol 36(2):189–194
136. Wykoff CC et al (2011) Preoperative evaluation for patients with choroidal/ciliary body melanomas: what is necessary? Am J Ophthalmol 151(6):921–924
137. Hendler K et al (2011) Trends in liver function tests: a comparison with serum tumor markers in metastatic uveal melanoma (part 2). Anticancer Res 31(1):351–357
138. Missotten GS et al (2007) S-100B protein and melanoma inhibitory activity protein in uveal melanoma screening. A comparison with liver function tests. Tumour Biol 28(2):63–69
139. Harbour JW (2012) The genetics of uveal melanoma: an emerging framework for targeted therapy. Pigment Cell Melanoma Res 25(2):171–181
140. Francken AB et al (2006) Detection of metastatic disease in patients with uveal melanoma using positron emission tomography. Eur J Surg Oncol 32(7):780–784

Chapter 22

A Prognostic Test to Predict the Risk of Metastasis in Uveal Melanoma Based on a 15-Gene Expression Profile

J. William Harbour

Abstract

Uveal (ocular) melanoma is an aggressive cancer that metastasizes in up to half of patients. Uveal melanoma spreads preferentially to the liver, and the metastatic disease is almost always fatal. There are no effective therapies for advanced metastatic disease, so the most promising strategy for improving survival is to detect metastasis at an earlier stage or to treat high-risk patients in an adjuvant setting. An accurate test for identifying high-risk patients would allow for such personalized management as well as for stratification of high-risk patients into clinical trials of adjuvant therapy.

We developed a gene expression profile (GEP) that distinguishes between primary uveal melanomas that have a low metastatic risk (class 1 tumors) and those with a high metastatic risk (class 2 tumors). We migrated the GEP from a high-density microarray platform to a 15-gene, qPCR-based assay that is now performed in a College of American Pathologists (CAP)-accredited Clinical Laboratory Improvement Amendments (CLIA)-certified laboratory on a routine clinical basis on very small samples obtained by fine needle aspiration and on archival formalin-fixed specimens. We collaborated with several centers to show that our specimen collection protocol was easily learned and performed and that it allowed samples to be safely and reliably transported from distant locations with a very low failure rate. Finally, we showed in a multicenter, prospective study that our GEP assay is highly accurate for predicting which patients will develop metastatic disease, and it was significantly superior to the previous gold standard, chromosome 3 testing for monosomy 3. This is the only prognostic test in uveal melanoma ever to undergo such extensive validation, and it is currently being used in a commercial format under the trade name DecisionDx-UM in over 100 centers in the USA and Canada.

Key words Uveal melanoma, Metastasis, Prognosis, Gene expression profiling, Support vector machine, Machine learning algorithm

1 Introduction

Uveal melanoma is the most common primary malignancy of the eye, with an incidence of about 1,200–1,500 new cases per year in the USA, and it accounts for about 5 % of all melanomas [1–4]. Uveal melanomas can arise anywhere in the uveal tract of the eye, composed of the iris, ciliary body, and choroid. Uveal melanomas rarely exhibit regional lymphatic spread, but, rather, they metastasize

Magdalena Thurin and Francesco M. Marincola (eds.), *Molecular Diagnostics for Melanoma: Methods and Protocols*, Methods in Molecular Biology, vol. 1102, DOI 10.1007/978-1-62703-727-3_22, © Springer Science+Business Media New York 2014

hematogenously to the liver and, to a lesser extent, other sites such as lung and bone [5]. Clinical and histopathologic features associated with poor prognosis include larger tumor size, ciliary body involvement, advanced patient age, epithelioid cell type, extracellular matrix patterning, and extraocular tumor invasion [6–10]. The mortality rate at 15-year diagnosis of the primary tumor is about 50 % [11], and median survival after detection of metastatic disease is about 9 months [12].

1.1 Chromosomal Alterations as Prognostic Markers

Several recurring chromosomal abnormalities in uveal melanoma have been used for prognostication, including loss of 1p, 3, 6q, 8p, and 9p and gain of 1q, 6p, and 8q. Various techniques have been used to detect these changes, including standard karyotyping [13–19], fluorescence in situ hybridization (FISH) [20, 21], comparative genomic hybridization (CGH) [22–28], spectral karyotyping [29], microsatellite analysis (MSA) [30, 31], multiplex ligation-dependent probe amplification (MLPA) [32], and single-nucleotide polymorphisms (SNPs) [33]. Loss of one copy of chromosome 3 (monosomy 3) occurs in almost half of uveal melanomas and is the most prognostically significant of these chromosomal markers [31, 34]. The prognostic accuracy of chromosome 3 status can be improved by including other chromosomal information, including 6p and 8q gain, as well as clinical and histopathologic information, which results in multiple combinations of prognostic groups [32].

1.2 Transition from Chromosomal Markers to Gene Expression Profiling

Cytogenetic alterations provided an important step towards the development of accurate prognostic markers for uveal melanoma, but they have a number of significant drawbacks that limit their value for routine clinical use. These methods were developed from uveal melanomas that were treated by enucleation, which provides a large amount of tumor tissue. However, about 90 % of uveal melanomas are treated not by enucleation but by radiotherapy, in which case the only opportunity to obtain tumor tissue is by needle biopsy. Unfortunately, the amount of tumor material obtained by needle biopsy is often insufficient for chromosomal assay techniques.

Further problems with chromosomal prognostic testing include sampling error resulting from intratumoral heterogeneity [32, 35] and the complicated combination of chromosomal changes and clinicopathologic information that are needed to maximize prognostic accuracy [32]. Thus, several groups explored the use of gene expression profile (GEP) as a potentially more robust prognostic and accurate method. Analysis of uveal melanomas using high-density microarrays showed that tumors with disomy 3 exhibited a different GEP than those with monosomy 3 [36]. Our group went on to show that GEP could classify UMs into two prognostically significant groups using unsupervised clustering techniques without regard to chromosomal status [2].

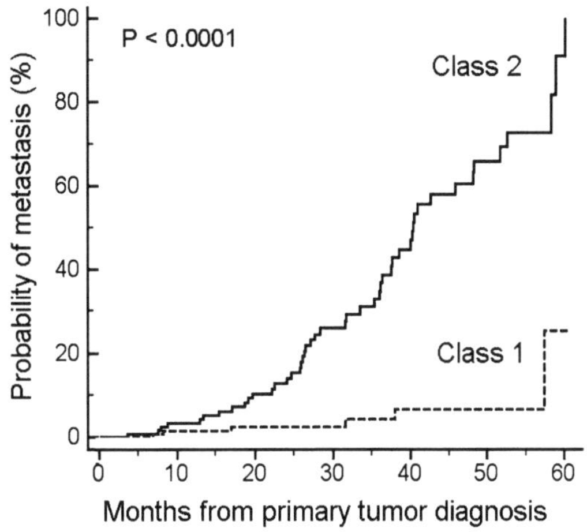

Fig. 1 Prognostic performance of the 15-gene assay. Kaplan–Meier survival plot of 334 uveal melanoma patients with up to 5-year follow-up

Class 1 tumors had a low risk and class 2 tumors had a high risk of metastasis (*see* Fig. 1). Notably, the prognostic accuracy of this GEP classification outperformed clinical, pathological, and cytogenetic prognostic indicators [37], and this has been confirmed by several independent groups [38, 39]. A likely reason for the superiority of GEP over cytogenetic methods for prognostication is that cytogenetic markers are often distributed heterogeneously throughout the tumor and are thus prone to sampling error. In contrast, GEP represents a functional "snapshot" of the tumor's microenvironment that is less variable across the tumor [40]. We migrated the GEP to an assay comprising 12 discriminating genes and 3 control genes performed on a microfluidics platform that could be used on a routine clinical basis on very small samples from fine needle biopsies [40]. The prognostic accuracy of this assay, and its superiority over chromosome 3 status for clinical prognostic testing, was recently validated in a prospective study involving ten centers across North America [41].

1.3 Biological Insights from GEP

Aside from its clinical value, gene expression profiling has provided important insights into the pathobiology of UM. The GEP of class 1 tumors closely resembles that of normal uveal melanocytes and low-grade uveal melanocytic tumors, whereas the GEP of class 2 tumors shows reduced expression of melanocytic genes and instead resembles the transcriptome of primitive neural/ectodermal stem cells [42, 43].

The 12 discriminating genes in the GEP assay are indicated in Table 1. Many of these genes have been previously shown to be associated with cancer [40].

Table 1
Genes included in the 15-gene expression profile

Gene symbol	Gene name
Up-regulated in class 2 uveal melanomas	
CDH1	E-cadherin
ECM1	Extracellular matrix protein 1
HTR2B	5-Hydroxytryptamine (serotonin) receptor 2B
RAB31	RAB31, member RAS oncogene family
Down-regulated in class 2 uveal melanomas	
EIF1B	Eukaryotic translation initiation factor 1B
FXR1	Fragile X mental retardation, autosomal homolog 1
ID2	Inhibitor of DNA binding 2
LMCD1	LIM and cysteine-rich domains 1
LTA4H	Leukotriene A4 hydrolase
MTUS1	Microtubule-associated tumor suppressor 1
ROBO1	Roundabout, axon guidance receptor, 1
SATB1	SATB homeobox 1
Control genes	
MRPS21	Mitochondrial ribosomal protein S21
RBM23	RNA-binding motif protein 23
SAP130	Sin3A-associated protein, 130 kDa

1.4 Class 2 Tumors and BAP1 Mutations

Our findings suggested that class 2 tumors have undergone mutations that lead to a loss of melanocyte cell identity and reversion to a stem-like phenotype. We used exome capture followed by next-generation sequencing to search for mutations that may be specifically associated with class 2 tumors [44]. We identified frequent inactivating mutations in the BRCA1-associated protein 1 (BAP1), located at chromosome 3p21.1, and loss of the other copy of chromosome 3, in the vast majority of class 2 tumors but in only one class 1 tumor which retained two copies of chromosome 3. BAP1 is a ubiquitin carboxy-terminal hydrolase that appears to play a major role in the developmental regulation of chromatin structure as a component of the Polycomb repressor complex PR-DUB [45]. We reported one uveal melanoma patient carrying a germline BAP1 mutation [44], and we identified another family with a germline BAP1 mutation in which uveal and cutaneous melanoma occurred in multiple family members (unpublished data). Subsequent to our report, there have been a growing number of cancers associated with somatic and germline BAP1 mutations, including uveal and cutaneous melanoma, mesothelioma, meningioma, lung cancer, breast cancer, and renal carcinoma [46–53]. Despite the strong correlation between BAP1 mutations and the class 2 signature, however, the latter continues to be much more accurate for clinical prognostic testing. As with chromosomal analysis, which suffers from intratumoral heterogeneity and consequent sampling error, BAP1 mutations can also be heterogeneously distributed within the tumor. Thus, we do not believe that either chromosomal analysis or BAP1 testing should replace the GEP assay for routine clinical use.

2 Materials

2.1 Tumor Tissue Preservation and RNA Isolation

1. Molecular Devices Picopure RNA Isolation Kit for fine needle aspiration biopsy (FNAB) (Molecular Devices, Sunnyvale, CA).
2. TRIzol RNA Isolation Reagent for Snap-Frozen Tumor Samples (Invitrogen, Carlsbad, CA).
3. RecoverAll Total Nucleic Acid Isolation Kit for Formalin-Fixed Paraffin-Embedded (FFPE) samples (Ambion, Austin, TX).
4. RNeasy Kit (Qiagen, Valencia, CA).
5. Microcentrifuge (Eppendorf 5415D or similar).
6. Nuclease-free pipette tips.
7. 0.5 ml microcentrifuge tubes (Applied Biosystems).

2.2 Real-Time PCR

1. cDNA synthesis reagents: High Capacity cDNA Reverse Transcription Kit (Applied Biosystems Inc.).
2. Pre-amplification reagents:
   (a) TaqMan® Pre-Amp Master Mix Kit.
   (b) 20× TaqMan® gene expression assays for the 12 discriminating genes and 3 control genes (Table 1).
3. Tris–EDTA buffer (10 mM Tris–HCl, 1 mM EDTA, pH 8.0).
4. RT-PCR reagents:
   (a) TaqMan® Gene Expression Master Mix.
   (b) TaqMan® Low Density Array Format 16 RT-PCR plate custom ordered to include the 12 discriminant genes and 3 control genes. The components of the TaqMan® Pre-Amp Mix Kit and Gene Expression Master Mix are the proprietary property of Applied Biosystems, Inc.
5. Centrifuge (Sorvall Legend T Plus with TTH-750 rotor).
6. RT-PCR instrument (7900HT Fast Real-Time PCR System).

2.3 Gene Expression Analysis and Class Assignment

1. Sequence Detection Systems (SDS) Software for 7900HT Fast Real-Time PCR System.
2. GIST Support Vector Machine learning algorithm software (http://www.chibi.ubc.ca/gist).

3 Methods

3.1 Preparation of RNA

3.1.1 Preparation of RNA from Needle Biopsy Samples

1. The preferred method of obtaining tumor tissue for the GEP assay is by FNAB (*see* **Note 1**). Once the sample is obtained in the needle hub, it is immediately handed off to an un-scrubbed assistant and expelled into an empty RNase-free tube in the operating room (*see* Fig. 2).
2. The needle is then placed in another RNase-free tube containing 200 μl of extraction buffer (XB) from the PicoPure® RNA isolation kit, which was drawn up into the needle hub to dislodge and collect additional tumor cells, and the XB is then transferred to the first (empty) tube.
3. The cap of the tube is closed, and the tube is flicked gently with the finger to suspend the tumor cells in the XB.
4. The collection tube is then snap frozen in liquid nitrogen prior to leaving the operating room.
5. For transport to the testing laboratory, tubes are placed on dry ice and mailed by overnight courier.
6. Once the specimen arrives in the laboratory, RNA is isolated using the PicoPure® kit (including the optional DNase step).
7. Pipet an equal volume of 70 % ethanol solution to the tube containing FNAB sample in extraction buffer by pipetting up and down ten times.
8. Pipet the mixture onto the membrane of the pre-cleansed purification column.
9. Spin at 100 × *g* for 2 min and immediately followed by a spin at 16,000 × *g* for 1 min.
10. Wash the column sequentially with wash buffer 1 and 2 and spin at 8,000 × *g* for 1 min. Follow with another wash with buffer 2, and spin at 16,000 × *g* to dry the column.
11. Elute RNA with 10–30 μl of DEPC-treated water or elution buffer (EB).
12. To remove genomic DNA from total RNA add 0.1 volume of 10× DNase I buffer and 0.5–1 μl of 2 U/μl DNase I to the RNA solution and incubate at 37 °C for 20–30 min.
13. Inactivate DNAse I with 0.1 volume of the DNAse inactivation reagent to the sample. Incubate in room temperature for 2 min, and spin at 10,000 × *g* for 1 min to pellet the DNase

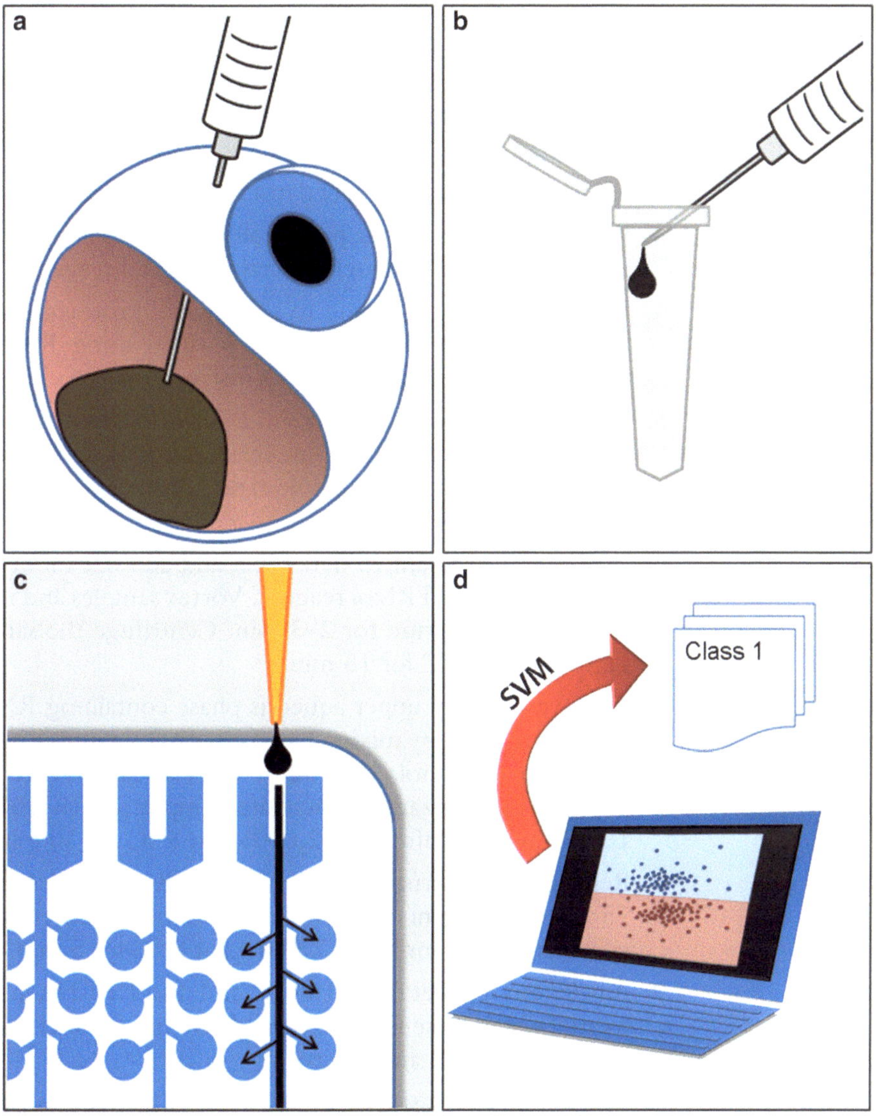

Fig. 2 Work flow for 15-gene expression profile prognostic assay. (**a**) A needle biopsy of the uveal melanoma is performed prior to plaque brachytherapy or immediately after enucleation (eye removal). (**b**) The needle biopsy aspirate is immediately expelled into an empty tube, and then the same needle is used to draw up 200 μl of extraction buffer, which is then expelled into the first tube containing the tumor sample. (**c**) RNA is isolated, converted to cDNA, pre-amplified, loaded onto TaqMan® Expression Assays on microfluidics cards, and subjected to PCR using the 7900HT Real-Time PCR System. (**d**) C_t values are calculated and analyzed using support vector machine (SVM), which compares new test samples to a validated training set of samples. SVM assigns each new sample to class 1 or class 2

inactivation reagent. RNA can be further purified using RNeasy column (Qiagen) or used for subsequent steps.

14. Determine the concentration of RNA samples using a Nanodrop Fluorospectrometer. This procedure usually yields about 100 ng to 1.5 μg total RNA per FNAB.

3.1.2 Preparation of RNA from Snap-Frozen Tumor Samples

1. For eyes that are undergoing enucleation, an alternative method for obtaining tumor samples is to open the globe immediately after the eye is removed and dissect a small piece of tumor tissue using a blade or a scissors.
2. The sample is wrapped in foil, immediately snap frozen in liquid nitrogen, and maintained in a frozen state (at least −80 °C).
3. When ready for analysis, part or all of the frozen tumor sample is thawed and immediately placed in TRIzol reagent.
4. RNA is isolated according to the TRIzol protocol, including the optional isolation step, and purified using RNeasy kits according to the manufacturer's instructions.
5. Homogenize tissue samples in 1 ml of TRIzol reagent per 50–100 mg of tissues and incubate at room temperature for 5 min to permit the complete tissue dissociation. Centrifuge to remove cell debris.
6. Transfer supernatant to new tube, and add 0.2 ml of chloroform per 1 ml or TRIzol reagent. Vortex samples and incubate at room temperature for 2–3 min. Centrifuge the samples at 12,000 × *g* at 8 °C for 15 min.
7. Remove carefully upper aqueous phase containing RNA, and precipitate RNA by mixing with isopropyl alcohol. Use 0.5 ml of isopropyl alcohol per 1 ml of TRIzol reagent used for the initial homogenization. Incubate samples at 15–30 °C for 10 min and centrifuge at 12,000 × *g* at 8 °C for 10 min.
8. Remove the supernatant, and wash the RNA pellet twice with 75 % ethanol (1 ml of ethanol per 1 ml of TRIzol reagent) by vortexing and spinning at 7,500 × *g* at 8 °C for 5 min.
9. Air-dry RNA pellet for 5–10 min, and dissolve RNA in DEPC-treated water. Take OD at 260 and 280 nm to determine sample concentration and purity.
10. RNA samples are stored at −80 °C and handled as described for the biopsy method.

3.1.3 Preparation of RNA from Formalin-Fixed Paraffin-Embedded Samples

1. The GEP assay can be reliably performed on FFPE samples that are up to 3 years old. For this method, five 10 μm sections are obtained from tissue blocks, and tumor tissue is scraped away from surrounding normal material using a dissecting microscope (laser capture microdissection is not necessary) and collected in RecoverAll™.
2. Total RNA is isolated using the RecoverAll™ Total Nucleic Acid Isolation kit following the manufacturer's protocol.
3. FFPE samples are deparaffinized using a series of xylene and ethanol washes. Tissue slices are placed in microcentrifuge tube, and 1 ml of xylene is added to the sample. Incubate the sample at 50 °C for 3 min to melt paraffin. Centrifuge at maximum speed at room temperature for 2 min.

4. Remove the xylene, and wash the pellet with 1 ml of ethanol by vortexing. Centrifuge at maximum speed at room temperature for 2 min. Repeat the washing step with 100 % ethanol. Remove the ethanol, and air-dry the pellet.
5. Next, the samples are subjected to a rigorous protease digestion. Add digestion buffer (100–200 μl) to each sample and 4 μl of Protease K. Incubate the sample in heat blocks at 50 °C for 15 min and then at 80 °C for 15 min.
6. Add isolation additive/ethanol mixture according to the volume of digestion buffer (e.g., 790–200 μl, respectively) and mix.
7. RNA is purified using filter cartridge methodology. Pipet the sample/ethanol mixture on the cartridge and centrifuge at 10,000 × g for 30 s. Discard the flow through, and wash the filter cartridge with 700 μl of wash 1 buffer followed by 500 μl of wash 2/3. Centrifuge at 10,000 × g for 30 s each time.
8. Final step includes an on-filter nuclease treatment with DNase mix containing 6 μl of 10× DNase buffer, 4 μl DNase, and 50 μl nuclease-free water at 22–25 °C for 30 min.
9. Filter cartridge is washed with 700 μl of wash 1 and centrifuged at 10,000 × g for 30 s. Repeat this step with wash 2/3. RNA is eluted into either water or the low-salt elusion solution. RNA samples are stored at −80 °C and handled as described for the biopsy method.

3.2 Real-Time PCR

1. RNA samples quantified using the Nanodrop 1000 spectrophotometer are converted to cDNA using the High Capacity cDNA Reverse Transcription kit from Applied Biosystems. Add 50 ng to 1 μg of RNA to the cDNA transcription step in a final reaction volume of 20 μl.
2. The reverse transcription reaction is performed in a 96-well plate using the 7900HT Real-Time PCR System.
3. Combine cDNA reactions with 0.2× pooled TaqMan assay mix containing equal volumes of each of the 15 TaqMan assays used to amplify discriminant and control genes and TaqMan® Pre-Amp Master Mix.
4. Pre-amplification is carried out for 14 cycles in a 96-well plate using the 7900HT system and immediately placed on ice following completion of cycling.
5. Dilute pre-amplified samples 20-fold into sterile TE buffer and store at −20 °C until needed.
6. Perform PCR step using the 7900HT Real-Time PCR System with Applied Biosystems TaqMan® Gene Expression Assays and Gene Expression Master Mix following the manufacturer's protocol.

7. Thaw, vortex, and centrifuge pre-amplified samples. Add an equal volume of 2× TaqMan® Gene Expression Master Mix to each reaction and mix thoroughly by vortexing. Centrifuge samples prior to loading to 96-well microfluidics plate.
8. TaqMan® Microfluidics Expression Arrays are custom ordered to include our 12 class discriminating genes, 3 endogenous control genes, and 18S rRNA as a manufacturer's control, and each sample is analyzed in triplicate.
9. Add 100 μl of reaction mix to each fill port of the custom microfluidics plate.
10. Centrifuge the array to dispense approximately 2 μl of pre-amplified reaction mix per well. Verify that all wells have uniform volume following centrifugation step. The plate is ready to be run on the 7900HT instrument.
11. SDSv2.3 software is used to control the 7900HT system, and samples undergo 40 cycles of amplification during the procedure.
12. C_t values are calculated using the manufacturer's software, and mean C_t values are calculated for all triplicate sets. ΔC_t values are calculated by subtracting the mean C_t of each discriminating gene from the geometric mean of the mean C_t values of the three endogenous control genes (*see* **Note 2**).
13. An "undetectable transcript" is defined as a transcript that exhibits no C_t value after 40 qPCR cycles. A "sample failure" is defined as a sample in which one or more endogenous control transcripts are undetectable after 40 qPCR cycles (*see* **Note 3**).

3.3 Analysis

1. We selected support vector machine (SVM) as the machine learning algorithm for this assay because it is a robust and widely accepted machine learning algorithm and because it outperformed other similar algorithms in our analyses.
2. SVM uses a training set of samples with known molecular class to assign new test samples. We have generated such a training set of samples from patients with very long follow-up.
3. SVM inputs the gene expression data of the training set as two sets of vectors (class 1 and class 2) in *n*-dimensional space and then constructs a hyperplane that maximizes the space between the two data sets [54]. SVM then classifies test samples by placing them on one or the other side of this hyperplane. The proximity of the sample to the hyperplane is inversely proportional to the discriminant score, which is a measure of confidence.

Initially, we were concerned that a low discriminant score may be associated with less accurate test results. However, this has not been the case. Nevertheless, we issue a reduced confidence warning if the score is below 0.1.

4 Notes

1. FNBA is typically performed in the operating room and may occur as an isolated procedure but more often is performed at the time of surgery for insertion of a radioactive plaque for brachytherapy or at the time of enucleation (eye removal). In the case of brachytherapy, the biopsy is performed immediately prior to attachment of the plaque to the surface of the eye. It is important to note that this assay has not been validated for tumors that were previously irradiated, which would be expected to alter global gene expression. In the case of enucleation, the biopsy is performed away from the operative field immediately after eye removal.
2. Since the amount of RNA in these samples is too low to evaluate for RNA quality using conventional electrophoretic methods, we have found it useful to use the geometric mean of the C_t values of the three endogenous controls as a measure of intact RNA template available for amplification in each sample. This is based on the assumption that the endogenous controls should be expressed at constant levels across all uveal melanomas, so a high C_t value should be a technical rather than biological aberration.
3. Sample failure in the prospective, multicenter study and on the current commercial platform is less than 5 % of samples, which is far superior to failure rates reported for all available chromosomal analytic platforms that have been subjected to peer review [41]. We found no relationship between sample failure and the concentration of RNA in the original sample as measured by NanoDrop, indicating that the GEP assay can detect RNA transcripts below the limits of the NanoDrop instrument. Rather, sample failure correlates with deviation from the SOPs for obtaining and processing samples. These deviations include failure to immediately snap freeze samples in the operating room and maintain them at −80 °C until analyzed and dilution of the 200 μl of extraction buffer with excess ocular fluid.

References

1. Harbour JW (2003) Clinical overview of uveal melanoma: introduction to tumors of the eye. In: Albert DM, Polans A (eds) Ocular oncology. Marcel Dekker, New York, pp 1–18
2. Onken MD, Worley LA, Ehlers JP, Harbour JW (2004) Gene expression profiling in uveal melanoma reveals two molecular classes and predicts metastatic death. Cancer Res 64:7205–7209
3. Egan KM, Seddon JM, Glynn RJ, Gragoudas ES, Albert DM (1988) Epidemiologic aspects of uveal melanoma. Surv Ophthalmol 32:239–251
4. Ramaiya KJ, Harbour JW (2007) Current management of uveal melanoma. Exp Rev Ophthalmol 2:939–946
5. Diener-West M, Reynolds SM, Agugliaro DJ, Caldwell R, Cumming K, Earle JD, Hawkins BS, Hayman JA, Jaiyesimi I, Jampol LM, Kirkwood JM, Koh WJ, Robertson DM, Shaw JM, Straatsma BR, Thoma J (2005)

Development of metastatic disease after enrollment in the COMS trials for treatment of choroidal melanoma: Collaborative Ocular Melanoma Study Group Report No. 26. Arch Ophthalmol 123:1639–1643
6. Augsburger JJ, Gamel JW (1990) Clinical prognostic factors in patients with posterior uveal malignant melanoma. Cancer 66:1596–1600
7. Gamel JW, McLean IW, Foster WD, Zimmerman LE (1978) Uveal melanomas: correlation of cytologic features with prognosis. Cancer 41:1897–1901
8. de la Cruz PO Jr, Spech CS, McLean IW (1990) Lymphocytic infiltration in uveal malignant melanoma. Cancer 65:112–115
9. Folberg R, Pe'er J, Gruman LM, Woolson RF, Jeng G, Montague PR, Moninger TO, Yi H, Moore KC (1992) The morphologic characteristics of tumor blood vessels as a marker of tumor progression in primary human uveal melanoma: a matched case-control study. Hum Pathol 23:1298–1305
10. Makitie T, Summanen P, Tarkkanen A, Kivela T (2001) Tumor-infiltrating macrophages (CD68(+) cells) and prognosis in malignant uveal melanoma. Invest Ophthalmol Vis Sci 42:1414–1421
11. Kujala E, Makitie T, Kivela T (2003) Very long-term prognosis of patients with malignant uveal melanoma. Invest Ophthalmol Vis Sci 44:4651–4659
12. Kath R, Hayungs J, Bornfeld N, Sauerwein W, Hoffken K, Seeber S (1993) Prognosis and treatment of disseminated uveal melanoma. Cancer 72:2219–2223
13. Griffin CA, Long PP, Schachat AP (1988) Trisomy 6p in an ocular melanoma. Cancer Genet Cytogenet 32:129–132
14. Horsman DE, Sroka H, Rootman J, White VA (1990) Monosomy 3 and isochromosome 8q in a uveal melanoma. Cancer Genet Cytogenet 45:249–253
15. Prescher G, Bornfeld N, Becher R (1990) Nonrandom chromosomal abnormalities in primary uveal melanoma. J Natl Cancer Inst 82:1765–1769
16. Sisley K, Rennie IG, Cottam DW, Potter AM, Potter CW, Rees RC (1990) Cytogenetic findings in six posterior uveal melanomas: involvement of chromosomes 3, 6, and 8. Genes Chromosomes Cancer 2:205–209
17. Wiltshire RN, Elner VM, Dennis T, Vine AK, Trent JM (1993) Cytogenetic analysis of posterior uveal melanoma. Cancer Genet Cytogenet 66:47–53
18. Singh AD, Boghosian-Sell L, Wary KK, Shields CL, De Potter P, Donoso LA, Shields JA, Cannizzaro LA (1994) Cytogenetic findings in primary uveal melanoma. Cancer Genet Cytogenet 72:109–115
19. Prescher G, Bornfeld N, Friedrichs W, Seeber S, Becher R (1995) Cytogenetics of twelve cases of uveal melanoma and patterns of nonrandom anomalies and isochromosome formation. Cancer Genet Cytogenet 80:40–46
20. McNamara M, Felix C, Davison EV, Fenton M, Kennedy SM (1997) Assessment of chromosome 3 copy number in ocular melanoma using fluorescence in situ hybridization. Cancer Genet Cytogenet 98:4–8
21. Patel KA, Edmondson ND, Talbot F, Parsons MA, Rennie IG, Sisley K (2001) Prediction of prognosis in patients with uveal melanoma using fluorescence in situ hybridisation. Br J Ophthalmol 85:1440–1444
22. Speicher MR, Prescher G, du Manoir S, Jauch A, Horsthemke B, Bornfeld N, Becher R, Cremer T (1994) Chromosomal gains and losses in uveal melanomas detected by comparative genomic hybridization. Cancer Res 54:3817–3823
23. Gordon KB, Thompson CT, Char DH, O'Brien JM, Kroll S, Ghazvini S, Gray JW (1994) Comparative genomic hybridization in the detection of DNA copy number abnormalities in uveal melanoma. Cancer Res 54:4764–4768
24. Ghazvini S, Char DH, Kroll S, Waldman FM, Pinkel D (1996) Comparative genomic hybridization analysis of archival formalin-fixed paraffin-embedded uveal melanomas. Cancer Genet Cytogenet 90:95–101
25. Aalto Y, Eriksson L, Seregard S, Larsson O, Knuutila S (2001) Concomitant loss of chromosome 3 and whole arm losses and gains of chromosome 1, 6, or 8 in metastasizing primary uveal melanoma. Invest Ophthalmol Vis Sci 42:313–317
26. Hughes S, Damato BE, Giddings I, Hiscott PS, Humphreys J, Houlston RS (2005) Microarray comparative genomic hybridisation analysis of intraocular uveal melanomas identifies distinctive imbalances associated with loss of chromosome 3. Br J Cancer 93:1191–1196
27. Kilic E, van Gils W, Lodder E, Beverloo HB, van Til ME, Mooy CM, Paridaens D, de Klein A, Luyten GP (2006) Clinical and cytogenetic analyses in uveal melanoma. Invest Ophthalmol Vis Sci 47:3703–3707
28. Ehlers JP, Worley L, Onken MD, Harbour JW (2008) Integrative genomic analysis of aneuploidy in uveal melanoma. Clin Cancer Res 14:115–122
29. Naus NC, van Drunen E, de Klein A, Luyten GP, Paridaens DA, Alers JC, Ksander BR, Beverloo HB, Slater RM (2001)

Characterization of complex chromosomal abnormalities in uveal melanoma by fluorescence in situ hybridization, spectral karyotyping, and comparative genomic hybridization. Genes Chromosomes Cancer 30:267–273

30. Tschentscher F, Prescher G, Zeschnigk M, Horsthemke B, Lohmann DR (2000) Identification of chromosomes 3, 6, and 8 aberrations in uveal melanoma by microsatellite analysis in comparison to comparative genomic hybridization. Cancer Genet Cytogenet 122:13–17
31. Scholes AG, Damato BE, Nunn J, Hiscott P, Grierson I, Field JK (2003) Monosomy 3 in uveal melanoma: correlation with clinical and histologic predictors of survival. Invest Ophthalmol Vis Sci 44:1008–1011
32. Damato B, Dopierala JA, Coupland SE (2010) Genotypic profiling of 452 choroidal melanomas with multiplex ligation-dependent probe amplification. Clin Cancer Res 16:6083–6092
33. Onken MD, Worley LA, Person E, Char DH, Bowcock AM, Harbour JW (2007) Loss of heterozygosity of chromosome 3 detected with single nucleotide polymorphisms is superior to monosomy 3 for predicting metastasis in uveal melanoma. Clin Cancer Res 13:2923–2927
34. Prescher G, Bornfeld N, Hirche H, Horsthemke B, Jockel KH, Becher R (1996) Prognostic implications of monosomy 3 in uveal melanoma. Lancet 347:1222–1225
35. Maat W, Jordanova ES, van Zelderen-Bhola SL, Barthen ER, Wessels HW, Schalij-Delfos NE, Jager MJ (2007) The heterogeneous distribution of monosomy 3 in uveal melanomas: implications for prognostication based on fine-needle aspiration biopsies. Arch Pathol Lab Med 131:91–96
36. Tschentscher F, Husing J, Holter T, Kruse E, Dresen IG, Jockel KH, Anastassiou G, Schilling H, Bornfeld N, Horsthemke B, Lohmann DR, Zeschnigk M (2003) Tumor classification based on gene expression profiling shows that uveal melanomas with and without monosomy 3 represent two distinct entities. Cancer Res 63:2578–2584
37. Worley LA, Onken MD, Person E, Robirds D, Branson J, Char DH, Perry A, Harbour JW (2007) Transcriptomic versus chromosomal prognostic markers and clinical outcome in uveal melanoma. Clin Cancer Res 13:1466–1471
38. Petrausch U, Martus P, Tonnies H, Bechrakis NE, Lenze D, Wansel S, Hummel M, Bornfeld N, Thiel E, Foerster MH, Keilholz U (2007) Significance of gene expression analysis in uveal melanoma in comparison to standard risk factors for risk assessment of subsequent metastases. Eye 22:997–1007
39. van Gils W, Lodder EM, Mensink HW, Kilic E, Naus NC, Bruggenwirth HT, van Ijcken W, Paridaens D, Luyten GP, de Klein A (2008) Gene expression profiling in uveal melanoma: two regions on 3p related to prognosis. Invest Ophthalmol Vis Sci 49:4254–4262
40. Onken MD, Worley LA, Tuscan MD, Harbour JW (2010) An accurate, clinically feasible multi-gene expression assay for predicting metastasis in uveal melanoma. J Mol Diagn 12:461–468
41. Onken M, Worley L, Char D, Augsburger J, Correa Z, Nudleman E, Aaberg TM Jr, Altaweel M, Bardenstein D, Finger P, Gallie B, Harocopos G, Hovland P, McGowan H, Milman T, Mruthyunjaya P, Simpson E, Smith M, Wilson D, Wirostko W, Harbour J (2012) Collaborative Ocular Oncology Group Report No. 1: prospective validation of a multi-gene prognostic assay in uveal melanoma. Ophthalmology 119(8):1596–1603. doi:10.1016/j.ophtha.2012.02.017
42. Onken MD, Ehlers JP, Worley LA, Makita J, Yokota Y, Harbour JW (2006) Functional gene expression analysis uncovers phenotypic switch in aggressive uveal melanomas. Cancer Res 66:4602–4609
43. Chang SH, Worley LA, Onken MD, Harbour JW (2008) Prognostic biomarkers in uveal melanoma: evidence for a stem cell-like phenotype associated with metastasis. Melanoma Res 18:191–200
44. Harbour JW, Onken MD, Roberson ED, Duan S, Cao L, Worley LA, Council ML, Matatall KA, Helms C, Bowcock AM (2010) Frequent mutation of BAP1 in metastasizing uveal melanomas. Science 330:1410–1413
45. Scheuermann JC, de Ayala Alonso AG, Oktaba K, Ly-Hartig N, McGinty RK, Fraterman S, Wilm M, Muir TW, Muller J (2010) Histone H2A deubiquitinase activity of the Polycomb repressive complex PR-DUB. Nature 465:243–247
46. Abdel-Rahman MH, Pilarski R, Cebulla CM, Massengill JB, Christopher BN, Boru G, Hovland P, Davidorf FH (2011) Germline BAP1 mutation predisposes to uveal melanoma, lung adenocarcinoma, meningioma, and other cancers. J Med Genet 48:856–859
47. Bott M, Brevet M, Taylor BS, Shimizu S, Ito T, Wang L, Creaney J, Lake RA, Zakowski MF, Reva B, Sander C, Delsite R, Powell S, Zhou Q, Shen R, Olshen A, Rusch V, Ladanyi M (2011) The nuclear deubiquitinase BAP1 is commonly inactivated by somatic mutations and 3p21.1 losses in malignant pleural mesothelioma. Nat Genet 43:668–672

48. Testa JR, Cheung M, Pei J, Below JE, Tan Y, Sementino E, Cox NJ, Dogan AU, Pass HI, Trusa S, Hesdorffer M, Nasu M, Powers A, Rivera Z, Comertpay S, Tanji M, Gaudino G, Yang H, Carbone M (2011) Germline BAP1 mutations predispose to malignant mesothelioma. Nat Genet 43:1022–1025
49. Wiesner T, Obenauf AC, Murali R, Fried I, Griewank KG, Ulz P, Windpassinger C, Wackernagel W, Loy S, Wolf I, Viale A, Lash AE, Pirun M, Socci ND, Rutten A, Palmedo G, Abramson D, Offit K, Ott A, Becker JC, Cerroni L, Kutzner H, Bastian BC, Speicher MR (2011) Germline mutations in BAP1 predispose to melanocytic tumors. Nat Genet 43:1018–1021
50. Njauw CN, Kim I, Piris A, Gabree M, Taylor M, Lane AM, Deangelis MM, Gragoudas E, Duncan LM, Tsao H (2012) Germline BAP1 inactivation is preferentially associated with metastatic ocular melanoma and cutaneous-ocular melanoma families. PLoS One 7(4):e35295. doi:10.1371/journal.pone.0035295
51. Pena-Llopis S, Vega-Rubin-de-Celis S, Liao A, Leng N, Pavia-Jimenez A, Wang S, Yamasaki T, Zhrebker L, Sivanand S, Spence P, Kinch L, Hambuch T, Jain S, Lotan Y, Margulis V, Sagalowsky AI, Summerour PB, Kabbani W, Wong SW, Grishin N, Laurent M, Xie XJ, Haudenschild CD, Ross MT, Bentley DR, Kapur P, Brugarolas J (2012) BAP1 loss defines a new class of renal cell carcinoma. Nat Genet 44(7):751–759. doi:10.1038/ng.2323
52. Wiesner T, Murali R, Fried I, Cerroni L, Busam K, Kutzner H, Bastian BC (2012) A distinct subset of atypical spitz tumors is characterized by BRAF mutation and loss of BAP1 expression. Am J Surg Pathol 36(6):818–830
53. Yoshikawa Y, Sato A, Tsujimura T, Emi M, Morinaga T, Fukuoka K, Yamada S, Murakami A, Kondo N, Matsumoto S, Okumura Y, Tanaka F, Hasegawa S, Nakano T, Hashimoto-Tamaoki T (2012) Frequent inactivation of the BAP1 gene in epithelioid-type malignant mesothelioma. Cancer Sci 103:868–874
54. Brown MP, Grundy WN, Lin D, Cristianini N, Sugnet CW, Furey TS, Ares M Jr, Haussler D (2000) Knowledge-based analysis of microarray gene expression data by using support vector machines. Proc Natl Acad Sci U S A 97:262–267

Chapter 23

Molecular Karyotyping for Detection of Prognostic Markers in Fine Needle Aspiration Biopsy Samples of Uveal Melanoma

Arupa Ganguly, Jennifer Richards-Yutz, and Kathryn G. Ewens

Abstract

Uveal melanoma is the most common cancer of the eye in which approximately 50 % of cases develop metastases that are fatal within 2–15 years. Thus it is critical to identify prognostic markers to select high-risk patients into an adjuvant treatment. Chromosomal copy number alterations have been associated with poor prognosis. Historically the gold standard for identifying chromosomal aberrations had been fluorescent in situ hybridization. But in recent years other techniques have been developed that allow very rapid molecular analysis for estimation of chromosomal copy number with finer resolution. These include microsatellite analysis, multiple ligation-dependent probe amplification, and, most recently, genome-wide single-nucleotide polymorphism array analysis. These various procedures have identified loss of all or part of chromosome 3 (monosomy), losses of 1p, 6q, or 8p, or gains of 6p or 8q which, together with tumor location, morphology, and size, can be used to accurately predict the risk of metastasis.

Key words Uveal melanoma, Chromosome aberrations, MSA, SNP array, MLPA, FISH

1 Introduction

Uveal melanoma (UM) is the most common cancer of the eye. The symptoms of UM include changes in vision, such as blurred vision, flashing lights, shadows, and cataracts. In many cases, no symptoms are noticed and the melanoma is diagnosed during a routine eye examination. UM is diagnosed in ~5–7 individuals per million per year. The average age at diagnosis for UM is in the fifties. Compared to melanoma of the skin, uveal melanomas are far less frequent. UM is distinct from most skin melanomas associated with ultraviolet exposure; however, it shares several similarities with other non-sun-exposed melanomas [1, 2].

Large UMs are usually treated by enucleation; however most of the smaller tumors (<10 mm in basal diameter) are treated by plaque radiotherapy, which is an eye-preserving surgery [3, 4]. Due to the high risk of liver metastasis, the standard of care

Magdalena Thurin and Francesco M. Marincola (eds.), *Molecular Diagnostics for Melanoma: Methods and Protocols*, Methods in Molecular Biology, vol. 1102, DOI 10.1007/978-1-62703-727-3_23, © Springer Science+Business Media New York 2014

following initial treatment with radiotherapy or enucleation includes routine liver function tests, CT scans, and MRI of the liver. However, since about 30–45 % of patients develop fatal metastases with 2–15 years [5, 6], the development of accurate, prognostic classifiers detectable on the primary tumor is of utmost importance for the clinical management, surveillance, and systemic therapy following initial treatment of UM.

1.1 Prognostic Markers of Uveal Melanoma

The pathology of UM sections suggested definite correlations between the cellular subtype of the tumor and prognosis. Thus, traditionally, UMs were classified as epithelioid cell type with poor prognosis and spindle cell type with a better prognosis. In reality, the tumors often have mixed cellularity and therefore have intermediate or undefined risk of spreading to other organs [7]. Numerous studies have also indicated a strong association between tumor size (largest basal diameter and thickness) and increased metastasis [8]. Cell morphology and tumor size on their own are not reliable predictors of future metastasis. But together with other factors such as ciliary body involvement, extra-ocular spread, and chromosomal gains and losses, a useful prognostic model can be established [9].

In the early 1990s, the first cytogenetic findings in UM were published which showed a high frequency of chromosome 3 monosomy as well as abnormalities in chromosomes 1, 6, and 8 [10–12]. Prescher et al. [13] next karyotyped 54 enucleated UM and found that 30 tumors (56 %) were monosomy for chromosome 3. More importantly, the data showed that by 3 years following treatment, 50 % of the patients with monosomy 3 showed metastasis whereas those with disomy 3 did not metastasize. The authors concluded that monosomy 3 was a significant predictor of poor survival [13]. Numerous studies following this observation have confirmed the original findings of the association between monosomy 3 and poor metastatic outcome. It also established that chromosome 1p-loss, 6q-loss, 8p-loss, and 8p-gain are correlated with poorer outcome, while 6p-gain appears to be correlated with better prognosis [14–18].

For the individuals with monosomy 3 and amplification of chromosome 8q, the prognosis is poor with a significantly increased risk of metastasis within approximately 2–5 years following initial treatment [15]. The results of chromosome testing provide individuals with an opportunity to decide to undergo more rigorous, routine screening and whether they want to participate in clinical trials and to plan how best to utilize the remaining disease-free years of life. However, this type of genetic testing includes a lack of exact information on the sensitivity of the test for determining the long-term risk of metastasis in individuals whose tumors are disomy 3 in conjunction with, or without, other chromosomal gains or losses.

1.2 Genetic Testing of UM Using DNA-Based Prognostic Markers

1.2.1 Fluorescent In Situ Hybridization

Since the early cytogenetic observations on UM, fluorescent in situ hybridization (FISH) analysis using probes that identify the centromere of chromosome 3 has been used as the gold standard for predicting copy number of chromosome 3 in UM samples [13, 19–21]. In 2002, a set of 40 uveal melanoma fine needle aspiration biopsies (FNABs) and the corresponding enucleated tumors were tested with FISH [22]. All biopsies were found to contain tumor cells, and FISH analyses of the samples were successful and concordant with the results from the tumor tissue in 99 % of cases. The authors demonstrated that the application of FISH to FNABs was a reliable method for assaying genetic prognostic parameters such as chromosome 3 loss and/or chromosome 8q gain.

A recent review of all publications using FISH for UM prognostication has been published [23]. It showed that there was significant variability in tissue sampling methods, selection of FISH probes, number of cells counted, and cutoff point used to determine monosomy 3 status, all of which have likely affected reported results. The reviewers emphasized that the clinical parameters and specific techniques employed to report FISH results should be specified so as to allow meta-analysis of published studies. The analysis showed that due to lack of standardized protocols, conclusions regarding the clinical utility of FISH were limited. However, FISH is a widely available, versatile technology and, when performed optimally, has the potential to be a valuable tool for determining the prognosis of uveal melanoma. One of the limitations of FISH analysis is that it requires cultured or growing cells which are often not feasible for small intraocular biopsy specimens [23].

1.2.2 Multiplex Ligation-Dependent Probe Amplification

To address the issue of chromosome gain, beyond loss of chromosome 3, Damato, Coupland, and colleagues have adopted multiplex ligation-dependent probe amplification (MLPA) for the routine clinical analysis of UM samples [14, 15, 24]. MLPA comprises a set of 43 probes, each hybridizing to a specific genomic sequence, utilizing a kit containing 12 control probes and 31 probes directed at 7 loci on chromosome 1, 13 on chromosome 3, 6 on chromosome 6, and 5 on chromosome 8 [14]. The probes have different lengths, so following amplification by polymerase chain reaction (PCR) they can be separated by gel electrophoresis and quantified by comparison with control sequences. A commercially available kit specifically designed for uveal melanoma (Salsa P027) is available from MRC-Holland, Amsterdam, Holland. Using MLPA, it was shown that, while monosomy for chromosome 3 is the strongest predictor of poor prognosis, additional chromosomal alterations including, but not limited to, chromosomes 1, 6, and 8 are associated with prognosis [14, 15, 24, 25]. Gain of chromosome 8q is significantly associated with earlier onset of metastasis, while changes involving chromosome 6p or 6q are associated with good or bad prognosis, respectively.

A series of publications support the use of MLPA for routine clinical prognostication, especially when the genetic data are considered together with clinical and histologic risk factors [14, 15, 24, 26]. The standard approach in these studies used correlation of MLPA results with survival using Kaplan–Meier analysis to create survival curves for time to metastasis-related death or using Cox univariate or multivariate analysis. The results demonstrated that metastatic death correlated most strongly with chromosome 3 loss and 8q gain ($P<0.001$ in Cox univariate analysis of both chromosomal abnormalities separately; chromosome 3 loss, $P=0.007$ and 8q-gain, $P<0.001$ in Cox multivariate analysis). Gain of chromosome 6p25 correlated with good survival (Cox univariate analysis, $P=0.003$). In addition, prediction of metastatic death was improved by considering equivocal chromosome 3 losses as abnormal and by taking into account multiple risk factors, such as 8q gains, tumor diameter, and histologic features indicative of high-grade malignancy [14].

1.2.3 Microsatellite Analysis

Microsatellite analysis (MSA)-based assays on tumor/normal paired samples are used to determine the loss of one copy of a chromosome pair based on loss of heterozygosity (LOH) or presence of both copies based on retention of heterozygosity (ROH). Accordingly, assays using highly polymorphic microsatellite markers have been used for evaluation of chromosome 3, 6, and 8 copy number in UM [27].

In our analysis of the applicability of MSA to identify chromosomal changes in UM, our objective was to obtain copy number profiles of chromosome 3 for a series of archived UM specimens. The main eligibility criterion for inclusion of any UM specimen in this study was the absence of any form of therapy to the eye prior to enucleation. In a series of 68 archived UM specimens, chromosome 3 copy number was inferred based on LOH or ROH of informative MSA markers in DNA isolated from tumor tissues. Depending on the presence of one or both alleles of each microsatellite marker tested, LOH along both p and q arms of chromosome 3 was inferred for 32 tumors and ROH was inferred for 16 tumors. In addition there was partial loss of the 3p, 3q, or both in 19 tumors, while DNA from one tumor did not yield enough signal.

(a) Chromosome 3 status of UM by analysis of FNAB samples.
   Most of the published work on genetic testing of UM has been performed on enucleated eyes in which a macroscopic sample of tumor was retrieved at the time of surgery and studied using one of several techniques described above. However, since the development of eye-sparing procedures such as plaque radiotherapy or charged particle radiotherapy, enucleation is typically reserved for eyes with large tumors. Currently, most eyes with UM are managed with these non-enucleation measures.

(b) Comparison of MSA data on tumor with FNAB samples.

We evaluated the consistency of MSA results obtained by analysis of DNA isolated from enucleated tumors that had corresponding FNAB samples using MSA results from a series of five "mock" FNAB samples, i.e., FNAB carried out on enucleated UM tumors after surgical resection. DNA was isolated from both the FNAB and enucleated tumor samples as well as matched blood samples, where the latter is considered to be the source of "normal" alleles, and subjected to MSA analysis. The results from two independent FNAB and tumor samples for the same tumor were highly concordant in three cases. However, in two cases we observed allelic imbalance (AI) in both FNAB and tumor samples. AI is defined as a difference in the ratio of the areas under the peaks for the two alleles of the microsatellite marker between the normal tissue and the FNAB/tumor that is indicative of tumor heterogeneity. In these two cases the presence of AI was consistent with the pathology reports for the tumor. In general, the results of the microsatellite assays were less consistent between FNAB and tumors when the pathology reports indicated mixed cellularity. In cases with AI in the FNAB and ROH in the second FNAB and/or in the tumor, the result was always interpreted as the presence of a subset of cells with LOH for that marker.

(c) MSA on a prospective series of UM FNAB samples.

After establishing that chromosome 3 profiles of FNAB and UM tumor were generally concordant, we evaluated the feasibility of testing a large cohort of 140 individuals with UM using microscopic sampling with FNAB prior to plaque radiotherapy. This was followed by DNA isolation and MSA as described above. We chose to use 6 microsatellite markers spanning chromosome 3 to analyze the FNAB samples (*see* Table 1 and Fig. 1); each marker set was done in triplicate to derive the mean and standard deviation for each measurement accurately. Figure 2 shows the results of MSA on two paired sets of DNAs isolated from blood and FNAB samples. As is evident, for the UM with disomy for chromosome 3, each marker has two alleles in both samples. In contrast, for the UM with monosomy for chromosome 3, the DNA from the blood displays two markers while that from the FNAB shows loss of one allele of each marker as indicated by the arrows.

The results of MSA on the 140 FNAB samples were subdivided into three categories. Forty-four samples had clear LOH for all markers tested on chromosome 3 (31 %), 76 had clear ROH (54 %), and 20 (14 %) yielded insufficient DNA for MSA [28]. Since then, the protocol for DNA isolation from FNAB has been modified, and the yield is close to 100 % using the protocol described in Sections 2.2 and 3.1 below.

Table 1
Description of the chromosome 3 markers used for MSA

Locus	Chromosome 3 location	Dye label	Heterozygosity	Allele size range (bp)
D3S1297	3p26.3	VIC	0.82	351–369
D3S1304	3p26.1	VIC	0.80	254–276
D3S1300	3p14.2	FAM	0.82	230–262
D3S1569	3q24	FAM	0.80	150–174
D3S1262	3q27.3	FAM	0.80	110–132
D3S1601	3q28	VIC	0.85	298–330

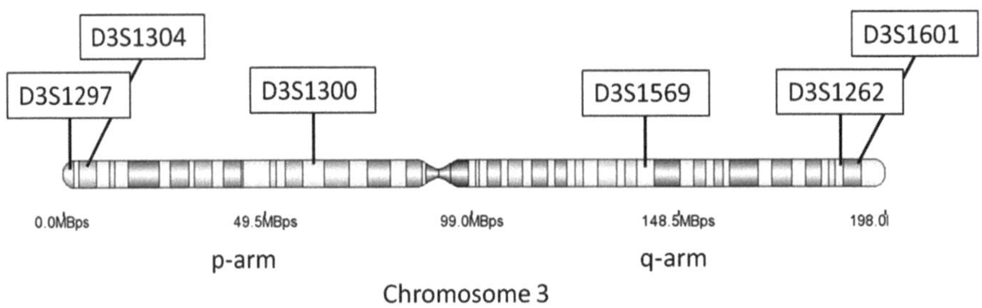

Fig. 1 Ideogram showing the p-arm and q-arm of chromosome 3, and the *boxes* with *lines* show the location on the chromosome of the six chromosome 3 markers used in the MSA

1.2.4 Single-Nucleotide Polymorphism

Currently, high-resolution whole-genome single-nucleotide polymorphism (SNP) arrays are routinely used for accurate estimation of chromosomal copy number loss and gain providing the benefit of molecular karyotyping of tumor samples without the need for culturing tumor cells [28, 29]. One benefit of analyses based on SNP arrays is the ability to unambiguously determine LOH and copy neutral duplication events. In addition, SNP arrays allow whole-genome profiling of tumor/FNAB DNA starting with as little as 250 ng of genomic DNA after optimization.

As a first step towards validation, we performed molecular karyotyping of UM samples by comparing the SNP genotype calls generated using DNA isolated from tumor or FNAB samples and matched peripheral blood lymphocytes of 100 UM patients. A single-array analysis was performed for each DNA sample (250 ng each) and hybridized to the SNP6.0 microarrays using the protocol defined by the manufacturer (Affymetrix, CA). The Affymetrix CNAT 4.0 and Genotype Console allows one to use "tumor-only" genotype, and cell intensity calls to be used to define LOH and to infer copy number

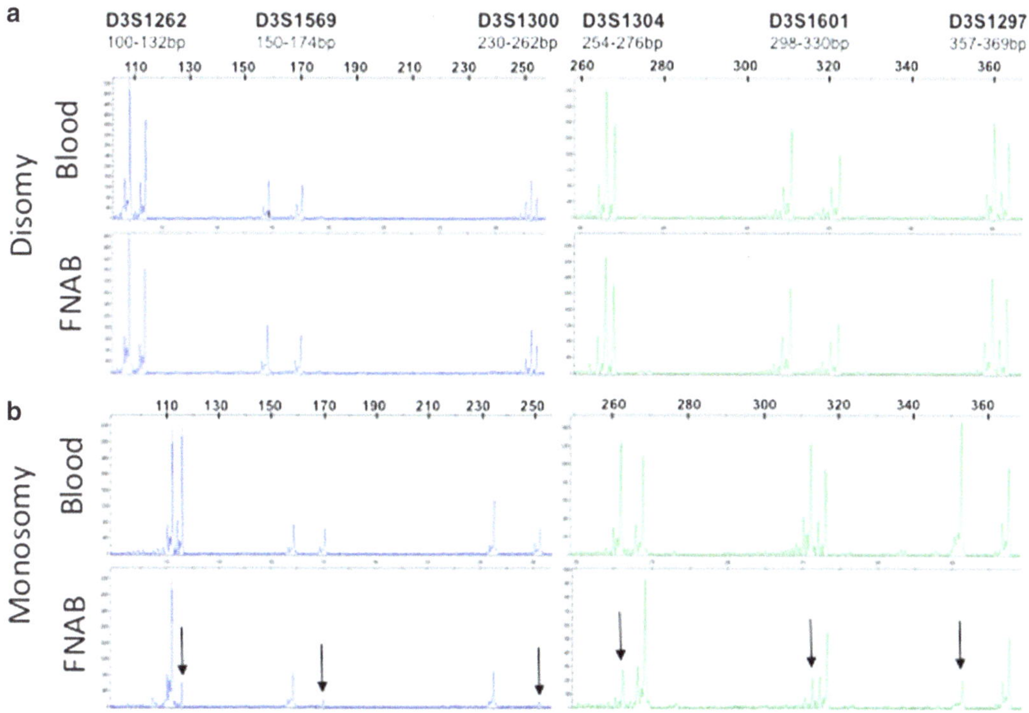

Fig. 2 GeneMapper plot showing allele heights for the six chromosome 3 microsatellite markers in a disomy (**a**) and monosomy (**b**) sample. Each *top panel* represents the results from blood, which is compared to the results from the matched FNAB sample *below*. The allele range for each marker is shown at the *top* represented by *black bar*. *Black arrows* in (**b**) indicate which allele has been lost

calls. An independent confirmation of this analysis data was obtained using dCHIP, a freely available software that allows inference of copy numbers and LOH for "tumor-only" samples [30].

With respect to quality assurance, two internal quality control measures are used. The call rate for all SNPs must be greater than 95 %, and zygosity of the SNPs on the X chromosome should identify correctly the gender of the individual.

We analyzed a series of 100 FNAB samples with SNP arrays. We observed monosomy 3 in 39 samples, partial monosomy for chromosome 3 in 6, amplification of 8q in 46, gain of 6p in 33, loss of 6p in 2, and loss of 6q in 18. Figure 3 shows the output that we obtain after copy number calls are made with Partek Genomics Suite (version 6.5). As is evident, the monosomy for chromosome 3 is indicated by copy number of 1 and complete LOH along the entire length of the chromosome. In addition, amplification of the q arm of chromosome 8 is clearly indicated.

Independent validation of the SNP array data for 20 FNAB samples was performed using the commercially available MLPA kits [14]. We used the kit according to instructions from the manufacturer and confirmed the SNP array results in all 20 cases tested.

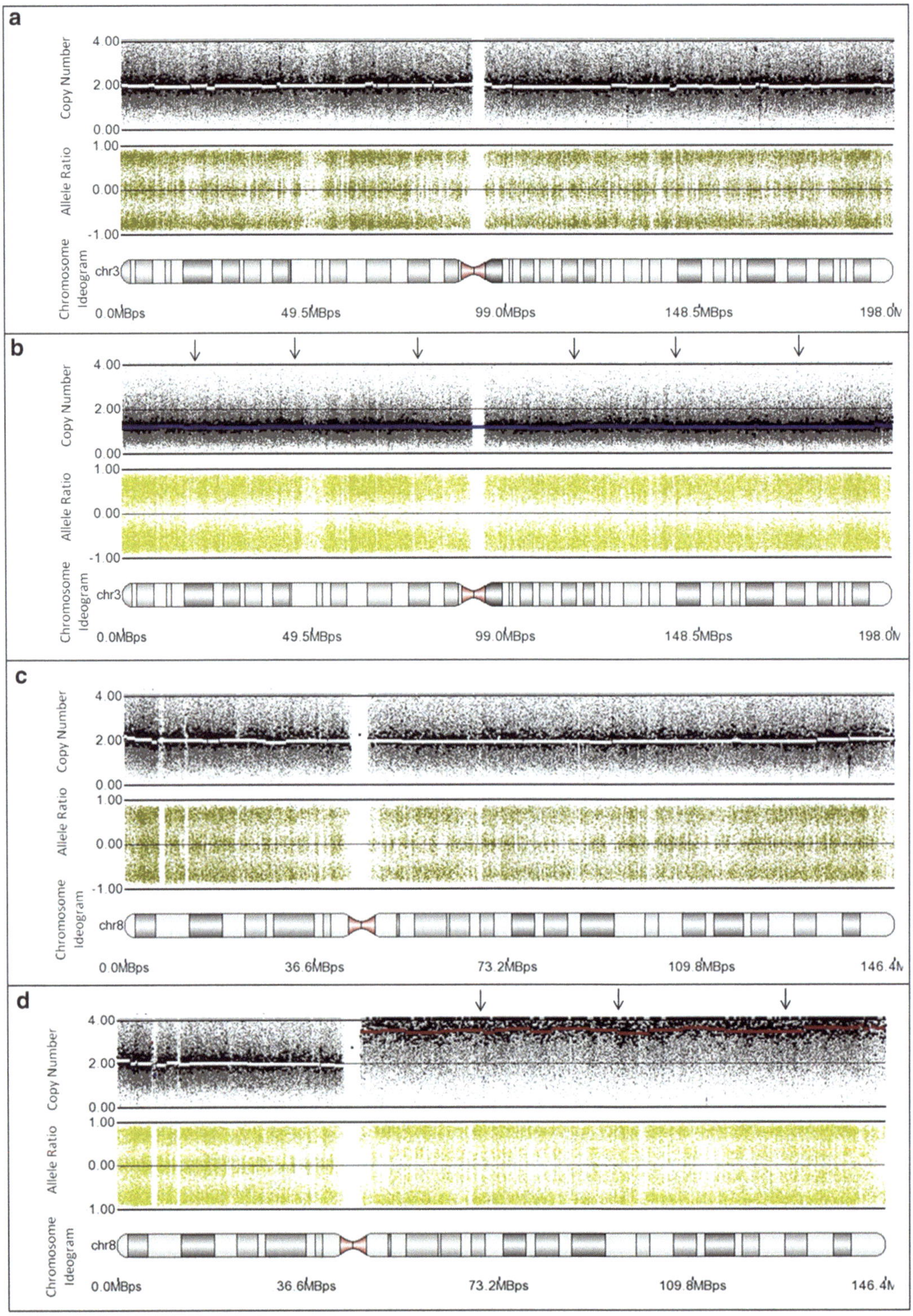

Fig. 3 Affymetrix SNP 6.0 copy number analysis from Partek. (**a**) and (**b**) show results from chromosome 3 and (**c**) and (**d**) show data from chromosome 8. The *top panel* depicts copy number (CN) with the average of the data points indicated by a *horizontal line* (a *white line* represents normal copy number, CN = 2; a *dark blue line* represents a loss; and *red line* represents a gain in CN). The *middle panel* depicts the data for the allele ratio. Data points at the *top* and *bottom* represent homozygous calls for SNPs, while data points in the *middle*

2 Materials

2.1 UM Samples

1. Hank's Balanced Solution for FNAB Collection (Gibco, Life Technologies).
2. Purple top EDTA vacutainer tubes for blood collection (BD Diagnostics) (*see* **Notes 1** and **2**).
3. FNAB from UM patients were submitted by Dr. Carol Shields from the Ocular Oncology Services of Wills Eye Hospital, Thomas Jefferson University, Philadelphia (*see* **Note 1**).

2.2 DNA Isolation Kits

1. Gentra Puregene Blood Kit (3 ml) (Qiagen) or the Gentra Puregene Blood Kit (1,000 ml) (Qiagen) for DNA isolation from blood.
2. QIAamp DNA Micro Kit (50) for processing FNAB samples (Qiagen).
3. DNeasy Blood & and Tissue Kit (50) for processing formalin fixed paraffin embedded (FFPE) and frozen tumor samples (Qiagen).

2.3 Microsatellite Analysis

1. PCR primer pairs for the microsatellite markers D3S1297, D3S1304, D3S1300, D3S1569, D3S1262, and D3S1601, where the forward primers for each pair are labeled with FAM (P/N 450005) or VIC (P/N 450007) dyes (Applied Biosystems) (Table 1).
2. A 10× primer mixture (50 μM) is prepared for D3S1297, D3S1304, D3S1300, D3S1569, D3S1262, and D3S1601 primer pairs. An equimolar mixture is prepared by mixing 50 μl of each primer (500 μM) and the final volume adjusted to 500 μl with Tris–EDTA (TE) buffer (10 mM Tris–HCl, pH 8.0, 1 mM EDTA (TEKnova)).
3. Multiplex PCR Kit containing polymerase master mix, water, and Q-solution (Qiagen).
4. GeneScan™ 500 ROX™ Size Standard, an internal lane size standard for fluorescence-based DNA electrophoresis system (Applied Biosystems).
5. Hi-Di™ Formamide to resuspend samples for capillary electrophoresis (Applied Biosystems).
6. Optical 96-well plate (Applied Biosystems).

Fig. 3 (continued) represent heterozygous calls. The *bottom panel* shows the chromosome ideogram, and the centromere is shown in *red*. (**a**) and (**c**) represent the normal pattern for their respective chromosomes. (**b**) depicts results for a sample which is monosomy for chromosome 3 (*blue line* indicated with *arrows*) and illustrates the corresponding absence in heterozygous calls in the allele ratio panel. (**d**) shows normal copy number for 8p but an amplification of 8q (*red line* indicated with *arrows*) with a decrease in heterozygous calls in the allele ratio panel

7. Micro-Amp Clear Adhesive film (Applied Biosystems).
8. Thermocycler, GeneAmp PCR System 2700 (Applied Biosystems).
9. ABI 3130xl Genetic Analyzer for multi-color fluorescence-based DNA analysis (Applied Biosystems).

2.4 Single-Nucleotide Polymorphism Arrays

1. SNP 6.0 arrays for SNP analysis (Affymetrix).
2. The Affymetrix® SNP 6 Core Reagent Kit (Affymetrix) provides the convenience of a complete solution in one comprehensive kit consisting of five sub-kits: Digest and Ligate Sub-kit, Affymetrix® Genome-Wide Human SNP Nsp/Sty Assay Kit 6.0, Hybridization Buffer Sub-kit, Hold and Stain Sub-kit, and Wash Sub-kit. The reagents are available for purchase as a complete kit or by individual sub-kits.
   (a) The Digest and Ligate Sub-kit contains the NspI and StyI enzymes used for digestion of genomic DNA as well as the specific adaptors for NspI- and StyI-digested DNA and T4 DNA ligase used to ligate the specific adaptors to the digested samples.
   (b) Affymetrix® Genome-Wide Human SNP Nsp/Sty Assay Kit 6.0 contains the TITANIUM™ DNA Amplification Kit used in the amplification of the ligated products along with the universal PCR primer 002. The reagents for fragmentation (GeneChip® fragmentation reagent and 10× fragmentation buffer) and labeling (30 mM GeneChip® DNA labeling reagent, 30 U/μL terminal deoxynucleotidyl transferase, 5× terminal deoxynucleotidyl transferase buffer) are also provided in this kit.
   (c) The Hybridization Buffer Sub-kit contains 2-(*N*-morpholino) ethanesulfonic acid (MES,12×; 1.25 M), Denhardt's Solution (50×), EDTA (0.5 M) , 165 μL Herring Sperm DNA (10 mg/mL), 0100 oligonucleotide control reagent, human Cot-1 DNA (1 mg/mL), Tween-20 (3 %), DMSO (100 %), and tetramethyl ammonium chloride (5 M) used for making the hybridization master mix.
3. Other reagents and materials:
   (a) Water (AccuGENE) (Lonza).
   (b) DNA Marker, All Purpose Hi-Lo (Bionexus).
   (c) Elution Buffer (EB) for elution of DNA after purification (Qiagen).
   (d) Absolute ethanol (for dilution to 75 %) (Sigma).
   (e) TBE gels, 2 and 4 % reliant precast (Lonza).
   (f) Thermocycler, GeneAmp PCR System 9700 (Applied Biosystems).

(g) Cooling chamber, double block (Diversified Biotech).
(h) Agencourt AMpure Magnetic Beads (60 ml) (Agencourt).
(i) MagnaRack (Invitrogen).
(j) Plate centrifuge, multipurpose (Eppendorf).
(k) GeneChip® Hybridization Oven 640 (Affymetrix).
(l) GeneChip® Fluidic Station 450 (Affymetrix).
(m) GeneChip® 3000 Scanner with 7G upgrade (Affymetrix).
(n) Eppendorf Safe-Lock Tubes (2.0 ml) (VWR).
(o) 96-well OD plates (for UV spectrometer) (E&K Scientific).
(p) Tough spots (1/2″) (Diversified Biotech).

2.5 Data Analysis Software

1. GeneMapper version 4.0 (Applied Biosystems) (url: http://www.icmb.utexas.edu/core/DNA/Information_Sheets/Genotype/GeneMapper_Microsatellite_Guide.PDF).
2. Genotyping Console Software (Affymetrix) (url: http://www.affymetrix.com/browse/level_seven_software_products_only.jsp?productId=131535&categoryId=35625 - 1_1).
3. dChip Software: Analysis and visualization of gene expression and SNP microarrays (url: http://biosun1.harvard.edu/complab/dchip/).
4. Partek Genomics Suite V6.5: Partek Inc., St Louis, MO (url: http://www.partek.com/).

3 Methods

Two different methods for evaluation of chromosome 3 copy number in FNAB samples are described in this protocol—MSA and SNP array. The methods are complementary and confirm the results of each platform independently. As the number of cells aspirated during FNAB can be highly variable, the advantage of the MSA method is in that it requires very little DNA (as small as 10 ng), whereas SNP array requires a larger amount of input DNA. Although SNP analysis provides more comprehensive characterization of genomic data, the MSA reliably provides the information on the chromosome 3 status in the absence of SNP array data. Thus a combination of both techniques should be used for prognostication of UM cases.

3.1 Genomic DNA Isolation

Genomic DNA is isolated from blood, FNAB, FFPE, and frozen tumor material using the specific commercial DNA isolation kits (Subheading 2.2 and *see* **Notes 1–3**) following the manufacturer's instructions.

3.2 Microsatellite Analysis

Genomic DNA, isolated from the blood, FNAB, FFPE, and frozen tumor samples, are used as templates for multiplex PCR amplification of microsatellite markers on chromosome 3 (*see* **Note 4**). The markers (Table 1) are amplified and analyzed following the manufacturer's instructions. The total number of PCR cycles is 30 for blood and tumor DNA and 37 for FNAB DNA. The amplification products are analyzed on a 3130xl Genetic Analyzer.

3.2.1 PCR Amplification and Fragment Size Analysis on ABI 3130xl (See Notes 5–9)

1. A total of six multiplex PCRs are performed per sample. Three PCR reactions use DNA that has been extracted from the blood sample and three use the DNA isolated from the corresponding FNAB or tumor section from one individual (FNAB, FFPE, or frozen tumor).
2. A 10× primer mixture (50 μM) (Subheading 2.3) is aliquoted into an 8-strip PCR tubes to be used in the following steps. The final volume is determined by the number of samples to be analyzed (final volume = number of samples × 2.2 μl which accounts for 10 % additional volume). Using a multichannel pipette, 2 μl of the mixture is drawn up and added to a clean 8-strip PCR tube. This is repeated until enough primer mixture has been aliquoted for the number of samples being run.
3. 4 μl of a 20 ng/μl dilution of DNA from blood or FNAB/tumor is added to each tube (80 ng total).
4. A master mix for multiplex PCR is prepared using the reagents provided in the Qiagen Multiplex PCR Kit in sufficient quantity for all samples plus 10 % additional. Thus, for 10 reactions, enough master mix is prepared for 11 reactions. For each reaction, the mix contains 2 μl water, 10 μl 2× Qiagen Multiplex PCR Master mix, and 2 μl Q-solution (5×) (total 14 μl).
5. 14 μl of this master mix is added to each tube which already contains the primers and DNA.
6. Tubes are capped, flicked, and given a quick spin in a microcentrifuge before placing them in a GeneAmp® 2700 PCR system and carrying out the PCR reaction using the following cycling protocol: 95 °C for 15 min; 94 °C for 30 s; 55 °C for 1 min 30 s; and 72 °C for 1 min 30 s. **Steps 1–4** are repeated for a total of 30 cycles (increased to 37 cycles if DNA is isolated from an FNAB sample) followed by 72 °C for 10 min and 4 °C hold.
7. After PCR, a 1:20 dilution of GS 500 ROX Size standard in Hi-Di Formamide is prepared. The volume of the diluted mix is adjusted such that there is enough for all samples plus 10 % additional, and 9 μl is aliquoted into each well of an optical 96-well plate (*see* **Note 5**).
8. 1 μl from each PCR reaction is added to each well. The plate is covered with a Micro-Amp Clear Adhesive film (Subheading 2.3).

9. The plate is given a quick spin at 1000 × *g* in a plate centrifuge for 1 min.
10. The plate is then incubated in a GeneAmp® 2700 PCR system at 95 °C for 5 min.
11. The optical 96-well plate is loaded onto the 3100xl Genetic Analyzer following the 3130xl User Guide.
12. The data is analyzed using GeneMapper version 4.0 (*see* **Notes 5–9**).
    (a) Data files (with file extension .fsa) are loaded into GeneMapper 4.0, and automatic binning is performed after assigning the panel with the allele size range bins according to Table 1.
    (b) Data for each sample is visually inspected to make sure that all alleles present have been called (*see* **Notes 6** and **7**).
    (c) Result of the normal tissue that is generated from analysis of matched blood DNA is compared against that of the FNAB/tumor sample, and a report to calculate LOH or ROH is generated as described below (*see* **Notes 8** and **9**).
13. The output from the ABI 3130xl instrument is analyzed using the allelic imbalance and LOH assessment tools included in the GeneMapper software (*see* **Note 9** and Fig. 2).

3.3 Single-Nucleotide Polymorphism

A single-array analysis is performed for each DNA sample (~160 ng each), and DNA is hybridized to the Affymetrix SNP 6.0 array using the protocol defined by the manufacturer (Affymetrix). In brief, the DNA samples are digested with NspI or StyI restriction enzymes, ligated to an adaptor, and amplified with a set of universal primers. The amplified DNA is then fragmented, labeled with a fluorescent dye, hybridized to the array, scanned, and analyzed.

3.3.1 SNP Array

In brief the protocol according to the instruction in the Affymetrix Genome-Wide Human SNP Nsp/Sty 6.0 User Guide (Genome-Wide Human SNP Nsp/Sty 6.0 User Guide) [31] is as follows:

1. Digestion using reagents from Affymetrix Digest and Ligate Sub-kit.
    (a) 8 μl of a 20 ng/μl dilution of FNAB or tumor sample is digested with NspI and StyI in separate reaction tubes. The reaction mixture contains 8.55 μl AccuGENE water, 2 μl 10× NEB buffer #2 or #3 (for respective restriction enzymes), 0.2 μl 100× BSA, and 1 μl NspI or StyI enzyme.
    (b) 11.75 μl of this mixture is added to each tube containing the DNA. This reaction is placed in a GeneAmp® PCR System 9700 thermocycler at 37 °C for 120 min and 65 °C for 20 min, with a 4 °C hold.

2. After the digestion reaction is complete, ligation of adaptors using T4 DNA ligase is performed: a mixture of T4 DNA ligase buffer (2.5 μl), NspI adaptor or StyI adaptor (0.75 μl), and 2 μl of T4 DNA ligase is assembled, and 5.25 μl is added to the reaction tubes containing the digested DNA. Ligation reaction thermocycler conditions are 16 °C for 180 min and 70 °C for 20 min, with a 4 °C hold.
3. When the ligation program is finished, the reactions are diluted with 75 μl of AccuGENE® water.
4. Next, 11 amplification reactions are assembled (six for NspI-digested and -ligated reactions and five for StyI-digested and -ligated reactions) (*see* **Notes 10** and **11**).
5. Since the PCR primer is universal to both adaptors, a single master mix is made for both NspI and StyI reactions using titanium Taq DNA polymerase from the assay kit.
6. 2 μl aliquot of a single PCR reaction out of the 6 NspI PCRs and one 2 μl aliquot from one out of the five StyI PCRs per sample are assessed on a 2 % agarose gel.
7. If successful amplification is observed for both PCR sets for each sample, all 11 PCR samples are pooled together into a single Eppendorf Safe-Lock 2.0 ml tube, and a modified purification procedure is used to purify the pooled PCRs.
   (a) One ml of AMpure magnetic beads is added to each pooled PCR product tube. Beads should be mixed thoroughly before addition to the samples.
   (b) After each tube is securely capped, the tubes are inverted ten times, incubated at room temperature for 10 min, and then centrifuged at 20,000 × g for 3 min.
   (c) After centrifugation, the tubes are placed in a magnetic stand and the supernatant is carefully pipetted out and discarded while leaving the tubes in the magnetic rack and the pellet behind.
   (d) 1 ml of freshly prepared 75 % ethanol is added to each sample, and tubes are capped and loaded into an adaptor and vortexed at 75 % power for 2 min.
   (e) The tubes are then centrifuged at 20,000 × g for 3 min. The tubes are placed back into the magnetic stand, and the supernatant is pipetted out. The samples are then spun again for 30 s at 20,000 × g and put back on the magnetic rack, and any remaining 75 % ethanol is removed.
   (f) Samples are allowed to dry uncapped for approximately 15 min, and 55 μl of Buffer EB (Qiagen) is added to each tube; the samples are vortexed at 75 % power for 10 min, making sure that the pellet is homogeneous slurry.
   (g) Samples are then spun at 20,000 × g for 5 min and placed in magnetic rack for 5–15 min or until all the magnetic beads are pulled to the side of the tube.

(h) 47 μl of eluted sample containing the DNA is carefully transferred into the appropriately labeled tube of a new 8-strip PCR tube.

(i) The concentrations of the samples are checked using 2 μl of sample in 198 μl of water. Use 2 μl of EB buffer in 198 μl of water for a blank. Concentrations should range between 4 and 6 mg/ml.

8. After proper concentrations are verified, fragmentation, quality control using 4 % TBE agarose gels, and labeling reactions are performed according to the Genome-Wide Human SNP Nsp/Sty 6.0 User Guide (*see* **Note 12**) [31].

3.3.2 SNP Array Hybridization and Data Analysis

1. Following target sample preparation as indicated above, the hybridization reaction is performed by preparing a hybridization master mix using reagents from the sub-kit and add the mix to each sample. Then, the samples are denatured at 95 °C for 10 min in a GeneAmp® PCR System 9700 thermal cycler. After denaturation, each sample is loaded onto a Genome-Wide Human SNP Array 6.0—one sample per array. The arrays are then placed into a hybridization oven that has been preheated to 50 °C, and samples are left to hybridize for 16–18 h. The oligonucleotide control reagent is added to patient samples to confirm successful hybridization.
2. Post hybridization washes and staining are done in the Affymetrix fluidics station 450.
3. Following the washing step, the arrays are scanned using a GeneChip® 3000 Scanner.
4. The data files with the file extension .cel are generated with Genotyping Console Software (Affymetrix *see* **Note 13**) and then imported into Partek Genomic Suite 6.5 for analysis using the copy number analysis workflow (*see* **Note 14** and Fig. 3).

4 Notes

1. The intraocular biopsy samples are collected immediately before plaque radiotherapy using FNAB. The samples are collected in Hank's balanced salt solution in a single pass in the operating room and refrigerated prior to analysis. This technique has been previously described [28]. A sample of blood is collected (purple top EDTA vacutainer tubes) at the time of treatment and refrigerated prior to shipment. For enucleated tumor tissue, 20 sections (5 μ thickness) are cut from archived FFPE samples for DNA isolation. When frozen tissue samples are available, 5–15 mg sections of the tumor tissue are used for DNA isolation.

2. CDC has standard guidelines and recommendations for prevention of exposure of laboratory workers to infectious agents present in blood and body fluid. Under these recommendations, blood and body fluids including biopsy samples of tumors of all human subjects are considered potentially infectious for blood-borne pathogens (HIV/AIDS, hepatitis B, hepatitis C). It is mandatory that workers use suitable barrier protection, which includes gloves, lab coats, and face shields for self-protection.
3. To reduce degradation of DNA, the stock should be stored in small aliquots at −20 °C. The working dilution of 20 ng/μl is stored separately from the stock, at −20 °C.
4. It is imperative to separate pre-PCR working area with the stock DNA solution from post-amplification reagents and analysis area to avoid cross contamination of the reagents.
5. For the MSA data analysis, the size standard should be examined to make sure that the correct sizes are assigned to the GS 500 ROX Size standard peaks.
6. If the size standard is correctly assigned but there are no allele peaks for the makers of the sample, the sample should be reloaded or the multiplex PCR should be repeated.
7. It is also imperative that the peak height for each allele is between 100 and 6,000 units. Too low or too high intensities give rise to incorrect ratios of the peak heights, which is critical for determination of loss or imbalance of one allele compared to the other. In such cases the samples should be rerun with proper dilutions.
8. Biopsy samples should share at least one allele for all six markers with the blood sample. This is a quality control check to avoid sample mix-up during setup of PCR products.
9. The threshold for LOH is set at <0.63 and >1.32 for comparing the ratios of peak heights for DNA isolated from normal blood and tumor tissue. AI is indicated when two peaks are present, but the ratio of the heights for the two peaks between tumor and normal samples is between 0.63 and 0.80 or 1.2 and 1.32. When DNA isolated from FNAB/tumor is analyzed without matched normal DNA, LOH is indicated by the presence of a single peak for all assayed markers, which is theoretically highly unlikely in a normal tissue. This is because the assay markers are chosen based on their high degree of heterogeneity in the Caucasian population. Similarly, AI is indicated when the ratio of the areas under the two peaks is <0.2 or >4.0 for all assayed markers. In addition, when DNA from normal tissue is analyzed and yields a single peak for a particular marker, it is recorded as uninformative.

10. For the FNAB samples, no changes are made to the Affymetrix SNP 6.0 array protocol, other than starting with 160 ng of DNA and performing 11 PCR reactions of Nsp and Sty (in the correct ratios) to achieve the required final pooled DNA quantity of 200 μg and the modified purification method to purify the 11 pooled PCRs.
11. The detailed protocol for purification of the 11 pooled PCRs included in this review is different from that included in the Genome-Wide Human SNP Nsp/Sty 6.0 User Guide [31]. The User Guide suggests seven PCRs all together for Nsp/Sty amplification and purification using a vacuum manifold. Due to the low DNA concentration of the FNAB samples, we have modified the protocol to perform 11 PCRs followed by pooling and purification using a MagnaRack.
12. It is very important that the thermocycler block be heated to 37 °C before samples are loaded for fragmentation.
13. Genotyping Console Software is the genotyping analysis software package designed to streamline whole-genome genotyping analysis and quality control for the Genome-Wide SNP 6.0 arrays. Genotyping Console's QC and visualization tools easily identify and segregate sample outliers. SNP cluster visualization provides a detailed look at the performance of SNPs of interest.
14. A genomic DNA positive control (Reference Genomic DNA 103) is provided in the Affymetrix Digest and Ligate Sub-kit. It can be used a routine experimental control and for troubleshooting if there are problems with the Affymetrix workflow.

References

1. Gaudi SM JL (2011) Molecular bases of cutaneous and uveal melanomas. Pathol Res Int. doi: 10.4061/2011/159421
2. van den Bosch T, Kilic E, Paridaens D, de Klein A (2010) Genetics of uveal melanoma and cutaneous melanoma: two of a kind? Dermatol Res Pract. doi:10.1155/2010/360136
3. Damato B (2004) Developments in the management of uveal melanoma. Clin Exp Ophthalmol 32:639–647
4. Shields J, Shields CL (2008) Posterior uveal melanoma. Clinical features. Lippincott, Williams and Wilkins, Philadelphia, PA
5. Kujala E, Mäkitie T, Kivelä T (2003) Very long-term prognosis of patients with malignant uveal melanoma. Invest Ophthalmol Vis Sci 44:4651–4659
6. Paul EV, Parnell BL, Fraker M (1962) Prognosis of malignant melanomas of the choroid and ciliary body. Int Ophthalmol Clin 12:387–402
7. Kincaid MC (1998) Uveal melanoma. Cancer Control 5:299–309
8. Damato B, Coupland SE (2009) A reappraisal of the significance of largest basal diameter of posterior uveal melanoma. Eye 23:2152–2162
9. Damato B, Eleuteri A, Taktak AFG, Coupland SE (2011) Estimating prognosis for survival after treatment of choroidal melanoma. Prog Retin Eye Res 30:285–295
10. Prescher G, Bornfeld N, Becher R (1990) Nonrandom chromosomal abnormalities in primary uveal melanoma. J Natl Cancer Inst 82:1765–1769
11. Sisley K, Cottam DW, Rennie IG, Parsons MA, Potter AM, Potter CW et al (1992) Non-random abnormalities of chromosomes 3, 6, and 8 associated with posterior uveal

melanoma. Genes Chromosomes Cancer 5: 197–200
12. Sisley KR, Rennie IG, Cottam DW, Potter AM, Potter CW, Rees RC (1990) Cytogenetic findings in six posterior uveal melanomas: involvement of chromosomes 3, 6, and 8. Genes Chromosomes Cancer 2:205–209
13. Prescher G, Bornfeld N, Hirche H, Horsthemke B, Jockel KH, Becher R (1996) Prognostic implications of monosomy 3 in uveal melanoma. Lancet 347:1222–1225
14. Damato B, Dopierala J, Klaasen A, van Dijk M, Sibbring J, Coupland SE (2009) Multiplex ligation-dependent probe amplification of uveal melanoma: correlation with metastatic death. Invest Ophthalmol Vis Sci 50:3048–3055
15. Damato B, Dopierala JA, Coupland SE (2010) Genotypic profiling of 452 choroidal melanomas with multiplex ligation-dependent probe amplification. Clin Cancer Res 16:6083–6092
16. Damato B, Duke C, Coupland SE, Hiscott P, Smith PA, Campbell I et al (2007) Cytogenetics of uveal melanoma: a 7-year clinical experience. Ophthalmology 114:1925–1931
17. Kilic E, Naus NC, van Gils W, Klaver CC, van Til ME, Verbiest MM et al (2005) Concurrent loss of chromosome arm 1p and chromosome 3 predicts a decreased disease-free survival in uveal melanoma patients. Invest Ophthalmol Vis Sci 46:2253–2257
18. van den Bosch T, van Beek JGM, Vaarwater J, Verdijk RM, Naus NC, Paridaens D et al (2012) Higher percentage of FISH-determined monosomy 3 and 8q amplification in uveal melanoma cells relate to poor patient prognosis. Invest Ophthalmol Vis Sci 53:2668–2674
19. Cross NA, Ganesh A, Parpia M, Murray AK, Rennie IG, Sisley K (2006) Multiple locations on chromosome 3 are the targets of specific deletions in uveal melanoma. Eye 20:476–481
20. Parrella P, Fazio VM, Gallo AP, Sidransky D, Merbs SL (2003) Fine mapping of chromosome 3 in uveal melanoma: identification of a minimal region of deletion on chromosomal arm 3p25.1-p25.2. Cancer Res 63:8507–8510
21. Tschentscher F, Prescher G, Horsman DE, White VA, Rieder H, Anastassiou G et al (2001) Partial deletions of the long and short arm of chromosome 3 point to two tumor suppressor genes in uveal melanoma. Cancer Res 61:3439–3442
22. Naus NC, Verhoeven ACA, van Drunen E, Slater R, Mooy CM, Paridaens DA et al (2002) Detection of genetic prognostic markers in uveal melanoma biopsies using fluorescence in situ hybridization. Clin Cancer Res 8:534–539
23. Aronow M, Sun Y, Saunthararajah Y, Biscotti C, Tubbs R, Triozzi P et al (2012) Monosomy 3 by FISH in uveal melanoma: variability in techniques and results. Surv Ophthalmol 57:463–473
24. Lake SL, Damato BE, Dopierala J, Baudo MM, Taktak AFG, Coupland SE (2011) Multiplex ligation-dependent probe amplification analysis of uveal melanoma with extraocular extension demonstrates heterogeneity of gross chromosomal abnormalities. Invest Ophthalmol Vis Sci 52:5559–5564
25. Vaarwater J, van den Bosch T, Mensink HW, van Kempen C, Verdijk RM, Naus NC et al (2012) Multiplex ligation-dependent probe amplification equals fluorescence in-situ hybridization for the identification of patients at risk for metastatic disease in uveal melanoma. Melanoma Res 22:30–37
26. Lake SL, Coupland SE, Taktak AFG, Damato BE (2010) Whole-genome microarray detects deletions and loss of heterozygosity of chromosome 3 occurring exclusively in metastasizing uveal melanoma. Invest Ophthalmol Vis Sci 51:4884–4891
27. Tschentscher F, Prescher G, Zeschnigk M, Horsthemke B, Lohmann DR (2000) Identification of chromosomes 3, 6, and 8 aberrations in uveal melanoma by microsatellite analysis in comparison to comparative genomic hybridization. Cancer Genet Cytogenet 122:13–17
28. Shields CL, Ganguly A, Materin MA, Teixeira L, Mashayekhi A, Swanson LA et al (2007) Chromosome 3 analysis of uveal melanoma using fine-needle aspiration biopsy at the time of plaque radiotherapy in 140 consecutive cases: the Deborah Iverson, MD, Lectureship. Arch Ophthalmol 125:1017–1024
29. Ewens KG, Kanetsky PA, Richards-Yutz J, Al-Dahmash S, De Luca, MC, Bianciotto CG et al (2013) Genomic profile of 320 uveal melanoma cases: Chromosome 8p-loss and metastatic outcome. Invest Ophthalmol Vis Sci 54:5721–5729
30. Lin M, Wei LJ, Sellers WR, Lieberfarb M, Wong WH, Li C (2004) dChipSNP: significance curve and clustering of SNP-array-based loss-of-heterozygosity data. Bioinformatics 20:1233–1240
31. Genome-Wide Human SNP Nsp/Sty 6.0 User Guide. http://www.affymetrix.com/support/technical/byproduct.affx?product=genomewidesnp_nsp_sty_assay

Part V

Emerging Markers/Targets in Melanoma

Chapter 24

ERBB4 Mutation Analysis: Emerging Molecular Target for Melanoma Treatment

Christopher Lau, Keith J. Killian, Yardena Samuels, and Udo Rudloff

Abstract

Recent sequencing efforts in melanoma have elucidated many previously unknown molecular pathways and biological mechanisms involved in melanoma development and progression and have yielded a number of promising targets for molecular therapy. As sequencing technologies have become more sophisticated and have revealed an ever-increasing complexity of the genetic landscape of melanoma, it has become clear that sequencing methods applied to clinical specimens have to reliably capture not only recurrent "hotspot" mutations like BRAFV600 and NRASQ61 or "mini-hotspot" mutations like exon 11 and 13 c-KIT but also heterogeneous somatic mutations dispersed across multiple functionally conserved regions of genes or entire genes. One such example in melanoma is the *ERBB4* receptor, or HER4, a member of the Erb receptor family, which has recently been shown to be a major oncogenic "driver" in melanoma. Mutated ERBB4 signaling activates both aberrant ERBB4 and PI3K-AKT signal transduction, mediates sensitivity to small-molecule inhibition with the dual-tyrosine kinase inhibitor lapatinib, and has recently also been implied in oncogenic glutamatergic signaling in melanoma. Mutations involving the ERBB4 gene act as "gain-of-function" mutations and predominantly involve the extracellular domains of the receptor. Additional sequencing efforts have recently identified recurrent mutations ("mini-hotspots") or mutation clusters which affect the regulation of, e.g., ligand binding, arrangement of extracellular domain alignment, or intramolecular tether formation.

In this chapter, we describe the methods used to determine the mutation status of all exons of the ERBB4 gene in clinical specimens obtained from patients afflicted by metastatic melanoma. Upon slight modifications, this protocol can also be used for mutational analysis of other oncogenes affected by "non-hotspot" mutations dispersed across multiple exons. This sequencing technique has successfully been applied within a clinical trial selecting patients with ERBB4-mutant melanoma for lapatinib treatment. With the increasing emergence of low-frequency oncogenes affected by heterogeneous activating mutations located in different exons and regions this method will provide a mean to translate the promise of recently obtained genetic knowledge into clinical genotype-directed targeted therapy trials.

Key words Metastatic melanoma, Genomic landscape, Somatic mutations, DNA isolation, Sanger sequencing, ERBB4 gene, Marker predictive for treatment, Mutation validation, Treatment target

Magdalena Thurin and Francesco M. Marincola (eds.), *Molecular Diagnostics for Melanoma: Methods and Protocols*, Methods in Molecular Biology, vol. 1102, DOI 10.1007/978-1-62703-727-3_24, © Springer Science+Business Media New York 2014

1 Introduction

Melanoma has become a "poster-child" during recent years for genetic discoveries and how such improved understanding of the dysfunctional genetic makeup of a solid organ cancer can translate into novel treatments for patients afflicted by this disease. It has been recognized early on that cutaneous malignant melanoma harbors as an environmentally caused solid organ cancer, a unique and complex mutation profile [1, 2]. Ultraviolet irradiation causes C→T and with less frequency CC→TT transitions, which give rise to a specific "UV mutational signature" in these skin cancers [3, 4]. UV mutational gene aberrations are more prevalent in melanoma arising from chronically sun-exposed areas (e.g., trunk, scalp) versus, e.g., acral melanomas. This unique mutation pattern suggests a "dose–response" relation of UV irradiation-induced skin damage and melanoma formation; however, recent whole-genome sequencing (WGS) efforts of acral melanoma have now also identified mutation patterns consistent with UV-induced DNA damage in melanomas arising in non-sun-exposed locations [5, 6]. Consistent with a causal function of UV irradiation-induced genetic changes, nearly all large-scale sequencing efforts carried out to date have found that melanoma, despite a large variation between individual tumors, harbors the largest number of genetic mutations (20–30 mutations/MB) among any solid organ cancer [1, 4, 7]. Interestingly, lung cancer, another environmentally induced malignancy, ranks second [7].

Since many of the large number of genetic variants identified in melanoma are "bystander" mutations and not involved in melanogenesis, the initial evaluation of newly discovered genetic variants is usually subject to a strict algorithm to determine if a particular mutation is a "driver" or a "passenger" mutation (reviewed in Walia et al. [7]). While there is no final agreement on the best approach to determine "driver" mutations without functional testing, the following three features are most commonly applied as surrogates for formal in vitro and in vivo testing:

1. "Hotspot" or cluster formation: One of the strongest indicators for a genetic variant to be a "driver" mutation is its detection at the same nucleotide or amino acid location in a larger specimen cohort. Such nonrandom, recurrent selection strongly suggests a growth advantage. Prime examples in melanoma are BRAFV600E, NRASQ61L, or K642E and L576P c-KIT mutations.
2. The N:S ratio: This ratio calculates the ratio of non-synonymous (NS) mutations which cause amino acid substitutions to synonymous (S) changes which do not. If a gene or a gene locus is more frequently affected by NS mutations than by S

mutations compared to the known background mutation frequency in a particular melanoma sample, it is more likely that these NS mutations are due to positive selection and represent "driver" mutations.

3. Biochemical impact of NS mutations: The functional impact of an NS mutation can be further validated by bioinformatic analysis of its impact on protein structure and function. For example, mutations affecting evolutionary conserved regions or functionally preserved domains like kinase or ligand-binding domains are more likely to be involved in cancer progression. The scale-invariant feature transform (SIFT) score is one of the most commonly used tools to rank the impact of amino acid changes on protein function.

Prior to the introduction of exomic and next-generation sequencing technologies, the genomic landscape of melanoma started to unfold with the extension of sequencing efforts from candidate genes onto whole candidate gene families [7]. The protein kinase family was the first gene family to be systematically interrogated using Sanger sequencing: since melanoma samples were underrepresented in the initial screening effort, a repeat genetic screen focusing on the protein tyrosine kinase family was carried out [1, 8]. The frequent involvement of activating mutations in tyrosine kinase genes in other cancers and the early success of targeting these mutated tyrosine kinase cancer genes with small-molecule inhibitors, like the L858R mutation-harboring non-small-cell lung cancer treated with erlotinib or gefitinib, provided a sound rationale for this effort [9, 10]. This sequencing effort yielded a number of new and therapeutically exploitable genes affected by oncogenic mutations, most notably the receptor tyrosine kinase ERBB4, or HER4, gene, a novel major oncogene in metastatic melanoma (Subheading 1.2). Other sequencing efforts directed against candidate gene families included screens in tyrosine phosphatases, matrix metalloproteinases, or the "A disintegrin and metalloproteinase" (ADAM) gene family [11–14]. While results of these sequencing efforts still await the identification of novel dysregulated targets and pathways which might become candidates for treatments, results of the recently completed sequencing of the coding regions of the G-protein-coupled receptor (GPCR) family have elucidated novel biological pathways involved in melanoma development and progression which might open new avenues for novel treatments in the future: using effective exon capture, the GPCRs GPR98 and GRM3 were frequently affected by somatic mutations in 27.5 and 16.3 % of cases in a cohort of 80 melanoma samples [15]. GRM3, which has a mutational hotspot at Glu870Lys found in four independent individuals, was shown in a number of in vitro and in vivo studies to function as an oncogenic driver mediating activation of the MAPK pathway [15].

The GRM3 receptor belongs to the metabotropic glutamate receptor family which is expressed in the brain and in gliomas [16]. Further findings from a recent exomic analysis performed by the same group showed that the *N*-methyl-d-aspartate (NMDA) receptor unit ε-1G GRIN2A, which belongs to the ionotropic glutamate receptor family, is affected in 25.2 % of cases by somatic mutations and functions as a tumor suppressor [17]. This independently discovered high mutation rate in both the GRM3 and GRIN2A receptors as well as previously identified mutated genes in melanoma which are involved in glutamate signalings strongly implies glutamate signaling as a novel mechanism in melanoma progression (reviewed in Prickett TD, Samuels Y. 2012) [16, 17]. Other genes involved in glutamate signal transduction and affected by somatic mutations include NRG-1-induced ERBB4 signaling, components of post-synaptic density complex (PSD complex) genes like PYK2, and PLCB4, a protein immediately downstream of NMDA receptors; or the ephrin receptors (in particular ephrin receptors B2 and B6) [18–20]. These genotyping results from multiple independent studies do open a plethora of potential novel therapeutic approaches which are not limited to direct downstream NDMA receptor signal transduction inhibition, like MEK inhibition, but for instance also include disruption or indirect manipulation of glutamate signaling using NMDA receptor agonists (glutamate analogs), inhibitors of metabotropic glutamate receptors like BAY 36-7620 or LY341495, or agents modulating the paracellular homeostasis of glutamate like riluzole [16, 21–23]. The recent exomic study also revealed a striking oncogenic hotspot in the TRAPP gene [17]. The Ser722Phe hotspot of the TRAPP gene, which regulates c-MYC- and E2F1-mediated transcription, was shown to function as a "gain-of-function" oncogene in melanoma. However, when extending this analysis onto additional specimens only 6 out of 167 (~4 %) melanomas harbored this mutation [17]. This increasing detection of low-frequency or "cancer-hill" genes, in recent candidate gene family and exomic sequencing efforts, is currently posing one of several unresolved problems with respect to clinical translation of these sequencing studies [24]. WGS on the other hand offers the unique advantage of integrating point mutations and genomic aberrations like amplifications, deletions, and chromosomal translocations into comprehensive maps of the entire tumor genome. The results of the first large-scale whole-genome analysis on 25 metastatic melanoma and matched normal specimens emphasize the comprehensiveness of the WGS approach: first, the study elegantly showed that the mutation rate in metastatic melanoma is more accurately determined as an average mutation rate of ~30 per MB with enrichment of C → T transitions consistent with UV-induced genetic changes and, secondly, identified several new genes affected by somatic mutations or chromosomal rearrangements [4]. One of the novel findings of the study is the discovery that different genetic mechanisms can lead to PREX2 dysregulation in melanoma. PREX2, a regulator of PTEN and the PI3K-Akt pathway, was found to harbor somatic mutations in 14 % of cases, and mutated variants of PREX2 functioned as tumor suppressors in an in vivo model of melanoma [4, 25]. Additionally, several rearrangements and chromosomal translocations at the PREX2 locus were identified suggesting a positive selection for PREX2 dysregulation on a genomic level, which, when combined with the findings of somatic PREX2 mutations, suggests that multiple different genetic causes of tumor-driving mechanism mediated by PREX2 exist in melanoma.

1.1 Mutations Within the Tyrosine Kinase Family in Melanoma

One of the early gene discoveries from candidate gene family sequencing with potential successful translation into the clinic stems from the genetic screen of the protein tyrosine kinase family in melanoma [8]. In the initial discovery set of 29 melanomas, 19 out of 86 tyrosine kinases were found to have mutations in the kinase domain-encoding exons [8]. Tyrosine kinase genes affected by kinase domain mutations in the initial screen were then comprehensively sequenced in an additional cohort of 79 specimens. The tyrosine kinase Erb receptor family member ERBB4, or HER4, was found to be the most frequently mutated gene affected by somatic mutations in 19 % of cases. Other frequently mutated genes included FLT3 in 10 %, PTK2B in 10 %, the ephrin receptor B2 and B6 genes in 9 %, and TIE2 in 8 %. The availability of additional independent mutation analyses obtained from additional specimens on different platforms now allows the buildup of detailed, in-depth mutation maps of melanoma oncogenes like recently performed for the BRAF, NRAS, and CDKN2A gene [26]. This allows both independent validation of initial sequencing results and, biologically more important, gives insight into positive selection of melanoma-driving genetic events when examining recurrence and location patterns or biophysical properties of the evolving somatic mutation pattern. The ERBB4 gene is a good example demonstrating the value of such comparative genetic screening. The mutational ERBB4 profile is quite different from other oncogenes including other ERBB receptor family members currently targeted in the clinic: to date, targeted therapy efforts focus predominantly on "hotspots" of oncogenes, e.g., vemurafenib or trametinib for BRAFV600 [27, 28], imatinib mesylate for c-KIT exon 11 and 13 mutations in melanoma [29], erlotinib or gefitinib for EGFR L858R mutations in lung cancer [10], or soon GDC-0941 for PI3KCA E545K, E542K (both exon 9), or H1047R (exon 20) mutations in breast or colon cancer [30, 31] to name a few. In the original genetic screen of melanoma samples, only the E452K mutation was found twice in the ERBB4 gene ("mini-hotspot"); all other identified mutations were spread across multiple different functional domains of the genes (*see* Fig. 1)

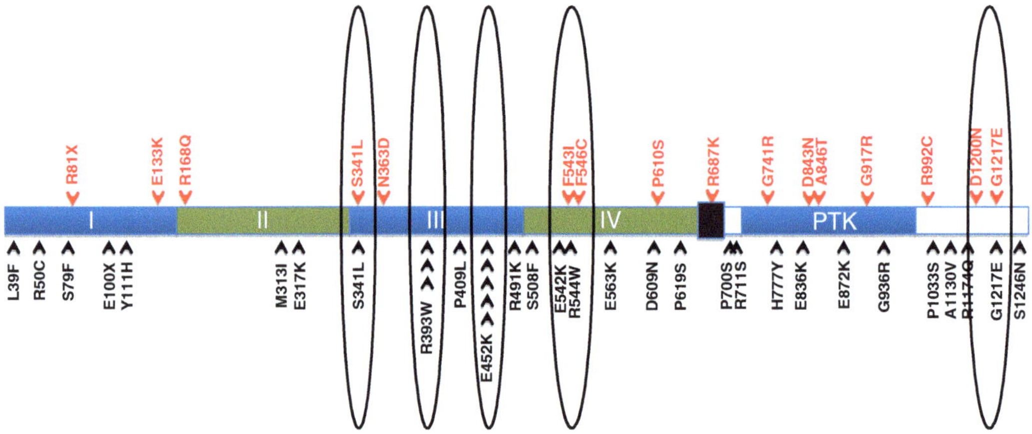

Fig. 1 Evolvement of clustering and the development of recurrence patterns ("mini-hotspot" mutations; *circles*) of somatic mutations affecting the ERBB4 gene in melanoma upon combining sequencing results from candidate gene family sequencing and exomic and whole-genome sequencing studies (previously identified mutations listed as *black arrows* on *bottom*, mutations identified as part of the NIH, Clinical Genomic Core profiling (clinical trial samples), listed in *red* on *top* (unpublished))

raising initially doubt about both the validity and future clinical applicability of these mutations as genetic markers. However, when adding recent findings from the above mentioned WGS efforts as well as sequencing results obtained from patients with metastatic melanoma enrolled onto a clinical trial (*NCI-11-C-0048*, NCT01264081; A Phase II Study of Lapatinib for the Treatment of Stage IV Melanoma Harboring ERBB4 Mutations (Subheading 1.3)) new patterns of recurrence as well as clustering of several of the originally identified missense mutations were identified indicating positive selection during melanoma progression [4, 17, 32, 33].

Thus, as the majority of cancer genes currently discovered have a dispersed mutation profile without a clear recurrence pattern a robust algorithm applicable to clinical specimens will be necessary in order for these findings to be used for targeted therapy approaches in the future. In this respect, the presented ERBB4 mutation testing method which was designed to capture all "non-hotspot" mutations in all 28 exons of the ERBB4 gene should be applicable to a wider number of newly discovered oncogenes affected by heterogeneous mutations dispersed across multiple regions.

1.2 Somatic Mutations in the ERBB4 Gene

The distribution pattern of mutations affecting the ERBB4 gene is unique and substantially different from the mutation profile of other members of the Erb receptor family, e.g., EGFR or HER2. While activating somatic mutations of the EGFR, and to a lesser degree the HER2 receptor, predominantly affect the kinase domain of the gene, the majority of ERBB4 mutations in melanoma, or in lung cancer, are located in exons encoding the extracellular domains of the receptor [34, 35]. This mutation profile appeared initially more consistent with that of a tumor-suppressor gene than an oncogene. However, thorough functional assessment of eight independent ERBB4 mutants showed that all examined ERBB4 gene mutations drive melanoma biology and function as a "gain-of-function" oncogene [8]. Studies on ERBB4 mutants included kinase assays showing an increase in basal ERBB4 autophosphorylation, increase in cell transformation ability, and increase in foci formation. Most importantly, loss of ERBB4 signaling led to selective cell death in cells harboring mutated, but not wild-type, ERBB4 receptors indicating true gain of function and "oncogene" addiction to mutated ERBB4 signaling in these melanomas. To explain the fact that all examined ERBB4 mutations, which are dispersed across various regions of the gene, cause the same phenotype of "oncogene addiction" to mutant ERBB4 signaling, a closer look at the structure–function relationship between location of these mutations and the functional impact of the induced amino acid changes onto the involved receptor domains was taken. The described S341L and R393W mutations of the ERBB4 receptor, for example, involve structurally highly conserved motifs of the receptor L2 domain [36, 37]. These amino acid alterations are likely to either directly alter the kinetics of ligand binding or expose differently charged residues due to a different arrangement of the helices or β sheets which indirectly enhance the affinity of the ligand to the receptor possibly leading to receptor activation and increased signal transduction. Another mechanism of how the identified ERBB4 mutations might cause receptor activation might be the release of the intramolecular "tether" of the inactive receptor leading to exposure of the dimerization domain and activation of ERB signaling [35]. The dimerization domain is facing in the non-active state of the receptor facing towards domain III/IV of the receptor. Ligand binding triggers a major rearrangement of all extracellular domains involving a 270° outward twist of the dimerization region of receptor domain II [35]. Multiple residues have been identified to mediate this tether: for instance, Arg405 in EGFR forms a salt bond with Glu293, and it is conceivable that R393W or the previously identified P409L mutation, which involves functionally homologous regions of the ERBB4 molecule involved in tether regulation, might alter the equilibrium towards a more open and consecutively active form of the receptor [35, 37].

While to date for many of the confirmed activating mutations like the C-terminal G1217E or the domain III E452K "mini-hotspots" no structural correlate has been identified, these mutations have potential clinical value (Subheading 1.3) and should not be disregarded. Considering the heterogeneity of both the actual genetic variants as well as their response to small-molecule inhibition genetic testing must employ a technique which captures all mutations in these oncogenes. As many other genes mediating tumor progression harbor a similar mutation profile like the ERBB4 gene, the presented sequencing strategy should be applicable to the rapidly enlarging pool of novel genes involved in melanoma progression.

1.3 Mutations in the ERBB4 Gene Predict Sensitivity to Treatment with the Lapatinib in Melanoma

The clinical importance of the described sequencing protocol for ERBB4 mutations stems from the exquisite sensitivity of melanomas harboring ERBB4 mutations to the dual-tyrosine kinase inhibitor lapatinib. Melanomas harboring ERBB4 mutations have 10–250-fold lower inhibitory 50 concentrations to lapatinib, a dual-EGFR/HER2 small-molecule inhibitor which also has activity against ERBB4, than melanomas with wild-type ERBB4 receptors. While the exact mechanism of lapatinib-mediated mutated ERBB4 signal inhibition remains to be elucidated, treatment of ERBB4 mutant melanoma leads to decreased ERBB4 receptor autophosphorylation, decreased Akt signaling, and induction of apoptosis. Melanomas harboring mutant ERBB4 showed a wide range of sensitivity to lapatinib suggesting possibly several different mechanisms to drug inhibition, for example inhibition of HER2 mutant ERBB4 heterodimer formation. Several key observations with respect to results of preclinical lapatinib testing in ERBB4 mutant cell lines emphasize the need to employ a comprehensive sequencing strategy: first, all identified ERBB4 mutations which mediated addiction to ERBB4 signaling and functioned as a gain-of-function oncogene also showed sensitivity to lapatinib confirming that the somatic mutation status of the ERBB4 gene is a suitable biomarker for selecting patients for lapatinib. Therefore, based on currently available data, no ERBB4 mutation should be missed in order to erroneously exclude patients from possible tyrosine kinase inhibitor treatment. Secondly, inhibition of cell growth in ERBB4 mutant melanomas was achieved at clinically achievable concentrations of lapatinib with the exception of melanomas harboring two or more synchronous mutations (e.g., melanoma 7T or 71T in the original report) [8]. While melanomas with multiple ERBB4 mutations still show sensitivity to lapatinib treatment, lapatinib is less active in these cases and patients with two or more mutations in their ERBB4 gene were excluded from the above phase II clinical trial. Overall, the heterogeneity of ERBB4 mutations, which do not form classical "hotspot" mutations, as well as a select sensitivity profile to lapatinib demand a sequencing method which reliably captures somatic mutations in any of the 28 exons of the ERBB4 gene and has a turnaround time which allows its use in patients frequently presenting with dire needs for additional treatment options. Subheading 3 describes a protocol which is optimized to perform such whole candidate gene sequencing. As for other clinical molecular pathology testing described in this series, a detailed histopathological review is required to confirm diagnosis of metastatic melanoma and actual harvesting of melanoma-harboring

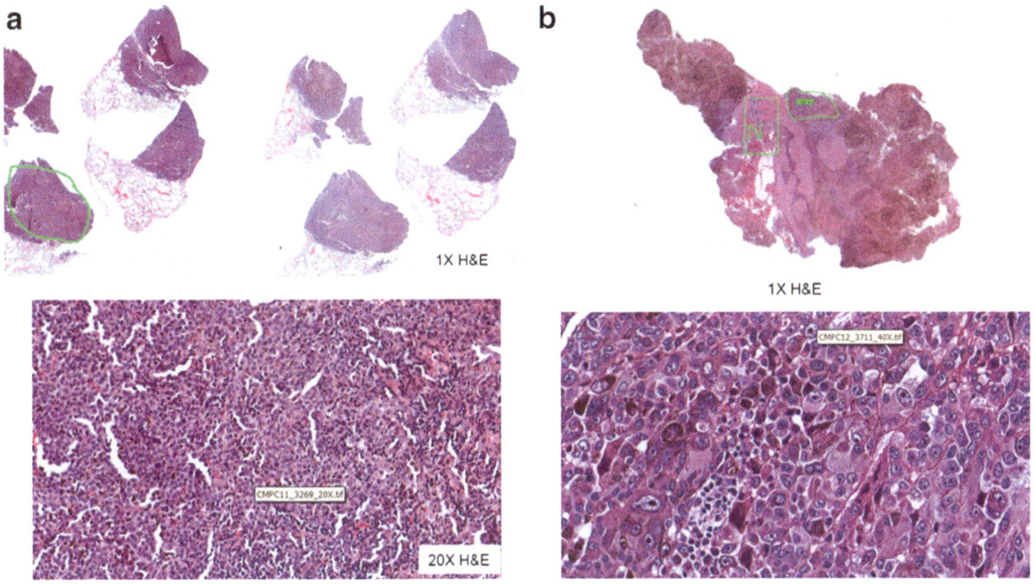

Fig. 2 Histopathological review and "macrodissection" of metastatic melanoma and matched normal tissue from surgically resected (**a**) lung metastasis and (**b**) brain metastasis

tissue. Figure 2 shows examples of histopathological reviews of metastatic lesions from the lung and brain prior to "macrodissection" and isolation of genomic DNA.

2 Materials

2.1 Equipment

1. ABI 3730 DNA Sequencer (Applied Biosystems).
2. Eppendorf Microcentrifuge or similar.
3. Eppendorf Thermomixer (24 × 2.0 mL).
4. Nanodrop Spectrophotometer ND-1000 to quantify and assess the quality of the DNAs.
5. VWR High-Speed Microplate Shaker.
6. DNA Engine Tetrad Thermal Cycler.
7. SORVALL Legend RT Plus Centrifuge.

2.2 Processing of Formalin-Fixed Paraffin-Embedded Tissue Blocks

1. Disposable biopsy punch with plunger (2 mm) (Miltex).
2. Ethyl alcohol (200 proof).
3. Micro tubes with screw cap (1.5 mL).
4. Sterile disposable safety scalpel.
5. Xylene substitute for deparafinizing formalin-fixed paraffin-embedded (FFPE) samples.
6. Tris–EDTA (TE) buffer (10 mM Tris-Cl, pH 7.5, 1 mM EDTA).

2.3 Genomic DNA Isolation

1. Proteinase K (600 AU/mL).
2. RNase A (7,000 U/mL).
3. QIAquick PCR Purification Kit contains QIAquick spin columns, Collection tubes, and PE Wash Buffer (Qiagen).
4. DNeasy Blood and Tissue Kit contains ATL tissue Lysis Buffer and AE Elution Buffer (Qiagen).
5. PM: Binding Buffer (Qiagen).

2.4 Array Comparative Genome Hybridization

1. Genomic DNA high-throughput ULS labeling kit (Agilent Technologies).
2. Oligo array comparative genome hybridization (aCGH)/ChiP-on-Chip Hybridization Kit (Agilent Technologies).
3. SurePrint G3 Hmn CGH 4x180K Oligo Microarray kit (Agilent Technologies).

2.5 Polymerase Chain Reaction (PCR Amplification) and PCR Cleanup

1. Titanium® Taq DNA Polymerase (Clontech).
2. MgCl2 solution (25 mM).
3. Nuclease-free water.
4. Exo-Sap It for cleanup of PCR products (USB/Affymetrix).
5. MicroAmp DNA/RNA/RNAse free adhesive film (Applied Biosystem).
6. 2 % Polyacrylamide gel.

2.6 Sanger Sequencing

1. Ultrapure deionized H_2O.
2. BigDye® Terminator v3.1 Cycle Sequencing Kit for PCR products including SAM solution (Applied Biosystems).
3. BigDye® Terminator v1.1, v3.1 5× Sequencing Buffer (Applied Biosystems).
4. Universal M13-F forward tgtaaaacgacggccagt and reverse M13-R caggaaacagctatgacc primers for DNA sequencing (IDT).
5. BigDye XTerminatorPurification Kit for DNA sequencing (Applied Biosystems).

3 Methods

3.1 Tissue Harvest of Metastatic Melanoma Deposits and Matched Normal

1. Manufacture Hematoxylin and Eosin (H&E)-stained slides from FFPE tissue blocks of metastatic melanoma lesions harvested surgically from any site.
2. Confirm diagnosis of melanoma, and select areas harboring tumor and normal surrounding tissue (*see* Fig. 2).
3. Using the marked H&E slide as a "template," microdissect corresponding areas of the FFPE block using a biopsy punch or scalpel.

4. Transfer paraffin cores to 1.5 mL micro tubes with screw caps and deparaffinize using xylene substitute. Add 1 mL of xylene substitute to each tube that contains the dissected specimen and incubate at 65 °C for 15 min.
5. Centrifuge tubes at maximum speed in an Eppendorf microcentrifuge for 1 min, and carefully discard the xylene substitute.
6. Repeat processes once for a total of two xylene substitute incubation steps. After removing most xylene substitute from each tube, wash residual xylene substitute away with two ethanol washes.
7. Add 1 mL of 100 % ethanol to each tube at room temperature, mix well, and centrifuge at maximum speed before discarding ethanol.
8. Repeat ethanol wash step once with 50 % ethanol (50 % 1× TE). After discarding most of the 50 % ethanol, leave tubes open at room temperature for 10 min to let residual ethanol evaporate.

3.2 Genomic DNA Extraction

1. Lyze the deparaffinized tissues in 100 μL of ATL lysis buffer and 20 μL of proteinase K at 65 °C overnight (18–24 h) in an Eppendorf thermo mixer.
2. Add an additional 20 μL of proteinase K on the next day, and continue the lysis at 65 °C overnight (additional 18–24 h) in the Eppendorf thermo mixer.
3. Inspect the specimens to ensure complete lysis.
4. If undigested tissues are observed, add an additional 20 μL of proteinase K and incubate at 65 °C for an additional 2–4 h or until the tissues are completely digested.
5. Remove the tubes from the thermo mixer, add 2 μL of RNAse A to the lysates, and incubate at room temperature for 5 min.
6. Add buffer PM, three times the volume, to the lysates and pipette mix.
7. Apply the mixture to the QIAquick columns and centrifuge at 9,300 × *g* in an Eppendorf microcentrifuge for 1 min.
8. Reapply the flow-through to the columns, repeat **step** 7 to increase DNA yield, and then discard the flow-through.
9. Add 720 μL of PE wash buffer to the columns, centrifuge at 16,100 × *g* for 1 min to purify DNA that are selectively bound to the Qiaquick silica-based membrane, and then discard flow-through.
10. Add 720 μL of 80 % ethanol, centrifuge at 16,100 × *g* for 1 min for an additional purification step, and then discard flow-through.
11. Transfer the columns to new collection tubes and centrifuge at 16,100 × *g* for 5 min.

12. Transfer the columns to pre-labeled 1.5 mL Eppendorf tubes and allow to air-dry with open caps for 5 min at room temperature to rid all residual ethanol.
13. Apply 70 μL 10 % buffer AE to the columns, wait for 2 min, and then centrifuge at 16,100 × *g* for 1 min to elute the bound DNA.
14. Reapply the eluted DNA to the columns, wait for 2 min, and then centrifuge at 16,100 × *g* for 1 min to increase DNA elution.
15. Measure the absorbance of the eluted DNAs at 230, 260, and 280 nm using NanoDrop to quantify and assess the quality of the DNAs.
16. (Optional) To determine the tumor fraction, label 500 μg of sample and reference genomic DNA using Agilent's Genomic DNA High-Throughput ULS Labeling Kit and hybridize to Agilent's SurePrint G3 Hmn CGH 4x180K Microarrays following the manufacturer's instructions. Analyze the results with software Nexus 6. Detection of gross chromosomal aberrations is indicative of satisfactory tumor fraction for the acceptance of a negative (wild type) ERBB4 mutation result.

3.3 PCR Amplification of 28 Exons of ERBB4 Gene

A total of 31 pairs of primers were custom designed to cover all 28 exons of the ERBB4 gene, including their splice junctions, using Primer3, a primer design software publically available online (http://frodo.wi.mit.edu/) (Table 1). The primers all contained tagged M13 forward or reverse sequences for downstream Sanger sequencing reaction (Subheading 2.5). An additional primer pair to amplify exon 15 of the BRAF gene was also included in the assay as an internal control.

1. Adjust sample DNAs and a positive control DNA control containing at least one previously identified variant to a DNA concentration of 10 ng/μL, and prepare a minimum total volume of 65 μL for each sample.
2. Aliquot 2 μL of normalized DNA into 32 wells (four columns) in a 96-well reaction plate for each sample and the positive control.
3. Aliquot 2 μL of PCR-grade water into 32 wells for the no-template control.
4. Aliquot 2 μL of 32 (2 μM) individual forward and reverse primer mixes into the separate wells for each sample and control.
5. Prepare reagent master mix containing the components listed in the table below, excluding DNA and primers, enough for all PCR reactions.
6. Aliquot 16 μL the reagent mix into each individual well.

Table 1
PCR primers used for ERBB4 sequencing

Gene	Exon	Primer name	[a]Forward primer	Primer name	[a]Reverse primer
ERBB4	1	ERBB4-X1b-F	GGGGATATGCCATTTGGAC	ERBB4-X1b-R	CGGAGTGCCAGAAGGAAC
ERBB4	2.1	ERBB4-X2.1c-F	TAAAGGTTATGTAATTTCACGTGTATC	ERBB4-X2.1c-R	GCTGGTTATCTCCAGGTTGC
ERBB4	2.2	ERBB4-X2.2c-F	AACAGCAGTACCGAGCCTTG	ERBB4-X2.2c-R	GCCACTGTCCATTCACAAAG
ERBB4	3	ERBB4-X3b-F	GGCAACTGTTTGTGTCTTTTCA	ERBB4-X3b-R	AAGCATATTTGCCATTTTGGA
ERBB4	4	ERBB4-X4b-F	TTCATCAACAAGCAGTTTGACA	ERBB4-X4b-R	TCGCCACATAGGGTAGAACA
ERBB4	5	ERBB4-X5-F	AAATCCTCATAAAGGAGCAGGAG	ERBB4-X5-R	CCAAAGCAAATCAACCACAAG
ERBB4	6	ERBB4-X6-F	TGAATTGAGTCAAAGACAGGGTG	ERBB4-X6-R	GGAATGACTTTGAGGAGGGC
ERBB4	7	ERBB4-X7b-F	TGAAAGTAATATTTGCTGTGTTGC	ERBB4-X7b-R	TTCTTTTGATTTCAAATAATGACCT
ERBB4	8	ERBB4-X8b-F	TGTTTTGAGCTTGTTTGCTGA	ERBB4-X8b-R	AAACCTTGTTATATAGGCCCAGTTC
ERBB4	9	ERBB4-X9b-F	TTGGCCAAAAATAAGTTTCTCAA	ERBB4-X9b-R	CACTTTGTAAAATAACTTGCACAAAAA
ERBB4	10	ERBB4-X10b-F	AAATTTGGCTACATCTCTTCTTGA	ERBB4-X10b-R	AAATTATATTGTTCATAGCGCAACA
ERBB4	11	ERBB4-X11-F	CCTTTCTCACTTCCCAACTTTC	ERBB4-X11-R	TACCTCACACCATCATCGGAG
ERBB4	12.1	ERBB4-X12.1c-F	TTCATGGTTCCGTTTTCTCA	ERBB4-X12.1c-R	AACACAGGTTGCTGTTGTCAG
ERBB4	12.2	ERBB4-X12.2c-F	AATCAGCGCAGGAAACATCT	ERBB4-X12.2c-R	GGTCCAAAGAAGAATGGGAAA
ERBB4	13	ERBB4-X13b-F	TCCCCTTGATTTTGGTGTTT	ERBB4-X13b-R	ATGAGGTGAAGGCAACCCTA
ERBB4	14	ERBB4-X14-F	TGATGCTCCTGGCACATAGAG	ERBB4-X14-R	CCCATGGCATCCTGTAAGTAG

(continued)

Table 1
(continued)

Gene	Exon	Primer name	[a]Forward primer	Primer name	[a]Reverse primer
ERBB4	15	ERBB4-X15c-F	GGAAATGACACCACTTTTCTTTTT	ERBB4-X15c-R	CCTTGGCCAGCAAGAATG
ERBB4	16	ERBB4-X16c-F	GGATGGAGAATGATGTTTTCTG	ERBB4-X16c-R	TGAGCGACAAAATGGAAACA
ERBB4	17	ERBB4-X17c-F	TTTTTCTCATTCTGGTTGTCAG	ERBB4-X17c-R	TCCCCAAACACATGAAGAGG
ERBB4	18	ERBB4-X18b-F	TTCTTCTTTCCGCTTTGCAG	ERBB4-X18b-R	TCCATTGGCTATTATTTTCTAAACA
ERBB4	19	ERBB4-X19b-F	TGTAACAGGTGCTAAATAAACATTTG	ERBB4-X19b-R	TGATTGCCTGGGTGTCTGTA
ERBB4	20	ERBB4-X20b-F	TTGAGTTGAAATCATGGTATTGC	ERBB4-X20b-R	TTCCATAGAAATTGACAGGCACT
ERBB4	21	ERBB4-X21b-F	GGGAAAACCTGGGCATTAAC	ERBB4-X21b-R	TCAAGCAAGATTGCTCTCAAAA
ERBB4	22	ERBB4-X22c-F	CCAGCCCAAAGACTCACATT	ERBB4-X22c-R	CAAGCTTTAATTCGCAAAGAAGA
ERBB4	23	ERBB4-X23b-F	TTGGTGTTTGGATTGACCTG	ERBB4-X23b-R	TGATGGTGATAACATTATTTTGCAG
ERBB4	24	ERBB4-X24-F	GAGTCGTTTCTTTCACTAGCTTGC	ERBB4-X24-R	TGTTTGTGGTCCTTTCCACAG
ERBB4	25	ERBB4-X25c-F	TGTGTCTGATGGGCAATCTT	ERBB4-X25c-R	TTATTTTGAAATGTTAGTGCTTATGAA
ERBB4	26	ERBB4-X26b-F	CCATCATTCCATTTTTCTTTCC	ERBB4-X26b-R	AAGCAAAGACCGAAAATCCT
ERBB4	27	ERBB4-X27b-F	ACAACGCCTTCTCTCCACAT	ERBB4-X27b-R	AATGGCGATCGTTTCTGAAT
ERBB4	28.1	ERBB4-X28.1c-F	TTTTCCAGAAACTAGAGGTTAGCTG	ERBB4-X28.1c-R	CAGGGTTGTCAAACGCTTTC
ERBB4	28.2	ERBB4-X28.2c-F	TGAAGAACAACATACTGTCAATGC	ERBB4-X28.2c-R	CAGGTGTGTCTCTCCACCTAAA
BRAF	15	BRAF-X15-F	TCATCCTAACACATTTCAAGCC	BRAF-X15-R	TTTGTGAATACTGGGAACTATGAAA

[a] *Note*: Every PCR primer contains a 5′ M13 forward (tgtaaaacgacggccagt) or reverse (caggaaacagctatgacc) tag

Reagent/material	Volume (μL)	Final concentration
10× Titanium Taq buffer	2	1×
50× dNTP mix (10 mM)	0.4	0.2 mM
50× Taq polymerase	0.4	1×
$MgCl_2$ (25 mM)	0.08	3.6 mM[a]
Genomic DNA (10 ng/μL)	2	1 ng/μL
Primer mix (2 μM)	2	0.2 μM
PCR-grade water	13.9	–
Total	20	

[a] *Note*: In addition to $MgCl_2$ in 10× buffer for final concentration of 3.6 mM

7. Seal the PCR plate with a PCR-compatible DNA/RNA/RNase-free adhesive film.
8. Lightly vortex the PCR plate for 5 s.
9. Centrifuge the 96-well reaction plates for 30 s at maximum speed of 600 × *g*.
10. Run the PCR reactions on a PTC-225 DNA Engine Tetrad Thermal Cycler with the following cycling conditions:

Step	Temperature	Time and cycles
1	95 °C	3 min
2	95 °C	30 s
3	61 °C	30 s
4	–	Repeat **steps 2–3** for a total of 5 cycles
5	95 °C	30 s
6	68 °C	1 min
7	–	Repeat **steps 5–6** for a total of 34 cycles
8	72 °C	5 min
9	4 °C	Hold

11. Upon completion of the PCR reaction, run 5 μL of each PCR amplification products on a 2 % gel electrophoresis.
12. Inspect gel image for the presence of single bands (expected size of 250–500 bp) indicative of successful PCR reactions (*see* **Note 1**).

3.4 PCR Product Cleanup

1. Add 6 μL of ExoSAP-IT into each remaining 15 μL of PCR products and pipette mix.
2. Seal the 96-well reaction plate and centrifuge for 30 s at maximum speed of 600 × g.
3. Incubate at 37 °C for 30 min to enzymatically degrade residual primers and dephosphorylate access dNTPs from the PCR step, and then incubate at 85 °C for 15 min to deactivate the *enzymes.*

3.5 Sequencing Reaction

1. Make 1:50 dilutions of the cleaned-up PCR products by adding 3 μL of the cleaned-up PCR products to 147 μL of 10 % buffer AE (*see* **Note 2**).
2. Aliquot 2 μL each of the diluted PCR products to two separate 96-well reaction plates, for both the forward and reverse sequencing reactions.
3. Each Sanger sequencing reaction would contain the following components:

Reagent/material	Volume (μL)	Final concentration
BigDye 3.1 (2.5×)	1	0.25×
BigDye buffer (5×)	1.5	0.75×
M13 F or R (10 μM)	0.32	320 nM
Cleaned-up PCR (1:50)	2	1:250
PCR-grade water	5.18	–
Total	10	

4. Run the sequencing reaction on the PTC-200 Peltier Thermal cycler with the following cycling conditions:

Step	Temperature	Time and cycles
1	96 °C	1 min
2	96 °C	10 s
3	50 °C	30 s
4	60 °C	4 min
5	–	Repeat **steps 2–4** for a total of 25 cycles
6	4 °C	Hold

3.6 Sanger Sequencing Reaction Purification

1. Purify the sequencing reaction products using the BigDye XTerminator Purification Kit by adding 45 μL of SAM Solution and 10 μL of BigDye XTerminator Solution to each well.
2. Seal the reaction plate, put it on a microplate shaker, and vortex for 30 min at 600 × g.
3. Centrifuge the plates at 1,000 × g for 2 min.

3.7 Capillary Electrophoresis

1. Load the centrifuged plates containing purified Sanger sequencing products on the Applied Biosystems 3730 DNA Analyzer for capillary electrophoresis following standard instrument protocol.
2. Wait for approximately 3 h for individual runs to complete.

3.8 Sequence Analysis

1. Move .abl sequence files that were generated into a designated folder.
2. Import the sequence files into the Variant Reporter software for subsequent sequence analysis.
3. Import ERBB4 reference sequence NM005235.2 and BRAF reference sequence NG_007873.2. 3. Use the default sequence quality and mixed base threshold for the automatic alignment and variant calling steps (*see* **Note 3**).
4. Click the Analyze button in the Variant Reporter software for alignment to reference and variant calling (*see* **Note 4**).
5. Manually inspect each aligned sequence trace and variant that was called.
6. Validate each variant by an additional validation assay starting from the PCR amplification step (*see* **Note 5**).

4 Notes

1. The agarose gel electrophoresis served as a quality control (QC) step for the PCR reaction. For any given PCR reaction, when a single visible band of expected size was absent or when multiple bands or smears appeared in the gel image, the individual PCR reaction would be repeated. When similar problems occur to all PCR products of a particular sample, the DNA would be re-extracted.
2. For the sequencing reactions, background noise within the sequence traces that reduce confidence in variant calling will result in repeat of the sequencing reaction. Unless the PCR failed QC, the original PCR products were used in the repeat sequencing reactions at three different dilutions: 1:25, 1:50, and 1:100.

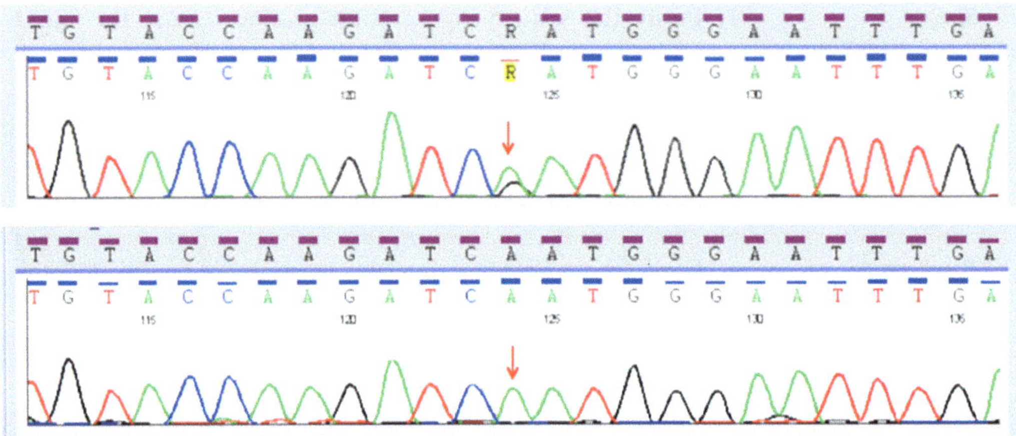

Fig. 3 Sanger sequencing traces for ERBB4 exon 9. *Top panel* shows the c.1185A>G p.N363D variant, and *lower panel* shows the matched normal tissue from the same patient. *Arrow* indicates the location of missense mutation

3. To avoid false-negative results due to insufficient tumor DNA fraction, a positive finding at the BRAFV600 hotspot, which should be found in ~50 % of melanoma cases, in addition to the evidence of positive copy number changes in the tumor genome which were almost always seen in melanoma cases, was used to confirm true negatives.
4. To determine if the identified variants were previously found in other cancers or if they were polymorphic genetic variations in the general population, they were searched against both the Catalogue of Somatic Mutations in Cancer (COSMIC) and the Single Nucleotide Polymorphism (dbSNP) databases. In addition, to determine whether they were somatic or germline variants, the assays starting from the PCR step were repeated using matched normal DNA samples for the particular ERBB4 exon harboring the identified variant (*see* Fig. 3).
5. To validate positive results when a variant is identified, an additional assay to confirm the result was run starting from the PCR amplification step. The positive result would be confirmed when the same variant was observed the second time.

Acknowledgement

Yardena Samuels is supported by the ERC (StG-335377).

References

1. Greenman C et al (2007) Patterns of somatic mutation in human cancer genomes. Nature 446(7132):153–158
2. Pleasance ED et al (2010) A comprehensive catalogue of somatic mutations from a human cancer genome. Nature 463(7278): 191–196
3. Drobetsky EA, Grosovsky AJ, Glickman BW (1987) The specificity of UV-induced mutations at an endogenous locus in mammalian cells. Proc Natl Acad Sci U S A 84(24): 9103–9107
4. Berger MF et al (2012) Melanoma genome sequencing reveals frequent PREX2 mutations. Nature 485(7399):502–506
5. Curtin JA et al (2005) Distinct sets of genetic alterations in melanoma. N Engl J Med 353(20):2135–2147
6. Turajlic S et al (2012) Whole genome sequencing of matched primary and metastatic acral melanomas. Genome Res 22(2):196–207
7. Walia V et al (2012) Delving into somatic variation in sporadic melanoma. Pigment Cell Melanoma Res 25(2):155–170
8. Prickett TD et al (2009) Analysis of the tyrosine kinome in melanoma reveals recurrent mutations in ERBB4. Nat Genet 41(10):1127–1132
9. Mok TS et al (2009) Gefitinib or carboplatin-paclitaxel in pulmonary adenocarcinoma. N Engl J Med 361(10):947–957
10. Rosell R et al (2009) Screening for epidermal growth factor receptor mutations in lung cancer. N Engl J Med 361(10):958–967
11. Solomon DA et al (2008) Mutational inactivation of PTPRD in glioblastoma multiforme and malignant melanoma. Cancer Res 68(24):10300–10306
12. Palavalli LH et al (2009) Analysis of the matrix metalloproteinase family reveals that MMP8 is often mutated in melanoma. Nat Genet 41(5):518–520
13. Wei X et al (2010) Mutational and functional analysis reveals ADAMTS18 metalloproteinase as a novel driver in melanoma. Mol Cancer Res 8(11):1513–1525
14. Wei X et al (2011) Analysis of the disintegrin-metalloproteinases family reveals ADAM29 and ADAM7 are often mutated in melanoma. Hum Mutat 32(6):E2148–E2175
15. Prickett TD et al (2011) Exon capture analysis of G protein-coupled receptors identifies activating mutations in GRM3 in melanoma. Nat Genet 43(11):1119–1126
16. Prickett TD, Samuels Y (2012) Molecular pathways: dysregulated glutamatergic signaling pathways in cancer. Clin Cancer Res 18(16):4240–4246
17. Wei X et al (2011) Exome sequencing identifies GRIN2A as frequently mutated in melanoma. Nat Genet 43(5):442–446
18. Hahn CG et al (2006) Altered neuregulin 1-erbB4 signaling contributes to NMDA receptor hypofunction in schizophrenia. Nat Med 12(7):824–828
19. Garcia RA, Vasudevan K, Buonanno A (2000) The neuregulin receptor ErbB-4 interacts with PDZ-containing proteins at neuronal synapses. Proc Natl Acad Sci U S A 97(7):3596–3601
20. Delint-Ramirez I et al (2010) In vivo composition of NMDA receptor signaling complexes differs between membrane subdomains and is modulated by PSD-95 and PSD-93. J Neurosci 30(24):8162–8170
21. D'Onofrio M et al (2003) Pharmacological blockade of mGlu2/3 metabotropic glutamate receptors reduces cell proliferation in cultured human glioma cells. J Neurochem 84(6):1288–1295
22. Namkoong J et al (2007) Metabotropic glutamate receptor 1 and glutamate signaling in human melanoma. Cancer Res 67(5): 2298–2305
23. Yip D et al (2009) A phase 0 trial of riluzole in patients with resectable stage III and IV melanoma. Clin Cancer Res 15(11):3896–3902
24. Wood LD et al (2007) The genomic landscapes of human breast and colorectal cancers. Science 318(5853):1108–1113
25. Fine B et al (2009) Activation of the PI3K pathway in cancer through inhibition of PTEN by exchange factor P-REX2a. Science 325(5945):1261–1265
26. Colombino M et al (2012) BRAF/NRAS mutation frequencies among primary tumors and metastases in patients with melanoma. J Clin Oncol 30(20):2522–2529
27. Chapman PB et al (2011) Improved survival with vemurafenib in melanoma with BRAF V600E mutation. N Engl J Med 364(26): 2507–2516
28. Flaherty KT et al (2012) Improved survival with MEK inhibition in BRAF-mutated melanoma. N Engl J Med 367(2):107–114
29. Guo J et al (2011) Phase II, open-label, single-arm trial of imatinib mesylate in patients with metastatic melanoma harboring c-Kit mutation or amplification. J Clin Oncol 29(21): 2904–2909
30. Samuels Y, Waldman T (2010) Oncogenic mutations of PIK3CA in human cancers. Curr Top Microbiol Immunol 347:21–41

31. Turke AB, Engelman JA (2010) PIKing the right patient. Clin Cancer Res 16(14):3523–3525
32. Dutton-Regester K et al (2012) A high-throughput panel for identifying clinically relevant mutation profiles in melanoma. Mol Cancer Ther 11(4):888–897
33. Wagle N et al (2011) Dissecting therapeutic resistance to RAF inhibition in melanoma by tumor genomic profiling. J Clin Oncol 29(22): 3085–3096
34. Molina-Vila MA et al (2009) Screening for EGFR mutations in lung cancer. Discov Med 8(43):181–184
35. Rudloff U, Samuels Y (2010) A growing family: adding mutated Erbb4 as a novel cancer target. Cell Cycle 9(8):1487–1503
36. Garrett TP et al (2002) Crystal structure of a truncated epidermal growth factor receptor extracellular domain bound to transforming growth factor alpha. Cell 110(6): 763–773
37. Ogiso H et al (2002) Crystal structure of the complex of human epidermal growth factor and receptor extracellular domains. Cell 110(6): 775–787

Chapter 25

Epigenetic Markers of Prognosis in Melanoma

Luca Sigalotti, Elisabetta Fratta, Giulia Parisi, Sandra Coral, and Michele Maio

Abstract

Prognostic molecular markers are urgently needed for allowing to discriminate the clinical course of disease of melanoma patients, which is highly heterogeneous and unpredictable also within a specific clinicopathological stage and substage of disease. Alterations in DNA methylation have been reported to be widely present in cutaneous melanoma, profoundly impacting its biology. In line with this notion, we have identified methylation markers as independent prognostic factors in stage IIIC melanoma patients. In this chapter we describe the measurement of the methylation of the *Long Interspersed Nucleotide Element-1* sequences in laser capture microdissected tumor tissues as a prognostic tool in stage III melanoma patients, which could help in achieving a more appropriate and patient-tailored clinical management of cutaneous melanoma.

Key words DNA methylation, Epigenetic, *Long Interspersed Nucleotide Element-1*, Repetitive elements, Methylation profiles, Prognosis

1 Introduction

The only currently established method to define prognosis of cutaneous melanoma (CM) patients remains the clinicopathological staging of the disease [1]. However, it is well known that the same clinicopathological staging category includes patients that may develop a quite different course of the disease, going from patients with a rather indolent and slowly evolving disease to those with a highly aggressive and rapidly progressing tumor. This important intra-stage heterogeneity in the clinical behavior of CM greatly hampers the possibility to provide the single patient with the most adequate clinical management, possibly leading to both under- or over-treatments. In this disappointing scenario, it is clearly of paramount importance to define reliable, well-characterized, and stable molecular markers that can allow the clinicians to finely dissect and predict the outcome of CM patients. The recent availability of high-throughput approaches has offered the possibility to instantly interrogate the whole genome of

Magdalena Thurin and Francesco M. Marincola (eds.), *Molecular Diagnostics for Melanoma: Methods and Protocols*, Methods in Molecular Biology, vol. 1102, DOI 10.1007/978-1-62703-727-3_25, © Springer Science+Business Media New York 2014

cancer cells, representing, in principle, terrific tools for the discovery of molecular indicators of prognosis as well as of response to therapy. Along this line, different prognostic molecular signatures have been identified through mRNA or microRNA profiling [2]. Unfortunately, a limited overlap between signatures published by different studies can be observed, possibly due to different causes, including tissue heterogeneity, different stages of disease examined, heterogeneous settings, noncanonical follow-up, and possibly individual variability in the transcriptomes of normal melanocytes [2]. This lack of overlap among published mRNA/miRNA signatures has impaired their transfer in the clinical practice to effectively improve the management of CM patients. Besides the promises offered by gene expression and miRNA profiling, the increasing awareness of the key role that epigenetic alterations have on the biology of CM cells is strongly supporting the potential utility of epigenetic determinants as candidates for identifying markers of prognosis and response to therapy in this malignancy. In particular, some characteristics of epigenetic markers render them particularly attractive for the final development of clinically applicable biomarkers, including (a) high stability in biologic samples, including FFPE tumor specimens; (b) limited susceptibility to tumor environmental factors; and (c) detectability in easily accessible body fluids (e.g., serum, plasma, sputum, urine) [3].

1.1 Epigenetics

"Epigenetics" refers to mitotically and meiotically heritable changes in gene expression that do not derive from alterations of the nucleotide sequence of DNA [4]. Epigenetic alterations are emerging as alternatives to mutations and chromosomal alterations in modifying gene expression and, as such, are being discovered to play a major role in the development of a variety of tumors [5]. The mediators of epigenetic inheritance include variations in the organization of chromatin, histone posttranslational modifications, and DNA methylation, the latter being the most widely studied epigenetic alteration in cancer, also thanks to the availability of simple and highly sensitive and specific measuring technologies [6].

In mammalian species, methylation is carried out by different DNA methyltransferase enzymes, which transfer a methyl group from *S*-adenosyl-methionine to the C5 position of the pyrimidine ring of cytosine residues within cytosine-guanine dinucleotides (CpG) [7]. The effect of DNA methylation is to act in cis by silencing the affected gene [8]. Various physiologic functions have been identified or proposed for DNA methylation, including (a) determination of the expression pattern of germline-specific genes; (b) establishment of genomic imprinting; (c) maintenance of balanced expression of X chromosome genes in females; (d) silencing of tissue-specific genes in cellular histotypes in which they should not be expressed; (e) maintenance of proper structure and integrity of chromosomes; and (f) provision of a defense system against mobile genetic elements like transposons [5, 9–11].

1.2 Melanoma Epigenetics

Aberrant DNA methylation was the first epigenetic mark to be associated with human cancer nearly 30 years ago [12]. Since that time, a number of cancer-related alterations in DNA methylation have been described, including genome-wide DNA hypomethylation and hypermethylation of tumor-suppressor genes (TSGs).

Aberrant DNA hypermethylation occurs in normally unmethylated promoters of many TSGs [13], resulting in the silencing of their expression. This mechanism of gene inactivation appears to be as efficient as gene mutation or deletion and results in the loss of essential tumor suppressor functions that are required for the tumorigenic process [14, 15]. So far, aberrant DNA hypermethylation in CM has been shown to result in the transcriptional silencing of at least 70 genes that are involved in essentially every known cancer-related pathway, such as cell cycle regulation, DNA repair, drug resistance, detoxification, apoptosis, tumor cell invasion, metastasis, angiogenesis, and immune recognition (for review *see* ref. 16). The most frequent and best characterized hypermethylated genes in CM are CDKN2A, RASSF1A, RAR-β2, and MGMT. CDKN2A encodes two overlapping proteins, p16INK4a and p14ARF, that act as tumor suppressors by negatively regulating cell cycle progression through the pRB and the p53 pathways, respectively [17]. Hypermethylation at CDKN2A locus could possibly contribute to the uncontrolled cell cycle progression of neoplastic cells by independently affecting both p16INK4a and p14ARF, which were found methylated in 27 and 57 % of metastatic CM samples, respectively [18]. RASSF1A is a Ras effector that interacts with Ras GTPases controlling several cellular events, including regulation of apoptosis, cellular growth, and microtubule dynamics during mitotic division. RASSF1A methylation is rare in stage I and II CM, still being detected in almost 50 % of stage IV CM, thus suggesting its inactivation to play a role in CM progression [19]. Aberrant methylation of the RAR-β2 gene is found in 70 % of CM lesions, leading to insensitivity to growth arrest, differentiation, and apoptotic signals triggered by retinoic acids [20]. Interestingly, the frequency of RAR-β2 promoter hypermethylation seems to be similar in primary as well as metastatic CM, thus indicating that RAR-β2 silencing might have a role in initial phases of melanocyte transformation [20]. MGMT gene hypermethylation, detected in 34 % of CM, associates with an impaired DNA repair capability of neoplastic cells [21] and in particular of alkyl-DNA adducts. Loss of MGMT activity may be advantageous in the tumorigenic process by providing neoplastic cells with increased mutation rates [21]. However, MGMT is also required for repairing alkyl-DNA adducts that are caused by, and mediate the efficacy of, alkylating chemotherapeutics. Accordingly, loss of MGMT expression by promoter methylation could be expected to sensitize neoplastic cells to alkylating drug-induced cell death as seen in glioma [21].

Besides gene-specific hypermethylation, genome-wide hypomethylation might contribute to tumorigenesis and cancer progression by promoting genomic instability, reactivating endogenous parasitic sequences, and inducing the expression of oncogenes. A large number of studies demonstrated that hypomethylation takes place predominantly in DNA repetitive elements of the genome [22, 23]. In this respect, the *Long Interspersed Nucleotide Element-1* (*LINE-1*) repetitive elements are the most well-documented repetitive elements displaying hypomethylation in various cancers. Consistently, Tellez et al. demonstrated that *LINE-1* methylation levels in CM cell lines were markedly reduced (mean = 36 %) as compared to normal human melanocytes (mean = 65 %). One additional outcome of overall genomic DNA hypomethylation in CM is the induction of the de novo expression of the cancer–testis antigens (CTA), immunogenic tumor-associated antigens. The biological significance of this gene re-expression for cancer cells continues to be poorly understood, but this phenomenon and the ability of CTA to generate both cellular and humoral immune responses in vivo identify them as ideal targets of immunotherapy for CM patients [24].

1.3 Emerging Potential Prognostic Methylation Markers in Melanoma

On the grounds of the above reported information, highlighting a key role of aberrant DNA methylation in molding CM biology, a growing number of studies have sought to evaluate the potential prognostic and predictive role of methylation markers in CM [16]. Different preliminary studies have reported the methylation of single genes/loci to have a potential in predicting survival or response to therapy in CM, although most of them have been conducted on cohorts of patients with heterogeneous stages of disease. Along this line, Lahtz and colleagues have recently reported that the methylation of the PI3K–AKT–mTOR pathway inhibitor *PTEN* represented an independent negative prognostic factor for overall survival (OS) in a cohort of 230 stage 0 to IV CM patients (multivariate Cox odds ratio = 1.75, $P = 0.014$) [25]. This observation might suggest an important role of aberrant epigenetic activation of the PI3K–AKT–mTOR pathway in the final outcome of the disease. As far as the prognostic clinical utility of PTEN methylation is concerned, the finding that it did not prove superior to the well-established prognostic markers of tumor thickness and ulceration [25] likely reduces its potential clinical impact as a single factor. Another example of prognostic methylation marker in CM is represented by the putative TSG TSLC1, which is thought to be involved in cell–cell contact and regulation of cell adhesion and motility. *TSLC1* methylation was significantly increased with advancing stages in 120 stage I to IV CM patients, being as well associated with a significantly poorer disease-related survival ($P = 0.03$, log-rank test) [26]. In contrast to the above-summarized associations between increased gene methylation and worse prognosis, the methylation of the "methylated in tumors" (*MINT*) locus *31* was recently shown to predict an improved disease-free survival and OS in the 25 stage III CM patients analyzed ($P = 0.047$ and $P = 0.013$, respectively). Since no established gene product is currently known for *MINT31*, the underlying biological cause of this association is still unknown [19].

Besides prognosis, initial studies have started to evaluate the predictive potential of aberrant methylation in CM. Until the most recent introduction of highly effective immunotherapeutic and targeted therapy approaches, the standard treatment for advanced CM has long relied on the use of alkylating agents such as dacarbazine and temozolomide. Accordingly, most of the predictive studies were focused on MGMT, which is involved in the repair/detoxification of the alkyl-DNA adducts caused by this class of drugs. Despite downregulation of MGMT by DNA methylation was convincingly shown to predict response to alkylating agents in glioma patients [21], results so far obtained on CM are contradictory. Indeed, though *MGMT* methylation significantly associated with increased response rates to combined treatment with temozolomide plus bevacizumab [27], most of the studies failed to demonstrate an association between *MGMT* methylation and response to alkylating drugs in CM [28, 29]. These disappointing results could be possibly linked to the overall low response rates of alkylating agents in CM and leave much room for improvement in identifying predictive methylation markers, especially those that would predict response to the most recent highly promising immunotherapeutic and targeted therapeutic agents (e.g., anti-CTLA-4, anti-PD1, anti-PDL1 immunostimulatory monoclonal antibodies, and small-molecule inhibitors of the RAF/MEK pathway). In this setting an important advantage of methylation markers in terms of potential clinical transferability could also come from their detectability in easily accessible body fluids. Indeed, the pioneering work by the group of Hoon identified circulating methylated *ER-α* and *RASSF1A* DNA as predictive markers of poor progression-free survival and OS in 50 stage IV CM patients treated with a biochemotherapy regimen of dacarbazine or temozolomide, cisplatin, vinblastine, interferon α-2b, interleukin-2, and tamoxifen [30, 31].

Overall, the above reported data are encouraging and strongly supportive of an important role of methylation markers in addressing prognosis and/or response to therapy in CM. However, most of these studies have several limitations that have impaired their immediate clinical usefulness and thus their swift transfer into the clinical environment. Among these are (a) the analysis of cohorts of patients including extremely heterogeneous stages of disease; (b) the investigation of only single or few genes; and (c) the a priori selection of the genes to be analyzed, usually based on data already available on other tumor types or focusing on the few genes that could be directly involved in pathways altered in CM. In particular, the different prognosis of patients according to their staging is well established, and studying cohorts of patients including different stages of disease dramatically hampers the possibility to answer the real current question: How can we discriminate prognosis/response to therapy in patients within the same stage or substage of disease? On the other hand, restricting the analysis to few selected genes may very likely overlook the impact of coordinate epigenetic alteration(s) on the biology and outcome of CM.

To address these issues, we have recently undertaken two separate but complementary approaches, both of which investigated the prognostic role of whole-genome DNA methylation in a clinicopathologically highly homogeneous cohort of substage IIIC CM patients. Specifically, we evaluated the prognostic value of (a) whole-genome DNA methylation profiles obtained by the Illumina Humanmethylation27 chip, which quantitatively interrogates the methylation of over 14,000 genomic loci [32], and (b) the methylation of the *LINE-1* repetitive sequences, used as a surrogate marker of the overall genomic DNA methylation content [33]. The studies took advantage of the availability of autologous short-term cultures of neoplastic cells from CM patients, which allowed us to define CM-specific methylation features, without the confounding interference of normal cells that are invariantly present at different extents in non-dissected tumor tissues.

1.4 Whole-Genome Methylation Profile as Promising Prognostic Marker in Melanoma

As far as Humanmethylation27 analysis is concerned, unsupervised K-means partitioning clustering allowed us to sort CM patients into two groups, based on the methylation profile of their neoplastic cells. These groups differed significantly for their global genomic methylation profile and were thus named low methylation (LM) and high methylation (HM). Interestingly enough, Kaplan–Meier analysis demonstrated an increased OS for LM as compared to HM patients ($P = 0.001$, log-rank = 10.2), with median OS of 31.5 and 10.4 months, respectively. Accordingly, the 5-year OS for LM-stage IIIC patients was 41.2 % as compared to 0 % for HM patients, and multivariate Cox regression analysis demonstrated that classification by methylation profile was the only predictor of OS (hazard ratio = 2.41, for HM; 95 % confidence interval: 1.02–5.70; $P = 0.045$) in the cohort of patients examined. In order to foster the application of these findings to the clinical routine, we simplified the whole-genome methylation profiles associated to the discovered prognostic classes by applying the nearest shrunken centroid classification algorithm. This approach led to the identification of a 17-gene methylation profile (methylation signature) that correctly assigned prognosis (overall error rate = 0) of stage IIIC patients and the size of which is reduced enough to be potentially utilizable in the routine clinical ascertainment of prognosis of CM patients [32].

1.5 Overall Genomic Methylation by LINE-1 Elements as Promising Prognostic Marker in Melanoma

Besides the above-reported detailed information offered by array methylation profiling, we asked whether a much simpler evaluation of genome-wide DNA methylation could still provide a highly effective factor able to predict survival of CM patients. Along this line, we focused on the *LINE-1* repetitive elements, which are a family of non-long terminal repeat retrotransposons that are the only autonomous transposable elements left in the human genome. The full-length *LINE-1* elements is about 6 kb long, though most of the genomic copies are not complete and working. Indeed, of more than 500,000 *LINE-1* copies present in the genome, only less than 100 are functional [34]. Irrespective of their functionality, and their possible influence on cell biology, their high copy number makes them account for about 17 % of the human genome [34], identifying them as attractive surrogates for the definition of the overall genomic DNA methylation content. Starting from these considerations, we measured *LINE-1* methylation in neoplastic cells from stage IIIC CM patients in the attempt to define whether it may provide a prognostic tool. To allow quantitative methylation measurements, genomic DNA was modified with sodium bisulfite which converts unmethylated, but not methylated, cytosines into uracil, allowing the methylation data to be read as primary DNA sequence differences. Indeed, following PCR and sequencing of bisulfite-modified DNA, methylated cytosines are read as cytosines, while unmethylated cytosines are read as thymines [35]. The evaluation of *LINE-1* methylation was then carried out at three CpG dinucleotides (CpG1, CpG2, and CpG3) on bisuilfite-modified genomic DNA by the quantitative sequencing approach termed pyrosequencing [35]. Interestingly, *LINE-1* elements were found to be homogeneously hypermethylated in normal cells (e.g., non-transformed melanocytes and peripheral blood mononuclear cells), while lower and heterogeneous levels of methylation characterized the short-term cultures of neoplastic cells from stage IIIC patients, offering the possibility to separate CM patients according to their tumor-specific *LINE-1* methylation. Association of *LINE-1* methylation status and OS of patients generated results that were highly concordant to those obtained by array-based whole-genome methylation profiling, strengthening the observation that patients with hypermethylated tumors have a worse prognosis. Indeed, Kaplan–Meier analyses demonstrated that *LINE-1* methylation of neoplastic cells above the median of the population (hypermethylation) significantly associated with a reduced OS in stage IIIC patients, with the strongest impact seen for CpG3 ($P=0.01$). Accordingly, patients with hypermethylated *LINE-1* had a worse median (11.5 months) and 5-year OS (7 %) as compared to *LINE-1* hypomethylated patients (31.9 months and 48 %, respectively). As seen for array-based methylation profiling, among all the variables examined by Cox regression analysis, *LINE-1* methylation was the only predictor of OS (hazard ratio = 2.63, for hypermethylated CpG3; 95 % confidence interval: 1.21–5.69; $P = 0.01$). Similar results were obtained when *LINE-1* methylation was measured by quantitative methylation-specific PCR (qMSP), which further improves the sensitivity of the analysis and was thus selected as the methodology of choice for the standard measurement of *LINE-1* methylation in any subsequent study.

The validation of the data obtained on autologous tumor tissues highlighted the need of performing the analysis on a highly purified population of neoplastic cells. Indeed, the variable presence of normal cells in the undissected tumor tissue may dramatically alter the CM-specific measurement of *LINE-1* methylation, leading to discordant values from those of short-term CM cell cultures. Accordingly, evaluation of methylation marks needs to be performed on surgical specimens that are constituted solely by neoplastic cells or on neoplastic cells purified from the surgical sample by either laser capture microdissection (LCM) or immunosorting.

In light of the information above, reporting a highly concordant prognostic value of *LINE-1* and whole-genome methylation profiling, the evaluation of *LINE-1* methylation currently appears more suited for a further evaluation and a swift translation into the clinical practice as prognostic molecular marker for CM patients. This is the result of both a simpler and more cost-effective technique as well as of the multi-copy nature of *LINE-1* elements, which dramatically improves sensitivity of detection making it particularly well suited for minimal amounts of neoplastic material as those obtained with LCM. Accordingly, the methodological section of the chapter specifically focuses on tumor-specific measurement of *LINE-1* methylation on LCM tumor cells by qMSP assays.

2 Materials

2.1 Isolation of CM Cells from Formalin-Fixed, Paraffin-Embedded Tissues (*See* Note 1)

1. Specimens for DNA analysis: Hematoxylin and eosin (H&E) (*see* **Note 2**)-stained sections on glass microscope slides obtained from formalin-fixed, paraffin-embedded (FFPE) tissues cut at 5 μm.
2. Automated LCM Instrument (ArcturusXT™ Microdissection System platform, Life Technologies).
3. LCM caps (Life Technologies).
4. Sterile Standard Pattern Forceps (Fine Science Tools).
5. Microcentrifuge tubes (0.2 ml) (Life Technologies).

2.2 Genomic DNA Extraction

1. QIAamp DNA Micro Kit for extraction of genomic DNA from LCM tissues (Qiagen).
2. Microcentrifuge tubes (1.5 ml) (Life Technologies).

3. Pipettes (2–20, 20–200, 100–1,000 μl) and plastic pipette tips (Rainin).
4. 96–100 % Ethanol.
5. Microcentrifuge (Eppendorf), thermal cycler (Veriti, Life Technologies), heating block (Stuart Scientific), or water bath (HAAKE).

2.3 Bisulfite Modification of Extracted DNA

1. EZ DNA Methylation-Gold Kit for complete bisulfite conversion of GC-rich DNA (Zymo Research).
2. Vortexer (Heidolph), thermal cycler (Veriti, Life Technologies).
3. Microcentrifuge tubes (0.2 ml), microcentrifuge tubes (1.5 ml), pipettes (2–20, 20–200, 100–1,000 μl), and plastic pipette tips (Rainin).
4. 96–100 % Ethanol.

2.4 Generation of LINE-1-Methylated and -Unmethylated Standards

1. EpiTect PCR Control DNA Set containing bisulfite converted methylated and unmethylated human control DNA (Qiagen).
2. Microcentrifuge tubes (0.2 ml) (Life Technologies), pipettes, and pipette tips (Rainin).
3. Thermal cycler (Veriti, Life Technologies).
4. Methylation-specific PCR (MSP) reagents: 10× PCR buffer (100 mM Tris–HCl pH 8.3, 500 mM KCl), 10 mM dNTP Mix and 50 mM $MgCl_2$ (Takara), 5 U/μl Platinum Taq DNA polymerase (Life Technologies).
5. MSP primers for *LINE-1*: Forward methylated primer (*LINE-1* M F) 5′-CGCGAGTCGAAGTAGGGC-3′, reverse methylated primer (*LINE-1* M R) 5′-ACCCGATTTTCCAAATACGACCG-3′, forward unmethylated primer (*LINE-1* U F) 5′-TGTGTGTGAGTTGAAGTAGGGT-3′, reverse unmethylated primer (*LINE-1* U R) 5′-ACCCAATTTTCCAAATACAACCATCA-3′ [35]. Primers are initially resuspended at a concentration of 100 pmol/μl in ultrapure water and then diluted at a concentration of 7.5 pmol/μl.
6. Electrophoresis reagents: Agarose (Lonza), ethidium bromide (Sigma), 6× loading buffer (30 % glycerol, 0.25 % Orange G), 100 bp ladder marker (Life Technologies).
7. Electrophoresis apparatus (Bio-rad).
8. UV transilluminator.
9. TOPO TA Cloning kit (Life Technologies).
10. Water bath, shaking and non-shaking incubator, ice bucket with ice.

11. LB medium and agar plates (for preparation refer to TOPO TA Cloning user manual).
12. Spreaders and tubes (5 ml) (International Pbi).
13. NucleoSpin Plasmid kit for purification of plasmid DNA (Macherey Nagel).
14. 96–100 % Ethanol.
15. Microcentrifuge (Eppendorf).
16. Spectrophotometer (Nanodrop, Thermo Scientific).
17. Sequencing reagents: ABI PRISM BigDye Terminator v3.1 Cycle Sequencing Kit, Hi-DiTM Formamide, and 5× Sequencing Buffer (Life Technologies).
18. Automated Sequencer for sequencing of the obtained construct (ABI PRISM 3100 Genetic Analyze, Life Technologies) (*see* **Note 3**).

2.5 Quantitative Methylation-Specific PCR Analysis of LINE-1

1. Microcentrifuge tubes (0.2 and 1.5 ml), pipettes (2–20, 20–200, 100–1,000 μl), and plastic pipette tips (Rainin).
2. Optical 96-well microtiter plates (Life Technologies).
3. Optical adhesive films (Life Technologies).
4. SYBR Green dye 2× mix (Life Technologies).
5. Real-time PCR instrument (ABI prism 7000 Sequence Detection System, Life Technologies).
6. LINE-1 primers for qMSP: *See* above (Subheading 2.4, **item 5**).
7. Buffer for standard curve preparation: 1 mM Tris–HCl, pH 8.3, 10 ng/μl Hind III digested Lambda DNA (Sigma).

3 Methods

3.1 Isolation of CM Cells from FFPE Tissues (*See* Note 4)

1. Isolate CM cells from H&E-stained FFPE tissue sections with an automated LCM apparatus using the infrared laser. Follow the procedures indicated in the instrument specifications (for a method *see* ref. 36).
2. Remove the optical-quality plastic support cap from the instrument.
3. At the bottom surface of the cap, locate the thermolabile polymer on which the CM cells have been captured, and gently peel it off from the edge using sterile nucleic acid-free forceps (*see* Fig. 1). Pay particular attention on not getting in contact with the captured neoplastic cells. Place the polymer on the bottom of a 0.2 ml microcentrifuge tube. The sample is ready for extraction of genomic DNA.

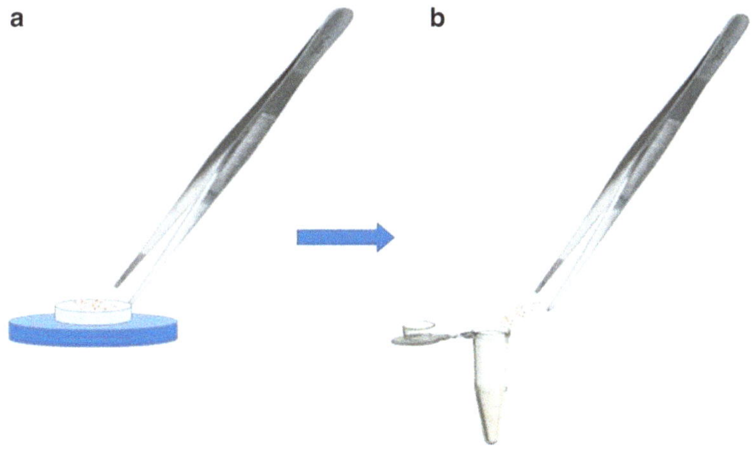

Fig. 1 Processing of laser capture microdissection caps for extraction of DNA. (**a**) After removing the plastic support cap from laser capture microdissection apparatus, peel off very carefully the polymer cell composite on the bottom surface of the cap with sterile standard pattern forceps. (**b**) Transfer gently the thermolabile polymer with adhering CM target cells on a 0.2 ml microcentrifuge tube, and proceed for DNA extraction

3.2 Extraction of Genomic DNA from LCM Tissues (See Note 5*)*

Genomic DNA is extracted from the LCM tissues obtained in Subheading 3.1 using the QIAamp DNA Micro Kit, following the manufacturer's protocol. Points to be considered in respect to the kit handbook are as follows:

1. Make sure that the polymer carrying the CM cells is fully submerged in the liquid phase after adding the 15 μl of buffer ATL and the 10 μl of proteinase K, as per the manufacturer's protocol.
2. Dissolve carrier RNA in buffer AE, according to the protocol instructions, and mix with buffer AL.
3. Since LCM has been performed on FFPE tissues, incubate the sample at 56 °C for 16 h in a thermal cycler with heated lid set to ≥65 °C.
4. Elute the purified DNA by applying 20 μl buffer AE to the center of the column.

3.3 Bisulfite Conversion of Genomic DNA

Genomic DNA from Subheading 3.2 is subjected to modification with sodium bisulfite using the EZ DNA Methylation-Gold Kit, according to the manufacturer's instructions. Below are recommendations to optimize the protocol:

1. After the addition of 200 μl of M desulfonation buffer to the column, incubate the sample at room temperature for 20 min.
2. Elute the bisulfite-converted DNA by adding 20 μl of M elution buffer to the column matrix.

Table 1
MSP mix setup

	Volume[a]	
Reagents	***MIX M***	***MIX U***
PCR buffer 10×	5.0 μl	5.0 μl
MgCl2 50 mM	3.0 μl	3.0 μl
dNTPs 10 mM	4.0 μl	4.0 μl
LINE-1 M F primer (7.5 pmol/μl)	1.0 μl	
LINE-1 M R primer (7.5 pmol/μl)	1.0 μl	
LINE-1 U F primer (7.5 pmol/μl)		1.0 μl
LINE-1 U F primer (7.5 pmol/μl)		1.0 μl
Platinum Taq DNA polymerase (5 U/μl)	0.25 μl	0.25 μl
ddH_2O	to 48 μl	to 48 μl

[a]Volumes are given for a single sample; in case of multiple samples, multiply each value for the total number of samples and add an extra 10 % volume for accounting losses during multiple pipetting

3.4 Preparation of LINE-1-Methylated and -Unmethylated Standards

1. Amplify *LINE-1*-methylated sequence (*LINE-1* M) and *LINE-1-unmethylated* sequence (*LINE-1* U) in two separate 0.2 ml microcentrifuge tubes, using as starting material 2 μl (20 ng) bisulfite-converted methylated human control DNA in tube 1 and 2 μl (20 ng) bisulfite-converted unmethylated human control DNA in tube 2. Set up *MIX M* and *MIX U* according to Table 1, and add 48 μl of *MIX M* in tube # 1 and 48 μl of *MIX U* in tube # 2. PCR amplification program consists of an initial denaturation step of 5 min at 95 °C, followed by 45 cycles of 15 s at 95 °C and 1 min at 60 °C.
2. Check the MSP products on 2 % agarose gel. If the PCR products migrate at the expected size (150 bp for both LINE-1 methylated and unmethylated) and no nonspecific bands or primer dimers are observed (*see* **Note 6**), proceed directly to **step 3**.
3. Clone the two MSP products (LINE-1 M and LINE-1 U standards) into plasmid vector pCR 2.1-TOPO, using the TOPO TA Cloning kit, following the manufacturer's instructions (*see* **Note 7**).
4. Isolate ten independent colonies for each transformation, separately inoculate each colony into 3 ml LB broth, and grow the cultures on constant agitation overnight at 37 °C.
5. Extract plasmid DNA from each culture using the NucleoSpin Plasmid kit.

6. Verify the sequence of the cloned PCR fragments by cycle sequencing the plasmids obtained in **step 5** above, using M13 forward primer and the ABI PRISM BigDye Terminator v3.1 Cycle Sequencing Kit. Reference methylated and unmethylated LINE-1 sequences are provided in Fig. 2. Plasmids containing verified LINE-1 U and M inserts are used as standards.
7. Quantify the concentration of the standards at Nanodrop Spectrophotometer. The number of molecules/μl is determined by applying the formula

   No. of molecules/μl = (STANDARD concentration (ng/μl)/(vector length + insert length) × 660) × N_A

   where vector length = 3,900 bp, insert length of LINE-1 M or LINE-1 U = 150 bp, 660 = base pair MW, and N_A = number of Avogadro (6.022×10^{23}).
8. Prepare serial dilutions 1:10 (from 5×10^4 to 5 molecules/μl) of standard curve for methylated and unmethylated target LINE-1 regions, using buffer for standard curve preparation (*see* **Notes 8** and **9**).

3.5 qMSP Analysis for the Methylation Levels of LINE-1 (See Note 10)

The qMSP technique is used for sensitive quantification of the methylation status of the sequence of interest. The technique relies on bisulfite treatment of genomic DNA, which results in the modification of the primary nucleotide sequence of the DNA according to the methylation status of cytosines. Indeed, bisulfite leads to the conversion of unmethylated cytosines to uracil, leaving unaltered methylated ones. This methylation-specific modification of the target DNA sequence is exploited to design two different primer pairs, one for the methylated and the other for the unmethylated sequence (Fig. 2). To increase the specificity of the amplification, primers are usually designed to have their 3′ end annealing to the potentially methylated CpG dinucleotides. Quantitative PCR reactions are run in parallel with the primers for methylated and for the unmethylated sequence, enabling to define the percentage of methylation of the target region (Fig. 2).

In addition to the test samples, each run must include methylated and unmethylated human control DNA (1 ng/μl dilution of EpiTect PCR Control DNA Set), a water blank, and the appropriate standards (5×10^4 to 5 molecules/μl of methylated or unmethylated plasmids, *see* Subheading 3.4 above). All samples, controls, and standards should be run in triplicates.

For *n* number of samples to be tested, follow Table 2 to prepare two separate qMSP master mixes in 1.5 ml tubes: *q MIX M*, for *LINE-1* methylated, and *q MIX U*, for unmethylated. Mix well by vortexing.

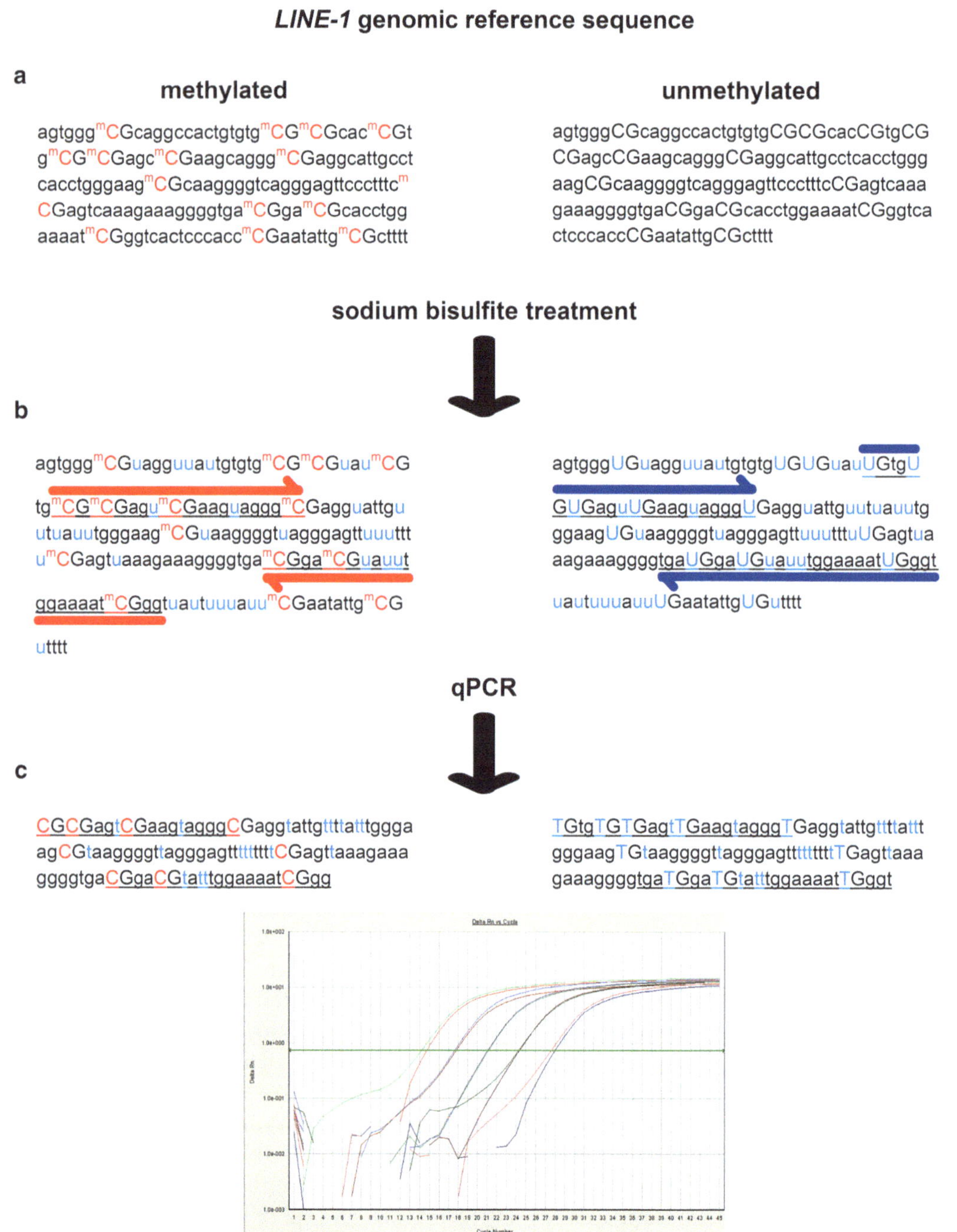

$$\% \ LINE\text{-}1 \text{ methylation} = \frac{\#\text{ of molecules from methylated } LINE\text{-}1 \text{ qPCR}}{\text{sum of } \#\text{ of molecules from methylated and unmethylated } LINE\text{-}1 \text{ qPCR}} \times 100$$

Fig. 2 Quantitative methylation-specific PCR for *LINE-1* sequences. (**a**) DNA methylation in mammalian genomes can be found only at cytosines (C) in the context of CpG dinucleotides. Reference *LINE-1* genomic DNA containing methylated (^{m}C, *left side*) or unmethylated (C, *right side*) are reported. (**b**) Sodium bisulfite

Table 2
qMSP mix setup

Reagents	Triplicate amount volume[a]	
	q MIX M	*q MIX U*
SYBR Green Mix 2×	37.5 μl	37.5 μl
LINE-1 M F primer (7.5 pmol/μl)	3.0 μl	
LINE-1 M R primer (7.5 pmol/μl)	3.0 μl	
LINE-1 U F primer (7.5 pmol/μl)		3.0 μl
LINE-1 U R primer (7.5 pmol/μl)		3.0 μl
ddH_2O	To 69 μl	To 69 μl

[a]Volumes are given for a single sample; in case of multiple samples, multiply each value for the total number of samples and add an extra 10 % volume for accounting losses during multiple pipetting

1. Prepare the final mix for each triplicate sample by transferring 69 μl of q MIX M to 0.2 ml tubes and by adding into each tube 6 μl of the appropriate test sample DNA or standard/control. Do the same for q MIX U. Mix well by vortexing.
2. Pipette 20 μl of the final mixes into each well of a 96-well microplate, and seal the plate with an optical-grade sealing tape.
3. Briefly centrifuge the plates to remove any drops and air bubbles.
4. Run the qMSP using the following program: 95 °C for 10 min, followed by 45 cycles of 15 s at 95 °C and 1 min at 60 °C. Set the fluorescence detection at the final step of each cycle repeat.
5. The threshold for determining the threshold cycle for each well must be set in the logarithmic phase of the amplification plot.
6. Establish the copy number of LINE-1-methylated or -unmethylated sequences in each sample by extrapolation of the respective standard curves. This is usually done automatically by the software when the run is set to absolute quantification using standard curves.

Fig. 2 (continued) treatment is carried out on genomic DNA to translate methylation data into primary sequence information: unmethylated cytosines are converted to uracil (U), while methylated cytosines remain unmodified. This methylation-specific sequence difference is exploited to design primers that specifically anneal to and amplify methylated (*LINE-1* M F and M R primers, *red arrows* on the *left side*) and unmethylated (*LINE-1* U F and U R primers, *blue arrows* on the *right side*) *LINE-1* sequences. (**c**) Absolute quantitative PCR is carried out in parallel using primers specific for the methylated or the unmethylated *LINE-1* sequences. The number of *LINE-1*-methylated or -unmethylated molecules in each test sample is obtained through extrapolation from the standard curves. Percent of *LINE-1* methylation is obtained as the number of methylated *LINE-1* molecules divided by the sum of the number of methylated and unmethyated *LINE-1* molecules × 100

7. Calculate the percentage of LINE-1 methylation as the ratio between methylated molecules and the sum of methylated and unmethylated molecules $(M/(M+U)) \times 100$.
8. CM cells are scored as hypomethylated or hypermethylated according to their LINE-1 methylation being < or ≥ the reference value. In our cohort of patients, this value has been selected as the median LINE-1 methylation of the analyzed population (i.e., 51.99 %). However, the specific value is amenable to further refinement based on the analysis of wider cohorts of stage III CM patients in order to identify the cutoff that could better separate good vs. bad prognosis patients.

4 Notes

1. In alternative to FFPE tissues, isolation of CM cells can be performed from frozen tissue sections using LCM, after correct sample preparation and staining (for a detailed procedure *see* ref. 36).
2. Besides H&E, LCM-compatible stainings are Wright-Giemsa, methylene blue, toluidine blue, and hematoxylin only.
3. Reagents are not required if plasmid DNA is sent to a sequencing facility.
4. If fresh tumor tissue from surgical lymph nodal resection is available, an alternative method for purifying CM cells can be recommended. After evaluating the presence of high-molecular-weight-melanoma-associated antigen (HMW-MAA)-positive cells in the metastatic lesion, through flow cytometry using an anti-HMW-MAA antibody (e.g., Anti-Melanoma MCSP-PE, Miltenyi Biotec), the protocol "Melanoma cell enrichment and detection kit-human" (Miltenyi Biotec) should be followed with minor changes. We recommend the following: (a) Perform the enzymatic digestion in 500 μl IMDM supplemented with 200 U/ml DNase I (molecular biology grade, e.g., Roche), without adding collagenase. Indeed collagenase cuts HMW-MAA molecule preventing the binding of anti-HMW-MAA antibody. (b) Push cells through a mesh screen (40 μm) on a 50 ml conical tube. Centrifuge cells at 300 × *g* and continue with the standard protocol, or store cell suspension in a mixed solution of 50 % FCS, 40 % RPMI, and 10 % DMSO at −80 °C for separation at a later time. (c) After the magnetic separation, wash the fraction of enriched CM cells for DNA analyses with 5–10 ml of saline solution. Count cells, centrifuge at 300 × *g* for 5′, resuspend cell pellet in 1 ml of saline solution, and put cell suspension in a 1.5 ml microcentrifuge tube. Centrifuge cells at 300 × *g* for 5′, discard supernatant, and freeze the pellet at −80 °C.

5. Alternatively, genomic DNA can be isolated from the frozen pellet of enriched CM cells (*see* **Note 4** above) by using QIAamp DNA Blood Mini Kit (Qiagen), following the manufacturer's instructions.
6. In case of presence of aspecific bands in the agarose gel, we recommend to gel purify the band containing the *LINE-1* M or U amplicon (e.g., Zymoclean Gel DNA Recovery Kit, Zymo Research).
7. For transformation of cloning reactions we use One Shot TOP10 Chemically Competent cells.
8. The presence of carrier λ DNA in buffer for standard curve preparation could help reducing loss of DNA in the very diluted solutions of *LINE-1* M and U standards.
9. Use at least 5 μl of plasmids containing verified *LINE-1* U and M inserts for performing the first dilution. Perform the subsequent serial dilutions diluting 50 μl standard in 450 μl buffer to reduce the impact on dilutions of pipetting errors. Dilution curves of methylated and unmethylated *LINE-1* standard are stored at −80 °C in single-use aliquots to ensure their preservation.
10. The plasmid pCR2.1-TOPO (empty vector, Life Technologies) should be used as an external reference to normalize the measurement of both *LINE-1* M and *LINE-1* U standard curves, prior to test the tumor samples. Briefly, after cloning and sequencing the *LINE-1* U and M standards, a qMSP analysis is performed with serial dilutions 1:10 (from 10^5 to 10^1 molecules) of pCR2.1-TOPO, used as standard curve of the assay, and of *LINE-1* M and *LINE-1* U, considered as samples, to assess their correct quantification, using primers pCR 2.1 1329 F 5′-AAGATGGATTGCACGCAGGT-3′ and pCR2.1 1409R 5′-AGCCGATTGTCTGTTGTGCC-3′.

References

1. Balch CM, Gershenwald JE, Soong SJ, Thompson JF, Atkins MB, Byrd DR, Buzaid AC, Cochran AJ, Coit DG, Ding S, Eggermont AM, Flaherty KT, Gimotty PA, Kirkwood JM, McMasters KM, Mihm MC Jr, Morton DL, Ross MI, Sober AJ, Sondak VK (2009) Final version of 2009 AJCC melanoma staging and classification. J Clin Oncol 27(36):6199–6206, doi:JCO.2009.23.4799 [pii] 10.1200/JCO.2009.23.4799
2. Tremante E, Ginebri A, Lo Monaco E, Frascione P, Di Filippo F, Terrenato I, Benevolo M, Mottolese M, Pescarmona E, Visca P, Natali PG, Giacomini P (2012) Melanoma molecular classes and prognosis in the postgenomic era. Lancet Oncol 13(5):e205–211. doi:10.1016/S1470-2045(12)70003-7
3. Carmona FJ, Esteller M (2011) Moving closer to a prognostic DNA methylation signature in colon cancer. Clin Cancer Res 17(6):1215–1217. doi:10.1158/1078-0432.CCR-10-3446
4. Wu C, Morris JR (2001) Genes, genetics, and epigenetics: a correspondence. Science 293(5532):1103–1105
5. Egger G, Liang G, Aparicio A, Jones PA (2004) Epigenetics in human disease and prospects for epigenetic therapy. Nature 429(6990):457–463
6. Kanwal R, Gupta S (2012) Epigenetic modifications in cancer. Clin Genet 81(4):303–311
7. Adams RL, Burdon RH (1982) DNA methylation in eukaryotes. CRC Crit Rev Biochem 13(4):349–384

8. Boyes J, Bird A (1991) DNA methylation inhibits transcription indirectly via a methyl-CpG binding protein. Cell 64(6):1123–1134
9. Futscher BW, Oshiro MM, Wozniak RJ, Holtan N, Hanigan CL, Duan H, Domann FE (2002) Role for DNA methylation in the control of cell type specific maspin expression. Nat Genet 31(2):175–179
10. Barlow DP (1995) Gametic imprinting in mammals. Science 270(5242):1610–1613
11. Goto T, Monk M (1998) Regulation of X-chromosome inactivation in development in mice and humans. Microbiol Mol Biol Rev 62(2):362–378
12. Feinberg AP, Vogelstein B (1983) Hypomethylation distinguishes genes of some human cancers from their normal counterparts. Nature 301(5895):89–92
13. Qu GZ, Ehrlich M (1999) Demethylation and expression of methylated plasmid DNA stably transfected into HeLa cells. Nucleic Acids Res 27(11):2332–2338
14. Herman JG, Baylin SB (2003) Gene silencing in cancer in association with promoter hypermethylation. N Engl J Med 349(21): 2042–2054
15. Jones PA (2002) DNA methylation and cancer. Oncogene 21(35):5358–5360
16. Sigalotti L, Covre A, Fratta E, Parisi G, Colizzi F, Rizzo A, Danielli R, Nicolay HJ, Coral S, Maio M (2010) Epigenetics of human cutaneous melanoma: setting the stage for new therapeutic strategies. J Transl Med 8:56
17. Palmieri G, Capone M, Ascierto ML, Gentilcore G, Stroncek DF, Casula M, Sini MC, Palla M, Mozzillo N, Ascierto PA (2009) Main roads to melanoma. J Transl Med 7:86
18. Freedberg DE, Rigas SH, Russak J, Gai W, Kaplow M, Osman I, Turner F, Randerson-Moor JA, Houghton A, Busam K, Timothy BD, Bastian BC, Newton-Bishop JA, Polsky D (2008) Frequent p16-independent inactivation of p14ARF in human melanoma. J Natl Cancer Inst 100(11):784–795
19. Tanemura A, Terando AM, Sim MS, van Hoesel AQ, de Maat MF, Morton DL, Hoon DS (2009) CpG island methylator phenotype predicts progression of malignant melanoma. Clin Cancer Res 15(5):1801–1807, doi:1078-0432.CCR-08-1361 [pii] 10.1158/1078-0432.CCR-08-1361
20. Hoon DS, Spugnardi M, Kuo C, Huang SK, Morton DL, Taback B (2004) Profiling epigenetic inactivation of tumor suppressor genes in tumors and plasma from cutaneous melanoma patients. Oncogene 23(22):4014–4022
21. Esteller M, Garcia-Foncillas J, Andion E, Goodman SN, Hidalgo OF, Vanaclocha V, Baylin SB, Herman JG (2000) Inactivation of the DNA-repair gene MGMT and the clinical response of gliomas to alkylating agents. N Engl J Med 343(19):1350–1354
22. Ehrlich M (2002) DNA methylation in cancer: too much, but also too little. Oncogene 21(35):5400–5413
23. Schulz WA, Elo JP, Florl AR, Pennanen S, Santourlidis S, Engers R, Buchardt M, Seifert HH, Visakorpi T (2002) Genomewide DNA hypomethylation is associated with alterations on chromosome 8 in prostate carcinoma. Genes Chromosomes Cancer 35(1):58–65
24. Fratta E, Sigalotti L, Colizzi F, Covre A, Nicolay HJ, Danielli R, Fonsatti E, Altomonte M, Calabro L, Coral S, Maio M (2010) Epigenetically regulated clonal heritability of CTA expression profiles in human melanoma. J Cell Physiol 223(2):352–358. doi:10.1002/jcp.22040
25. Lahtz C, Stranzenbach R, Fiedler E, Helmbold P, Dammann RH (2010) Methylation of PTEN as a prognostic factor in malignant melanoma of the skin. J Invest Dermatol 130(2):620–622, doi:jid2009226 [pii] 10.1038/jid.2009.226
26. You Y, Ma L, You M, Li X, Wang S, Li H, Wu D, Yang H, Li ZY (2010) TSLC1 gene silencing in cutaneous melanoma. Melanoma Res 20(3):179–183. doi:10.1097/CMR.0b013e32833413c0
27. Schraml P, von Teichman A, Mihic-Probst D, Simcock M, Ochsenbein A, Dummer R, Michielin O, Seifert B, Schlappi M, Moch H, von Moos R (2012) Predictive value of the MGMT promoter methylation status in metastatic melanoma patients receiving first-line temozolomide plus bevacizumab in the trial SAKK 50/07. Oncol Rep 28(2):654–658. doi:10.3892/or.2012.1826
28. Rietschel P, Wolchok JD, Krown S, Gerst S, Jungbluth AA, Busam K, Smith K, Orlow I, Panageas K, Chapman PB (2008) Phase II study of extended-dose temozolomide in patients with melanoma. J Clin Oncol 26(14):2299–2304. doi:10.1200/JCO.2007.14.5292
29. Hassel JC, Sucker A, Edler L, Kurzen H, Moll I, Stresemann C, Spieth K, Mauch C, Rass K, Dummer R, Schadendorf D (2010) MGMT gene promoter methylation correlates with tolerance of temozolomide treatment in melanoma but not with clinical outcome. Br J Cancer 103(6):820–826. doi:10.1038/sj.bjc.6605796
30. Mori T, Martinez SR, O'Day SJ, Morton DL, Umetani N, Kitago M, Tanemura A, Nguyen SL, Tran AN, Wang HJ, Hoon DS (2006) Estrogen receptor-alpha methylation predicts melanoma progression. Cancer Res 66(13):6692–6698, doi:66/13/6692 [pii] 10.1158/0008-5472.CAN-06-0801

31. Mori T, O'Day SJ, Umetani N, Martinez SR, Kitago M, Koyanagi K, Kuo C, Takeshima TL, Milford R, Wang HJ, Vu VD, Nguyen SL, Hoon DS (2005) Predictive utility of circulating methylated DNA in serum of melanoma patients receiving biochemotherapy. J Clin Oncol 23(36):9351–9358, doi:23/36/9351 [pii] 10.1200/JCO.2005.02.9876
32. Sigalotti L, Covre A, Fratta E, Parisi G, Sonego P, Colizzi F, Coral S, Massarut S, Kirkwood JM, Maio M (2012) Whole genome methylation profiles as independent markers of survival in stage iiic melanoma patients. J Transl Med 10(1):185. doi:10.1186/1479-5876-10-185
33. Sigalotti L, Fratta E, Bidoli E, Covre A, Parisi G, Colizzi F, Coral S, Massarut S, Kirkwood JM, Maio M (2011) Methylation levels of the "Long Interspersed Nucleotide Element-1" repetitive sequences predict survival of melanoma patients. J Transl Med 9(1):78. doi:10.1186/1479-5876-9-78
34. Cordaux R, Batzer MA (2009) The impact of retrotransposons on human genome evolution. Nat Rev Genet 10(10):691–703. doi:10.1038/nrg2640
35. Iacopetta B, Grieu F, Phillips M, Ruszkiewicz A, Moore J, Minamoto T, Kawakami K (2007) Methylation levels of LINE-1 repeats and CpG island loci are inversely related in normal colonic mucosa. Cancer Sci 98(9):1454–1460. doi:10.1111/j.1349-7006.2007.00548.x
36. Espina V, Wulfkuhle JD, Calvert VS, VanMeter A, Zhou W, Coukos G, Geho DH, Petricoin EF III, Liotta LA (2006) Laser-capture microdissection. NatProtoc 1(2):586–603

Chapter 26

Isolation of Melanoma Cell Subpopulations Using Negative Selection

Ana Slipicevic, Rajasekharan Somasundaram, Katrin Sproesser, and Meenhard Herlyn

Abstract

Melanomas are phenotypically and functionally heterogeneous tumors comprising of distinct subpopulations that drive disease progression and are responsible for resistance to therapy. Identification and characterization of such subpopulations are highly important to develop novel targeted therapies. However, this can be a challenging task as there is a lack of clearly defined markers to distinguish the melanoma subpopulations from a general tumor cell population. Also, there is a lack of optimal isolation methods and functional assays that can fully recapitulate their phenotype. Here we describe a method for isolating tumor cells from fresh human tumor tissue specimens using an antibody coupled magnetic bead sorting technique that is well established in our laboratory. Thus, melanoma cells are enriched by negative cell sorting and elimination of non-tumor cell population such as erythrocytes, leukocytes, and endothelial cells. Enriched unmodified tumor cells can be further used for phenotypic and functional characterization of melanoma subpopulations.

Key words Subpopulations, Tumor cell isolation, Magnetic beads, Tumorigenic potential

1 Introduction

Melanoma like other solid tumors is a highly heterogeneous cancer with complex cellular biology and distinct intra- and inter-tumoral differences. Melanoma is composed of tumor-cell subpopulations that contribute to tumor initiation, self-renewal, tumor maintenance, progression, and resistance to therapy. This phenotypic and functional heterogeneity among tumor cells develops during progression and can be partially explained by cancer development models. In the traditional clonal evolution model a substantial proportion of cells in a tumor have the potential to drive disease progression [1, 2]. As an alternative, the cancer stem cell (CSC) model argues that tumor growth is primarily driven by selective proliferation of a rare population of highly tumorigenic cells that

Magdalena Thurin and Francesco M. Marincola (eds.), *Molecular Diagnostics for Melanoma: Methods and Protocols*, Methods in Molecular Biology, vol. 1102, DOI 10.1007/978-1-62703-727-3_26,

have self-renewal capacity and produce all major cells population that are less or non-tumorigenic [3–5]. However, an increasing number of evidence suggests that melanoma cell heterogeneity and progression cannot fully be explained by either of these models but rather through a novel cell plasticity model [6–9]. According to this model the plasticity of cancer cells allows them to switch between more or less malignant states that are phenotypically distinct. Moreover, these differences are a direct response to environmental factors or stress, including therapy. Therapy resistance is attributed to phenotypic and functional changes in subpopulations that are fully reversible. Thus, a better understanding of tumor heterogeneity and subpopulations is required to target them and further improve current therapies. Several markers associated with phenotypically distinct subpopulations of cancer stem cell-like characteristics are reported in melanoma. The most extensively studied markers so far are described below.

1.1 Markers Defining Melanoma Cell Subpopulations

1. *ABC transporters.* ATP-binding cassette (ABC) transporters are a large family of transmembrane proteins that use ATP hydrolysis for translocation of numerous substrates across extracellular and intracellular membranes [10]. Some of the members of this family, including ABCB5, ABCB8, and ABCG2, are expressed in various cancers including melanoma and are often associated with chemoresistance [11, 12]. Expression of ABCB5 increases during melanoma progression and a subpopulation of melanoma cells with high expression of ABCB5, are shown to possess tumor-initiating properties [13]. ABCB5+ cells have the ability to form heterogeneous tumors with respect to ABCB5 expression. These cells also expressed markers such as CD133, CD166, and Nestin that are generally present in undifferentiated tumors. Targeting ABCB5 cell subpopulations by anti-ABCB5 antibodies resulted in almost complete inhibition of tumor growth in mouse xenograft model. ABCG2 is co-expressed in a chemoresistant CD133+ melanoma subpopulation with high aggressive potential in vivo [14, 15] In addition to ABCB5 and ABCG2, an in vitro study has shown the presence of an ABCB8+ melanoma subpopulation that is resistant to doxorubicin [16]. However, expression of ABCB8 in melanoma patient tumor-tissue samples remains to be confirmed.
2. *CD20*, encoded by the MS4A1 gene, is a transmembrane protein, expressed at the B-cell surface and is involved in Ca2+ channeling, proliferation and differentiation of B cells [17, 18]. Genetic profiling of melanoma tumors showed that CD20 expression is associated with a more aggressive tumor phenotype [19]. Our previous studies have demonstrated that a small subpopulation of melanoma cells express CD20 when grown as tumor spheroids under in vitro culture conditions

[20]. These cells had the ability to differentiate into multiple cell lineages including melanocytes, adipocytes, chondrocytes, and osteoblasts and to initiate tumors in mice, indicating cancer stem-like features. Recently, Schmidt et al. showed that targeting of a small population of melanoma cells expressing CD20 in a mouse xenograft model, using engineered T cells with redirected specificity for CD20, led to complete and lasting inhibition of tumor growth [21]. Furthermore, advanced melanoma patients treated with rituximab, an anti-CD20 antibody, in an adjuvant setting, remained disease free during 42 months of observation [22, 23]. Even though the function of CD20 in melanoma cells is poorly understood and CD20 positive cells represent a very small subpopulation (<2 %), these data suggests that CD20+ cells are an interesting therapeutic target.

3. *CD133/prominin-1* is a transmembrane glycoprotein expressed by several types of undifferentiated cells including hematopoietic and fetal brain stem cells as well as endothelial progenitor and prostate epithelial cells [24]. CD133 has been identified as a marker of brain tumor-initiating cells and is expressed in other solid cancers including, liver, lung, pancreas, prostate, breast, and colon carcinomas [25–29]. In addition, it is frequently found in drug-resistant tumor subpopulations of breast cancer, glioma, and lung cancer after chemotherapy [26, 30, 31]. Scattered expression of CD133 has been detected in both benign nevi and melanomas but in addition to other stem-cell markers like CD166 and Nestin, its expression was increased in primary and metastatic melanomas compared to benign nevi [32–34]. Early studies of CD133+ melanoma cells showed that only these cells were capable of forming tumors in immune deficient NOD/SCID mice, thus assigning tumor-initiating properties to CD133+ subpopulation [14]. In the cultured melanoma cell line WM115, most cells expresses high levels of CD133 under adherent culture conditions. Cultivation of these cells as non-adherent spheroids or injection in mice led to loss of CD133+ cells, which suggests that expression of CD133 is dependent on environmental stimuli. CD133 expressing subpopulations often show co-expression of Nestin, a type VI intermediate filament protein highly expressed in stem cells of neural crest origin, and associated with dedifferentiation and more aggressive behavior in melanoma [33, 35, 36]. However, co-expression of Nestin might be expected since melanocytes share common lineage with neural crest cells. Two recent studies have provided additional data supporting the use of CD133 as a marker of more aggressive melanomas. Sharma et al. showed that CD133 mRNA level strongly and negatively correlates with clinical outcome and could be a potential predictor of poor prognosis in high-risk melanoma. The CD133+ subpopulation was able to repopulate and form tumors

in vivo while CD113- cells failed to form tumors under same conditions. Furthermore, in primary cell cultures these distinct subpopulations maintained their CD133 status for up to 8 passages [37]. Data from Lai et al. suggest that the CD133+ subpopulation in melanoma can contribute to perivascular niche morphogenesis and tumorigenicity through vasculogenic mimicry [38]. However, other studies with several cancer types, including melanoma, showed that the CD133- subpopulations can have tumor-initiating properties making further characterization of CD133+ subpopulation warranted [29, 39–41].

4. *CD271/NGFR/p75 neurotrophin receptor* is a transmembrane protein, which functions as a receptor for the neurotrophins growth factors that stimulate neuronal cells to survive and differentiate. In addition to being expressed in neural-crest-derived tissues, CD271 has been found in several types of cancer including melanoma. Several studies have addressed the possibility that CD271 might be a marker of melanoma initiating cells. Boiko et al. showed that the CD271+ melanoma subpopulations derived from patients' tissues was more tumorigenic and aggressive when transplanted in immunodeficient NOD/SCID IL2Rγ null (NSG) mice than the CD271- subpopulation [42]. Furthermore, CD271+ cells had lost several melanoma-associated antigens including MART1, MAGE, and Tyrosinase. Expression of CD271 also correlated with higher metastatic potential and poor prognosis in patients. In contrast to these studies, Held et al. showed that a CD34+/CD271- subpopulation of melanoma cells had greater ability to establish new tumors than CD34+/CD271+ [43]. Recently Quintana et al. demonstrated that both CD271+ and CD271- cells have similar capacity to form tumors. As was discussed for CD133, these discrepancies have to be addressed before drawing any conclusions about the utilization of CD271 as a marker for a tumor-initiating subpopulation in melanoma.

5. *JARID1B.* Our group have previously identified histone demethylase jumonji ARID (JARID, also referred as lysine demethylase 5 [KDM5]) 1B, which regulate gene expression and transcriptional activities, as a possible marker of a tumor-initiating subpopulation in melanoma [9]. Cells with high expression of JARID1B are rare and represent only ~1–5 % of the total cell population. They are slow cycling and have stem-like or tumor-initiating properties with aggressive growth potential. JARID1B+ cells are essential for long-term tumor growth of xenografts in immunodeficient mice and can give rise to heterogeneous progeny suggesting that JARID1B might provide tumor maintenance functions for melanomas. JARID1A, a close homolog of JARID1B, is required for drug resistance in non-small-cell lung cancer cells [44], suggesting that slow cycling subpopulations need to be selectively targeted.

1.2 The Challenges and Uncertainty of Subpopulations Markers Studies

Earlier studies of human melanomas transplanted into nude mice suggested that only one in a million cells is capable of forming tumors, supporting the cancer stem cell hypothesis of melanoma propagation [13]. However, using a NSG mouse model, Quintana et al. demonstrated that from total unselected melanoma cells, as many as 30 % can be tumorigenic [40]. This frequency was comparable both between cells obtained directly from patients or xenografts as well as between primary versus metastasis derived cells while there was no correlation between tumorigenic cell frequency and tumor growth rate or aggressiveness. Similar findings were also reported with mouse models of melanoma [43]. In our own studies we find that melanoma xenografts can develop from a single cell derived from either patient samples or cell lines. Quintana et al. subdivided melanomas into 50 subpopulations based on the differences in surface marker expression, including CD133, ABCB5, and CD271, and have not found any subpopulations that lacks the ability to form a phenotypically heterogeneous tumor when injected into NSG mice. Thus, there is an overwhelming evidence suggesting that certain phenotypic and functional features of tumorigenic cells can be transiently and reversibly turned on and off [9, 45].

It has been discussed whether the reported discrepancies between the studies might be due to methodological issues. More permissive conditions, including the degree of immunodeficiency in recipient mice, extracellular environment provided by Matrigel and assay duration might have contributed to tumor take rate. However, one might reason that if the tumor cells did not possess tumor-initiating capabilities, they would not gain these properties from exposure to Matrigel or subcutaneous tissues of the mice as the normal human melanocytes were unable to grow under identical conditions. This underlines the difficulties in defining therapeutically relevant subpopulations based solely on the expression of a surface marker. From a therapeutic standpoint our efforts should be focused on characterizing all cells because all have intrinsic tumorigenic potential regardless of the assay used.

1.3 Method for the Isolation and Purification of Unmodified Tumor Cells from Human Melanomas

The subpopulation markers identified by studying established cell cultures ultimately need to be validated in patient derived material. Unfortunately, the amount of patient tumor material is often limited and the tumor tissue often contains necrotic debris as well as a mixture of normal cells including hematopoietic cells, endothelial cells and fibroblasts which collectively can account for up to 50 % of all cells. Obtaining high purity and sufficient cell numbers from patient samples is often challenging due to the small size. Most isolation and purification methods can damage tumor cells which can further influence results of downstream applications. One potential method of tumor cell isolation is direct antibody labeling of cell surface markers followed by Fluorescence Activated

Cell Sorting (FACS) sorting. However, FACS sorting can be harsh on the cells and requires extensive washing steps which results in cell loss. For this reason, we have adapted a method that relies on magnetic bead cell-sorting. We have applied a negative isolation approach by using an antibody cocktail to remove all unwanted cells such as endothelial cells (CD31), hematopoietic (nucleated) cells (CD45), and red blood cells (hTER119) from the tumor tissue sample, leaving only enriched and unmodified tumor cells for use in downstream assays. Because fibroblasts and melanoma cells share their markers, we have not attempted to remove fibroblasts. The amount of available tissue and the nature of the downstream application should be considered while deciding which method to use.

2 Materials

2.1 Enzymatic Digestion Media

1. Collagenase IV (2,000 U/ml, Worthington Biochemicals) dissolved in 1× HBSS with 5 mM $CaCl_2$ to a final concentration of 200 U/ml, (stored in aliquots at −20 °C).
2. DNase I stock (4,000 U/mg) (10× stock Sigma-Aldrich) dissolved in 1× HBSS (stored in aliquots at −20 °C).
3. 0.05 % Trypsin–ethylenediamine tetraacetic acid (EDTA) (Gibco®, Life Technologies).

2.2 Melanoma Cells Preparation and Sorting

1. Leibovitz's L15 Media without phenol red (132 ml) (Gibco®, Life Technologies) (150 ml); 1× Penicillin–streptomycin (Penn/Strep); 1 mg/ml Bovine serum albumin (BSA) (150 mg, tissue culture grade); 4-(2-Hydroxyethyl) piperazine-1-ethanesulfonic acid (HEPES) (10 mM, pH 7.4 (1.5 ml of a 1 M stock), and 10 % sterile deionized water (15 ml).
2. Wash buffer: Hank's buffered salt solution (HBSS) (Gibco®, Life Technologies), 2 % FBS (Hyclone), 1× Penn/Strep (Gibco®, Life Technologies).
3. Sterile petri dishes (100×20 mm, Corning).
4. Sterile centrifuge Falcon tubes (50 ml, BD Biosciences).
5. Falcon cell strainer to obtain single cell suspension by removing clumps and debris from clinical samples prior to analysis (40 μm, BD Biosciences).
6. Dynabeads® Antibody Coupling Kit (Life Technologies) that allows for coupling of antibodies to bead surface. All antibody–beads coupling reactions are performed as described in the manufacturer's protocol.
7. Antibodies used for negative selection to purify melanoma: CD31 (Platelet endothelial cell adhesion molecule, PECAM-1),

CD41 (integrin alpha chain 2b), and TER119 (erythroid cell marker). We have used 25 μg of respective antibodies per 1 mg magnetic beads. We have used self-generated antibodies against human CD31, CD45, and hTER119 for cost efficiency. Commercial antibodies are available, Red blood specific antibody hTER119 can be replaced with Anti-human Glycophorin A/CD235a-antibody (R&D Systems Inc.).

Alternatively, pre-coupled beads with antibodies CD31, CD41, and hTER119 Dynabeads® are available (Life Technologies).

2.3 Fluorescein Activated Cell Sorting (FACS)

1. Hank's buffered salt solution (HBSS) (Gibco®, Life Technologies), 2 % FBS (Hyclone), 1× Penn/Strep (Gibco®, Life Technologies).
2. Fluorescein isothiocyanate (FITC) conjugated melanoma specific antibody anti-CD146 (melanoma cell adhesion molecule, MCAM), clone P1H12 (BD-Pharmingen).
3. Isotype-matched IgG antibody control for background staining (clone MOPC-21, BD-Pharmingen).
4. LSR II Flow Cytometer (BD Biosciences) used for FACS analysis.

2.4 Reagents for Clonogenicity Studies

1. *Tu 2 % medium for melanoma cell culture:* 80 % MCDB153 basal medium (Sigma-Aldrich) and 20 % Leibovitz's L15 medium(Sigma-Aldrich) supplemented with 2 % FBS (Hyclone); 5 μg/ml Insulin (Sigma-Aldrich) and 1.68 mM CaCl2 (Sigma-Aldrich).
2. Matrigel basement membrane matrix (BD Matrigel™, BD Biosciences).

3 Methods

3.1 Tumor Tissue Dissociation into Single Cell Suspension

1. Wash tumor sample three times in Leibovitz's L15 Medium at room temperature to remove and discard any visible associated fat and connective tissue (*see* **Note 1**).
2. Place the tumor tissue in a sterile petri dish and finely mince the tissue into very small pieces (as small as possible) using a scalpel blade at room temperature.
3. Transfer the tissue fragments into a sterile 50 ml centrifuge tube containing 10 ml of enzymatic digestion medium per gram of tumor tissue. Place the tube in the incubator or water bath with vigorous triturating every 5 min at 37 °C for 20 min.
4. Following incubation, add cold wash HBSS medium up to 50 ml, spin down cells at 300 × *g* at 4 °C for 4 min. Aspirate the supernatant after centrifugation.

5. Resuspend the cell pellet in 5 ml of 0.05 % trypsin–0.5 mM EDTA and DNase solution (100 U/ml) by gentle shaking (*not* by pipetting) and incubate at 37 °C for 2 min (*see* **Note 2**).
6. In order to remove trypsin and resuspend the disaggregated tumor cells add cold staining medium up to 50 ml. Filter through a 40 μm cell strainer in order to obtain a single cell tumor suspension.
7. Spin the cells down at 300 × *g* at 4 °C for 4 min, aspirate the supernatant and resuspend the cells in an adequate volume of staining medium.
8. Perform a viability count using hemocytometer and Trypan Blue dead-cell discrimination dye. Adjust the concentration of the cells to 1×10^6 cells/ml (*see* **Note 3**).

3.2 Negative Selection to Enrich for Melanoma Cells Using Magnetic Beads

Melanoma cells are enriched by negative selection by depletion of endothelial cells, hematopoietic (nucleated) cells and red blood cells using magnetic bead separation technique.

1. To each well of a 24-well plate add 100 μl cell suspension at 1×10^6 cells/ml obtained after tumor tissue dissociation, 50 μl of each of the antibody-conjugated bead solution (anti-CD31, anti-CD45, and hTER19) and 10 μl FBS (*see* **Note 4**).
2. Incubate the plate on wet ice for 3 h with gentle manual rotation every hour.
3. Transfer the cells into a 1.5 ml microcentrifuge tube and place the tube on a magnet for 2 min in order to separate the cells (Fig. 1a).
4. While keeping the tube on the magnetic rack transfer the unbound tumor cells to a new sterile tube (Fig. 1b).
5. Perform a viability count using hemocytometer and Trypan Blue dead-cell discrimination dye.
6. Following enrichment purity of tumor cells is confirmed by FACS analysis using FITC conjugated mouse anti-human CD146 antibody. to evaluate the yield and the purity of the melanoma cells. FITC conjugated mouse IgG1, κ isotype antibody is used as control antibody. At this stage the cells can be used for further characterization and downstream assays (*see* **Note 5**).

3.3 Flow Cytometry Analysis of Purified Melanoma Cells

1. 6×10^5 cells from purified melanoma cell suspension are divided into 3 new tubes. Samples are centrifuged at 300 × *g*, aspirated, and resuspended in 50 μl of HBSS medium containing 2 % FBS.
2. Add 5 μl of FITC-conjugated CD146 antibody or 2.5 μl/ml FITC-conjugated mouse IgG1, κ isotype a control antibody to tube 1 and 2. Cells in the third tube are resuspended in 50 μl

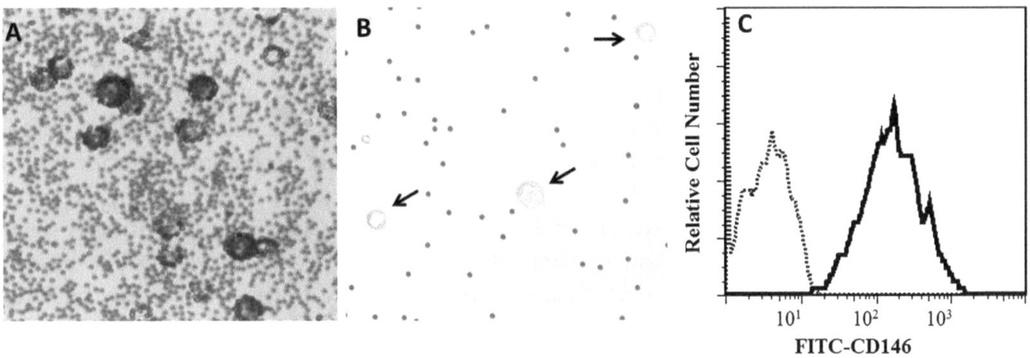

Fig. 1 (**a**) Suspension obtained after magnetic separation containing endothelial (CD31), hematopoietic (CD45), and red blood cells (hTER119) bound to magnetic beds and (**b**) Suspension containing unmodified tumor cells after separation. (**c**) Flow-cytometric analysis of CD146 expression on purified melanoma tumor cell suspension as seen in (**b**). *Dashed line* histogram represents Mouse IgG1, κ Isotype Control antibody. Fluorescence histograms were derived from gated events based on negative PI staining and the forward and side light-scatter characteristics of viable single cells

of HBSS containing 2 % FBS for unstained control cells. The cells are incubated in dark at 4 °C for 30 min.

3. Centrifuge cells at 300×*g* for 5 min, aspirate supernatant, and resuspend cells in 500 μl HBSS, 2 % FBS with 1 μg/ml propidium iodide for discrimination of life/dead cells. Transfer samples to FACS machine-compatible, sterile 5 ml round bottom tubes. During flow-cytometric analysis dead cells are excluded based on positive propidium iodide, while any potential doublets or apoptotic cells are excluded based on side and forward scatter (Fig. 1c).

4 Notes

1. Melanoma tissues are obtained in accordance with consent procedures approved by the Internal Review Boards of The Wistar Institute and Hospital of University of Pennsylvania. To obtain the maximum amount of viable cells and minimize the interference with surface marker expression it is critical that fresh tumor tissue is processed as soon as possible following the surgical procedure. Tumor tissue usually is obtained within 1–2 h after surgical removal.
2. Exposure of the tumor cells to trypsin should be minimized in order to reduce cell surface damage and loss of cell surface markers.
3. At this stage it is useful to assess viability of the cells in the suspension by carrying out a Trypan Blue dye exclusion test. Since magnetic beads can stick to dead cells nonspecifically.

Slow-speed centrifugation at $200 \times g$ might be used to remove dead cells debris prior to cell–antibody–bead coupling.

4. Antibody–beads coupling reactions are performed using Dynabeads® Antibody Coupling Kit as described in the manufacturer's protocol. This step must be completed prior to the start of the experiment. The prepared beads can be prepared and stored at 4 °C until needed. During cell–antibody–bead incubation total volume of 260 μl per well should not be exceeded. Smaller volumes allow better interaction between cells and antibody-conjugated beads. Optimization of these conditions was performed using established in vitro melanoma cell culture where cells were counted before and after the magnetic beat sorting using anti-CD146 bound beads. Using this procedure we found that exceeding 1×10^5 cells per well results in low binding efficiency of antibody-conjugated beads. At this optimal cell–bead ratio >95 % of the cells were pull down.
5. After assessing viability and cell numbers by counting, cells can be directly used for further selection based on any melanoma cell surface marker of interest (CD20, ABCB5, CD133, etc.) using positive selection with antibody bound to the beads; in clonogenic assays; for the assessment of tumorigenic potential in immunodeficient mouse models or molecular analysis of RNA, gene expression, etc. [9, 20].

Clonogenicity of the purified melanoma cells can be evaluated using limiting dilution assay by distributing cells in 96-well plates in vitro. The presence of single cells is confirmed visually by inspecting each well microscopically. Cells are supplemented with fresh Human Embryonic Stem Cells (hESC) medium every second day and examined for formation of spheres [20]. For in vivo tumorigenicity studies, sorted cells are resuspended in melanoma Tu 2 % medium with 25 % Matrigel basement membrane matrix (BD Matrigel™, BD Biosciences) and single cell is injected into NSG mice. Single cell for injection is isolated by limiting dilution seeding of the cells in a 96-well plate. Injection of the single cell is performed by drawing the cell into a syringe containing Matrigel and visually confirming that the cell has been removed from the well [9].

References

1. Nowell PC (1976) The clonal evolution of tumor cell populations. Science 194:23–28
2. Fearon ER, Vogelstein B (1990) A genetic model for colorectal tumorigenesis. Cell 61:759–767
3. Dick JE (2008) Stem cell concepts renew cancer research. Blood 112:4793–4807
4. Lobo NA, Shimono Y, Qian D, Clarke MF (2007) The biology of cancer stem cells. Annu Rev Cell Dev Biol 23:675–699
5. Reya T, Morrison SJ, Clarke MF, Weissman IL (2001) Stem cells, cancer, and cancer stem cells. Nature 414:105–111
6. Gupta PB, Onder TT, Jiang G et al (2009) Identification of selective inhibitors of cancer stem cells by high-throughput screening. Cell 138:645–659
7. Mani SA, Guo W, Liao MJ et al (2008) The epithelial-mesenchymal transition generates cells with properties of stem cells. Cell 133:704–715

8. Marusyk A, Polyak K (2010) Tumor heterogeneity: causes and consequences. Biochim Biophys Acta 1805:105–117
9. Roesch A, Fukunaga-Kalabis M, Schmidt EC et al (2010) A temporarily distinct subpopulation of slow-cycling melanoma cells is required for continuous tumor growth. Cell 141:583–594
10. Jones PM, George AM (2004) The ABC transporter structure and mechanism: perspectives on recent research. Cell Mol Life Sci 61:682–699
11. Dean M, Fojo T, Bates S (2005) Tumour stem cells and drug resistance. Nat Rev Cancer 5:275–284
12. Szakacs G, Annereau JP, Lababidi S et al (2004) Predicting drug sensitivity and resistance: profiling ABC transporter genes in cancer cells. Cancer Cell 6:129–137
13. Schatton T, Murphy GF, Frank NY et al (2008) Identification of cells initiating human melanomas. Nature 451:345–349
14. Monzani E, Facchetti F, Galmozzi E et al (2007) Melanoma contains CD133 and ABCG2 positive cells with enhanced tumourigenic potential. Eur J Cancer 43:935–946
15. Taghizadeh R, Noh M, Huh YH et al (2011) CXCR6, a newly defined biomarker of tissue-specific stem cell asymmetric self-renewal, identifies more aggressive human melanoma cancer stem cells. PLoS One 5:e15183
16. Elliott AM, Al-Hajj MA (2009) ABCB8 mediates doxorubicin resistance in melanoma cells by protecting the mitochondrial genome. Mol Cancer Res 7:79–87
17. Somasundaram R, Villanueva J, Herlyn M (2011) Will engineered T cells expressing CD20 scFv eradicate Melanoma? Mol Ther 19:638–640
18. Tedder TF, Engel P (1994) CD20: a regulator of cell-cycle progression of B lymphocytes. Immunol Today 15:450–454
19. Bittner M, Meltzer P, Chen Y et al (2000) Molecular classification of cutaneous malignant melanoma by gene expression profiling. Nature 406:536–540
20. Fang D, Nguyen TK, Leishear K et al (2005) A tumorigenic subpopulation with stem cell properties in melanomas. Cancer Res 65:9328–9337
21. Schmidt P, Kopecky C, Hombach A, Zigrino P, Mauch C, Abken H (2011) Eradication of melanomas by targeted elimination of a minor subset of tumor cells. Proc Natl Acad Sci U S A 108:2474–2479
22. Pinc A, Somasundaram R, Wagner C et al (2012) Targeting CD20 in melanoma patients at high risk of disease recurrence. Mol Ther 20(5):1056–1062
23. Schlaak M, Schmidt P, Bangard C, Kurschat P, Mauch C, Abken H (2012) Regression of metastatic melanoma in a patient by antibody targeting of cancer stem cells. Oncotarget 3:22–30
24. Neuzil J, Stantic M, Zobalova R et al (2007) Tumour-initiating cells vs. cancer "stem" cells and CD133: what's in the name? Biochem Biophys Res Commun 355:855–859
25. Dembinski JL, Krauss S (2009) Characterization and functional analysis of a slow cycling stem cell-like subpopulation in pancreas adenocarcinoma. Clin Exp Metastasis 26(7):611–623
26. Liu G, Yuan X, Zeng Z et al (2006) Analysis of gene expression and chemoresistance of CD133+ cancer stem cells in glioblastoma. Mol Cancer 5:67
27. Ricci-Vitiani L, Lombardi DG, Pilozzi E et al (2007) Identification and expansion of human colon-cancer-initiating cells. Nature 445: 111–115
28. Salmaggi A, Boiardi A, Gelati M et al (2006) Glioblastoma-derived tumorospheres identify a population of tumor stem-like cells with angiogenic potential and enhanced multidrug resistance phenotype. Glia 54:850–860
29. Shmelkov SV, Butler JM, Hooper AT et al (2008) CD133 expression is not restricted to stem cells, and both CD133+ and CD133- metastatic colon cancer cells initiate tumors. J Clin Invest 118:2111–2120
30. Levina V, Marrangoni AM, DeMarco R, Gorelik E, Lokshin AE (2008) Drug-selected human lung cancer stem cells: cytokine network, tumorigenic and metastatic properties. PLoS One 3:e3077
31. Visvader JE, Lindeman GJ (2008) Cancer stem cells in solid tumours: accumulating evidence and unresolved questions. Nat Rev Cancer 8:755–768
32. Frank NY, Margaryan A, Huang Y et al (2005) ABCB5-mediated doxorubicin transport and chemoresistance in human malignant melanoma. Cancer Res 65:4320–4333
33. Klein WM, Wu BP, Zhao S, Wu H, Klein-Szanto AJ, Tahan SR (2007) Increased expression of stem cell markers in malignant melanoma. Mod Pathol 20:102–107
34. Rappa G, Fodstad O, Lorico A (2008) The stem cell-associated antigen CD133 (Prominin-1) is a molecular therapeutic target for metastatic melanoma. Stem Cells 26:3008–3017

35. Piras F, Perra MT, Murtas D et al (2010) The stem cell marker nestin predicts poor prognosis in human melanoma. Oncol Rep 23:17–24
36. Fusi A, Reichelt U, Busse A et al (2011) Expression of the stem cell markers nestin and CD133 on circulating melanoma cells. J Invest Dermatol 131:487–494
37. Sharma BK, Manglik V, O'Connell M et al (2012) Clonal dominance of CD133+ subset population as risk factor in tumor progression and disease recurrence of human cutaneous melanoma. Int J Oncol 41(5):1570–1576
38. Lai CY, Schwartz BE, Hsu MY (2012) CD133+ Melanoma subpopulations contribute to perivascular niche morphogenesis and tumorigenicity through vasculogenic mimicry. Cancer Res 72(19):5111–5118
39. Wang J, Sakariassen PO, Tsinkalovsky O et al (2008) CD133 negative glioma cells form tumors in nude rats and give rise to CD133 positive cells. Int J Cancer 122:761–768
40. Quintana E, Shackleton M, Foster HR et al (2010) Phenotypic heterogeneity among tumorigenic melanoma cells from patients that is reversible and not hierarchically organized. Cancer Cell 18:510–523
41. Joo KM, Kim SY, Jin X et al (2008) Clinical and biological implications of CD133-positive and CD133-negative cells in glioblastomas. Lab Invest 88:808–815
42. Boiko AD, Razorenova OV, van de Rijn M et al (2010) Human melanoma-initiating cells express neural crest nerve growth factor receptor CD271. Nature 466:133–137
43. Held MA, Curley DP, Dankort D, McMahon M, Muthusamy V, Bosenberg MW (2010) Characterization of melanoma cells capable of propagating tumors from a single cell. Cancer Res 70:388–397
44. Sharma SV, Lee DY, Li B et al (2010) A chromatin-mediated reversible drug-tolerant state in cancer cell subpopulations. Cell 141: 69–80
45. Magee JA, Piskounova E, Morrison SJ (2012) Cancer stem cells: impact, heterogeneity, and uncertainty. Cancer Cell 21:283–296

Chapter 27

Circulating Tumor Cells as Prognostic Biomarkers in Cutaneous Melanoma Patients

Eiji Kiyohara, Keisuke Hata, Stella Lam, and Dave S.B. Hoon

Abstract

Detection of circulating tumor cells (CTC) in peripheral blood has been investigated for its prognostic ability, and its potential to measure the effectiveness of treatment(s) in patients with melanoma. However, a highly sensitive and specific assay is required to detect CTC in patients' blood. We have developed a multimarker quantitative real-time reverse transcriptase polymerase chain reaction (RT-qPCR) assay for detecting CTC directly from peripheral blood specimens without the need of separating CTC from leukocytes (PBL). We selected and optimized four mRNA biomarkers (MART-1/Melan-A, MAGE-A3, PAX3, and GalNAc-T) for detection and prediction of clinical outcome in melanoma patients. Our protocol has both high sensitivity and specificity for CTC in blood specimens—detecting approximately one to five melanoma cells in 10^7 PBL. We have demonstrated the significance of this assay for serial bleed assessment of CTC in clinical trials and for daily clinical usage.

Key words Circulating tumor cells, CTC, Melanoma, Quantitative real-time RT-PCR

1 Introduction

To date, the American Joint Committee on Cancer (AJCC) staging criteria are commonly used for the staging of primary and metastatic melanoma in clinical settings [1], and making decisions for patient management. The presence of metastases to regional lymph nodes and/or distant organs can be used to predict prognosis and treatment stratification [2]. However, more precise and predictive approaches, such as blood biomarkers, to assess real-time metastasis process are increasing in demand in order to better monitor patients, predict recurrences earlier and assess tumor progression. To date, there are no effective blood biomarkers for melanoma, except for serum lactate dehydrogenase (LDH) in stage IV melanoma (AJCC staging manual 7th edition) that offers a relatively limited prognostic value. To overcome this challenge, we have developed and verified an assay in multiple clinical settings and trials for detecting

Magdalena Thurin and Francesco M. Marincola (eds.), *Molecular Diagnostics for Melanoma: Methods and Protocols*, Methods in Molecular Biology, vol. 1102, DOI 10.1007/978-1-62703-727-3_27, © Springer Science+Business Media New York 2014

specific mRNA biomarkers expressed by circulating tumor cells (CTC) using quantitative real-time polymerase chain reaction (RT-qPCR) directly from peripheral blood leukocytes (PBL) fraction without the need to isolate CTC. We have shown that specific CTC mRNA biomarkers can be used as surrogate predictors of treatment outcome in a single institute, domestic (USA) setting, and international multicenter clinical trials [3, 4].

The features of our established CTC assay are multifold: (1) using a mRNA based multimarker assay optimized for CTC detection, (2) detecting mRNA directly from PBL fractions without the need of isolating CTCs, (3) ability to quantify mRNA levels for assessed biomarkers, (4) eliminating tedious enrichment steps making it more logistically feasible for clinical laboratories, (5) logistically practical for multicenter studies (domestic and international), (6) ability to store blood specimen mRNA for short or long-term to repeat results for verification, (7) application to any type of body fluid (bone marrow, cerebral spinal fluid, pleural/peritoneal fluids, and (8) substitution, deletion, and/or addition of other CTC specific mRNA biomarkers in assay runs. Any CTC detection methods with a single biomarker or nonquantitative assays have limitations in terms of the sensitivity and specificity due to the heterogeneity of cutaneous melanoma [5]. In order to maximize the sensitivity and specificity in detecting CTCs, we carefully screened and assessed for a correlation with clinical disease outcome in phase II trials, and selected four mRNA biomarkers that were frequently expressed in circulating melanoma cells, but not in the normal background levels of the PBLs. These mRNA biomarkers include: (1) MART-1/Melan-A, melanoma antigen recognized by T cells-1; (2) MAGE-A3, melanoma antigen gene-A3 family; (3) PAX3, paired box homeotic gene transcription factor 3; and (4) GalNAc-T, $\beta 1 \rightarrow 4$-*N*-acetylgalactosaminyl transferase. MART-1 is a major melanocyte differentiation antigen that is exclusive to and expressed in >90 % of melanoma cells [4]. MAGE-3 is expressed in malignant cells of different embryonic origin, and is found in >60 % of melanomas [4, 5]. PAX3 is a transcription factor and potential stem cell gene in cutaneous melanoma [4, 6, 7]. GalNAc-T is a key enzyme involved in the biosynthesis of gangliosides GM2 and GD2, which are highly expressed in metastatic melanomas [4, 8]. Traditionally known melanogenesis genes, such as tyrosinase, gp100, and microphthalmia associated transcription factor (MITF), were not used in this study because of their limited prognostic utility, and mostly due to the false positive results when assayed in control PBLs. Meta-analysis of 53 studies, including 5,433 patients with TNM stage I to IV cutaneous and uveal melanoma, suggest that CTC might have prognostic value in melanoma patients [9]. However, problems of past studies with CTC detection have been technical issues, including different CTC isolation techniques, poor assay sensitivity, lack of quantitative tests, biomarker specificity, sample size, and different patient cohorts assessed.

Multiple studies using various CTC enrichment techniques with specific antibodies provide evidence that the number of circulating tumor cells is an independent predictor of progression-free and overall survival in patients with epithelial malignancies [10], but are limited in terms of antibody sensitivity and specificity. We previously reported a CTC enrichment assay in melanoma using multiple antibodies targeting melanoma cell-surface antigens that demonstrate potential clinical usefulness of employing an enrichment step for detecting CTCs from blood of melanoma patients [7, 11]. However, in this study, by carefully selecting four optimized CTC biomarkers, we eliminated the CTC enrichment steps and simplified the overall procedure, while maintaining effectiveness, for large-scale international clinical trials. Importantly, this approach overcomes the need for applying multiple antibodies for CTC enrichment due to heterogeneity of melanoma. We have assessed CTC enrichment with antibody-coated magnetic bead parallel to the direct CTC assay to verify the latter assay accuracy. The direct CTC assay requires minimal processing time of blood specimens, which is logistically feasible in most clinical and hospital laboratories. In terms of sensitivity, we have shown that the RT-qPCR assay can detect approximately one to five melanoma cells in 10^7 PBLs (will vary for mRNA biomarker depending on the cell line expression level in spiking experiments) [12]. This approach has allowed us to conduct multicenter trials not only in the USA, but internationally, as demonstrated successfully by our group [3, 4, 8, 12]. We have reported that a specific panel of CTC biomarker expressions could predict disease outcome in patients from phase II and III clinical trials of adjuvant immunotherapy [3, 5] and biochemotherapy [4]. Figure 1 is from a recent representative international CTC clinical phase III trial study analyzed by our assay for melanoma stage IV patients pre- and during randomized adjuvant melanoma cell vaccine and BCG therapy trial [3]. In this trial, CTC biomarker detection on both pretreatment and serial bleed specimens was significantly associated with both overall survival (*see* Fig. 1) and disease-free survival after complete metastasectomy.

2 Materials

Any enzymes should be used from the freezer just before preparing mixture.

2.1 PBL Isolation

1. Plastic tubes (15 mL).
2. Disposable sterile serological pipettes (10 mL).
3. Sterile Pasteur pipettes.
4. BD Vacutainer Tubes with 3.2 % buffered sodium citrate (BD) for blood specimen collection.
5. Purescript® RBC lysis solution (Gentra).
6. 1× Phosphate-buffered saline, (PBS, pH 7.4).

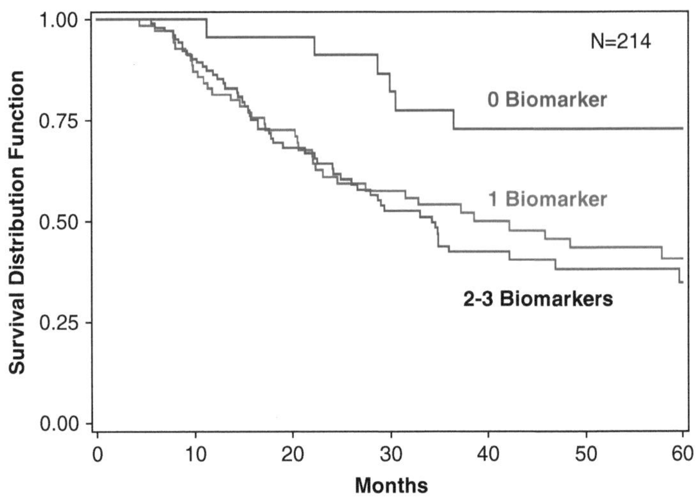

Fig. 1 Kaplan–Meier survival curves based on serial bleed specimens from the international phase III clinical trial of adjuvant melanoma cell vaccine plus BCG for melanoma stage IV patients pre and during adjuvant treatment CTC analysis. Blood specimens, which were collected before treatment (baseline), month 1 and 3, were analyzed by three mRNA biomarkers (MART-1, MAGE3, and PAX3). Overall survival was significantly worse for patients with >0 mRNA positive CTC biomarkers than those with no positive mRNA CTC biomarkers ($P = 0.012$). Reprinted with permission from Hoshimoto et al. [3]

2.2 RNA Extraction

1. Microcentrifuge tubes (1.5 mL).
2. TRI Reagent® for tissue homogenization (Molecular Research Center, Inc.).
3. Phase Separation Reagent: 1-bromo-3-chloro-propane (BCP) for RNA isolation (Molecular Research Center, Inc.).
4. 2-Propanol (isopropanol) (Fisher Scientific).
5. Ethyl alcohol (EtOH) 200 proof, ACS/USP grade.
6. RNA secure™ resuspension solution® (Life Technology).

2.3 RNA Quantification

1. Quanti-iT™ Ribogreen® RNA assay kit (Invitrogen).
2. Costar clear polystyrene 96-well plates (Fisher Scientific).
3. TE buffer (10 mM Tris–Cl, pH 7.5, 1 mM EDTA).

2.4 Reverse Transcription (RT)

1. First strand buffer (5×, VWR), stored at −30 °C.
2. 10 mM dNTPs (Roche Diagnostic), stored at −30 °C.
3. Oligo (dt) primer 333 ng/μL (Gene Link), stored at −30 °C.
4. RNasin (VWR) 20–40 u/μL, stored at −30 °C.
5. Moloney Murine Leukemia Virus (M-MLV) RT (VWR) 200 u/μL, stored at −30 °C.

Table 1
PCR primers

Designation	Name	Sequence	Amplicon size
Housekeeping 1	GAPDH	Forward: 5′-GGG TGT GAA CCA TGA GAA GT Reverse: 5′-GAC TGT GGT CAT GAG TCC T Probe (FAM): 5′-CAG CAA TGC CTC CTG CAC CAC CAA	136
CTC Marker 1	MART 1	Forward: 5′-AAA ACT GTG AAC CTG TGG TT Reverse: 5′-ATG TCT CAG GTG TCT CGC Probe (FAM): 5′-ATG AGA AAC TCT CTG CAG AAC AGT CA	110
CTC Marker 2	MAGE A3	Forward: 5′-AGG AGA AGA TCT GCC AGT GG Reverse: 5′-AGT GCT GAC TCC TCT GCT CA Probe (FAM): 5′-AGC TCC TGC CCA CAC TCC CGC CTG T	105
CTC Marker 3	PAX3	Forward: 5′-CAA TGG CCT CTC ACC TCA G Reverse: 5′-TGG TGG TAG GTT CCA GAC C Probe (FAM): 5′-CCA GAC TGA TTA CGC GCT CTC CC	116
CTC Marker 4	GalNAc-T	Reverse: 5′-CCA ACA CAG CAG ACA CAG TC Forward: 5′-GAT GTT GTA CTG GGC TCC CT Probe (FAM): 5′-ATG AGG CTG CTT TCA CTA TCC GCA	131

6. Molecular bio grade H2O, stored at room temperature.
7. PCR microtubes (0.6 mL), stored at room temperature.
8. Set heat blocks at the following temperatures: 70 °C, 37 °C, and 95 °C.

2.5 Polymerase Chain Reaction

1. PCR thermocycler (CFX96 Touch Real-Time PCR Detection System).
2. PCR primers (Integrated DNA Technologies) (*see* Table 1).
3. AccuQuant qPCR custom superMix w/ROX (2× , Quanta Biosciences, Inc): The formulation is 40 mM Tris pH 8.4, 100 mM KCl, 10 mM magnesium chloride, 0.4 mM dATP, 0.4 mM dCTP, 0.4 mM dGTP, 0.8 mM dUTP, 2× ROX reference dye, proprietary stabilizers and enhancers, 100 u/mL iTaq polymerase.

3 Methods

3.1 PBL and CTCs Isolation

1. Collect 9.0 mL peripheral blood into two tubes containing sodium citrate (4.5 mL) (pale blue top) (*see* **Notes 1** and **2**).
2. Fill each 15 mL tube with 10 mL Purescript RBC Lysis Solution (PLS), using a sterile 10 mL serological pipette.
3. Transfer 2 mL blood into 15 mL tubes and gently invert the tubes containing blood and PLS.
4. Incubate on their sides at 22–25 °C for 15 min.
5. Centrifuge at 300×*g* at 22–25 °C for 10 min (*see* **Note 3**).
6. Aspirate the supernatant. Avoid aspirating any part of the PBL white pellet.
7. Transfer 10 mL of RBC lysis buffer to one of the two 15 mL tubes containing the PBL and CTCs, using a new 10 mL pipette.
8. Pipette up and down carefully to resuspend the pellet well (*see* **Note 4**).
9. Transfer the entire volume of RBC lysis solution to the second 15 mL tube containing the PBL/CTCs.
10. Pipette up and down to combine the content of both tubes.
11. Centrifuge at 300×*g* at 22–25 °C for 5 min.
12. Aspirate the supernatant. Avoid aspirating any part of the white pellet containing PBL/CTCs.
13. Transfer 10 mL of PBS to the pellet with a new 10 mL serological pipette. Wash the pellet by pipetting up and down the solution.
14. Centrifuge at 300×*g* at 22–25 °C for 5 min.
15. Aspirate the supernatant. Avoid aspirating any part of the white pellet containing PBL/CTCs.
16. Immediately proceed to the RNA extraction step.

3.2 RNA Extraction

1. Transfer 1-mL of TRI Reagent to 15 mL tube containing PBL/CTCs pellet. Homogenize and lyse the PBL/CTCs thoroughly via pipetting (*see* **Note 5**).
2. Transfer contents to new 1.5-mL microcentrifuge tube.
3. Add 100 μL of the phase separation reagent (BCP) to the homogenate in the 1.5 mL microcentrifuge tube and vortex for 15–20 s.
4. Incubate the homogenized solution at 22–25 °C for 5 min.
5. Centrifuge at 17,000×*g* and 4 °C for 15 min.
6. Prepare a new 1.5 mL microcentrifuge Eppendorf tube (DNA/RNA free) for each specimen. Add 600 μL of isopropanol to the tubes, cap tightly, and set aside at room temperature.

7. Following centrifugation, gently transfer the top aqueous (RNA) layer into the isopropanol-containing 1.5 mL microcentrifuge tube (*see* **Note 6**).
8. Invert the tubes up and down 4 or 5 times to mix well and then store the samples overnight at −30 °C.
9. The following day, centrifuge the tube at 17,000 × *g* at 4 °C for 20 min. A white RNA pellet should be visible at the bottom of the microcentrifuge tube.
10. Decant the supernatant and remove excess isopropanol with a 200-μL pipettor.
11. Apply 1-mL of cold 75 % EtOH to the pellet. Perform a quick vortex to dislodge the pellet.
12. Centrifuge the tube at 17,000 × *g* and 4 °C for 5 min.
13. Decant the supernatant and remove excess EtOH with a 200-μL pipettor.
14. Dry the pellet using speed vacuuming for 2 min at room temperature (*see* **Note 7**).
15. Resuspend the dry pellet with 42 μL of pre-heated (60 °C for 10 min) RNA secure.
16. Incubate samples at 60 °C for 10 min.
17. The RNA can be used either immediately, or stored temporarily in RNA secure in 1.5-mL microcentrifuge tubes at −30 °C for 3–6 months or at −80 °C for up to 1 year.

3.3 RNA Quantification

Mix 2 μl RNA with 98 μl of 1× TE buffer according to Quanti-IT Ribogreen RNA assay kit's protocol.

3.4 Reverse Transcription

1. Label the cDNA samples with 0.6 mL PCR microtube.
2. For multimarker assay, add 5 μg RNA (5× assay) which is diluted in to 57.5 μL by molecular grade H_2O (*see* **Notes 8** and **9**).
3. Incubate the samples at 70 °C for 5 min.
4. Incubate the samples on ice for at least 5 min.
5. Prepare the following 42.5 μL RT-cocktail (5× assay) on ice; Mix 20 μL of 5× first strand buffer, 10 μL of 10 mM dNTPs, 10 μL of Oligo(dt) primer (333 ng/μL), 2.5 μL of RNasin (20–40 u/μL), and 5 μL of M-MLV RT (200 u/μL), for each well (*see* **Note 10**).
6. Add the 42.5 μL RT-cocktail volume to each 57.5 μL sample.
7. Incubate the samples at 37 °C for at least 2 h.
8. Incubate the samples at 95 °C for 5 min.
9. Transfer the samples on ice for 5 min.
10. Store the cDNA samples (100 μL) at −30 °C (*see* **Note 11**).

3.5 Polymerase Chain Reaction

1. Prepare 20 μl of PCR cocktail on ice; Mix 12.5 μL of QuantaBiosciences's supermix, 0.50 μL of forward primers, 0.50 μL of reverse primers (*see* Table 1), 0.15 μL of probe, and 6.35 μL of H_2O, for each well (see **Note 12**).
2. Distribute 20 μl of PCR cocktail into the 96-well plate on ice.
3. Add 5 μL cDNA template to each designated well. For PCR reagent control, add 5 μL of H_2O in place of cDNA.
4. Add standards to the designated wells in duplicates (*see* **Note 13**).
5. Seal the microplate with the microplate sealer.
6. Centrifuge the microplate at 400×*g* at 22–25 °C for 1 min (*see* **Note 14**).
7. Load the plate into the PCR thermocycler.
8. Program the thermocycler as follows: hold at 95 °C for 5 min, followed by 45 cycles of denaturation at 95 °C for 30 s, annealing at the following temperature for 30 s (55 °C; GAPDH, 55 °C; MART-1, 58 °C; MAGE-A3, 62 °C for PAX3 and GalNAc-T) and extension at 72 °C for 30 s, followed by final extension at 72 °C for 5 min (*see* **Notes 15–18**).

4 Notes

1. Before blood is collected, discard the first 1–2 mL of blood to prevent contamination with skin cells. Blood specimens should be kept at 20–25 °C and processed within 24 h of collection time.
2. All blood isolation should be performed inside sterile laminar-flow HEPA filter hood.
3. Avoid hard breaking of the centrifuge to keep PBL and CTCs pellet at the bottom of the tubes.
4. Avoid producing air bubbles.
5. Wipe pipettors with bleach-dampened paper towels and dry off the bleach.
6. Draw the top aqueous carefully without touching the organic/pink layer from the phase-separated sample in the 1.5-mL tube by 200 μL pipettor. If you touch and draw the organic/pink layer, it is better to discard the organic/pink layer.
7. Careful not to overdry the RNA pellet.
8. A total 1× volume equals to 11.5 μL.
9. Controls include as follows for all assay runs: 2 well-characterized melanoma cell lines for individual biomarker as positive controls, normal donor PBLs from healthy volunteers as negative controls, and RT reagent control (H_2O + reagent). Master bank for cell lines needs to be established for consistency of specific gene mRNA expression.

10. 8.5 μL RT-cocktail (1× assay) consists of the following volumes; Mix 4 μL of 5× first strand buffer, 2 μL of 10 mM dNTPs, 2 μL of Oligo(dt) primer (333 ng/μL), 0.5 μL of RNasin (20–40 u/μL), and 1 μL of M-MLV RT (200 u/μL), for each well.
11. The cDNA easily degrades if not stored properly, especially if there are several freeze & thaw cycles.
12. PCR reagent controls must be verified for individual lots and stored under General Laboratory Protocol (GLP) conditions. PCR primers should be used within 6 months from the synthesis date.
13. A standard curve for each assay is generated with tenfold serial dilutions of the specific gene plasmid templates (10^7–10^2 copies) [4].
14. Make sure that there are no bubbles at the bottom of the wells.
15. Several melanoma cell lines were run to establish positive controls at no later than PCR cycle #25. Normal PBLs were utilized for negative controls.
16. Glyceraldehyde-3-phosphate dehydrogenase (GAPDH) is used as an internal control. If the quantification cycle (Cq) value of GAPDH is higher than 30, the sample is excluded from the analysis.
17. All samples are assessed in triplicates, and the mean threshold values (Cq) are used to determine the patients' status. Cutoff threshold cycle for all biomarkers is 42. Any one-marker expressed by the CTC was set to establish a patient's positive PCR overall specimen status.
18. All studies must be under well-documented Standard Operating Procedures (SOP) and under GLP conditions.

Acknowledgements

This study was supported by Dr. Miriam & Sheldon G. Adelson Medical Research Foundation, Leslie and Susan Gonda (Goldshmied) Foundation (Los Angeles, CA), Ruth and Martin H. Weil Fund (Los Angeles, CA), and Grant No. P01 CA012582 Project II and Core from the National Institutes of Health/National Cancer Institute, USA. This work was supported in part by the fund from Japan Society for the Promotion of Science (JSPS) for the "Institutional Program for Young Researcher Overseas Visits."

References

1. Balch CM, Gershenwald JE, Soong SJ et al (2009) Final version of 2009 AJCC melanoma staging and classification. J Clin Oncol 27(36):6199–6206
2. AJCC Cancer Staging Manual (2010) In: Edge S, Byrd D, Compton C et al. (eds) 7th edn. Springer, NewYork, NY
3. Hoshimoto S, Faries MB, Morton DL et al (2011) Assessment of prognostic circulating tumor cells in a phase III trial of adjuvant immunotherapy after complete resection of stage IV melanoma. Ann Surg 255(2): 357–362

4. Koyanagi K, O'Day SJ, Gonzalez R et al (2005) Serial monitoring of circulating melanoma cells during neoadjuvant biochemotherapy for stage III melanoma: outcome prediction in a multicenter trial. J Clin Oncol 23(31):8057–8064
5. Hoon DS, Bostick P, Kuo C et al (2000) Molecular markers in blood as surrogate prognostic indicators of melanoma recurrence. Cancer Res 60(8):2253–2257
6. Nicholl MB, Elashoff D, Takeuchi H et al (2010) Molecular upstaging based on paraffin-embedded sentinel lymph nodes: ten-year follow-up confirms prognostic utility in melanoma patients. Ann Surg 253(1):116–122
7. Takeuchi H, Morton DL, Kuo C et al (2004) Prognostic significance of molecular upstaging of paraffin-embedded sentinel lymph nodes in melanoma patients. J Clin Oncol 22(13):2671–2680
8. Koyanagi K, O'Day SJ, Boasberg P et al (2010) Serial monitoring of circulating tumor cells predicts outcome of induction biochemotherapy plus maintenance biotherapy for metastatic melanoma. Clin Cancer Res 16(8): 2402–2408
9. Mocellin S, Hoon D, Ambrosi A et al (2006) The prognostic value of circulating tumor cells in patients with melanoma: a systematic review and meta-analysis. Clin Cancer Res 12(15): 4605–4613
10. Cristofanilli M, Budd GT, Ellis MJ et al (2004) Circulating tumor cells, disease progression, and survival in metastatic breast cancer. N Engl J Med 351(8):781–791
11. Kitago M, Koyanagi K, Nakamura T et al (2009) mRNA expression and BRAF mutation in circulating melanoma cells isolated from peripheral blood with high molecular weight melanoma-associated antigen-specific monoclonal antibody beads. Clin Chem 55(4):757–764
12. Koyanagi K, Kuo C, Nakagawa T et al (2005) Multimarker quantitative real-time PCR detection of circulating melanoma cells in peripheral blood: relation to disease stage in melanoma patients. Clin Chem 51(6):981–988

Chapter 28

Detection of Chondroitin Sulfate Proteoglycan 4 (CSPG4) in Melanoma

Yangyang Wang, Francesco Sabbatino, Xinhui Wang, and Soldano Ferrone

Abstract

The tumor antigen chondroitin sulfate proteoglycan 4 (CSPG4) appears to be a useful biomarker to identify melanoma cells and an attractive target to apply antibody-based immunotherapy for the treatment of melanoma. Here we described the reverse transcription-polymerase chain reaction (RT-PCR) method and the immunohistochemical (IHC) staining method to detect the expression of CSPG4 in melanoma cells and tissues.

Key words CSPG4, Melanoma, RT-PCR, IHC staining

1 Introduction

A large body of clinical evidence has convincingly shown that tumor antigen (TA)-specific monoclonal antibodies (mAb) can be effective in the treatment of various types of malignant diseases [1]. These clinical results are mediated by immunological and non-immunological mechanisms. The latter ones include the ability of TA-specific mAb to modulate signaling pathways associated with apoptosis, proliferation, survival, and migration of malignant cells [2, 3], while the former ones include the ability of TA-specific mAb to mediate complement- and cell-dependent lysis of tumor cells as well as to trigger or enhance a TA-specific T cell immune response [4–7].

In light of this information we have focused our studies on the membrane bound chondroitin sulfate proteoglycan 4 (CSPG4), a TA we had identified on human melanoma cells in the late 1970s–early 1980s, utilizing mouse mAb elicited with human melanoma cells [8, 9]. We named this antigen high molecular weight-melanoma associated antigen (HMW-MAA), because of the apparent restriction of its

Magdalena Thurin and Francesco M. Marincola (eds.), *Molecular Diagnostics for Melanoma: Methods and Protocols*, Methods in Molecular Biology, vol. 1102, DOI 10.1007/978-1-62703-727-3_28,

expression to melanoma cells in the initial studies and because of its large molecular size. CSPG4 consists of two components which share the same polypeptide moiety, but differ in the extent of glycosylation and chondroitin sulfate bound to it: the smaller and larger subunit have an approximate molecular weight (m.w.) of 260 and >440 kD, respectively.

CSPG4 has been the focus of our studies for the last 30 years, since this TA meets most, if not all the criteria required to be an attractive target of mAb-based immunotherapy. First, CSPG4 is highly expressed on malignant cells in various types of cancer and therefore is readily available to be targeted by antibodies. It is noteworthy that no effective therapy is available for most, if not all the types of cancer which express CSPG4. They include malignant melanoma, glioma, head and neck cancer, triple negative breast cancer, mesothelioma, chordoma, chondrosarcoma, and osteosarcoma [8–11]. Therefore the development of an effective CSPG4-targeted, mAb-based therapy would fulfill an unmet clinical need. Second, CSPG4 is expressed not only on differentiated cancer cells, but also on cancer initiating cells (CICs) at least in the tumor types we have analyzed [12]. They include malignant melanoma, head and neck cancer, and triple negative breast cancer. Therefore CSPG4 is expected to mediate the targeting not only of differentiated cancer cells, but also of CICs. According to the cancer stem cell theory [13, 14], CICs which are chemo- and radio-resistant and are tumorigenic in immunodeficient mice play a crucial role in metastatic spread and disease recurrence. Therefore these cells have to be eradicated in order to "cure" a malignant disease. Third, CSPG4 has limited heterogeneity in its expression both within a malignant tumor and among multiple metastases present in a patient; these findings are paralleled by the rather homogeneous expression of CSPG4 in cell lines. However it is noteworthy that there is molecular and cellular heterogeneity in the expression of mAb defined CSPG4 epitopes. This heterogeneity is likely to reflect variability in the extent of glycosylation of the polypeptide moiety of CSPG4, since carbohydrates have been shown to play an important role in the expression of the epitopes recognized by most of the human and mouse mAb which have been described in the literature and which have been characterized by us [15, 16]. A practical implication of this heterogeneity is the potential occurrence of false-negative results when tumor cells or pools of CSPG4 molecules are tested with a single CSPG4-specific mAb. Fourth, CSPG4 expression is stable as indicated by the limited changes in the percentage of stained tumor cells and in the staining intensity when CSPG4 expression by cell lines cultured in vitro for up to 6 months is monitored at monthly intervals by staining with mAb and flow-cytometric analysis. These in vitro findings are paralleled by the lack of marked changes in the expression level of CSPG4 we have observed in metastases removed at different times from a few patients with melanoma and stained with mAb. In addition we are aware of only one patient in whom induction of CSPG4-specific antibodies by active specific immunotherapy was associated with CSPG4 loss in one metastatic lesion. The very low frequency of CSPG4 loss when melanoma cells are exposed to selective pressure is compatible with a crucial role of CSPG4 in the biology of melanoma cells. As a result loss of CSPG4 may be incompatible with survival of melanoma cells. In this regard, several lines of evidence indicate that CSPG4 plays an important role in the proliferation, survival, and migration of malignant cells as it is involved with the related signaling pathways. These functional properties of CSPG4 provide a mechanism for the ability of CSPG4-specific mAb to inhibit the in vitro growth and migration of human malignant cells which express CSPG4 and their growth and metastatic spread in immunodeficient mice [10, 17]. Lastly CSPG4 has a restricted distribution in normal tissues [17]. This distribution may account for the lack of side effects when CSPG4-specific antibodies have been induced in patients by active specific immunotherapy [18, 19] or CSPG4-specific mAb have been administered to patients [8, 9].

CSPG4 is expressed in 80 % melanoma including various subtypes of cutaneous melanoma with the exception of acral lentiginous melanoma. In the latter subtype CSPG4 has a low expression in primary lesions, but has a high expression in metastatic lesions. CSPG4 is also commonly expressed in uveal melanoma. This distribution of CSPG4 has been taken as evidence to suggest its role in the metastatic spread of melanoma cells.

In summary, CSPG4 expression is associated with the metastatic potential of melanoma cells and at least in acral lentiginous melanoma with the disease aggressions. In addition, in vitro and in vivo studies suggest that targeting CSPG4 with antibodies reduces tumor growth. The clinical significance of these findings is suggested by the association between induction of CSPG4-specific antibodies by active specific immunotherapy and statistically significant increase in melanoma patients' survival. These data suggest that CSPG4 represents a prognostic marker associated with melanoma progression in acral lentiginous melanoma and potentially a marker to identify melanoma patients to be treated with CSPG4 targeted therapy. The tests described in this chapter could be useful for validation studies to determine clinical validity and utility of CSPG4 as a prognostic marker and a potential therapy target.

2 Materials

2.1 Patient Lesions

Lesions of melanocytic origin were obtained from patients who had undergone surgery. The diagnosis of melanoma lesions was based on histopathologic characteristics. Normal tissue microarray (Cat#FBN401) was purchased from US Biomax, Inc.

2.2 Cell Lines

1. The human melanoma M21 cell line [20] which expresses CSPG4 is used as a source of RNA for detection of CSPG4 by RT-PCR. The human melanoma cell line M14 [21], used as the negative control for CSPG4 expression. These cell lines are maintained in complete medium (CM) at 37 °C in a humidified 5 % CO_2 incubator.
2. The M14 cell line stably transfected with CSPG4 is used as the CSPG4-expressing cell line, M14/CSPG4 [21]. The M14/CSPG4 cell line is maintained in CM supplemented with 400 μg/mL geneticin (G418) (Life Technologies Corporation) at 37 °C in a humidified 5 % CO_2 incubator.

2.3 Solutions and Reagents for Cell Culture

1. Complete medium (CM): RPMI 1640 medium (Corning Incorporated), supplemented with 10 % Fetal Bovine Serum (FBS) (PAA Laboratories Inc.).
2. Geneticin (G418) (50 mg/mL; Life Technologies).
3. Phosphate buffered saline (PBS, pH 7.2–7.4).
4. Protease-free cell detachment solution: Dissolve 0.186 g of Ethylenediaminetetraacetic Acid, Disodium Salt Dihydrate (EDTA) in 500 mL of PBS.

2.4 Solutions and Reagents for Reverse Transcription-Polymerase Chain Reaction (RT-PCR)

1. TRIzol® Reagent (Life Technologies).
2. Chloroform (Thermo Fisher Scientific Inc.).
3. RNase-free water (Promega Corp.).
4. 75 % Ethanol (EtOH) in Milli-Q water.
5. Oligo $(dT)_{12-18}$ primer (500 μg/mL) (Life Technologies).
6. 10 mM dNTP Mix (Life Technologies).
7. M-MLV Reverse Transcriptase kit (M-MLV RT) (Life Technologies): Contains 40,000 U of M-MLV RT (200 U/μL); 5× First-Strand Buffer [250 mM Tris–HCl (pH 8.3), 375 mM KCl, 15 mM $MgCl_2$]; and 0.1 M DTT.
8. Taq DNA Polymerase kit (Life Technologies): Contains 100 U of Taq DNA polymerase (5 U/μL); 10× PCR buffer [200 mM Tris–HCl (pH 8.4), 500 mM KCl, Minus Mg]; and 50 mM $MgCl_2$.
9. Primers: CSPG4 forward primer (10 μM) (5′-TGGCCTTCACTGTCACTGTCC-3′); CSPG4 reverse primer (10 μM) (5′-CACTTGCTTCTGGGCCGTCACTCG-3′) [22]; β-actin forward primer (10 μM)(5′-CGTCTTCCCCTCCATCG-3′); and β-actin reverse primer (10 μM) (5′-CTCGTTAATGTCACGCAC-3′).
10. RNase/DNase-free PCR tubes (Thermo Fisher Scientific Inc.).
11. Gene Amp PCR System 9700 (Applied Biosystems).
12. AlphaImager™ 2200 Documentation System (Imgen Technologies).

2.5 Solutions and Reagents for Immunohistochemical (IHC) Staining of Tissue Sections

1. Fisher Protocol 10 % Buffered Formalin (10 % NBF) (Thermo Fisher Scientific Inc.).
2. 4 % paraformaldehyde (PFA) in PBS: Add 4 g of PFA to 80 mL of PBS in a 250 mL flask. Stir and heat the mixture up to 60 °C for at least 1 hour (h) and then allow it to cool down to room temperature. Bring the final volume to 100 mL with PBS.
3. 3 % hydrogen peroxide (H_2O_2) in Milli-Q water.
4. Antigen retrieval buffer: Dissolve 0.372 g EDTA in 800 mL of Milli-Q water in a 1.5 L flask. Add 0.63 mL of Tween 20. Adjust pH of the solution to 8.0 with 1 N NaOH. Bring the final volume of the solution to 1 l with Milli-Q water.
5. Tris-Buffered Saline with 0.1 % Tween 20 (TBS-T): Dissolve 8 g of NaCl, 0.2 g of KCl, and 3 g of Tris Base in 800 mL of Milli-Q water in a 1.5 L flask. Add 1 mL of Tween 20. Adjust pH of the solution to 7.4 using 36 % HCl. Bring the final volume of the solution to 1 L with Milli-Q water.
6. Blocking buffer A: Add 1 g of bovine serum albumin (BSA) (Thermo Fisher Scientific Inc.) and 5 mL of normal horse serum (NHS) (Thermo Fisher Scientific Inc.) to 100 mL of PBS.
7. Blocking buffer B: Add 1 g of BSA and 5 mL of NHS to 100 mL of TBS-T.
8. ABC solution: Dispense1 drop (about 50 μL) from each of the two bottles containing reagents A and B of the VECTASTAIN® ABC Elite Kit (Vector Laboratories, Inc.) in 10 mL of PBS. The mixture should stand for more than 30 min at room temperature before use.
9. Detection solution: Dispense 1 drop (around 50 μL) from the bottle containing Dako Liquid DAB (Dako North America, Inc.) in 1 mL of Substrate Chromogen System (Dako North America, Inc.) right before use.
10. Xylene (Thermo Fisher Scientific Inc.).
11. 70 % EtOH in Milli-Q water.
12. 90 % EtOH in Milli-Q water.
13. Mayer's Hematoxylin (Lillie's modification) (Dako North America, Inc.).
14. Depex Mounting Medium (Electron Microscopy Sciences).
15. Thermo Scientific HM 325 Manual Rotary Microtome (Thermo Fisher Scientific Inc.).
16. Optimum Cutting Temperature (OCT) Compound to embed cell lines prior to cryostat sectioning (VWR Corp.).
17. Tissue-TekCryomold Molds/Adapters (Sakura Finetek) for preparation of specimen blocks (VWR Corp.).
18. ImmEdge Hydrophobic Barrier Pen (Vector Laboratories, Inc.) to mark tissue section.

Table 1
mAb used in IHC staining of melanoma tissue sections

mAb	Isotype	Specificity
763.74	Mouse IgGl	CSPG4
VF1-TP41.2	Mouse IgGl	CSPG4
VT80.12	Mouse IgGl	CSPG4
D2.8.5-C4B8	Mouse IgGl	CSPG4
225.28	Mouse IgG2a	CSPG4
MK2-23	Mouse IgGl	An idiotope of the CSPG4-specific mAb 763.74
F3-C25	Mouse IgG2a	An idiotope of the HLA class II antigen-specific mAb CR11-462

2.6 Antibodies

1. The monoclonal antibodies (mAb) (Table 1) D2.8.5-C4B8, 763.74, VF1-TP41.2, VT80.12, all IgG1, and the mAb 225.28, an IgG2a, specific for distinct and spatially distant epitopes of CSPG4 [8, 12, 23, 24], the isotype-matched anti-idiotypic mAb MK2-23, an IgG1 [25], which recognizes an idiotope of the CSPG4-specific mAb 763.74, and the isotype-matched anti-idiotypic mAb F3-C25, an IgG2a [26], which recognizes an idiotope of the HLA class II antigen-specific mAb CR11-462 were developed and characterized as described previously.
2. mAb were purified either from mouse ascitic fluid or from spent medium of mAb producing hybridomas as described [27].
3. Dako EnVision+ System—HRP Labelled Polymer Anti-mouse is purchased from Dako North America, Inc.

3 Methods

3.1 Reverse Transcription-Polymerase Chain Reaction (RT-PCR) (Fig. 1)

3.1.1 Total RNA Extraction

1. Detach M21, M14, and M14/CSPG4 cells from one T-25 flask using 3 mL of cell Protease-free cell detachment solution; following a 3–5 min incubation at room temperature, add 10 mL of CM. Transfer the cell suspension to a sterile 15 mL falcon tube and centrifuge it at 307 ×*g* at room temperature for 4 min.
2. Remove medium, resuspend cells in 10 mL of PBS, and centrifuge tube at 307 ×*g* at room temperature for 4 min.
3. Remove PBS and lyse cells of each cell line with 1 mL of TRIzol® Reagent by pipetting cells up and down ten times at room temperature (*see* **Note 1**).
4. Incubate samples at room temperature for 5 min.
5. Add 0.2 mL of chloroform. Cap tubes securely.

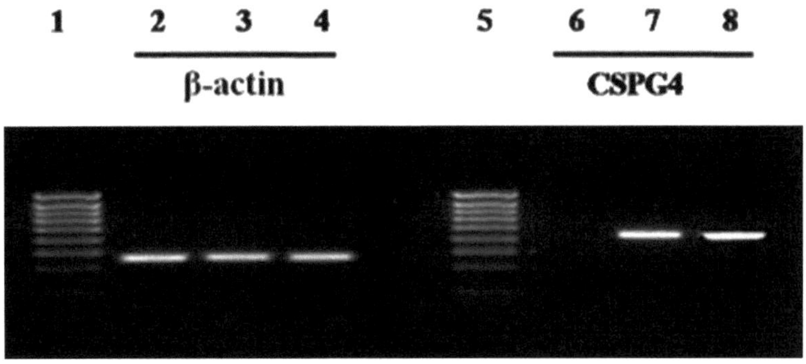

Fig. 1 Analysis of molecular characteristics of CSPG4 synthesized by cultured human melanoma cells M21. RT-PCR was performed on total RNA extracted from M21 cells (*lanes 4* and *8*) to amplify the CSPG4 cDNA, which generated a 439 bp fragment. The PCR product was analyzed using a 1.5 % agarose gel. The melanoma cell line M14, which does not express CSPG4 (*lanes 2* and *6*), and M14/CSPG4, which expresses CSPG4 following stable transfection with CSPG4 encoding plasmid DNA (*lanes 3* and *7*) were used as controls. The housekeeping gene β-actin (*lanes 2, 3,* and *4*) was used as an internal control of RT-PCR. *Lanes 1* and *5* show the DNA molecular markers

6. Shake tubes vigorously for 15 s.
7. Incubate tubes at room temperature for 3 min.
8. Centrifuge tubes at 12,000 × *g* at 4 °C for 15 min.
9. Carefully transfer aqueous phase (clear phase) to an RNase-free microfuge tube (*see* **Note 2**).
10. Add 500 μL of 100 % isopropanol.
11. Incubate tubes at room temperature for 10 min.
12. Centrifuge tubes at 12,000 × *g* for at 4 °C 10 min.
13. Discard supernatant carefully.
14. Add 1 mL of 75 % EtOH, vortex tubes for 10 s, and centrifuge them at 12,000 × *g* for at 4 °C 10 min.
15. Remove EtOH and add 1 mL of 75 % EtOH, vortex tubes for 10 s, and centrifuge them at 12,000 × *g* at 4 °C for 10 min.
16. Remove EtOH and allow RNA pellets to air-dry (*see* **Note 3**).
17. Add 30 μL of RNase-free water to RNA pellets and incubate tubes at 60 °C for 10 min.
18. Measure RNA concentration by Bio-Rad Smart Spec™ 3000 spectrophotometer (Bio-Rad Laboratories, Inc.) (*see* **Note 4**). Adjust RNA concentration to 0.5 μg/μL using RNase-free water.

3.1.2 First-Strand cDNA Synthesis Using M-MLV RT

1. Add 1 μL of 500 μg/mL oligo $(dT)_{12-18}$ primer, 1 μL of RNA (from RNA extraction), 1 μL of 10 mMdNTP Mix, and 9 μL of RNase-free water to a 0.2 mL RNase/DNase-free PCR

tube. There are total three tubes, and each tube contains RNA from one of the melanoma cell lines M21, M14, and M14/CSPG4.

2. Heat mixture to 65 °C for 5 min and chill on ice within 10 s.
3. Centrifuge tubes at 12,000 × *g* for 10 s and add 4 μL of 5× First-Strand Buffer and 2 μL of 0.1 M DTT to each tube.
4. Mix contents in each tube gently by pipetting five times and incubate each tube at 37 °C for 2 min.
5. Add 1 μL of M-MLV RT to each tube and incubate each tube at 37 °C for 50 min.
6. Heat the mixture at 70 °C for 15 min to stop the reaction.

3.1.3 Polymerase Chain Reaction (PCR)

1. Add 5 μL of 10× PCR buffer, 2 μL of 50 mM $MgCl_2$, 1 μL of 10 mM dNTP Mix, 1 μL of 10 μM forward primer and 1 μL of 10 μM reverse primer, 0.5 μL of Taq DNA polymerase, 1 μL of cDNA (from first-strand reaction) and 38.5 μL of autoclaved distilled water to a 0.2 mL RNase/DNase-free PCR tube. Layer 1–2 drops (~50 μL) of silicone oil over the reaction in each tube (*see* **Notes 5** and **6**).
2. In a Gene Amp PCR System 9700 heat the above cDNA mixture at 95 °C for 5 min prior to performing PCR under the following cycling conditions for 35 cycles: 94 °C for 30 s (denaturation), 58 °C for 1 min (annealing) and 72 °C for 1 min (extension), with a final extension of 10 min at 72 °C.
3. Electrophorese the resulting PCR products using a 1.5 % agarose gel with ethidium bromide.
4. Image the gel with AlphaImager™ 2200 Documentation System.

3.2 Immunohistochemical (IHC) Staining of Melanoma Tissue Sections

3.2.1 Preparation of Sections from Pelleted Cells Utilized as a Negative and a Positive Control for CSPG4 Expression. All Steps Are Performed at Room Temperature or as Specifically Indicated

1. Detach M14 and M14/CSPG4 cells from one T-175 flask using 10 mL of protease-free cell detachment solution; following a 3–5 min incubation, add 30 mL of CM. Transfer the cell suspension to a sterile 50 mL falcon tube and centrifuge it at 307 × *g* for 4 min (*see* **Note 7**).
2. Remove medium, resuspend cells in 30 mL of PBS, and centrifuge tube at 307 × *g* for 4 min.
3. Preparation of cell pellet-derived sections to be used as controls for IHC staining of frozen sections: add 3 mL of Optimum Cutting Temperature (OCT) Compound to cell pellet in a Tissue-TekCryomold Molds/Adapters (Sakura Finetek). Freeze it for 24 h at −80 °C and cut 8 μM tissue sections using a Thermo Scientific cryostat.
4. Preparation of cell pellet-derived sections to be used as controls for IHC staining of FFPE sections: Resuspend pelleted

cells in 30 mL of 10 % NBF for 24 h. Embed fixed cell pellet to make a paraffin embedded block in an automatic paraffin block maker. Cut 5 μM tissue sections of cell pellet blocks using a Manual Rotary Microtome.

3.2.2 IHC Staining of Frozen Melanoma Tissue Sections with CSPG4-Specific Mouse mAb or Mouse mAb Pool. All Steps Are Performed at Room Temperature or as Specifically Indicated (see Note 8*)*

1. Fix tissue sections using 4 % PFA in PBS for 20 min.
2. Wash tissue sections in PBS three times for 5 min each time.
3. Circumscribe tissue sections with ImmEdge Hydrophobic Barrier Pen.
4. Wash tissue sections in PBS twice for 5 min each time.
5. Apply 3 % H_2O_2 to tissue sections for 20 min.
6. Wash tissue sections in PBS twice for 5 min each time.
7. Incubate tissue sections with blocking buffer A for 30 min in a moist chamber.
8. Incubate tissue sections overnight at 4 °C with CSPG4-specific mAb: 225.28, mAb 763.74, mAbVF1-TP41.2, and/or mAb VT80.12 (*see* **Note 9**). mAb F3-C25 is used as a specificity control for mAb 225.28 and mAb MK2-23 is used as a specificity control for other CSPG4-specific mAb. The final concentration of individual mAb is 5 μg/mL in blocking buffer A when used as single mAb or when used in the mAb pool.
9. Wash tissue sections in PBS five times for 5 min each time.
10. Incubate tissue sections with Dako EnVision+ System—HRP Labelled Polymer Anti-mouse for 30 min in a moist chamber.
11. Wash tissue sections in PBS three times for 5 min each time.
12. Apply detection solution to tissue sections for 5 min (*see* **Note 10**).
13. Immerse tissue sections in Milli-Q water for 3 min.
14. Counterstain slides with Mayer's Hematoxylin (Lillie's modification) for 30 s.
15. Wash tissue sections with running water for 10 min.
16. To dehydrate tissue sections, incubate them in 70, 90, and 100 % EtOH. Each incubation is for 30 s. Then incubate tissue sections in xylene for 20 min.
17. Mount coverslip using Depex Mounting Medium.

3.2.3 IHC Staining of FFPE Melanoma Tissue Sections with CSPG4-Specific Mouse mAb or mAb Pool (Fig. 2). All Steps Are Performed at Room Temperature or as Specifically Indicated (see Note 8*)*

1. To deparaffinize/hydrate tissue sections, incubate them in xylene for 20 min. Then incubate tissue sections in 100, 90, and 70 % EtOH. Each incubation is for 30 s.
2. Wash tissue sections twice in Milli-Q water for 5 min each time.
3. Boil samples for 20 min in a slide jar containing 100 mL antigen retrieval buffer, and then cool down for 40 min (*see* **Note 11**).

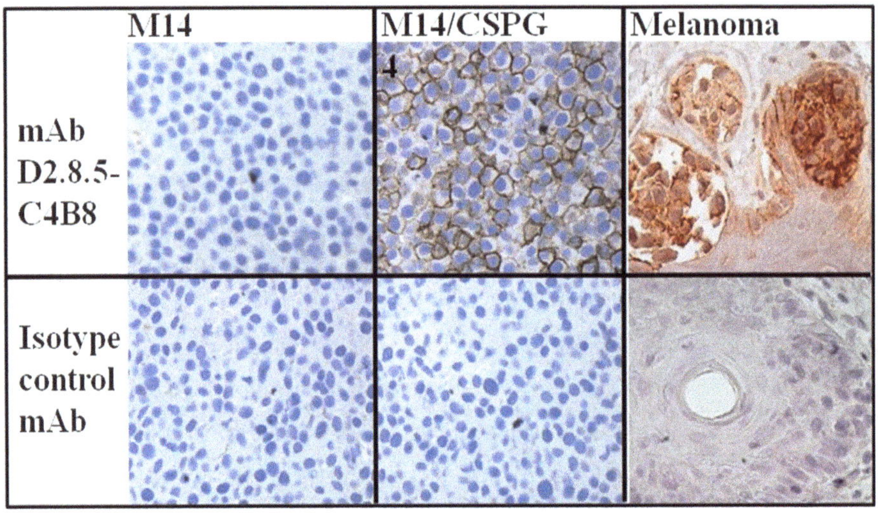

Fig. 2 IHC staining with CSPG4-specific mAb D2.8.5-C4B8 of an FFPE human melanoma tissue section. Strong CSPG4 staining of a human melanoma tissue section by mAb D2.8.5-C4B8 is shown. Cytoplasmic and membrane staining of the cell pellet positive control (M14/HMW) is shown. No staining of the cell pellet negative control (M14) is detected. The isotype-matched mAb MK2-23 is used as a specificity control

4. Wash tissue sections once in Milli-Q water for 3 min each time.
5. Circumscribe tissue section with ImmEdge Hydrophobic Barrier Pen.
6. Incubate slides in 3 % H_2O_2 for 20 min.
7. Wash tissue sections twice in TBS-T for 5 min each time.
8. Incubate slides with blocking buffer B for 30 min in a moist chamber.
9. Incubate tissue sections overnight at 4 °C with CSPG4-specific mAb: D2.8.5-C4B8, mAb 763.74, mAbVF1-TP41.2 and/or mAb VT80.12 (*see* **Note 9**). mAb MK2-23 is used as a specificity control for all CSPG4-specific mAb. The final concentration of individual mAb is 4 μg/mL in blocking buffer B.
10. Wash tissue sections five times in TBS-T for 5 min each time.
11. Incubate slides with Dako EnVision+ System—HRP Labelled Polymer Anti-mouse for 45 min in a moist chamber.
12. Wash tissue sections three times in TBS-T for 5 min each time.
13. Apply detection solution to tissue sections for 5 min (*see* **Note 10**).
14. Immerse tissue sections in Milli-Q water for 3 min.
15. Counterstain slides with Mayer's Hematoxylin (Lillie's modification) for 30 s.
16. Wash tissue sections with running water for 10 min each time.

17. To dehydrate tissue sections, incubate them in 70, 90, and 100 % EtOH. Each incubation is for 30 s. Then incubate tissue sections in xylene for 20 min.
18. Mount coverslip using Depex Mounting Medium.

3.2.4 Score the IHC Staining

1. Cytoplasmic and/or membrane staining is considered positive for CSPG4. The percentage of stained tumor cells is determined in 5 randomly chosen fields of the tissue sections. The staining intensity is graded by semiquantitative analysis by two investigators and categorized on a scale of 0, 1, 2 or 3+ representing negative, weak, intermediate, or strong staining intensity.
2. The average of the percentage of stained tumor cells and of the staining intensity in the five fields is utilized to calculate the IHC staining score. The IHC staining score is calculated by multiplying the staining intensity score value of 0–3 by the percentage of CSPG4 positive tumor cells for a final score of 0–300. Tumors with a score of at least of 200 are considered positive; those with a score of 100–199 are considered heterogeneous and those with a score less than 100 are considered negative.

4 Notes

1. During the RNA isolation all tubes and tips should be kept in a RNase-free condition to avoid RNA degradation.
2. The mixture separates into a lower red phenol–chloroform phase, an interphase, and a colorless upper aqueous phase. RNA remains exclusively in the aqueous phase. The upper aqueous phase is around 50 % of the total volume. Avoid drawing any of the interphase or organic layer into the pipette when removing the aqueous phase.
3. Do not allow RNA to dry completely, because the pellet can lose solubility.
4. The A_{260}–A_{280} ratio of extracted RNA should be above 1.8.
5. The addition of silicone oil to the PCR is not necessary in thermal cyclers equipped with a heated lid.
6. M14 and M14/CSPG4 RNA should be used each time as a negative and positive control, respectively, when performing RT-PCR for CSPG4. β-actin gene is amplified as endogenous control for RT-PCR.
7. When preparing cell pellet sections, Trypsin should be used to detach cells since CSPG4 is sensitive to Trypsin. M14 and M14/CSPG4 cell pellet-derived sections should be used each time as a negative and a positive control, respectively when performing IHC staining for CSPG4 expression.

These cell pellet-derived sections should also be used to optimize mAb concentration for IHC staining. The optimal mAb concentration is that which gives the strongest specific antigen staining with the lowest nonspecific background. After determining the optimum titer/dilution of the primary antibody, the secondary antibody dilution should be optimized.

8. Drying of tissue sections at each step should be avoided.
9. Because of the cellular and molecular heterogeneity in the expression of CSPG4 epitopes recognized by mAb, IHC staining of tissue sections should utilize a pool of mAb recognizing distinct CSPG4 epitopes and not single mAb to avoid false-negative results.
10. The incubation time following the addition of the detection solution in general ranges between 2 and 5 min. In each experiment this time has to be selected by monitoring the staining of the positive control and lack of background staining in the negative control.
11. For the antigen retrieval of FFPE sections, the tissue sections should be indirectly heated, not directly boiled. The slide jar containing tissue sections and antigen retrieval buffer should be heated in a 1,000 mL beaker with 500 mL of boiling Milli-Q water.

Acknowledgements

This work was supported by Susan G. Komen for the Cure Postdoctoral Fellowship Grant # KG111486; and by R01 CA110249 and R01-1CA138188 grants awarded by the National Cancer Institute.

References

1. Campoli M, Ferrone S (2009) Immunotherapy of malignant disease: the coming age of therapeutic monoclonal antibodies. In: DeVita V, Hellman S, Rosenberg S (eds) Cancer: principles and practice of oncology. Lippincott Williams and Wilkins, New York, NY, pp 1–18
2. Arteaga CL, Sliwkowski MX, Osborne CK, Perez EA, Puglisi F, Gianni L (2011) Treatment of HER2-positive breast cancer: current status and future perspectives. Nat Rev Clin Oncol 9:16–32
3. Seshacharyulu P, Ponnusamy MP, Haridas D, Jain M, Ganti AK, Batra SK (2012) Targeting the EGFR signaling pathway in cancer therapy. Expert Opin Ther Targets 16:15–31
4. Guermonprez P, Valladeau J, Zitvogel L, Thery C, Amigorena S (2002) Antigen presentation and T cell stimulation by dendritic cells. Ann Rev Immunol 20:621–667
5. Clynes R (2006) Antitumor antibodies in the treatment of cancer: Fc receptors link opsonic antibody with cellular immunity. Hematol Oncol Clin North Am 20:585–612
6. Boross P, Leusen JH (2012) Mechanisms of action of CD20 antibodies. Am J Cancer Res 2:676–690
7. Okroj M, Österborg A, Blom AM (2013) Effector mechanisms of anti-CD20 monoclonal antibodies in B cell malignancies. Cancer Treat Rev 39:632–639
8. Campoli MR, Chang CC, Kageshita T, Wang X, McCarthy JB, Ferrone S (2004) Human high molecular weight-melanoma-associated antigen (HMW-MAA): a melanoma cell surface

chondroitin sulfate proteoglycan (MSCP) with biological and clinical significance. Crit Rev Immunol 24:267–296
9. Campoli M, Ferrone S, Wang X (2010) Functional and clinical relevance of chondroitin sulfate proteoglycan 4. Adv Canc Res 109:73–121
10. Wang X, Osada T, Wang Y, Yu L, Sakakura K, Katayama A et al (2010) CSPG4 protein as a new target for the antibody-based immunotherapy of triple-negative breast cancer. J Natl Canc Inst 102:1496–1512
11. Rivera Z, Ferrone S, Wang X, Jube S, Yang H, Pass HI et al (2012) CSPG4 as a target of antibody-based immunotherapy for malignant mesothelioma. Clin Cancer Res 18:5352–5363
12. Wang X, Wang Y, Yu L, Sakakura K, Visus C, Schwab JH et al (2010) CSPG4 in cancer: multiple roles. Curr Mol Med 10:419–429
13. Marsden CG, Wright MJ, Pochampally R, Rowan BG (2009) Breast tumor-initiating cells isolated from patient core biopsies for study of hormone action. Meth Mol Biol 590:363–375
14. Visvader JE (2011) Cells of origin in cancer. Nature 469:314–322
15. Morgan AC Jr, Woodhouse C, Bartholemew R, Schroff R (1986) Human melanoma-associated antigens: analysis of antigenic heterogeneity by molecular, serologic and flow-cytometric approaches. Mol Immunol 23:193–200
16. Ziai MR, Imberti L, Nicotra MR, Badaracco G, Segatto O, Natali PG et al (1987) Analysis with monoclonal antibodies of the molecular and cellular heterogeneity of human high molecular weight melanoma associated antigen. Cancer Res 47:2474–2480
17. Wang X, Katayama A, Wang Y, Yu L, Favoino E, Sakakura K et al (2011) Functional characterization of an scFv-Fc antibody that immunotherapeutically targets the common cancer cell surface proteoglycan CSPG4. Cancer Res 71:7410–7422
18. Mittelman A, Chen ZJ, Yang H, Wong GY, Ferrone S (1992) Human high molecular weight melanoma-associated antigen (HMW-MAA) mimicry by mouse anti-idiotypic monoclonal antibody MK2-23: induction of humoral anti-HMW-MAA immunity and prolongation of survival in patients with stage IV melanoma. Proc Natl Acad Sci U S A 89:466–470
19. Mittelman A, Chen GZ, Wong GY, Liu C, Hirai S, Ferrone S (1995) Human high molecular weight-melanoma associated antigen mimicry by mouse anti-idiotypic monoclonal antibody MK2-23: modulation of the immunogenicity in patients with malignant melanoma. Clin Canc Res 1:705–713
20. McCabe RP, Quaranta V, Frugis L, Ferrone S, Reisfeld RA (1979) A radioimmunometric antibody-binding assay for evaluation of xenoantisera to melanoma-associated antigens. J Natl Cancer Inst 62:455–463
21. Luo W, Hsu JC, Tsao CY, Ko E, Wang X, Ferrone S (2005) Differential immunogenicity of two peptides isolated by high molecular weight-melanoma-associated antigen-specific monoclonal antibodies with different affinities. J Immunol 174:7104–7110
22. Luo W, Wang X, Kageshita T, Wakasugi S, Karpf AR, Ferrone S (2006) Regulation of high molecular weight-melanoma associated antigen (HMW-MAA) gene expression by promoter DNA methylation in human melanoma cells. Oncogene 25:2873–2884
23. Chen ZJ, Yang H, Kageshita T, Ferrone S (1991) Human high-molecular-weight melanoma-associated antigen mimicry by mouse antiidiotypic monoclonal antibody TK7-371. Cancer Res 51:4790–4797
24. Wilson BS, Imai K, Natali PG, Ferrone S (1981) Distribution and molecular characterization of a cell-surface and a cytoplasmic antigen detectable in human melanoma cells with monoclonal antibodies. Int J Cancer 28:293–300
25. Kusama M, Kageshita T, Chen ZJ, Ferrone S (1989) Characterization of syngeneic antiidiotypic monoclonal antibodies to murine anti-human high molecular weight melanoma-associated antigen monoclonal antibodies. J Immunol 143:3844–3852
26. Perosa F, Ferrone S (1988) Syngeneic antiidiotypic monoclonal antibodies to the murine anti-HLA-DR, DP monoclonal antibody CR11–462. Hum Immunol 23:255–269
27. Temponi M, Kageshita T, Perosa F, Ono R, Okada H, Ferrone S (1989) Purification of murine IgG monoclonal antibodies by precipitation with caprylic acid: comparison with other methods of purification. Hybridoma 8:85–95

Chapter 29

Targeting Damage-Associated Molecular Pattern Molecules (DAMPs) and DAMP Receptors in Melanoma

Brian A. Boone and Michael T. Lotze

Abstract

Damage-associated molecular pattern molecules (DAMPs) are proteins released from cells under stress due to nutrient deprivation, hypoxia, trauma, or treatment with chemotherapy, among a variety of other causes. When released, DAMPs activate innate immunity, providing a pathway to a systemic inflammatory response in the absence of infection. By regulating inflammation in the tumor microenvironment, promoting angiogenesis, and increasing autophagy with evasion of apoptosis, DAMPs facilitate cancer growth. DAMPs and DAMP receptors have a key role in melanoma pathogenesis. Due to their crucial role in the development of melanoma and chemoresistance, DAMPs represent intriguing targets at a time when novel treatments are desperately needed.

Key words Damage-associated molecular pattern molecules, DAMPs, DAMP receptors, RAGE, HMGB1, S100

1 Damage-Associated Molecular Pattern Molecules (DAMPs)

Pathogen-associated molecular pattern molecules (PAMPs), such as gram-negative derived lipopolysaccharide (LPS), induce systemic inflammation in response to infection. Widespread systemic inflammatory responses are also seen following traumatic injury and in non-pathogen-associated disease processes, suggesting that other signals exist to cause widespread innate immune activation in the absence of infection. In addition to PAMPs, there are additional proteins that can be secreted by cells to induce an inflammatory response following cellular injury, allowing the immune system to respond to damage/stress/"danger" not only from pathogens, but also toxins, mechanical damage, and in the setting of carcinogenesis [1]. Because these proteins are released in high levels by injured cells, and in consilience with so-called PAMPs or

Magdalena Thurin and Francesco M. Marincola (eds.), *Molecular Diagnostics for Melanoma: Methods and Protocols*, Methods in Molecular Biology, vol. 1102, DOI 10.1007/978-1-62703-727-3_29,

Pathogen-Associated Molecular Pattern molecules, they are termed damage-associated molecular pattern molecules (DAMPs) [2]. When cells undergo apoptotic cell death, there is a deliberate, scheduled process that results in clearance of cellular debris by phagocytosis and uptake by adjoining epithelial cells, resulting in minimal immune activation. However, cells that are injured, or die by necrosis, release factors, DAMPs, communicating to the host that cellular injury has occurred, activating an immune response and mobilizing repair mechanisms. The best studied DAMPs include HMGB1, the S100 family of molecules, heat shock proteins, uric acid, heparin sulfate, and ATP. Many DAMPs are found in the cytosol and result in significant immune response when released into the extracellular space by damaged cells, however not all DAMPs are intracellular. Hyaluronic acid in the extracellular matrix and complement in the plasma also serve as DAMPs. Additional molecules that are recognized as DAMPs are listed in Table 1. DAMPs signal through pathogen recognition receptors (PRRs) in a manner similar to PAMPs, including the Toll-like receptor family and the receptor for advanced glycation end products (RAGE). Additional DAMP receptors are listed in Table 2. DAMPs have been characterized in several disease processes including diabetes, cardiovascular disease, trauma, neurodegenerative disease, rheumatoid arthritis, and several cancers.

Table 1
A comprehensive list of recognized damage-associated molecular pattern molecules (DAMPs)

Damage-associated molecule patterns (DAMPs)	
HMGB1	Heparan sulfate
S100	Hyaluronic acid
Uric acid	Galectin
Heat shock protein	Cathelicidin
Complement	Defensins
RNA	Annexins
DNA	Nucleolin
ATP	Thymosins
Amyloid	

Table 2
A list of recognized DAMP receptors

DAMP receptors
RAGE
TLR 2
TLR 4
TIM-3
CD 24/Siglec 10
P2X7
TREM1

2 DAMPs in Melanoma

Chronic inflammation in the tumor microenvironment plays a key role in cancer pathogenesis. In melanoma, chronic inflammation is thought to result in a complex network of immunosuppression that allows malignant cells to escape immune surveillance. A better understanding of the pathways involved in the induction of chronic inflammation in melanoma is therefore of critical importance as mortality from the disease continues to increase. Several DAMPs have been implicated in the pathogenesis of melanoma. While several of these molecules have been established as prognostic markers, particularly in the case of S-100, research into how these molecules interact with immune cells in the tumor microenvironment and contribute to chronic inflammation is of critical importance. Additionally, several DAMPs represent therapeutic targets in melanoma at a time when novel therapies are desperately needed.

2.1 S100B and Related Proteins

The S100 protein family is made up of EF-hand calcium-binding proteins consisting of over 20 members [3]. The protein complex was named S100 because of its solubility in 100 % ammonium sulfate solution. S100 proteins have a broad range of functions, including extensive involvement in cell signaling, differentiation, motility, and transcriptional regulation. Several members of the S100 family are recognized as DAMPs and S100 proteins bind to the DAMP receptor RAGE [4].

S100 proteins are upregulated in a number of cancers [5]. S100 A2 and A6 are expressed at a high level in benign nevi and absent in malignant melanoma, suggesting a role in tumor suppression for melanoma [6]. S100A4 is expressed in malignant melanoma and is associated with a poor prognosis [7]. However, the focus of research for the study of S100 proteins in melanoma has been on S100B, which has been extensively evaluated as a prognostic marker. S100B has also been evaluated as a marker to determine lymph node status, to monitor response to treatment and for post treatment surveillance.

A likely mechanism for S100B role in melanoma tumorigenesis lies in its interaction with p53. S100B binds to p53 and inhibits its phosphorylation by protein kinase C, subsequently inhibiting p53 function, resulting in decreased apoptosis [8, 9]. Due to the close association of S100B and related proteins with melanoma, these proteins represent a novel treatment target for malignant melanoma. Based on the effects S100B has on p53 as previously described, prevention of the S100B/p53 complex formation could potentially restore the tumor suppressor and pro-apoptotic function of p53 in melanoma. The use of small interference RNA (siRNA) to inhibit S100B improves survival and restores p53 levels in melanoma cancer cells, demonstrating this concept [10]. A computer-aided drug design study to search for small molecule inhibitors of S100B identified 7 compounds that bind to S100B, 5 of which subsequently inhibited growth of primary melanoma cells [11]. One inhibitor, the FDA approved drug pentamidine isethionate, was discovered to bind S100B at the p53 binding site. Further study of pentamidine in melanoma by an independent group confirmed that pentamidine had growth inhibitory activity in human melanoma cells taken from 18 clinical tumors [12]. A phase II trial is reportedly underway (www.clinicaltrials.gov Identifier: NCT00729807) with anticipated completion in 2010, however there have been no updates on the trial since December 2009.

Targeting the transcription factors that regulate S100B represents an alternative method of targeting the DAMP in melanoma. The transcription factor HOCXII and SRC-1, its coactivator have been described in regulation of S100B and are significantly elevated in malignant melanoma tumors [13]. S100B expression was found to be dependent on both HOCXII and SRC-1 in melanoma cells. The authors demonstrated that the drug dasatinib, an Src/Abl inhibitor, inhibits S100B production in melanoma by targeting the HOXCII–SRC-1 interaction and preventing HOXCII binding to the S100B promoter. Preclinical trials of dasatinib in melanoma demonstrated inhibited growth in three of the five melanoma cell lines tested and as well as synergistic effects with the chemotherapy temozolomide. In this study, dasatinib induced apoptosis consistent with S100B inhibition and restoration of wild type p53 [14]. A Phase II trial of dasatinib in 39 patients demonstrated a significant amount of toxicity, requiring frequent dose reduction and/or interruption. Additionally disappointing was the response rate of only 5 % and median progression free survival limited to 8 weeks [15]. However, the authors noted improved response rates in patients with c-kit mutations and speculated that biomarker-based selection of patients for dasatinib might identify those patients most likely to respond to therapy. Additionally, administering dasatinib in combination with chemotherapy may improve response and survival.

There are several other novel treatments targeting S100 proteins that are less extensively studied and which require further development. Given elevated levels of S100A4 in melanoma and the association of S100A4 with poor prognosis, S100A is another target for melanoma therapy. Hofmeister et al. developed HLA-A1-restricted peptide epitopes to S100A4 capable of generating a T cell response and demonstrated cytotoxicity of S100A4 positive cells [16]. Such a strategy that generates an immune response to S100 proteins could bypass the antitumor immunosuppression seen in melanoma.

Another potential target of S100 protein family is the utilization of vitamin D analogs. The vitamin D analog Calcipotriol suppresses inflammation associated with S100A proteins that are involved in psoriasis [17]. Decreased vitamin D3 is a hypothesized risk factor for malignant melanoma, suggesting a potential role for treatment of vitamin D analogs in melanoma [18]. This potential treatment has not yet been evaluated for melanoma.

2.2 HMGB1

High mobility group box 1 (HMGB1) is a highly conserved nuclear protein and is well established as the prototypical DAMP. The protein was initially named HMG due to its rapid mobility on electrophoresis gels over 30 years ago [19]. The HMGB family consists of 3 members, HMGB1, HMGB2, and HMGB3, with HMGB4 only expressed during embryogenesis. HGMB1 is a 215-AA, 30 kDa protein and binds to DNA via two DNA-binding HMG boxes, the A-box (aa1-79) and the B-box (aa89-163), in addition to a negatively charged, acidic carboxyl terminal tail. HMGB2 has remarkably similar biologic activities as that of HMGB1 and is expressed at lower levels in hematopoietic cells; HMGB3 is primarily expressed in the testes.

HMGB1 has a two-fold function based on its location (Fig. 1). Inside the cell, HMGB1 functions as a DNA chaperone, participating in DNA replication, transcription and repair, and interacts with several transcription factors [20]. When HGMB1 is released extracellularly, either actively during infection or passively in response to cellular stress or necrosis, it binds RAGE, TLR 2, TLR 4, TLR9, TIM3, and CD24/Siglec 10 resulting in immune cell migration, activation, proliferation and differentiation. This inflammatory response serves as a "danger" signal, activating innate immunity in response to cellular stress. Extracellular HMGB1 results in endothelial cell activation, stromagenesis, recruitment and activation of innate immune cells and eventually leads to a chronic inflammatory state.

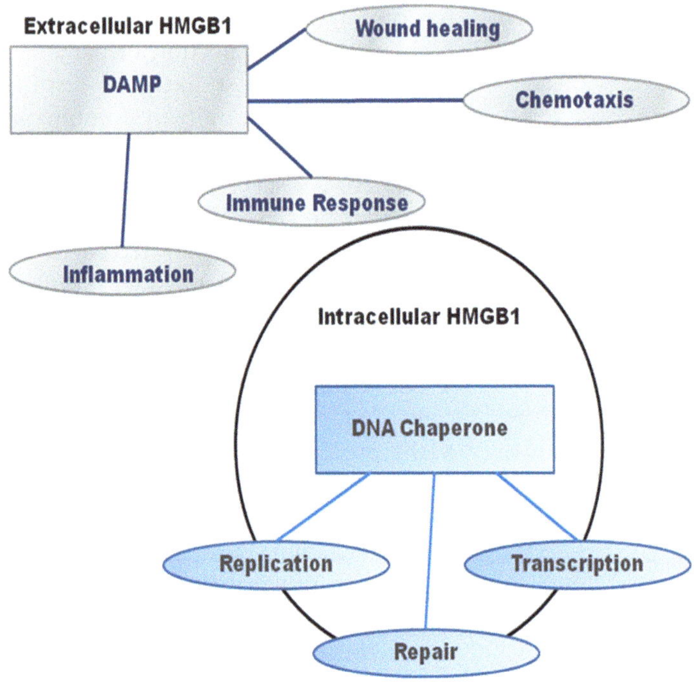

Fig. 1 HMGB 1 function based on location. HMGB1 has distinct roles based on its location. When HGMB1 is released outside the cell as a DAMP in response to cellular stress, inflammation and subsequent repair processes ensue. However, Intracellularly HMGB1 serves as a DNA chaperone, participating in DNA replication, transcription, and repair. Figure adapted from Tang et al. [20]

HMGB1 is intimately involved in development of several cancers and has roles in each of the hallmarks of cancer; including ability for replication, self-sufficient growth, angiogenesis, evasion of apoptosis, inflammation, tissue invasion and metastasis, and insensitivity to growth inhibitors (Fig. 2) [21]. The chronic inflammatory state that HMGB1 promotes in the tumor microenvironment leads to tumor cell survival, growth, and metastases. HMGB1 effects on carcinogenesis have also been demonstrated in melanoma. HMGB1 moves from the nucleus to the cytosol in human melanoma cells treated with NK and T cells and is ultimately released into the tumor microenvironment upon cytolysis [22]. In addition to serving as a danger signal following release after tumor treatment, HMGB1 contributes to development of melanoma through its interaction with melanoma inhibitory activity (MIA). MIA is a protein found in high levels in malignant melanoma but low levels in benign nevi that has been associated to increase further with melanoma progression [23]. HMGB1 regulates MIA expression by binding the highly conserved region (HCR) promoter element, demonstrating that it is an important regulator of melanoma progression [24]. Because of its multifactorial role in the development

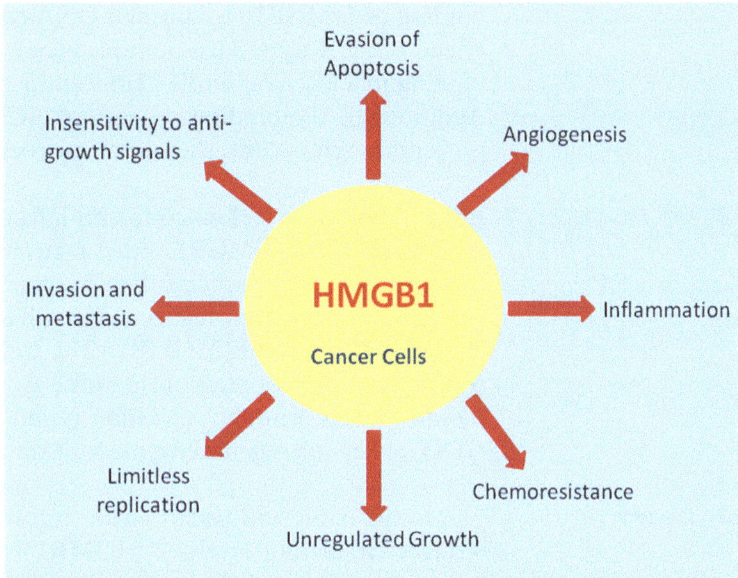

Fig. 2 HGMB1 promotes tumor growth in the tumor microenvironment. HMGB1 promotes each of the hallmarks of cancer, including ability for unregulated growth, angiogenesis, inflammation in the tumor microenvironment, resulting in development of locally invasive cancer and promoting metastases. Figure adapted from Tang et al. [21]

of melanoma, HGMB1 represents a novel treatment target in malignant melanoma. Fortunately, there are several treatments which target HGMB1 and its effects.

2.2.1 Platinum-Based Chemotherapy

The administration of platinum-based chemotherapy in melanoma has several advantages compared with other chemotherapeutic agents because this class of drugs limits the contribution of HMGB1 to melanoma progression. Oxaliplatin, which leads to predominately apoptotic cell death, results in retention of HMGB1 in the nucleus longer than other cytotoxic agents in melanoma cells [25]. This DAMP sequestration decreased chemotherapy-associated inflammation in the tumor microenvironment and may play a role in the clinical efficacy of platinum based chemotherapy. Additionally, it makes platinating agents the ideal agent to be combined with immunotherapeutic strategies because the sequestration of HMGB1 diminishes the antitumor immunosuppression in the tumor microenvironment. Several studies evaluating cisplatin in melanoma suggest a possible mechanism of HMGB1 sequestration by platinating agents. Cisplatin exerts its effects by damaging DNA, resulting in formation of DNA intrastrand cross-links which unwind and bend DNA. Because of its intracellular role as a DNA chaperone, HMGB1 binds to DNA altered by cisplatin. This tight binding of HMGB1 to damaged DNA correlates to the antitumor effects of the drug and has multiple beneficial effects [26]. HGMB1 binding may also play a role in preventing repair of damaged DNA. Additionally, the binding sequesters HGMB1 inside the nucleus, preventing release into the tumor microenvironment.

2.2.2 Ethyl Pyruvate

Ethyl pyruvate is a low-cost, anti-inflammatory compound that inhibits release of HMGB1. Ethyl pyruvate has been demonstrated to protective role in ischemia reperfusion injury, hemorrhagic shock and sepsis by preventing release of HMGB1 from the cell and decreasing levels of circulating HGMB1 [27]. In melanoma, ethyl pyruvate results in tumor suppression in vitro, as well as in in vivo isograft mouse models, through inhibition of indoleamine 2,3-dioxygenase (IDO), a key tolerogenic enzyme for many human tumors [28].

2.2.3 Quercetin

Quercetin is an antioxidant with anti-inflammatory effects that reduces circulating levels of HGMB1 in animal models of LPS induced sepsis by inhibiting its release [29]. Additionally, quercetin mediates down-regulation of mutant p53, suggesting a role as an anticancer treatment. Quercetin has lethal effects on melanoma cells and sensitizes cells to chemotherapy [30].

2.3 Galectins

Galectins are a family of proteins that share a unique carbohydrate recognition domain allowing them to bind to glycosylated proteins [31]. Galectins play a role in development of cancer and resistance to therapy by binding to cell surface molecules to initiate cell adhesion and eventual metastasis, as well as through signal transduction, apoptosis, and angiogenesis. Galectin-3 is expressed in human melanoma cells and correlates with disease outcome [32]. Galectin-1 has several roles promoting cancer growth and metastasis (Fig. 3). Galectin-1 has proangiogenic effects and is released under hypoxic conditions [33]. Additionally, galectin-1 promotes resistance to therapy [34] and evasion of host immune response by inducing apoptosis of activated T cells.

Because galectins contribute to melanoma carcinogenesis via multiple diverse pathways, targeting galectin in melanoma has intriguing therapeutic potential. Silencing galectin-3 in melanoma cells using siRNA significantly reduced the tumorigenic and metastatic potential of the cells, reinforcing their key role in carcinogenesis [35]. Citrus pectin is a complex polysaccharide capable of binding Galectin-3 that can also be used to target galectins in melanoma. pH modified citrus pectin inhibited melanoma cell adhesion to laminin and anchorage independent growth [36]. Citrus pectin also decreased metastases in an in vivo tumor lung metastases model [37]. Tumor growth, angiogenesis, and spontaneous metastases were significantly lower in mice given oral modified pectin [38]. Further study into targeting galectin in melanoma is warranted.

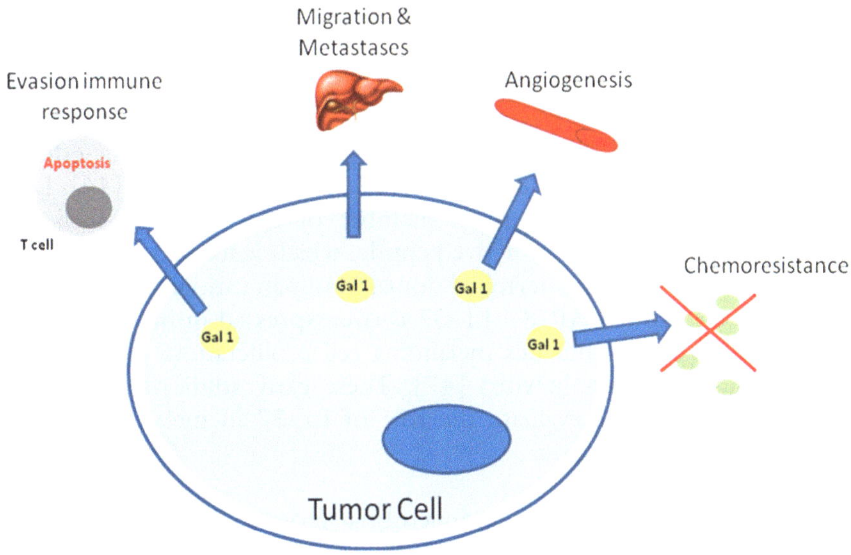

Fig. 3 Galectin-1 promotes tumor growth and metastases by several mechanisms including evasion from immunosurveillance, angiogenesis, chemoresistance, and cell migration and metastasis. Figure adapted from Lefranc et al. [34]

2.4 Heat Shock Protein

The heat shock proteins (HSPs) are a highly conserved protein family induced by stress named after their relative molecular mass. HSPs are molecular chaperones with crucial roles in protein stabilization and folding, contributing to carcinogenesis through increased angiogenesis and promotion of invasion and metastasis [39]. HSPs are upregulated in melanoma and correlate with prognosis [40].

Due to their chaperone function and ability to present tumor-associated antigens to antigen presenting cells, heat shock proteins represent a novel opportunity to improve anticancer vaccines [41]. HSP-based vaccines and vaccine adjuncts have been utilized in clinical trials of melanoma with phase I/II studies demonstrating an HSP vaccine to be safe and effective [42]; however, a Phase III study failed to show survival benefit on intention to treat analysis [43].

Development of inhibitors of HSP represents another novel treatment of melanoma utilizing DAMP targets. A selective inhibitor of HSP-90, SNX-2112, inhibits the growth of melanoma cells in vitro and induced apoptosis. The inhibitor also had growth inhibitory effects in a xenograft mouse model of melanoma [44].

2.5 Others DAMPS in Melanoma

2.5.1 ATP

Extracellular ATP is also a DAMP implicated in melanoma. Large amounts of ATP in the cytoplasm are released into the extracellular space in response to cellular stress or damage. ATP is released from melanoma cells in response to y-irradiation, suggesting DAMP release may be implicated in response to and resistance to radiation therapy [45]. Further exploration into the role of extracellular ATP in melanoma pathogenesis and potential treatment implications is warranted.

2.5.2 Cathelicidin

Cathelicidins are highly conserved antimicrobial peptides that are characterized as DAMPS. They have chemotactic effects on neutrophils, monocytes, T cells, and macrophages [46]. LL-37 is the only characterized member of the human cathelicidin family. LL-37 is the active peptide, which is formed by proteolysis of the inactive C-terminal domain Human cationic antimicrobial protein 18 (hCAP18). LL-37 is overexpressed in human melanoma cells and stimulates melanoma cell proliferation, migration, and invasiveness in vitro [47]. These early studies suggest future work should evaluate the role of LL-37 in melanoma treatment and progression.

2.5.3 Defensins

Defensins are antimicrobrial proteins that are chemotactic when released in response to stress [48]. Defensins have a role in mammalian pigmentation, but their precise role in melanoma pathogenesis remains undiscovered [49]. Harnessing the properties of defensins to promote antitumor NK and T cell responses is yet another mechanism utilizing DAMPs to treat melanoma. Vaccination with β-defensin 2 decreased the growth of implanted B16 melanoma cells and promoted the infiltration of T cells, NK cells, and macrophages, suggesting the potential for development of immunotherapy using defensins [50].

2.5.4 Nucleolin

Nucleolin is a RNA-binding protein that has broad function including DNA replication and repair, mRNA stability, and ribosome biosynthesis [51]. Abnormal patterns of nuclear positivity of nucleolin are present in melanoma, yet absent in benign lesions [52]. Additionally, the percentage of abnormal patterns was higher in primary melanoma than dysplastic nevi and higher in melanoma metastases than in primary disease. The abnormal patterns correlated with prognosis second only to thickness in predicting survival. These results suggest nucleolin may be useful as a biomarker or potential target for primary and metastatic melanoma.

3 DAMP Receptors in Melanoma

3.1 Receptor for Advanced Glycation End Products (RAGE)

The receptor for advanced glycation end products (RAGE) is the prototypical DAMP receptor. RAGE is a member of the immunoglobulin super family encoded in the Class III region of the major histocompatibility complex. RAGE plays a crucial role in regulating inflammation, metabolism, and autophagic/apoptotic flux in the setting of stress [53]. RAGE ligands include a large number of DAMPs (Fig. 4).

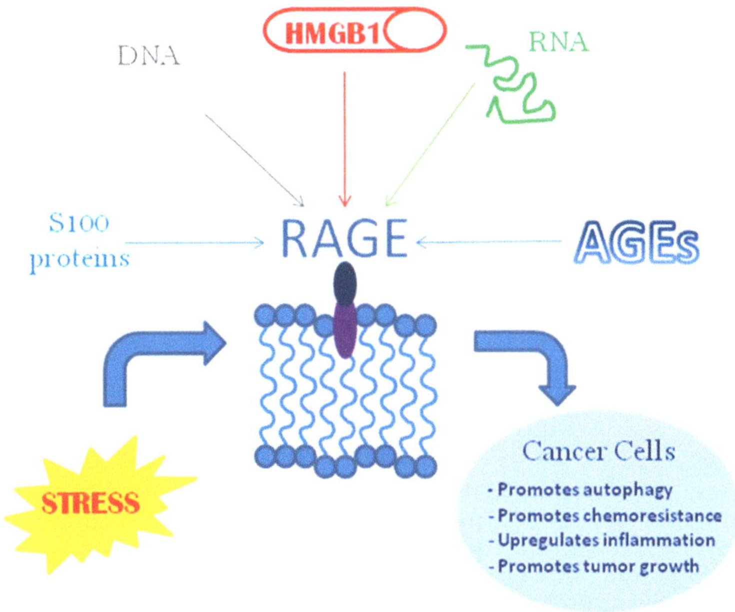

Fig. 4 RAGE ligands. Cellular stress leads to upregulation of RAGE as well as several DAMPs which serve as RAGE ligands. This binding interaction facilitates cancer cell growth by stimulating autophagy, promoting chemoresistance, and increasing inflammation in the tumor microenvironment. Figure adapted from Sims et al. [79]

RAGE has been detected in melanoma tissue and human melanoma cells [54]. In survey of 40 human melanoma tumor samples, RAGE showed slightly increased transcription in Stage IV melanoma [55]. RAGE transcription levels had relatively low variance compared to S100 protein transcription levels. Additionally, soluble RAGE (sRAGE), which is a RAGE antagonist, is under expressed in melanoma compared to normal skin.

Advanced glycation end products (AGEs), which bind RAGE, are formed in sun exposed skin and generate oxygen radicals thought to be involved in melanoma carcinogenesis [56]. AGEs stimulate the growth, migration, and invasion of human melanoma cells in vitro [57]. Tumor formation in melanoma cell xenografts in athymic mice was prevented by treatment with anti-RAGE antibodies. When mice with significant tumor burden were treated, anti-RAGE antibodies resulted in prolonged survival and decreased formation of spontaneous pulmonary metastasis compared to untreated animals. These studies suggest that RAGE has a role in pathogenesis of melanoma and it is a potential target for treatment, with promising results in preliminary in vivo studies.

A COOH-terminal motif of HMGB1 has been identified as being responsible for binding to RAGE, which effectively blocks RAGE and inhibits downstream functions. Administration of this peptide resulted in decreased migration of fibrosarcoma cells and inhibited formation of pulmonary metastases in an in vivo model. While this binding motif has not been studied in melanoma, the study demonstrates that RAGE inhibition results in therapeutic effects and similar results would likely be discovered in melanoma models.

RAGE is typically expressed in a membrane-bound form; however, protelytic cleavage and alternative mRNA splicing can result in a soluble isoform that lacks transmembrane and cytoplasmic domains, known as soluble RAGE (sRAGE) [53]. sRAGE acts as a decoy receptor by binding DAMPs and antagonizing RAGE, making it a potential therapeutic tool against RAGE induced chronic inflammation and carcinogenesis [58]. While administration of sRAGE has been shown to suppress the growth of tumor cells in animal studies, it has not been evaluated specifically in melanoma [59]. The preliminary success of sRAGE in suppressing tumor growth suggests that blocking RAGE may have therapeutic benefit in melanoma and other cancers. Small antagonistic peptides have been designed and when administered in vivo results in reduced growth and metastasis of pancreatic and glioma tumors [60]. The use of antagonist peptides against RAGE have not been evaluated for treatment of melanoma, but this is a novel treatment that warrants further investigation.

3.2 TIM-3

T cell immunoglobulin and muc domain-3 (TIM-3) was first identified as a receptor on T helper type 1 cells that when bound by galectin-9 resulted in apoptosis [61]. TIM-3 is now known to be expressed on a variety of immune cells and contributes to chronic inflammation. TIM-3 is bound by several DAMP ligands in addition to galectin, including HMGB1. It is the binding of HGMB1 but not galectin-9 that regulates regulation receptor-mediated innate immune response [62].

TIM-3 is expressed in melanoma cells at higher levels than melanocytes and thought to play a key role in local immunosuppression and metastasis formation in melanoma [63]. TIM-3 is upregulated on mast cells found in tumor following TGF-β administration, suggesting that TIM-3 is important for tumor immunosuppression, as TGF-β is known to inhibit T-cell proliferation and drives conversion from CD4+CD25- T cells to CD4+CD25+ T regulatory cells. Administration of TLR 4 ligand results in upregulation of TIM-3 expression in tumor-associated endothelial cells, suggesting the receptor plays a role in communication between the tumor and endothelial cells [64]. TIM-3 activates the NF-κB pathway in melanoma cells, which promoted proliferation and diminished apoptosis. Additionally, TIM-3 was found to increase tumor cell metastatic potential. Upregulation of TIM-3 is associated with tumor-antigen specific CD8+ T cell dysfunction, resulting in decreases of IFN-y, TNF, and IL-2 and contribute to the tumor immune escape seen in melanoma [65].

Targeting TIM-3 has been demonstrated to be effective in treating melanoma in preclinical studies. Monoclonal antibody blockade or deletion of TIM-3 enhanced the antitumor effects of plasmid DNA in a model of melanoma subcutaneous tumors by overcoming TIM-3-mediated suppression of the innate immune response to treatment [62]. Additionally, TIM-3 blockade enhanced the effects of chemotherapy, suggesting TIM-3 inhibition could have a synergistic role in combination with current treatment regimens.

3.3 Toll- Like Receptors (TLRs)

Toll- like receptors (TLRs) were initially discovered in *Drosophila* in the 1980s. Activation of Toll pathway resulted in antimicrobial peptides that were essential for defense against pathogens, given that *Drosophila* lack an adaptive immune response. TLRs are pattern recognition receptors crucial for defense against invading pathogens, however there is extensive evidence that TLRs, particularly TLR 2 and TLR 4, are DAMP receptors that respond to nonmicrobial endogenous danger signals [66, 67].

TLRs play in a role in melanoma in addition to several other cancers. TLR 2, 3, 4, 7, and 9 have all been showed to be expressed in human melanocytes [68, 69]. TLR 4 has an important function in murine skin tumorigenesis by promoting a chronic inflammatory state that is HMGB1 dependent [70]. The precise role of TLRs in cancer is incompletely understood and there is significant debate regarding whether treatment should target TLR agonists or antagonists [71, 72]. Despite having been shown to regulate tumor immunosuppressive properties, TLR 4 has been suggested to have a beneficial role in promoting antitumor immunity in melanoma in preliminary studies [73–75]. Much of the work on TLR in melanoma has been on agonist for TLR 7 and 9, which have resulted in several clinical trials suggesting TLR agonists can stimulate innate immune response to treat tumor [76]. In contrast, blocking TLR 2 resulted in a reduction of pulmonary metastases and increased the survival in a mouse melanoma model [77]. TLR 2 blockade in combination with TLR 9 agonists result in synergistic suppression of melanoma metastases in animal models, with treatment resulting in increased infiltration of NK and cytotoxic T cells and decreases in T regulatory cells [78]. This study suggests that utilizing TLR 2 antagonist in combination with TLR 9 agonists promotes antitumor response by eliminating immunosuppressive factors in the tumor environment.

4 Conclusions

DAMPs play a critical role in melanoma carcinogenesis and progression to metastases. Therapeutic targeting of DAMPs and DAMP receptors has tremendous potential at a time when novel therapies are desperately needed. A number of targets have been identified and found to be effective in preliminary preclinical models. Further work to characterize the role of DAMPs in melanoma progression and further explore avenues for targeting DAMPs in clinical treatment of melanoma is warranted.

References

1. Matzinger P (2002) The danger model: a renewed sense of self. Science 296:301–305
2. Lotze MT, Zeh HJ, Rubartelli A et al (2007) The grateful dead: damage-associated molecular pattern molecules and reduction/oxidation regulate immunity. Immunol Rev 220:60–81
3. Marenholz I, Heizmann CW, Fritz G (2004) S100 proteins in mouse and man: from evolution to function and pathology (including an update of the nomenclature). Biochem Biophys Res Commun 322:1111–1122
4. Leclerc E, Fritz G, Vetter SW, Heizmann CW (2009) Binding of S100 proteins to RAGE: an update. Biochim Biophys Acta 1793: 993–1007
5. Ilg EC, Schafer BW, Heizmann CW (1996) Expression pattern of S100 calcium-binding proteins in human tumors. Int J Cancer 68: 325–332
6. Maelandsmo GM, Florenes VA, Mellingsaeter T et al (1997) Differential expression patterns of S100A2, S100A4 and S100A6 during progression of human malignant melanoma. Int J Cancer 74:464–469
7. Helfman DM, Kim EJ, Lukanidin E, Grigorian M (2005) The metastasis associated protein S100A4: role in tumour progression and metastasis. Br J Cancer 92:1955–1958
8. Baudier J, Delphin C, Grunwald D et al (1992) Characterization of the tumor suppressor protein p53 as a protein kinase C substrate and a S100b-binding protein. Proc Natl Acad Sci U S A 89:11627–11631
9. Lin J, Yang Q, Wilder PT et al (2010) The calcium-binding protein S100B down-regulates p53 and apoptosis in malignant melanoma. J Biol Chem 285:27487–27498
10. Lin J, Yang Q, Yan Z et al (2004) Inhibiting S100B restores p53 levels in primary malignant melanoma cancer cells. J Biol Chem 279: 34071–34077
11. Markowitz J, Chen I, Gitti R et al (2004) Identification and characterization of small molecule inhibitors of the calcium-dependent S100B-p53 tumor suppressor interaction. J Med Chem 47:5085–5093
12. Smith J, Stewart BJ, Glaysher S et al (2010) The effect of pentamidine on melanoma ex vivo. Anticancer Drugs 21:181–185
13. deBlacam C, Byrne C, Hughes E et al (2011) HOXC11-SRC-1 regulation of S100beta in cutaneous melanoma: new targets for the kinase inhibitor dasatinib. Br J Cancer 105: 118–123
14. Eustace AJ, Crown J, Clynes M, O'Donovan N (2008) Preclinical evaluation of dasatinib, a potent Src kinase inhibitor, in melanoma cell lines. J Transl Med 6:53
15. Kluger HM, Dudek AZ, McCann C et al (2011) A phase 2 trial of dasatinib in advanced melanoma. Cancer 117:2202–2208
16. Hofmeister-Mueller V, Vetter-Kauczok CS, Ullrich R et al (2009) Immunogenicity of HLA-A1-restricted peptides derived from S100A4 (metastasin 1) in melanoma patients. Cancer Immunol Immunother 58:1265–1273
17. Hegyi Z, Zwicker S, Bureik D et al (2012) Vitamin D analog calcipotriol suppresses the Th17 cytokine-induced proinflammatory S100 "alarmins" psoriasin (S100A7) and koebnerisin (S100A15) in psoriasis. J Invest Dermatol 132:1416–1424
18. Godar DE, Landry RJ, Lucas AD (2009) Increased UVA exposures and decreased cutaneous vitamin D(3) levels may be responsible for the increasing incidence of melanoma. Med Hypotheses 72:434–443
19. Goodwin GH, Johns EW (1977) The isolation and purification of the high mobility group (HMG) nonhistone chromosomal proteins. Methods Cell Biol 16:257–267
20. Tang D, Kang R, Zeh HJ 3rd, Lotze MT (2011) High-mobility group box 1, oxidative stress, and disease. Antioxid Redox Signal 14:1315–1335
21. Tang D, Kang R, Zeh HJ 3rd, Lotze MT (2010) High-mobility group box 1 and cancer. Biochim Biophys Acta 1799:131–140
22. Ito N, DeMarco RA, Mailliard RB et al (2007) Cytolytic cells induce HMGB1 release from melanoma cell lines. J Leukoc Biol 81:75–83
23. Perez RP, Zhang P, Bosserhoff AK et al (2000) Expression of melanoma inhibitory activity in melanoma and nonmelanoma tissue specimens. Hum Pathol 31:1381–1388
24. Poser I, Golob M, Buettner R, Bosserhoff AK (2003) Upregulation of HMG1 leads to melanoma inhibitory activity expression in malignant melanoma cells and contributes to their malignancy phenotype. Mol Cell Biol 23: 2991–2998
25. Dong Xda E, Ito N, Lotze MT et al (2007) High mobility group box I (HMGB1) release

from tumor cells after treatment: implications for development of targeted chemoimmunotherapy. J Immunother 30:596–606
26. Pasheva EA, Ugrinova I, Spassovska NC, Pashev IG (2002) The binding affinity of HMG1 protein to DNA modified by cis-platin and its analogs correlates with their antitumor activity. Int J Biochem Cell Biol 34:87–92
27. Ulloa L, Ochani M, Yang H et al (2002) Ethyl pyruvate prevents lethality in mice with established lethal sepsis and systemic inflammation. Proc Natl Acad Sci U S A 99:12351–12356
28. Muller AJ, DuHadaway JB, Jaller D et al (2010) Immunotherapeutic suppression of indoleamine 2,3-dioxygenase and tumor growth with ethyl pyruvate. Cancer Res 70:1845–1853
29. Tang D, Kang R, Xiao W et al (2009) Quercetin prevents LPS-induced high-mobility group box 1 release and proinflammatory function. Am J Respir Cell Mol Biol 41:651–660
30. Rosner K, Ropke C, Pless V, Skovgaard GL (2006) Late type apoptosis and apoptosis free lethal effect of quercetin in human melanoma. Biosci Biotechnol Biochem 70:2169–2177
31. Camby I, Le Mercier M, Lefranc F, Kiss R (2006) Galectin-1: a small protein with major functions. Glycobiology 16:137R–157R
32. Vereecken P, Debray C, Petein M et al (2005) Expression of galectin-3 in primary and metastatic melanoma: immunohistochemical studies on human lesions and nude mice xenograft tumors. Arch Dermatol Res 296:353–358
33. Le QT, Shi G, Cao H et al (2005) Galectin-1: a link between tumor hypoxia and tumor immune privilege. J Clin Oncol 23:8932–8941
34. Lefranc F, Mathieu V, Kiss R (2011) Galectin-1-mediated biochemical controls of melanoma and glioma aggressive behavior. World J Biol Chem 2:193–201
35. Mourad-Zeidan AA, Melnikova VO, Wang H et al (2008) Expression profiling of Galectin-3-depleted melanoma cells reveals its major role in melanoma cell plasticity and vasculogenic mimicry. Am J Pathol 173:1839–1852
36. Inohara H, Raz A (1994) Effects of natural complex carbohydrate (citrus pectin) on murine melanoma cell properties related to galectin-3 functions. Glycoconj J 11:527–532
37. Platt D, Raz A (1992) Modulation of the lung colonization of B16-F1 melanoma cells by citrus pectin. J Natl Cancer Inst 84:438–442
38. Nangia-Makker P, Hogan V, Honjo Y et al (2002) Inhibition of human cancer cell growth and metastasis in nude mice by oral intake of modified citrus pectin. J Natl Cancer Inst 94: 1854–1862
39. Calderwood SK, Khaleque MA, Sawyer DB, Ciocca DR (2006) Heat shock proteins in cancer: chaperones of tumorigenesis. Trends Biochem Sci 31:164–172
40. Shipp C, Weide B, Derhovanessian E, Pawelec G (2012) Hsps are up-regulated in melanoma tissue and correlate with patient clinical parameters. Cell Stress Chaperones 18(2):145–154
41. Ciocca DR, Cayado-Gutierrez N, Maccioni M, Cuello-Carrion FD (2012) Heat shock proteins (HSPs) based anti-cancer vaccines. Curr Mol Med 12(9):1183–1197
42. Pilla L, Patuzzo R, Rivoltini L et al (2006) A phase II trial of vaccination with autologous, tumor-derived heat-shock protein peptide complexes Gp96, in combination with GM-CSF and interferon-alpha in metastatic melanoma patients. Cancer Immunol Immunother 55:958–968
43. Testori A, Richards J, Whitman E et al (2008) Phase III comparison of vitespen, an autologous tumor-derived heat shock protein gp96 peptide complex vaccine, with physician's choice of treatment for stage IV melanoma: the C-100-21 Study Group. J Clin Oncol 26:955–962
44. Liu KS, Ding WC, Wang SX et al (2012) The heat shock protein 90 inhibitor SNX-2112 inhibits B16 melanoma cell growth in vitro and in vivo. Oncol Rep 27:1904–1910
45. Ohshima Y, Tsukimoto M, Takenouchi T et al (2010) gamma-Irradiation induces P2X(7) receptor-dependent ATP release from B16 melanoma cells. Biochim Biophys Acta 1800: 40–46
46. Zanetti M (2004) Cathelicidins, multifunctional peptides of the innate immunity. J Leukoc Biol 75:39–48
47. Kim JE, Kim HJ, Choi JM et al (2010) The antimicrobial peptide human cationic antimicrobial protein-18/cathelicidin LL-37 as a putative growth factor for malignant melanoma. Br J Dermatol 163:959–967
48. Territo MC, Ganz T, Selsted ME, Lehrer R (1989) Monocyte-chemotactic activity of defensins from human neutrophils. J Clin Invest 84:2017–2020
49. Fernandez LP, Milne RL, Pita G et al (2009) Human beta-defensins (HBD1 and HBD3) and malignant melanoma susceptibility. Melanoma Res 19:340–341
50. Mei HF, Jin XB, Zhu JY et al (2012) Beta-defensin 2 as an adjuvant promotes anti-melanoma immune responses and inhibits the growth of implanted murine melanoma in vivo. PLoS One 7:e31328
51. Abdelmohsen K, Gorospe M (2012) RNA-binding protein nucleolin in disease. RNA Biol 9(6):799–808
52. Mourmouras V, Cevenini G, Cosci E et al (2009) Nucleolin protein expression in cutaneous melanocytic lesions. J Cutan Pathol 36: 637–646
53. Sparvero LJ, Asafu-Adjei D, Kang R et al (2009) RAGE (receptor for advanced glycation

endproducts), RAGE ligands, and their role in cancer and inflammation. J Transl Med 7:17
54. Eichmuller S, Usener D, Jochim A, Schadendorf D (2002) mRNA expression of tumor-associated antigens in melanoma tissues and cell lines. Exp Dermatol 11:292–301
55. Leclerc E, Heizmann CW, Vetter SW (2009) RAGE and S100 protein transcription levels are highly variable in human melanoma tumors and cells. Gen Physiol Biophys 28 Spec No Focus:F65–F75
56. Masaki H, Okano Y, Sakurai H (1999) Generation of active oxygen species from advanced glycation end-products (AGEs) during ultraviolet light A (UVA) irradiation and a possible mechanism for cell damaging. Biochim Biophys Acta 1428:45–56
57. Abe R, Shimizu T, Sugawara H et al (2004) Regulation of human melanoma growth and metastasis by AGE-AGE receptor interactions. J Invest Dermatol 122:461–467
58. Raucci A, Cugusi S, Antonelli A et al (2008) A soluble form of the receptor for advanced glycation endproducts (RAGE) is produced by proteolytic cleavage of the membrane-bound form by the sheddase a disintegrin and metalloprotease 10 (ADAM10). FASEB J 22: 3716–3727
59. Taguchi A, Blood DC, del Toro G et al (2000) Blockade of RAGE-amphoterin signalling suppresses tumour growth and metastases. Nature 405:354–360
60. Arumugam T, Ramachandran V, Gomez SB et al (2012) S100P-derived RAGE antagonistic peptide reduces tumor growth and metastasis. Clin Cancer Res 18:4356–4364
61. Zhu C, Anderson AC, Schubart A et al (2005) The Tim-3 ligand galectin-9 negatively regulates T helper type 1 immunity. Nat Immunol 6:1245–1252
62. Chiba S, Baghdadi M, Akiba H et al (2012) Tumor-infiltrating DCs suppress nucleic acid-mediated innate immune responses through interactions between the receptor TIM-3 and the alarmin HMGB1. Nat Immunol 13:832–842
63. Wiener Z, Kohalmi B, Pocza P et al (2007) TIM-3 is expressed in melanoma cells and is upregulated in TGF-beta stimulated mast cells. J Invest Dermatol 127:906–914
64. Wu FH, Yuan Y, Li D et al (2010) Endothelial cell-expressed Tim-3 facilitates metastasis of melanoma cells by activating the NF-kappaB pathway. Oncol Rep 24:693–699
65. Fourcade J, Sun Z, Benallaoua M et al (2010) Upregulation of Tim-3 and PD-1 expression is associated with tumor antigen-specific CD8+ T cell dysfunction in melanoma patients. J Exp Med 207:2175–2186
66. Yu M, Wang H, Ding A et al (2006) HMGB1 signals through toll-like receptor (TLR) 4 and TLR2. Shock 26:174–179
67. Park JS, Svetkauskaite D, He Q et al (2004) Involvement of toll-like receptors 2 and 4 in cellular activation by high mobility group box 1 protein. J Biol Chem 279:7370–7377
68. Saint-Jean M, Knol AC, Nguyen JM et al (2011) TLR expression in human melanoma cells. Eur J Dermatol 21:899–905
69. Yu N, Zhang S, Zuo F et al (2009) Cultured human melanocytes express functional toll-like receptors 2-4, 7 and 9. J Dermatol Sci 56: 113–120
70. Mittal D, Saccheri F, Venereau E et al (2010) TLR4-mediated skin carcinogenesis is dependent on immune and radioresistant cells. EMBO J 29:2242–2252
71. Matijevic T, Pavelic J (2010) Toll-like receptors: cost or benefit for cancer? Curr Pharm Des 16:1081–1090
72. Huang B, Zhao J, Unkeless JC et al (2008) TLR signaling by tumor and immune cells: a double-edged sword. Oncogene 27:218–224
73. Nunez NG, Andreani V, Crespo MI et al (2012) IFNbeta produced by TLR4-activated tumor cells is involved in improving the antitumoral immune response. Cancer Res 72:592–603
74. Tittarelli A, Gonzalez FE, Pereda C et al (2012) Toll-like receptor 4 gene polymorphism influences dendritic cell in vitro function and clinical outcomes in vaccinated melanoma patients. Cancer Immunol Immunother 61(11):2067–2077
75. Zhu XM, Yao YM, Liang HP et al (2011) High mobility group box-1 protein regulate immunosuppression of regulatory T cells through toll-like receptor 4. Cytokine 54: 296–304
76. Pashenkov M, Goess G, Wagner C et al (2006) Phase II trial of a toll-like receptor 9-activating oligonucleotide in patients with metastatic melanoma. J Clin Oncol 24:5716–5724
77. Yang HZ, Cui B, Liu HZ et al (2009) Blocking TLR2 activity attenuates pulmonary metastases of tumor. PLoS One 4:e6520
78. Yan J, Hua F, Liu HZ et al (2012) Simultaneous TLR2 inhibition and TLR9 activation synergistically suppress tumor metastasis in mice. Acta Pharmacol Sin 33:503–512
79. Sims GP, Rowe DC, Rietdijk ST et al (2010) HMGB1 and RAGE in inflammation and cancer. Annu Rev Immunol 28:367–388

Chapter 30

The Clinical Use of PET/CT in the Evaluation of Melanoma

Khun Visith Keu and Andrei H. Iagaru

Abstract

Positron emission tomography combined with computed tomography (PET/CT) has emerged in the last decade as a dominant imaging modality used for staging, monitoring response and surveillance of various cancers, including melanoma. Using 2-deoxy-2-(^{18}F)fluoro-D-glucose (^{18}F-FDG) as the radiopharmaceutical, PET/CT has demonstrated its efficacy and its utility in the management of patients with advanced melanoma. Nonetheless, challenges remain in the early stage evaluation of melanoma and in the development of novel radiotracers to better characterize lesions found on PET/CT. This chapter focuses on the advantages and limitations of this imaging modality in melanoma. We also detail and describe the approach to perform ^{18}F-FDG PET/CT, the methods to accurately quantify lesions, as well as the pearls/pitfalls of image interpretation. Finally, an overview of preclinical and investigational clinical radiopharmaceuticals is presented.

Key words PET/CT, FDG, Melanoma, Molecular imaging

1 Introduction

The incidence of cancer has increased dramatically in the past decades, becoming the first leading cause of death in many high-income countries and soon, in every other regions of the world, irrespective of level of resource [1]. The global rise of cancer incidence is also reflected in malignant melanoma: in the USA alone, the number of new cases has increased from 55,100 in 2004 to 68,000 cases in 2010 [2, 3]. While representing only 10 % of all skin cancers detected, malignant melanoma causes as much as two-thirds of all death related to skin diseases [4]. Therefore, accurate staging is critical for identification of potentially resectable distant lesions, to avoid unnecessary surgery when curative intent is not possible and to assure appropriate treatment.

During initial staging, patients with melanoma often underwent a technique called lymphoscintigraphy that is used for the detection of a sentinel node. Since nodal micro-metastasis is not uncommon and the lymphatic drainage is frequently unpredictable,

Magdalena Thurin and Francesco M. Marincola (eds.), *Molecular Diagnostics for Melanoma: Methods and Protocols*, Methods in Molecular Biology, vol. 1102, DOI 10.1007/978-1-62703-727-3_30, © Springer Science+Business Media New York 2014

this technique is a valuable adjunct to clinical evaluation [5, 6]. It involves an injection of colloids around the primary tumor or scar from biopsy. These particles then migrate along the lymphatic vessels before getting trapped in a sentinel node upstream. In addition to lymphoscintigraphy, other nuclear medicine and molecular imaging methods have a role in the initial evaluation of melanoma, for monitoring therapy and for surveillance. Other examinations, such as whole body bone scintigraphy have not been used successfully in melanoma because of its low yield in early stages and the predominant lytic pattern of bone metastasis seen in this disease, since this technique is more sensitive for blastic lesions that show high bone remodeling [7]. A whole body survey to evaluate the extent of malignancy was achieved during the pre-PET era with gallium-67 citrate (^{67}Ga-citrate) or technetium-99 m sestamibi (^{99m}Tc-sestamibi), but these agents failed to stage accurately cancer for many reasons, including their inability to localize the lesions precisely within an anatomic structure, the high radiation dosimetry (with ^{67}Ga-citrate) and their inaccuracy comparing to other available imaging techniques [8]. The evaluation of melanoma and other cancers had changed dramatically since the addition of metabolic imaging using PET. Unlike the anatomic imaging methods such as computed tomography (CT), magnetic resonance imaging (MRI) or ultrasound (US), PET imaging offers another perspective to evaluate disease by measuring the metabolic or functional pathway of the disease. The most widely used radiotracer is 2-deoxy-2-(^{18}F) fluoro-D-glucose (^{18}F-FDG), which exploits the glucose metabolism that is up-regulated in most cancer cells [9]. Although distant metastases can be better assessed with ^{18}F-FDG PET, the role of this modality for the evaluation of loco-regional extent of disease remains uncertain. Lymphoscintigraphy followed by biopsy evaluates better nodal micro-invasion and this technique is well implemented in the management of melanoma patients. Ongoing research investigates other metabolic pathways and receptors that may identify earlier and more accurately melanoma lesions.

1.1 PET/CT Technology

PET is a molecular imaging modality that evaluates the biodistribution of a radioactive substance that is injected in non-pharmacological doses into living organisms. PET imaging is an effective technique that is highly sensitive to assay quantitatively in vivo the biochemical and functional mechanisms of various pathological processes, including cancer. This modality is noninvasive, like other anatomical approaches; however, PET has the capability to detect substance at the level 10^{-11}–10^{-12} M comparing to 10^{-3}–10^{-5} M for MRI [10].

PET technology was described by Michael E. Phelps and Edward J. Hoffman in 1973 [11]. Over the past 40 years, this technology has kept improving and most of the accomplishments have been related to the fast development of computers, electronics, semi-conductor devices, and scintillating crystals during the early

1990s. Modern PET scanners combined with CT are now much faster, efficient, and reliable: they can evaluate the whole body from vertex to toes in less than 30 min while providing excellent combined anatomical and functional images. Because of their intrinsic physical characteristics related to crystals and electronics, PET scanners are affected by the partial volume effect, which is defined as a loss of apparent activity within a region of interest or object. This occurs when the lesion to be imaged is less than two times the full width at half maximum (FHWM), which is a measure of the spatial resolution of the system. The FWHM of a modern clinical PET scanner is approximately 4–6 mm [12–14]. The resultant is that the activity within the lesion is underestimated, which can reduce the potential for lesion detection and quantification. With an ideal scanner, all lesions of different sizes that have the same concentration of radiopharmaceutical will have the same intensity on PET images. Unfortunately, this effect degrades the signal intensity when the lesion is below 15–20 mm. The partial volume effect can be corrected by multiple methods, but this is beyond the scope of this book.

Nowadays, all manufacturers offer their PET scanners equipped with a CT scan allowing for concurrent anatomical imaging: these machines are referred as combined PET/CT scanners. The CT component provides essential information for attenuation correction of PET images and also helps to localize the metabolic foci seen on PET within an anatomic structure [15]. These images are obtained sequentially starting with a CT study and following with a PET acquisition (Fig. 1). Diagnostic CT scans with or without intravenous injection of contrast agent can be done as part of the PET/CT appointment. The combination of both technologies provides excellent images and has become an important tool for clinicians in evaluating and staging cancer: it improves the accuracy of the interpretation and also the confidence of the readers.

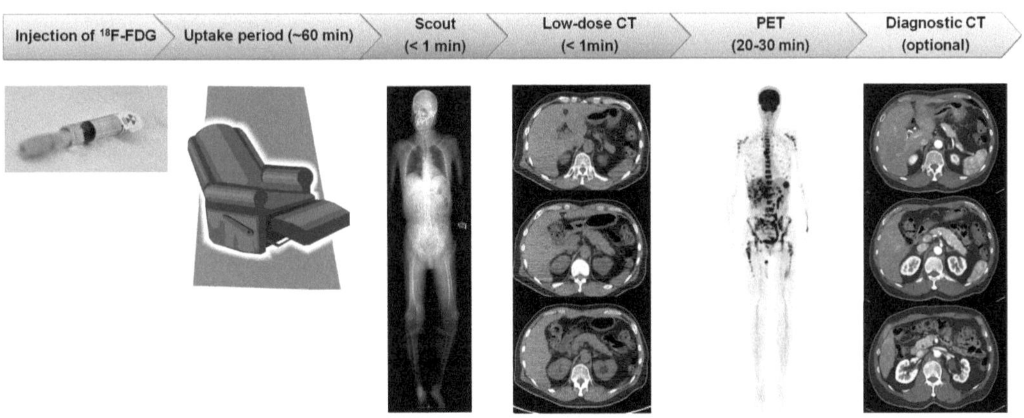

Fig. 1 Procedure timeline for a PET/CT examination. From Stanford University Medical Center

In melanoma, the integrated modality PET/CT has proven its superiority over PET or CT alone for N- and M-staging [16].

1.1.1 ^{18}F-FDG

A PET/CT scanner by itself cannot provide any metabolic images unless the patient is injected with a radiopharmaceutical that will emit photons from organs or lesions that will be detected by the arrays of scintillating crystals. A radiopharmaceutical consists of two or three components generally (Fig. 2). The first one is the radioisotope that emits photons during the decay process. The most commonly used clinical radioisotopes are ^{18}F, ^{11}C, ^{13}N, and ^{68}Ga. The second component is a molecule that interrogates the metabolic pathway of interest. Sometimes, a third component is a linker between the molecule of interest and the radioisotope, such as a bifunctional chelator (e.g., DOTA) [17]. All compounds used with PET scanners are positron emitters that produce two distinct photons of 511 keV energy at 180° apart. These photons are detected by opposite scintillating crystals [15]. Each isotope has a half-life that limits its use or the availability for different centers. The half-life is the period of time for an isotope to decay or to decrease by 50 % of its previous radioactive quantity: an ideal radioisotope would have a half-life long enough for the labeling process with the molecule of interest and for scanning, but relatively short that the time of residence in the patient is reduced to the minimum to avoid unnecessary radiation exposure. The most widely used radiotracer is fluorine-18 (^{18}F) with a half-life of 109.8 min.

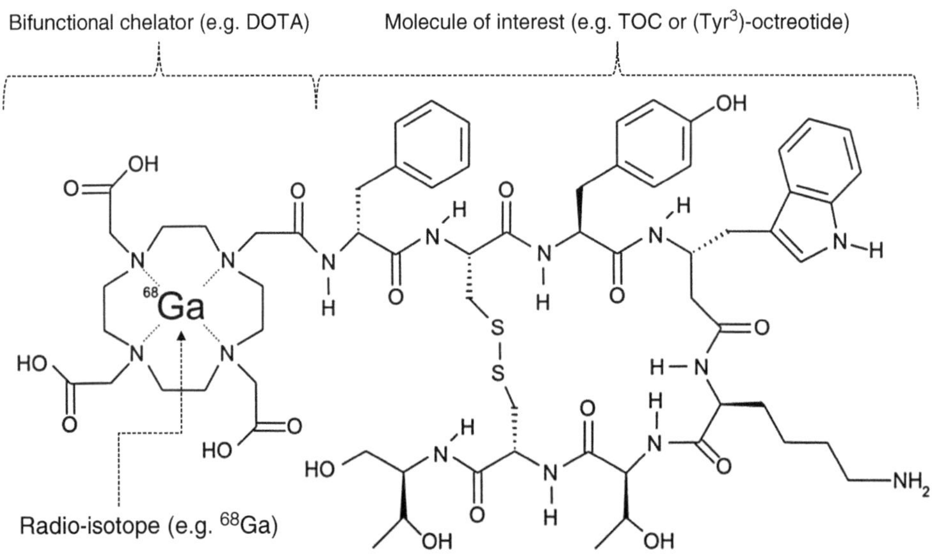

Fig. 2 This radiopharmaceutical is used for diagnosis of neuroendocrine tumors: the molecule comprises a large peptide, (Tyr3)-octreotide or TOC, that is linked to the radioisotope 68Ga (half-life: 68 min) by the bifunctional chelator agent DOTA. It is known as 68Ga-DOTATOC, a somatostatin receptor agent used with PET/CT. Image from Wikipedia

Carbon-11 is a very interesting isotope since the labeling with this tracer is much more convenient than ^{18}F and it can be incorporated in almost any natural molecule through a covalent bond, without altering its biological properties [17]. Most radioisotopes used in PET are produced by a particle accelerator, called a cyclotron, which is often installed in research or large academic institutions. Because of its very short half-life (20 min), carbon-11 compounds are rarely used outside of these environments. Fluorine-18 is also produced in a similar manner, but its longer half-life allows the transportation to distant sites as far as 2–3 h by plane.

The most commonly used clinical radiotracer in oncology is ^{18}F-FDG. The first synthesis of ^{18}F-FDG was carried out in Brookhaven National Laboratory by Wolf et al. in 1976 [18]. Since the discovery, several improvements in the synthesis lead to better production yields. Nowadays, the multistep production of $^{18F-}$FDG is automated in most locations: the computerized controlled syntheses on module reduce the radioactive exposure to workers and limit human errors. The commonly precursor molecule for the production of ^{18}F-FDG is 1,3,4,6-O-Acetyl-2-O-trifluoromethanesulfonyl-beta-D-mannopyranose (mannose triflate) [19]. The similar structure of ^{18}F-FDG to glucose explains its affinity with glucose transporter-1 (GLUT-1) and to a lesser extent, glucose transporter-3 (GLUT-3). Once the ^{18}F-FDG is injected intravenously, it will be transported across the cell membrane of organs or lesions with over expression of GLUT-1 [20]. Inside the cell, ^{18}F-FDG behaves like a glucose molecule, getting phosphorylated by hexokinase-6. However, ^{18}F-FDG-6-phosphate formed cannot further metabolized down the glucose pathway since it lacks the hydroxyl (-OH) on 2' position such as in the glucose structure. ^{18}F-FDG-6-phosphate can be dephosphorylated by glucose-6-phosphatase and then pump out by the cell, but this metabolic pathway is generally down-regulated in cancer cells comparing to its counterpart, hexokinase-6 (Fig. 3) [9, 21]. Therefore, once phosphorylated, ^{18}F-FDG-6-phosphate is metabolically trapped in the cytoplasm. In cancer cells, the aerobic glycolysis is up-regulated because of the Warburg effect, which in consequence explains the increase demands of glucose for these cells [22]. Besides the up-regulation of GLUT transporters and hexokinase-6, the down-regulation of glucose-6-phosphatase in cancer cells, ^{18}F-FDG uptake mechanisms comprise other factors, such as the number of viable cells (e.g., necrotic masses do not accumulate in the center), the cell density (e.g., mucinous tumor tends to accumulate less), the blood flow to the tissue, the index of mitosis or proliferation rate, and the presence of inflammatory cells [21, 23, 24]. PET/CT data represents a static image ("snapshot") of a dynamic process and it relies on the assumption that ^{18}F-FDG uptake is virtually complete and no other enzymatic processes are undergoing (such as glucose-6-phosphatase).

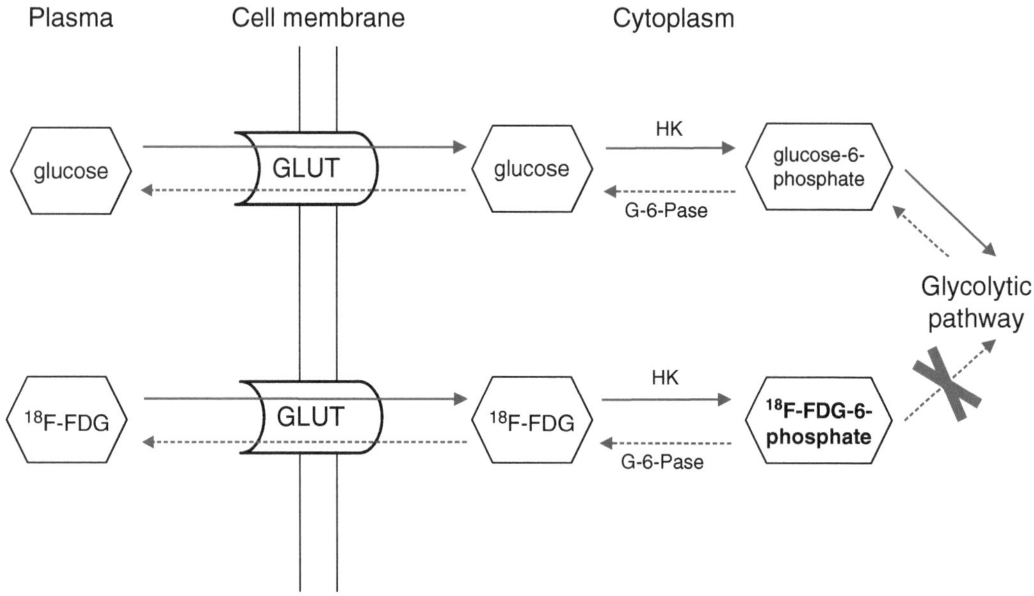

Fig. 3 Like the natural glucose molecule, ^{18}F-FDG enters the cell membrane via facilitated glucose transporter (GLUT): in tumors cells, the enzyme hexokinase (HK) is up-regulated comparing to its counterpart glucose-6-phosphatase (G-6-Pase). However, ^{18}F-FDG-6-phosphate formed cannot further metabolized down the glycolytic pathway (Krebs cycle) since it lacks the hydroxyl (–OH) on 2′ position such as in the glucose structure. Ultimately, ^{18}F-FDG-6-phosphate is metabolically trapped and accumulates over time. *From Stanford University Medical Center*

The normal biodistribution of ^{18}F-FDG is shown in Fig. 4. It is taken up avidly by the brain, which the only substrate is glucose. The radiotracer is excreted by the kidneys into the bladder, which explains the intense uptake. Physiological uptake is also seen in salivary glands, the liver, the spleen, the gonads, and the gastrointestinal tracts. Cardiac uptake is variable since the organ can sustains with free fatty acids, glucose, or lactate: no factors can really predict the pattern of uptake [25].

1.1.2 The Role of ^{18}F-FDG PET/CT in Melanoma

^{18}F-FDG is mostly used in oncological applications [26]. The results from the National Oncologic PET Registry (NOPR) lead to recommendations regarding the use of ^{18}F-FDG for different cancers: over the years, the indications became broader as more studies demonstrated the advantages of this imaging technique [27]. However, the initial local evaluation of superficial melanoma is technically unfeasible because of the partial volume effect and the inherent poor spatial resolution of a PET/CT system. PET scanners can detect at best a lesion of 5 mm on the skin surface, if partial volume effect is not taking into consideration. In theory, CT has a better spatial resolution, but for superficial cutaneous lesions the findings are rather nonspecific. In primary melanoma thicker than >4 mm (T4), a prospective study by Maubec and colleagues failed to prove the utility of ^{18}F-FDG PET in the primary

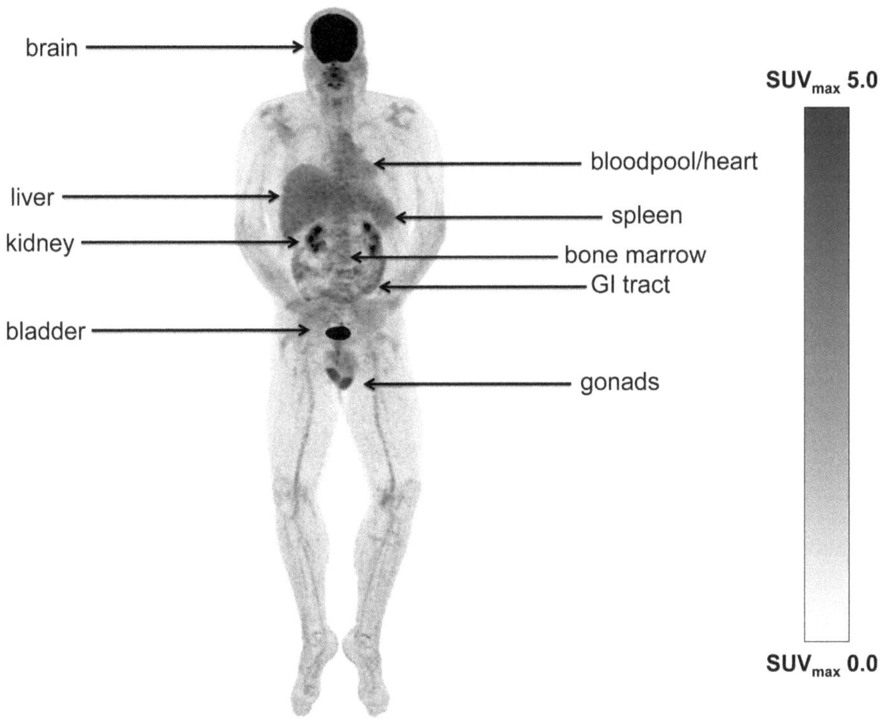

Fig. 4 The normal biodistribution of ^{18}F-FDG is shown on this maximum-intensity-projection image. Physiological uptake is seen in the brain, the bloodpool (vessels and heart), the liver, the spleen, the gastrointestinal (GI) tract, the kidneys, the bladder, the gonads, and the bone marrow. *From Stanford University Medical Center*

workup, with 0 % sensitivity, but 92 % specificity for regional microscopic lymph nodes. Furthermore, in their cohort PET failed to identify a primary melanoma of 1.5 cm diameter and 5 mm thickness [28]. In stage I, II, or III, initial investigations have shown that ^{18}F-FDG PET is an insensitive indicator of occult regional lymph node metastases because the tumor burden in the study population (4.3 mm^3) is far below the expected spatial resolution of modern PET scanners (spatial resolution of approximately 5 mm or a tumor volume of approximately 65 mm^3) [29]. A more recent study did not reveal any better performance for detecting regional lymph node metastases in malignant melanoma: for stage I or II, this modality yield a sensitivity of 14.3 %, specificity of 94.7 % and a positive predictive value of 50 % [30]. A study by Horn and colleagues revealed also that ^{18}F-FDG PET cannot be recommended as a routine investigation for patients with malignant melanoma even in the setting of positive sentinel node biopsy (sensitivity of 50 % and specificity of 31 %) [31]. However, this modality plays an important role when palpable lymph nodes are present: both PET and CT have proven to upstage the patients in 27 % and 24 % of cases respectively, in the series by Bastiaannet and colleagues [32]. Moreover, treatment was changed in 19 % of their patients.

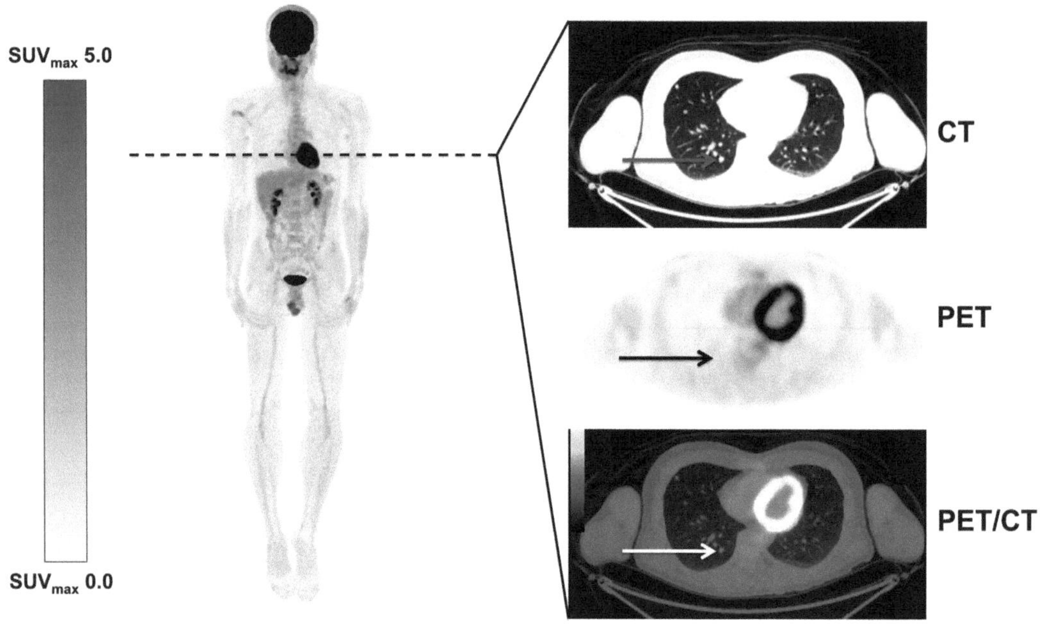

Fig. 5 A thirty-nine-year-old male with known right orbital melanoma treated surgically followed by adjuvant chemotherapy. The surveillance ^{18}F-FDG PET/CT was negative based on PET only (**a**), but the low-dose CT revealed multiple small pulmonary nodules (transaxial CT image in **b**). Follow-up biopsy of the largest lesion—5 mm–(*arrows*) was concordant with metastatic melanoma. This example clearly proves the advantage of a combined PET/CT scanner. *From Stanford University Medical Center*

Aukema and colleagues have shown similar results in a prospective study and that overall survival at 2 years was correlated with PET/CT findings [33]. As is the case with other malignancies, ^{18}F-FDG shows remarkable results in the evaluation of distant metastases: a meta-analysis evolving 28 studies and 2,905 patients concluded that PET is useful for the initial staging of patients with cutaneous malignant melanoma, especially as adjunctive role in stages III and IV, to help detect deep soft-tissue lesions, lymph nodes, and visceral metastases [34]. The pooled estimated sensitivity and specificity were 83 and 85 %; it was also suggested in 8 studies that ^{18}F-FDG altered the patients' management in 33 % of cases. Despite the fact that PEt alone is known to miss small lung metastasis, the CT component of modern PET/CT scanners increases the accurate detection of pulmonary nodules (Fig. 5) [16, 35].

The role of imaging in the evaluation of local and regional recurrence remains controversial. Some studies suggest that ^{18}F-FDG PET/CT or any total body imaging might not be beneficial. A few authors recommend instead proper physical examination, but recent evidence suggested the superiority of ultrasound in assessing loco-regional sites [36, 37]. Since distant recurrence occurs in the first 2–3 years, it appears justified to perform ^{18}F-FDG PET/CT in these subgroups of patients. Researchers have previously shown the important role of ^{18}F-FDG PET/CT

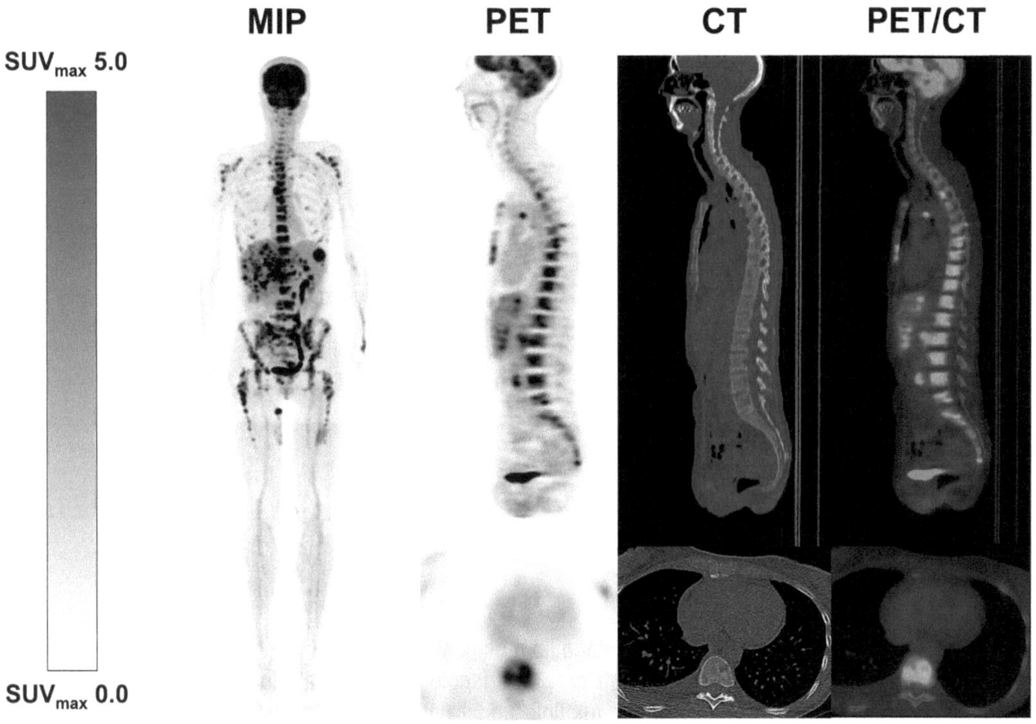

Fig. 6 A fifty-one-year-old female with known stage IVc melanoma of the right thigh, treated with interferon and partial liver lobectomy. On follow-up, she complained of bone pain and her liver enzymes were disturbed. This surveillance ^{18}F-FDG PET/CT demonstrated widespread disease within the axial skeleton (lytic lesions), liver, mediastinal and retroperitoneal nodes, and spleen. *From Stanford University Medical Center*

for the detection of residual/recurrent melanoma with a sensitivity of 89.3 % and a specificity of 88 % [38]. For follow-up, ^{18}F-FDG PET/CT certainly helps to confirm or rule out the possibility of recurrence (Fig. 6). Its main advantage is a rapid survey of the whole body to identify all possible sites of metastasis and avoiding metastectomy of an apparent solitary lesion [39]. A large meta-analysis in 2011 from 74 studies containing 10,528 patients, confirmed also the superiority of PET/CT over other modalities for the detection of distant metastases in both staging and surveillance of melanoma patients (Fig. 7) [37].

1.1.3 Practical Considerations of ^{18}F-FDG PET/CT Scanning

^{18}F-FDG doses are made locally in large academic centers or are delivered to smaller institutions by external providers in the local area. The quantity injected differs largely across centers [26]. Differences related to hardware (crystals and electronics), but also the reconstruction algorithms or scanning protocols, explain this discrepancy. For example in busy clinics, one would prefer injecting a little more ^{18}F-FDG in order to scan faster. Also, the rapid advances of PET/CT hardware and reconstruction algorithm in the past decade allow for faster image acquisition or for less radiotracer being injected, while maintaining the same image quality.

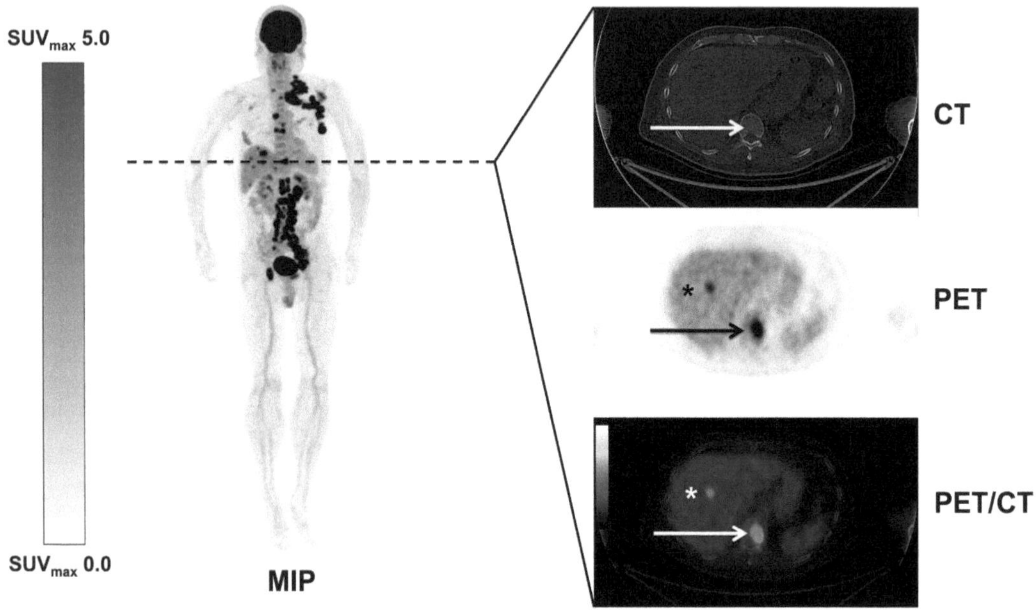

Fig. 7 A sixty-six-year-old male with known stage IIb melanoma of the left calf, treated 5 years ago. He was referred for enlarged lymph nodes in the left cervical triangle and bilateral inguinal regions. The ^{18}F-FDG maximum-intensity-projection (MIP) showed multiple nodal uptake above and below the diaphragm, liver lesions (*asterisk*), and several bone lesions (*arrows* on transaxial images). At first glance, a primary lymphoma was suspected, but biopsy confirmed later widespread metastatic melanoma. *From Stanford University Medical Center*

Nonetheless, guidelines do exist to help achieving global standard for ^{18}F-FDG PET/CT imaging. The Society of Nuclear Medicine recommends an administration between 370 and 740 MBq (10–20 mCi) of ^{18}F-FDG depending on the camera model, the duration of imaging and the reconstruction algorithms [40]. The European Association of Nuclear Medicine provides the most complete recommendation on the proper dosage; it is all in the balance between ^{18}F-FDG activity and duration of the scan [41]. With ALARA principle (As Low As Reasonably Achievable) in mind, reducing activity should be favored but longer scan could be uncomfortable for the patients with more risks of motion artifacts. Depending on the PET/CT system, the dosage can be calculated as follow:

^{18}F-FDG in MBq for 2D scans with bed overlap of <25 % = 27.5 × weight*/(min/bed)

^{18}F-FDG in MBq for 3D scans with bed overlap of <25 % = 13.8 × weight*/(min/bed)

^{18}F-FDG in MBq for 3D scans with bed overlap of 50 % = 6.9 × weight*/(min/bed)

*Weights are in kilograms

In heavier patients (>90 kg), these equations would assume a larger dose: a study had shown that increasing scanning time is preferable than increasing the dose in this setting, while larger dose will not necessarily improve the image quality [42]. A maximum dose has also been suggested, limited to 530 MBq. In modern scanners, the duration of imaging can be set differently so areas outside of the thorax or the abdomen, with less attenuation, can be scanned faster (up to 50 % less time comparing to the trunk).

With an average dose of 370 MBq (10.0 mCi) of ^{18}F-FDG, the patient is exposed to 6–8 mSv (0.6–0.8 rem), which is the equivalent of 2–3 years of natural background radiation in the US [41, 43]. CT acquired during the same study will expose the patient to an extra 1–20 mSv (0.1–2.0 rem), depending on the intended protocol used for attenuation correction and localization of PET lesions only (low dose-CT) or for diagnostic purposes with one or multiple phases (and with or without intravenous contrast-enhanced media). The CT acquisition parameters for low dose CT are generally as follow: kilovoltage (100–120 kVp or 130–140 kVp for larger patients) [44], tube current-rotation (10–120 mAs) [45, 46], slice thickness (2.5–5.0 mm), a 512 × 512 matrix size, and a smooth filter. Many strategies exist for reducing more substantially radiation dose to the patients, for example, newer iterative reconstruction algorithms or tube current modulation, which will change the dose based on the attenuation along the *z*-axis [44]. Many experts recommend that if contrast media is used intravenously, this should be performed after the PET acquisition since the dense material could cause artifact reconstruction or affect PET quantification [47]. For oral agents, high concentration of barium or iodine could create the same problems: dilution of the material or using negative contrast media is recommended instead [41].

PET data should be reconstructed with all proper corrections, such as detector efficiency (normalization), system dead time, random coincidence, scatter, attenuation, and physical decay [41]. The most effective and robust method is the iterative reconstruction which include the maximum-likelihood (ML) or ordered subset expectation-maximization (OSEM) algorithms which handle more efficiently the noise profile and reducing significantly the streaks artifacts related to filtered backprojection algorithm (FBP) [48]. Since potential artifacts caused by CT attenuation could alter the interpretation, it is desirable to perform data reconstruction without attenuation correction to resolve these issues. These two datasets (with and without attenuation correction) should be interpret together in all axes (transaxial, sagittal, and coronal) with also the maximum-intensity-projection (MIP) (Fig. 8). The EANM guidelines suggest some indicative settings for reconstruction depending on the system used [41]. For Siemens/CTI or GE systems, the product of iterations and subsets should be larger than 50 (e.g., 2 iterations × 32 subsets; or 4 iterations × 20 subsets); a 5 mm FHWM

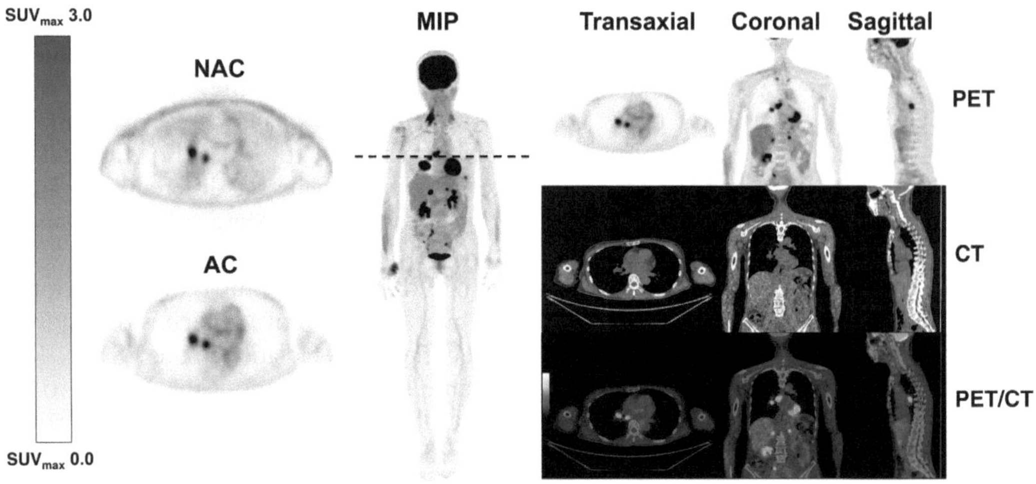

Fig. 8 A sixty-five-year-old female with known stage IIIb nasal melanoma, treated 2 year ago for right cervical nodes recurrence. This ^{18}F-FDG PET/CT surveillance scan demonstrated lung lesions, right hilar nodes, adrenals metastasis, and one left lytic rib lesion. The study can be viewed with non-attenuated correction (NAC) or attenuated correction (AC) slices; with the maximum-intensity-projection (MIP); and within all axes (transaxial–coronal–sagittal). *From Stanford University Medical Center*

Gaussian filter should be applied; the matrix size are generally from 128 × 128 up to 256 × 256. For Philips systems, they proceed differently with a reconstruction named LOR-RAMLA (Line of Response—Row-Action Maximum-Likelihood algorithm), which is also an iterative process, but fewer configurations are possible on site. The normal filter should however be applied with a matrix size of 144 × 144. There is no general consensus on how the reconstruction algorithms should be applied in clinics; however, they should meet the quality control specification from the National Electrical Manufacturers Association (NEMA) NU 2 standards.

1.1.4 Semi-quantification of PET Images Using Standardized Uptake Values (SUV)

Generally, conventional nuclear medicine and radiology examinations are interpreted visually, without any quantification aid. In current practice, PET findings are reported to clinicians qualitatively and quantitatively. Although quantification can be a major adjunct tool to visual interpretation, it is mainly employed for comparison of scans intra-patient (e.g., monitoring response to therapy) or inter-patient (e.g., evaluation of degrees of pathology). The most widely used and simplest equation is the standardized uptake value (SUV) maximum or mean corrected for body weight (BW) [49]:

SUV_{WB} = [Activity in the voxel (kBq/ml)/Activity injected (this activity is corrected for the physical decay of the radiotracer at the time of scanning) (kBq)] × BW (kg)

SUV is not an absolute value, but a relative measurement of the uptake of radiotracer in the tissue comparing to the rest of the body. This assumes that if ^{18}F-FDG is evenly distributed in the whole body, the SUV in normal tissue would be equal to 1. Instead of body weight, the injected dose may also be corrected for the ideal body weight (IBW), the lean body weight (LBW) or the body surface area (BSA). These values could be obtained with these equations [49]:

IBW (in kg) = 45.5 + 0.91(height in cm − 152)

LBW (in kg) = 1.07 (weight in kg) − 148(weight in kg/height in cm)^2

BSA (in m^2) = (weight in kg])$^{0.425}$ × (height in cm)$^{0.725}$ × 0.007184

These values will allow calculating a SUV value corrected, as follow:

SUV_{IBW} = [Activity in the voxel (kBq/ml)/Activity injected (this activity is corrected for the physical decay of the radiotracer at the time of scanning) (kBq)] × IBW (kg)

SUV_{LBW} = [Activity in the voxel (kBq/ml)/Activity injected (this activity is corrected for the physical decay of the radiotracer at the time of scanning) (kBq)] × LBW (kg)

SUV_{BSA} = [Activity in the voxel (kBq/ml)/Activity injected (this activity is corrected for the physical decay of the radiotracer at the time of scanning) (kBq)] × BSA (kg)

SUV_{LBW} seems to better represent the clinical outcome or at least better represent the effective biodistribution of ^{18}F-FDG. The uptake of this radiotracer is very low otherwise in the fat compartment: in consequence, in overweight or obese patient the volume of distribution of ^{18}F-FDG will overestimate and potentially increase the SUV values in tumors (Fig. 9). Moreover, since body weight could fluctuate and since fat is generally the compartment which will lose volume after chemotherapy, studies have suggested that SUV_{LBW} should be replacing the SUV_{BW} [49]. As for SUV_{IBW} and SUV_{BSA}, a study had shown that these methods are less effective for clinical routine application [49]. Quantification is primordial in PET/CT, the SUV varies not only with the body weight or the dose injected, but it is influenced by many factors: blood glucose level, uptake period, patient motion, scan acquisition parameters, reconstruction parameters, synchronization of clock between dose calibrator and scanners, etc. [50]. Therefore, to ensure a valid and confident measurement of the SUV between consecutive studies, patients should be scan on the same scanner, using the similar acquisition and reconstruction settings, receiving the same dose of ^{18}F-FDG, having the same uptake period of time before scanning, and probably using SUV_{LBW} for comparison. Their weight should be measured on the same day of the scan with an accredited balance that is checked at least annually.

1.1.5 Patient Preparation

^{18}F-FDG PET/CT is an excellent tool for oncology. As is the case with all other imaging techniques, scanning the patient in the most appropriate settings will ensure the most accurate evaluation. Thus, the preparation should aim at reducing false-positive

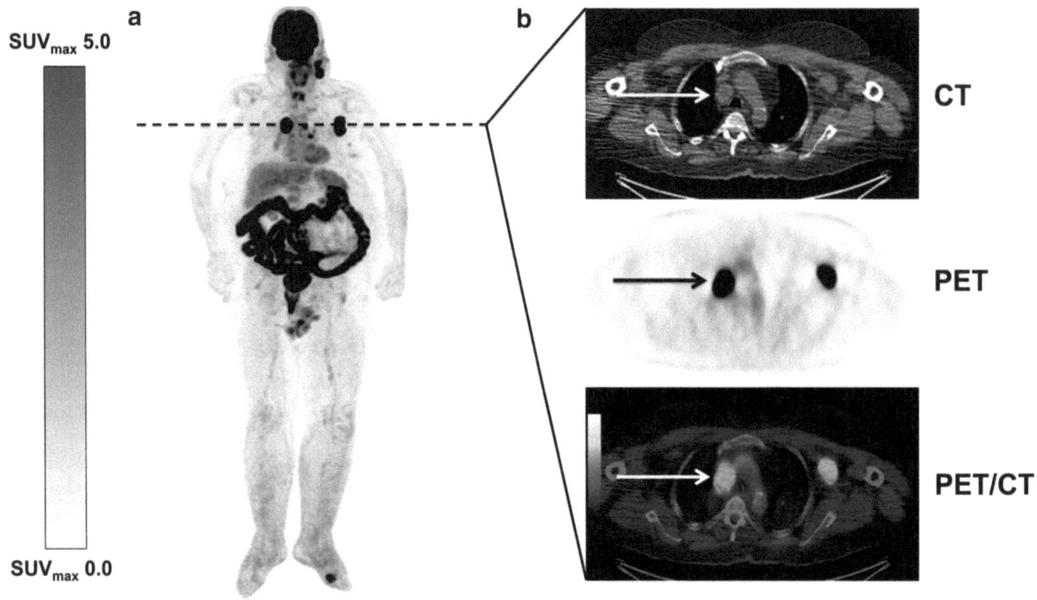

Fig. 9 A sixty-six-year-old female with known stage IIIc melanoma of the scalp, treated 3 years ago. A [18F]-FDG PET/CT surveillance scan was performed and demonstrated recurrence (**a**) in the left cervical, left axillary, and mediastinal nodes: the intense intestinal uptake was related to diabetic medications (non-pathological). The right paratracheal node (*arrows*) shown in transaxial view (**b**) has a SUVmax of 37.7 (corrected for body weight) versus 22.5 (corrected for lean body weight). *From Stanford University Medical Center*

findings and maximizing uptake in cancer lesions. One of the most important factors that the referring physician should be aware of is the timing of the scan. Indeed, any acute disease or state that might confound the interpretation of the scan needs to be addressed and/or discussed with the PET/CT clinics. This includes, but is not limited to the topics discussed below [40, 41, 50, 51].

Acute infection, particularly in the area of interest: any bacterial or fungal infections are known to cause false-positive findings, and to a lesser extent with parasitic or viral infection. For example, an acute pneumonia will likely mask any possible metastases within that lung lobe and contiguous inflammatory nodes in the lung hilum and the mediastinum can be misinterpreted as metastatic disease. In general, it is suggested to wait approximately 1 week after the infection has resolved before scanning the patient.

Any surgical procedures, including superficial biopsies disrupt the homeostasis of the area of concern by creating foci of inflammation or resolving inflammation (scars). They are well known to cause multiples false-positive findings. In the literature, some groups suggest to wait at least 4 weeks for a major procedure and 2 weeks for any type of biopsy.

Because of possible stunning of cancer cells by chemotherapy drugs, false-negative findings are common if scanning is performed to early. Most guidelines and studies suggest waiting about 10–14 days [41].

Radiotherapy is known to cause inflammation within and around the targeted area. On ^{18}F-FDG PET/CT, these areas are represented by moderate uptake which can be difficult to differentiate from residual disease. Time to scan from the end of radiotherapy varies considerably between studies: it has been suggested that after 12 weeks, PET/CT can be performed while avoiding most of the post-treatment inflammatory changes [52].

Once the PET/CT scan is scheduled, the patient needs to follow several instructions. The purpose of patient preparation is to reduce the uptake in physiological or benign structures while increasing the uptake in target lesions [41]. The patients are asked to fast 6–8 h prior to the injection time of ^{18}F-FDG: any meals or liquids containing sugar must be avoided because an excess of unlabeled glucose will saturated the trans-membranous glucose transporters (GLUT) and therefore reduce the uptake of radiotracer in cancer cells [41, 53]. Many studies have shown the significant reduction of uptake in tumors when scans were done under glucose loading state as opposed to a fasting state within the same patient [54, 55]. The fasting state is important to maintain a low level on endogenous insulin until the time of ^{18}F-FDG injection. Hyperinsulinemia affects the uptake since the radiotracer is driven into the skeletal and cardiac muscles after translocation of GLUT-4 receptors. These mechanisms clearly reduce the availability of ^{18}F-FDG for cancer cells and also impact the visual interpretation of images: it results in decreasing the detection rate and the quantification [53].

In practice, patients scheduled to undergo PET/CT scanning in the morning should not eat after midnight and for those whore are scheduled in the afternoon can have a light breakfast. Patients with intravenous access or parenteral nutrition should not have glucose in their solution/fluid 4 h prior to the scan. Patients with diabetic mellitus type II taking oral medication should continue their regular prescription drugs while complying with the previous fasting recommendations. For patients with diabetes mellitus type I or insulin-dependent type II, the preparation is a little more cumbersome. The glucose level should be under control prior to ^{18}F-FDG PET/CT. Patients may have a normal breakfast very early in the morning with subsequent injection of normal insulin. Their scan should however be scheduled late in the morning (e.g., 11 a.m.), so that the insulin levels return to normal). The appropriate protocol for these patients varies from center to center. Referring physicians and patients are encouraged to address these issues with PET/CT clinics prior to scheduling. Before injecting ^{18}F-FDG, the blood glucose level is always measured. A value from 100 to 150 mg/dl is required at the time of injection. Above 150 mg/dl, the patient should be rescheduled [40].

Patients are allowed to drink water during the fasting time and they are also encouraged to drink about 0.5–1.0 l within the hour before the examination: a well hydrated patient will allow the technologist to get a better vein access for the injection of radiotracer, dilute the ^{18}F-FDG concentration in urine (less reconstruction artifact or blurring of surrounding structures) and help with radiation safety [53, 56]. The patient needs to avoid strenuous exercise 24–48 h before the scan: skeletal muscle uptake is often seen in patients who trained or lifted weights few days before the ^{18}F-FDG PET/CT [57, 58]. The patients can take their regular medications as prescribed.

A proper intravenous access is important when injecting a radiopharmaceutical so the risk of dose infiltration is reduced to the minimum. When it does happen, unnecessary radiation exposure results at the injection site. A portion of the dose is not distributed across the body which theoretically reduces the number of ^{18}F-FDG molecule for cancer cells, so the uptake and quantification can be erroneous. Finally, the infiltration dose can be reabsorbed locally by the lymphatic route and accumulated in non-malignant nodes upstream [59]. While this false-positive finding is well known in the literature, technologists and physicians should be aware of it. In melanoma patients, this is even more important since the primary tumor can be localized on an extremity and the drainage is unpredictable in one third of the patients [6]. When the primary tumor is located on the upper trunk, the injection could be made at the level of the foot or the ankle. Another approach is to inject in the antecubital fossa contralateral to the lesion. The IV catheter should remain in place throughout the whole scan. It is left in place for the potential injection of pain medication, sedation drugs or other type of drugs, if necessary. A previous placed catheter or any indwelling port is usually not used for the injection to avoid the risk of contamination.

Patients should be kept warm once they arrived in the clinic, optimally for 30–60 min before the injection of ^{18}F-FDG and during the uptake period to reduce the accumulation of radiotracer in brown adipose tissue (BAT) or brown fat [41, 60]. The latter plays a role in thermogenesis and can be dramatically activated in a cold or anxious patient [61, 62]. The brown fat activation could be a source of false-positive findings (lowering specificity) or it could masquerade other lesions in the surrounding (lowering sensitivity). Preventing BAT uptake is ensured by keeping the patient in thermo-neutral conditions (e.g., warm blankets, same temperature across the department, avoid cold air from air conditioning) or by administrating medications prior to the examination. These include benzodiazepines, beta-adrenergic blocking agents, reserpine or fentanyl [61, 63, 64].

Breast-feeding women can undergo ^{18}F-FDG PET/CT scanning: the residual radioactivity from the patient will not pass through the breast milk [65]. Radiation exposure to babies will result from close proximity to the mothers and this is the reason to recommend discontinuing direct breast-feeding for 16–24 h (pumping and nursing is encouraged).

1.1.6 Other Technical Considerations

After the radiopharmaceutical injection, the patient is instructed to rest and lie quietly for approximately 60 min. During this waiting period, the patient should avoid talking, excessive movement, and walking, in order to minimize ^{18}F-FDG uptake in the muscles. The waiting area should be relaxing, comfortable, and warm (to avoid brown fat activation).

A total whole-body PET/CT from vertex to toes is advisable to avoid missing any potential lesions in melanoma patients. This imaging protocol requires longer acquisition times, which may reduce the comfort of the patient and may not be suitable in busy clinics. Moreover, several studies recommend performing total body scans only in patients with known local (or previous) primary or metastatic disease in the legs or the scalp. Otherwise, a routine skull base to upper thigh scan may be sufficient [66, 67]. Nevertheless, the improving hardware and software allow for faster image acquisition without comprising the image quality [12–14]. If lesions are suspected in the abdomen and pelvis, the use of oral contrast may be beneficial. In these cases, the patients are asked to ingest oral contrast solution during the uptake period of ^{18}F-FDG at time 0 and 30 min after the injection of radiotracer, and a few minutes before starting the scan. The physician can also choose to hydrate more intravenously and/or to administrate furosemide, a loop diuretic, since lesions in the pelvis area can be hidden by intense ^{18}F-FDG excretion in the bladder.

For advanced stage malignant melanoma, a recent study by Pfluger and colleagues did not demonstrate the superiority of contrast-enhanced CT (CECT) versus non-enhanced low-dose CT (NECT) when combined with ^{18}F-FDG. From 232 lesions analyzed and 151 proven to be metastases, they concluded that the sensitivity and specificity for PET/CECT was 100 and 93 % comparing to 97 and 93 %, respectively for PET/NECT [68]. Therefore, it appears that there is no real advantage from performing an intravenous injection of contrast media. Proceeding with PET/NECT reduces the radiation exposure and avoids the potential side-effects of contrast agents. However, if CECT is required, a qualified physician should assess the indications and contraindications before performing the scan, including but not limited to interaction with medications or pertinent medical history of kidneys function.

1.1.7 Advantages of ^{18}F-FDG PET/CT

The main advantage is the ability to survey the whole body in one examination with the injection of a single radiopharmaceutical. It combines two different technologies that together are cost-effective for the healthcare system and beneficial for the patient [69, 70].

This modality is useful for evaluating the extent of disease in melanoma patients with high risk factors and for detecting recurrence [37, 39, 69]. Since biochemical/metabolic changes occur earlier than anatomical changes, PET has the potential to detect earlier foci of recurrence than CT or MRI [10]. Moreover, it could monitor therapy response when systemic agents are used or identify site for biopsy to avoid area of necrosis.

1.1.8 Limitations and Pitfalls of ^{18}F-FDG PET/CT

^{18}F-FDG PET/CT is limited by its spatial resolution for the detection of small lesions. In consequence, there is no clear role for screening or evaluation of the local cutaneous tumor. Nodal micro-metastases are not well evaluated, and therefore the nodal staging of melanoma patients must include sentinel node mapping with ^{99m}Tc-sulfur colloid [5, 71]. Evaluation of small pulmonary nodules (<10 mm) is limited by the limits of spatial resolution and the breathing motion artifacts (these are even more aggravated in the basal segments of the lungs) [72, 73]. There are also numerous causes of abnormal nonmalignant ^{18}F-FDG uptake. These include inflammatory processes such as post-surgical, post-biopsy, post-radiation, or post-chemotherapy inflammation, acute or chronic infections, site of cutaneous injections (e.g., low-molecular weighted heparin, insulin, interferon), granulomatous diseases, organs inflammation (e.g., gastritis, esophagitis, vasculitis, atherosclerosis), noninfected grafts, etc. [40, 41, 51, 74, 75]. Besides inflammation, ^{18}F-FDG uptake has been described in benign conditions such as ipsilateral nodes after dose infiltration at the injection site, brown fat tissue, muscles, thymus (physiological or post-chemotherapy), benign neoplasms (e.g., Warthin's tumor, adrenal adenoma, Paget's disease, enchondroma), bone marrow activation following granulocyte/macrophage colony stimulating factor injection (GM-CSF), etc. [40, 41, 51, 57, 61, 63, 75–77]. ^{18}F-FDG PET/CT has limited use for the evaluation of brain metastases because of the underlying high physiological activity in the cerebrum. Therefore, brain MRI is the modality of choice.

1.2 Recent Advances and Future Directions

1.2.1 Radiopharmaceuticals

Given the highly advertised potential advantages of personalized medicine, efforts are focused on increasing knowledge and improving patient treatments, thus ameliorating the chance of success while minimizing side effects. Deeper understanding of molecular biology of cancer has certainly helped in looking for better-targeted molecules for treatment as well as for imaging. These findings or opportunities in research lead to novel radiopharmaceuticals that can be more sensitive and/or more specific than ^{18}F-FDG. For advanced melanoma, ^{18}F-FDG PET/CT is an excellent imaging modality [78]. However, the management of patients in stage I or II is not really impacted by this technique and as previously mentioned, its accuracy in evaluating regional metastases is surpassed by the sentinel node biopsy [28, 79]. Therefore, there is a need to find targeted and more specific radiotracers that may have better affinity for melanoma cells in order to improve the detection of lesions. Besides ^{18}F-FDG, no other compounds are actually used in clinics or accepted by the FDA, but many publications mainly in murine models have shown potential use of new tracers.

Different groups have tried to label α-melanocyte-stimulating hormone peptide analogues, targeting the melanocortin 1 receptor (MC1R) that is overexpressed in human melanoma cells. Nonspecific bindings, high accumulation of peptides in kidneys, slow uptake or inefficient retention in human tumors, are the major challenges and problems that are needed to overcome. Nevertheless, these preclinical data provide good results regarding the detection of disease, mainly because of the high target-to-background ratios comparing to ^{18}F-FDG. Cantorias and colleagues evaluated the potential role of ^{68}Ga-DOTA-Re(Arg11)CCMSH given to B16/F1 melanoma-bearing C57 mice, which resulted in good images with a high tumor-to-non target organ ratios at an early time point (i.e., at 1 h biodistribution: tumor–blood, 14.3; tumor–muscle, 89.6; tumor–skin, 12.3) and fast clearance of the labeled peptide from kidney and other healthy tissues [80]. This may have a potential role in early detection of melanoma metastasis. Another group leading by Wei et al. explored the use of ^{111}In-, ^{86}Y-, and ^{68}Ga-labeled CHX-A″-Re(Arg(11))CCMSH peptide in B16/F1 melanoma-bearing mice [81]. Melanoma tumor uptake and imaging were exhibited and the investigators concluded that the facile radiolabeling properties of CHX-A″-Re(Arg(11))CCMSH allows it to be employed as a melanoma imaging agent with little or no purification after ^{111}In, ^{86}Y, and ^{68}Ga labeling. One group have experimented the labeling of metallopeptides using ^{18}F as the radioisotope: Cheng's group evaluated ^{18}F-FP-RMSH-1 in mice bearing B16F10 tumors and the image quality was good at 1 and 2 h (Fig. 10) [82]. The ratio of tumor to background or normal organ were high for C57BL/6 mice bearing B16F10 murine tumors (high MC1R expression) comparing to Fox Chase SCID mice bearing A375M human tumors (expressing a low density of MC1 receptors). These results are very promising for a near future PET probe for imaging MC1R positive melanoma.

Another approach to image melanoma is targeting the formation of melanin: one of the major substrate is tyrosine which is an amino acid that is transformed into dihydroxyphenylalanine (DOPA) after entering the cell membrane. A study by Dimitrakopoulou-Strauss and colleagues evaluated the use of ^{18}F-DOPA in metastatic melanoma and the mechanism of uptake to determine whether is related to metabolism ^{18}F-FDG or perfusion ^{15}O-water [83]. They concluded that ^{18}F-DOPA could help in identifying viable metastatic lesions in patients with negative ^{18}F-FDG. Since the synthesis of ^{18}F-DOPA is difficult and expensive, its use is thus limited for research purposes [84].

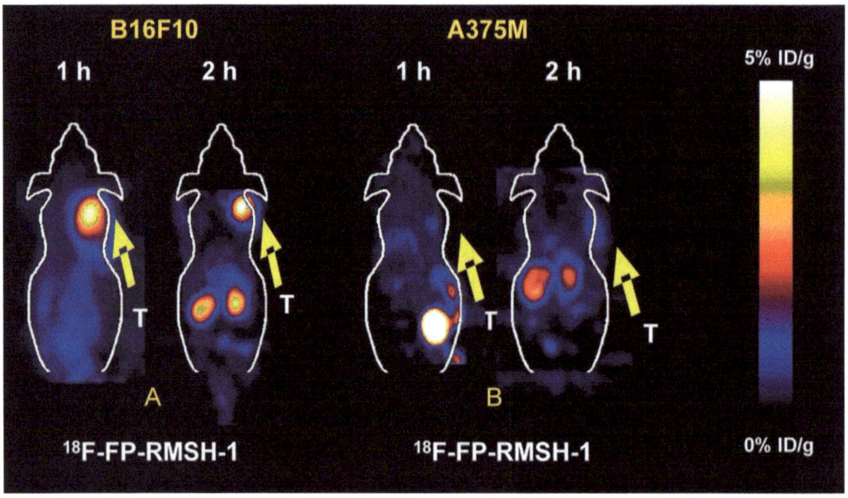

Fig. 10 Coronal small-animal PET images at 1 and 2 h after tail vein injection of ^{18}F-FP-RMSH-1 in mice bearing B16F10 tumors with high MC1R expression (**a**) comparing to A375M tumors with low MC1R expression (**b**). These tumors are located on the right shoulder of mice (represented by letter T). *Courtesy of Professor Zhen Cheng at MIPS Stanford University*

Part of the strategy in anticancer therapy is drugs targeting angiogenesis: in the attempt of growing and evading, cancer cells are seeking for nutrients with the development of new vessels. It has been shown that integrins such as $\alpha_v\beta_3$ play an important role in the regulation of tumor growth and maybe the disruption of extracellular matrix. This subtype of integrins is highly expressed in the endothelial cells of new vessels. The use of tracers targeting this receptor can evaluate the expression of $\alpha_v\beta_3$ for the selection of appropriate patients that could undergo anti-angiogenesis treatment. Beer and colleagues described and evaluated the role of ^{18}F-galacto-RGD in human with different type of cancers [85]. Results showed significant uptake within tumor lesions and they highly correlated to immunochemistry findings of $\alpha_v\beta_3$ receptors and microvessel density. Therefore, the investigators concluded that this PET probe could potentially use as biomarkers for angiogenesis and used for personalizing drug therapy. Miao's group has recently evaluated a labeled ^{99m}Tc hybrid designed peptide RGD conjugated with alpha-melanocyte stimulating hormone that targeted both melanocortin-1 (MC1) and $\alpha_v\beta_3$ integrin receptors [86]. This novel hybrid peptide proves to behave superiorly than ^{99m}Tc-labeled α-MSH or RGD peptide alone: flank M21 human melanoma tumors in study were clearly visualized and this molecule can potentially be used as a dual-receptor-targeting imaging probe for melanoma detection.

DNA synthesis proliferation agent has been also explored for the staging of melanoma patients: 3-^{18}F-fluoro-3-deoxy-L-thymidine (^{18}F-FLT) has been investigated by Cobben et al. and they concluded that this agent may have a potential use in clinical stage III [87]. However, this study was not compared to ^{18}F-FDG which is the actual standard care for advanced stage melanoma. A more recent study from Czernin's group evaluated the role ^{18}F-FDG as a metabolism agent and ^{18}F-FLT as a cell replication agent, in the evaluation of patients with advanced melanoma receiving the CTLA4-blocking antibody tremelimumab [88]. Only ^{18}F-FLT allows mapping and noninvasive imaging of cell proliferation in secondary lymphoid organs after CTLA4 blockade. There were however no difference in the evaluation of metastatic lesion. The role of this radiotracer in the management of melanoma needs further investigations.

An important feature of cancer cells is their rapid growing in a hostile environment with poorly organized vasculature that leads to areas of inefficient oxygenation and perfusion. Hypoxia in these regions is a negative prognostic and plays a central role in tumor progression, chemoresistance, and radioresistance [89]. Despite the development of hypoxia agents, only few studies are evaluating melanoma. Wyss and colleagues have shown that an established hypoxia PET tracer ^{18}F-fluoromisonidazole (^{18}F-FMISO) can be used to clearly visualize hypoxic regions in 10 out of 11 experimental tumor models, including B16 melanoma tumors in syngeneic Balb/c mice [90].

The field of antibody engineering has accelerated in the past few years and different investigators have shown the potential use of these targeted biomarkers as imaging agents with better binding specificity, but also as therapeutic agents [91]. Labeling with a beta-minus emitter, these new molecules could be an attractive agents for radio-immunotherapy [92, 93]. Revskaya and colleagues have demonstrated that melanin-binding IgM mAbs labeled with ^{188}Re was more effective in slowing tumor growth in mice than chemotherapy with dacarbazine, but the administration of chemotherapy followed by ^{188}Re was more effective than either modality alone [93]. This novel approach for melanoma looks promising and reflected the trends into a more personalized medicine.

1.3 Hardware and Techniques

Improvements in the past decade have also involved the hardware. Counting rates, precision, and image contrast are much improved. For example, faster crystals and electronics allow most modern state-of-the-art PET/CT to incorporate point spread function and time-of-flight technology information into the reconstruction algorithms, consequently improving the detection of smaller lesions (better contrast and less noise) and the quantification (Fig. 11) [12–14]. These techniques could potentially be an important asset in the evaluation of small (<1 cm) lesions.

Once detected on diagnostic scans, the remaining challenge is localizing precisely these small structures during surgery. Intraoperative handheld devices might play a key role: they are used by surgeons during the sentinel lymph node dissection in patients with melanoma and breast cancer. New design and crystals

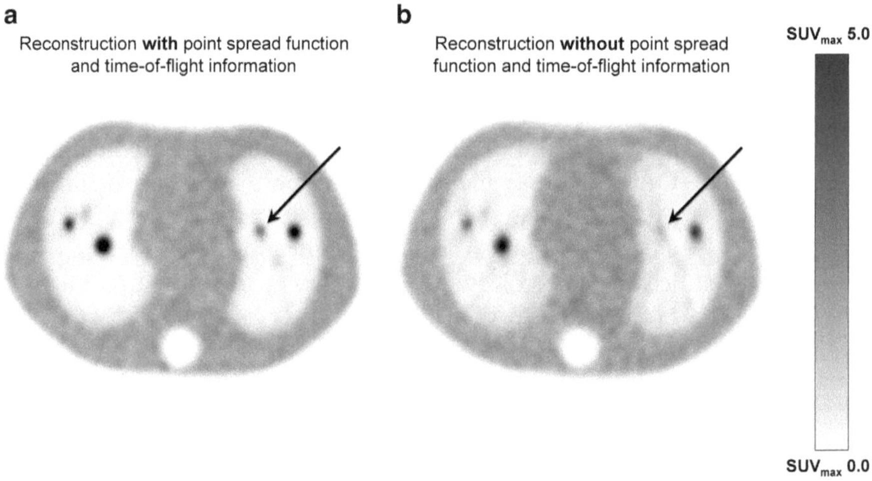

Fig. 11 Transaxial images of an Anthropomorphic Torso Phantom™ obtained on a GE Healthcare Discovery™ 690 PET/CT scanner with (**a**) and without (**b**) point spread function and time-of-flight information. Lesions on image (**a**) have a better contrast and are better defined comparing to those on image (**b**) for example, a 6 mm diameter lesion (*arrow*) is clearly visible on image A. *From Stanford University Medical Center*

used for the production of these new probes allow the detection of high-energy photons from PET tracers. Povoski and colleagues described an innovative multimodality approach of perioperative ^{18}F-FDG PET/CT imaging by using an intraoperative PET hand-held imaging device and intraoperative ultrasound for tumor localization and verification of resection of all sites of hypermetabolic tumor foci in a case of occult recurrent metastatic melanoma [94]. They concluded that this technique could potentially impact patient care, since it would aid significantly in the immediate, real-time intraoperative verification of complete removal of all hypermetabolic activity within the surgical resection field. A retrospective study by Franc and colleagues evaluated intraoperative imaging in patients with suspicion of recurrent melanoma. They found 8 of the 19 surgical specimens to have increased ^{18}F-FDG uptake using the high-energy probe and missed only one lesion, yielding a sensitivity of 89 % (8 of 9) and a specificity of 100 % (10 of 10) [95]. While further experiments are needed, these studies demonstrate the new possibilities for improving surgical procedures.

PET/MRI is a new emergent modality that integrates the evaluation of metabolic and anatomic imaging simultaneously. This novel modality reduces dramatically the ionizing radiation to the patients since MRI technology is based on non-ionizing radiofrequency signals to produce images [96]. For T-staging, none of the actual imaging modalities, including PET or MRI, could evaluate or screen patients at risk of melanoma. For N-staging,

^{18}F-FDG PET/CT has proven its superiority to CT or MRI, while the latter accuracy seems to be at least as equal to whole-body CT [97, 98]. Recent studies have shown that whole-body MRI might be as accurate to ^{18}F-FDG PET/CT when using different combination of conventional sequences with diffusion weighted MRI: however, multiple sequences mean longer acquisition [99, 100]. But clearly, the main advantage of MRI is associated with its better contrast of soft-tissue which resides in better detection of metastases in organs and brain [98]. PET/MRI is on its early milestone, but the few around the world sites that experience this modality in clinical settings are encouraged by the initial results and expected this modality will become a 1-stop-shop whole-body N- and M-staging tool in high-risk patients with melanoma (AJCC stages > III) [96].

References

1. Bray F, Jemal A, Grey N, Ferlay J, Forman D (2012) Global cancer transitions according to the human development index (2008–2030): a population-based study. Lancet Oncol 13(8):790–801. doi:10.1016/s1470-2045(12)70211-5
2. Jemal A, Tiwari RC, Murray T, Ghafoor A, Samuels A, Ward E, Feuer EJ, Thun MJ (2004) Cancer statistics, 2004. CA Cancer J Clin 54(1):8–29
3. Jemal A, Siegel R, Xu J, Ward E (2010) Cancer statistics, 2010. Ca 60(5):277–300
4. Linos E, Swetter SM, Cockburn MG, Colditz GA, Clarke CA (2009) Increasing burden of melanoma in the United States. J Invest Dermatol 129(7):1666–1674. doi:10.1038/jid.2008.423
5. Uren RF, Thompson JF, Howman-Giles R, Chung DK (2006) The role of lymphoscintigraphy in the detection of lymph node drainage in melanoma. Surg Oncol Clin N Am 15(2):285–300. doi:10.1016/j.soc.2005.12.006
6. Statius Muller MG, Hennipman FA, van Leeuwen PA, Pijpers R, Vuylsteke RJ, Meijer S (2002) Unpredictability of lymphatic drainage patterns in melanoma patients. Eur J Nucl Med Mol Imaging 29(2):255–261
7. Elias Brountzos IP, Dimitrios Bafaloukos, Dimitrios Kelekis (2001) Bone metastases from malignant melanoma: a retrospective review and analysis of 28 cases. Radiol Oncol 35:209–214
8. Kalff V, Hicks RJ, Ware RE, Greer B, Binns DS, Hogg A (2002) Evaluation of high-risk melanoma: comparison of [18F]FDG PET and high-dose 67Ga SPET. Eur J Nucl Med Mol Imaging 29(4):506–515. doi:10.1007/s00259-001-0735-8
9. Gatenby RA, Gillies RJ (2004) Why do cancers have high aerobic glycolysis? Nat Rev Cancer 4(11):891–899. doi:10.1038/nrc1478
10. James ML, Gambhir SS (2012) A molecular imaging primer: modalities, imaging agents, and applications. Physiol Rev 92(2):897–965
11. Nutt R (2002) The history of positron emission tomography. Mol Imaging Biol 4(1):11
12. Surti S, Kuhn A, Werner ME, Perkins AE, Kolthammer J, Karp JS (2007) Performance of Philips Gemini TF PET/CT scanner with special consideration for its time-of-flight imaging capabilities. J Nucl Med 48(3):471–480
13. Bettinardi V, Presotto L, Rapisarda E, Picchio M, Gianolli L, Gilardi MC (2011) Physical performance of the new hybrid PETCT discovery-690. Med Phys 38(10):5394–5411. doi:10.1118/1.3635220
14. Jakoby BW, Bercier Y, Conti M, Casey ME, Bendriem B, Townsend DW (2011) Physical and clinical performance of the mCT time-of-flight PET/CT scanner. Phys Med Biol 56(8):2375–2389. doi:10.1088/0031-9155/56/8/004
15. Basu S, Kwee TC, Surti S, Akin EA, Yoo D, Alavi A (2011) Fundamentals of PET and PET/CT imaging. Ann N Y Acad Sci 1228:1–18. doi:10.1111/j.1749-6632.2011.06077.x
16. Reinhardt MJ, Joe AY, Jaeger U, Huber A, Matthies A, Bucerius J, Roedel R, Strunk H, Bieber T, Biersack HJ, Tuting T (2006) Diagnostic performance of whole body dual modality 18F-FDG PET/CT imaging for

N- and M-staging of malignant melanoma: experience with 250 consecutive patients. J Clin Oncol 24(7):1178–1187. doi:10.1200/jco.2005.03.5634

17. Vallabhajosula S, Solnes L, Vallabhajosula B (2011) A broad overview of positron emission tomography radiopharmaceuticals and clinical applications: what is new? Semin Nucl Med 41(4):246–264. doi:10.1053/j.semnuclmed.2011.02.003
18. Ido T, Wan CN, Casella V, Fowler JS, Wolf AP, Reivich M, Kuhl DE (1978) Labeled 2-deoxy-D-glucose analogs. 18F-labeled 2-deoxy-2-fluoro-D-glucose, 2-deoxy-2-fluoro-D-mannose and 14C-2-deoxy-2-fluoro-D-glucose. J Labelled Comp Rad 14(2):175–183. doi:10.1002/jlcr.2580140204
19. Yu S (2006) Review of F-FDG synthesis and quality control. Biomed Imaging Interv J 2(4):e57. doi:10.2349/biij.2.4.e57
20. Macheda ML, Rogers S, Best JD (2005) Molecular and cellular regulation of glucose transporter (GLUT) proteins in cancer. J Cell Physiol 202(3):654–662. doi:10.1002/jcp.20166
21. Buck AK, Reske SN (2004) Cellular origin and molecular mechanisms of 18F-FDG uptake: is there a contribution of the endothelium? J Nucl Med 45(3):461–463
22. Warburg O (1956) On the origin of cancer cells. Science 123(3191):309–314
23. Berger KL, Nicholson SA, Dehdashti F, Siegel BA (2000) FDG PET evaluation of mucinous neoplasms. Am J Roentgenol 174(4):1005–1008
24. Bos R, van der Hoeven JJM, van der Wall E, van der Groep P, van Diest PJ, Comans EFI, Joshi U, Semenza GL, Hoekstra OS, Lammertsma AA, Molthoff CFM (2002) Biologic correlates of 18fluorodeoxyglucose uptake in human breast cancer measured by positron emission tomography. J Clin Oncol 20(2):379–387. doi:10.1200/jco.20.2.379
25. Kaneta T, Hakamatsuka T, Takanami K, Yamada T, Takase K, Sato A, Higano S, Kinomura S, Fukuda H, Takahashi S, Yamada S (2006) Evaluation of the relationship between physiological FDG uptake in the heart and age, blood glucose level, fasting period, and hospitalization. Ann Nucl Med 20(3):203–208
26. Beyer T, Czernin J, Freudenberg LS (2011) Variations in clinical PET/CT operations: results of an international survey of active PET/CT users. J Nucl Med 52(2):303–310. doi:10.2967/jnumed.110.079624
27. Hillner BE, Siegel BA, Shields AF, Liu D, Gareen IF, Hanna L, Stine SH, Coleman RE (2009) The impact of positron emission tomography (PET) on expected management during cancer treatment: findings of the national oncologic PET registry. Cancer 115(2):410–418. doi:10.1002/cncr.24000
28. Maubec E, Lumbroso J, Masson F, Suciu V, Kolb F, Mamelle G, Cavalcanti A, Boitier F, Spatz A, Auperin A, Leboulleux S, Avril MF (2007) F-18 fluorodeoxy-D-glucose positron emission tomography scan in the initial evaluation of patients with a primary melanoma thicker than 4 mm. Melanoma Res 17(3):147–154. doi:10.1097/CMR.0b013e32815c10b0
29. Wagner JD, Schauwecker D, Davidson D, Coleman JJ III, Saxman S, Hutchins G, Love C, Hayes JT (1999) Prospective study of fluorodeoxyglucose-positron emission tomography imaging of lymph node basins in melanoma patients undergoing sentinel node biopsy. J Clin Oncol 17(5):1508
30. Singh B, Ezziddin S, Palmedo H, Reinhardt M, Strunk H, Tuting T, Biersack HJ, Ahmadzadehfar H (2008) Preoperative 18F-FDG-PET/CT imaging and sentinel node biopsy in the detection of regional lymph node metastases in malignant melanoma. Melanoma Res 18(5):346–352. doi:10.1097/CMR.0b013e32830b363b
31. Horn J, Sjostrand H, Lock-Andersen J, Loft A (2010) PET scanning for malignant melanoma and positive sentinel node diagnostics. Ugeskr Laeger 172(15):1126–1130
32. Bastiaannet E, Wobbes T, Hoekstra OS, van der Jagt EJ, Brouwers AH, Koelemij R, de Klerk JM, Oyen WJ, Meijer S, Hoekstra HJ (2009) Prospective comparison of [18F]fluorodeoxyglucose positron emission tomography and computed tomography in patients with melanoma with palpable lymph node metastases: diagnostic accuracy and impact on treatment. J Clin Oncol 27(28):4774–4780. doi:10.1200/jco.2008.20.1822
33. Aukema TS, Valdes Olmos RA, Wouters MW, Klop WM, Kroon BB, Vogel WV, Nieweg OE (2010) Utility of preoperative 18F-FDG PET/CT and brain MRI in melanoma patients with palpable lymph node metastases. Ann Surg Oncol 17(10):2773–2778. doi:10.1245/s10434-010-1088-y
34. Krug B, Crott R, Lonneux M, Baurain JF, Pirson AS, Vander Borght T (2008) Role of PET in the initial staging of cutaneous malignant melanoma: systematic review. Radiology 249(3):836–844. doi:10.1148/radiol.2493080240
35. Strobel K, Dummer R, Husarik DB, Perez Lago M, Hany TF, Steinert HC (2007) High-risk melanoma: accuracy of FDG PET/CT with added CT morphologic information for

detection of metastases. Radiology 244(2):566–574. doi:10.1148/radiol.2442061099
36. Ho Shon I, Chung DKV, Saw RPM, Thompson J (2008) Guidelines for imaging in cutaneous melanoma. Nucl Med Commun 29(10):877–879
37. Xing Y, Bronstein Y, Ross MI, Askew RL, Lee JE, Gershenwald JE, Royal R, Cormier JN (2011) Contemporary diagnostic imaging modalities for the staging and surveillance of melanoma patients: a meta-analysis. J Natl Cancer Inst 103(2):129–142. doi:10.1093/jnci/djq455
38. Iagaru A, Quon A, Johnson D, Gambhir SS, McDougall IR (2007) 2-Deoxy-2-[F-18] fluoro-D-glucose positron emission tomography/computed tomography in the management of melanoma. Mol Imaging Biol 9(1):50–57. doi:10.1007/s11307-006-0065-0
39. Ho Shon IA, Chung DK, Saw RP, Thompson JF (2008) Imaging in cutaneous melanoma. Nucl Med Commun 29(10):847–876. doi:10.1097/MNM.0b013e32830439fb
40. Delbeke D, Coleman RE, Guiberteau MJ, Brown ML, Royal HD, Siegel BA, Townsend DW, Berland LL, Parker JA, Hubner K, Stabin MG, Zubal G, Kachelriess M, Cronin V, Holbrook S (2006) Procedure guideline for tumor imaging with 18F-FDG PET/CT 1.0. J Nucl Med 47(5):885–895
41. Boellaard R, O'Doherty M, Weber W, Mottaghy F, Lonsdale M, Stroobants S, Oyen WJG, Kotzerke J, Hoekstra O, Pruim J, Marsden P, Tatsch K, Hoekstra C, Visser E, Arends B, Verzijlbergen F, Zijlstra J, Comans EFI, Lammertsma A, Paans A, Willemsen A, Beyer T, Bockisch A, Schaefer Prokop C, Delbeke D, Baum R, Chiti A, Krause B (2010) FDG PET and PET/CT: EANM procedure guidelines for tumour PET imaging: version 1.0. Eur J Nucl Med Mol Imaging 37(1):181–200
42. Masuda Y, Kondo C, Matsuo Y, Uetani M, Kusakabe K (2009) Comparison of imaging protocols for 18F-FDG PET/CT in overweight patients: optimizing scan duration versus administered dose. J Nucl Med 50(6):844–848. doi:10.2967/jnumed.108.060590
43. ICRP (2008) Radiation dose to patients from radiopharmaceuticals. Addendum 3 to ICRP Publication 53. ICRP Publication 106. Approved by the Commission in October 2007. Ann ICRP 38(1–2):1–197. doi:10.1016/j.icrp.2008.08.003
44. Dougeni E, Faulkner K, Panayiotakis G (2012) A review of patient dose and optimisation methods in adult and paediatric CT scanning. Eur J Radiol 81(4):e665–e683. doi:10.1016/j.ejrad.2011.05.025
45. Kumar S, Pandey AK, Sharma P, Malhotra A, Kumar R (2012) Optimization of the CT acquisition protocol to reduce patient dose without compromising the diagnostic quality for PET-CT: a phantom study. Nucl Med Commun 33(2):164–170. doi:10.1097/MNM.0b013e32834e0993
46. Xia T, Alessio AM, De Man B, Manjeshwar R, Asma E, Kinahan PE (2012) Ultra-low dose CT attenuation correction for PET/CT. Phys Med Biol 57(2):309–328. doi:10.1088/0031-9155/57/2/309
47. McKeown C, Dempsey MF, Gillen G, Paterson C (2012) Quantitative analysis shows that contrast medium in positron emission tomography/computed tomography may cause significant artefacts. Nucl Med Commun 33(8):864–871. doi:10.1097/MNM.0b013e3283531d45
48. El Fakhri G, Santos PA, Badawi RD, Holdsworth CH, Van Den Abbeele AD, Kijewski MF (2007) Impact of acquisition geometry, image processing, and patient size on lesion detection in whole-body 18F-FDG PET. J Nucl Med 48(12):1951–1960. doi:10.2967/jnumed.108.007369
49. Sugawara Y, Zasadny KR, Neuhoff AW, Wahl RL (1999) Reevaluation of the standardized uptake value for FDG: variations with body weight and methods for correction. Radiology 213(2):521–525
50. Boellaard R (2009) Standards for PET image acquisition and quantitative data analysis. J Nucl Med 50(Suppl 1):11S–20S. doi:10.2967/jnumed.108.057182
51. Culverwell AD, Scarsbrook AF, Chowdhury FU (2011) False-positive uptake on 2-[18F]-fluoro-2-deoxy-D-glucose (FDG) positron-emission tomography/computed tomography (PET/CT) in oncological imaging. Clin Radiol 66(4):366–382. doi:10.1016/j.crad.2010.12.004
52. Schöder H, Fury M, Lee N, Kraus D (2009) PET monitoring of therapy response in head and neck squamous cell carcinoma. J Nucl Med 50(Suppl 1):74S–88S. doi:10.2967/jnumed.108.057208
53. Vriens D, Visser E, Lioe-Fee G-O, Oyen W (2010) Methodological considerations in quantification of oncological FDG PET studies. Eur J Nucl Med Mol Imaging 37(7):1408–1425. doi:10.1007/s00259-009-1306-7
54. Lindholm P, Minn H, Leskinen-Kallio S, Bergman J, Ruotsalainen U, Joensuu H (1993) Influence of the blood glucose concentration on FDG uptake in cancer—a PET study. J Nucl Med 34(1):1–6

55. Langen K-J, Braun U, Kops ER, Herzog H, Kuwert T, Nebeling B, Feinendegen LE (1993) The influence of plasma glucose levels on fluorine-18-fluorodeoxyglucose uptake in bronchial carcinomas. J Nucl Med 34(3):355–359
56. Ceriani L, Suriano S, Ruberto T, Giovanella L (2011) Could different hydration protocols affect the quality of 18F-FDG PET/CT images? J Nucl Med Technol 39(2):77–82. doi:10.2967/jnmt.110.081265
57. Jackson RS, Schlarman TC, Hubble WL, Osman MM (2006) Prevalence and patterns of physiologic muscle uptake detected with whole-body 18F-FDG PET. J Nucl Med Technol 34(1):29–33
58. Costelloe CM, Murphy WA, Chasen BA (2009) Musculoskeletal pitfalls in 18F-FDG PET/CT: pictorial review. Am J Roentgenol 193(3 Supplement):WS1–WS13. doi:10.2214/ajr.07.7138
59. Osman MM, Muzaffar R, Altinyay ME, Teymouri C (2011) FDG dose extravasations in PET/CT: frequency and impact on SUV measurements. Front Oncol 1:41. doi:10.3389/fonc.2011.00041
60. Garcia CA, Van Nostrand D, Atkins F, Acio E, Butler C, Esposito G, Kulkarni K, Majd M (2006) Reduction of brown fat 2-deoxy-2-[F-18]fluoro-D-glucose uptake by controlling environmental temperature prior to positron emission tomography scan. Mol Imaging Biol 8(1):24–29. doi:10.1007/s11307-005-0030-3
61. Tatsumi M, Engles JM, Ishimori T, Nicely O, Cohade C, Wahl RL (2004) Intense (18) F-FDG uptake in brown fat can be reduced pharmacologically. J Nucl Med 45(7): 1189–1193
62. Ouellet V, Labb S, Blondin D, Phoenix S, Gurin B, Haman F, Turcotte E, Richard D, Carpentier A (2012) Brown adipose tissue oxidative metabolism contributes to energy expenditure during acute cold exposure in humans. J Clin Invest 122(2):545–552
63. Gelfand MJ, O'Hara SM, Curtwright LA, Maclean JR (2005) Pre-medication to block [(18)F]FDG uptake in the brown adipose tissue of pediatric and adolescent patients. Pediatr Radiol 35(10):984–990. doi:10.1007/s00247-005-1505-8
64. Williams G, Kolodny GM (2008) Method for decreasing uptake of 18F-FDG by hypermetabolic brown adipose tissue on PET. AJR Am J Roentgenol 190(5):1406–1409. doi:10.2214/ajr.07.3205
65. Hicks RJ, Binns D, Stabin MG (2001) Pattern of uptake and excretion of (18)F-FDG in the lactating breast. J Nucl Med 42(8): 1238–1242
66. Niederkohr RD, Rosenberg J, Shabo G, Quon A (2007) Clinical value of including the head and lower extremities in 18F-FDG PET/CT imaging for patients with malignant melanoma. Nucl Med Commun 28(9): 688–695. doi:10.1097/MNM.0b013e32827420cc
67. Querellou S, Keromnes N, Abgral R, Sassolas B, Le Roux PY, Cavarec MB, Le Duc-Pennec A, Couturier O, Salaun PY (2010) Clinical and therapeutic impact of 18F-FDG PET/CT whole-body acquisition including lower limbs in patients with malignant melanoma. Nucl Med Commun 31(9):766–772. doi:10.1097/MNM.0b013e32833cb8b7
68. Pfluger T, Melzer HI, Schneider V, Fougere CL, Coppenrath E, Berking C, Bartenstein P, Weiss M (2011) PET/CT in malignant melanoma: contrast-enhanced CT versus plain low-dose CT. Eur J Nucl Med Mol Imaging 38(5):822–831. doi:10.1007/s00259-010-1702-z
69. Krug B, Crott R, Roch I, Lonneux M, Beguin C, Baurain JF, Pirson AS, Vander Borght T (2010) Cost-effectiveness analysis of FDG PET-CT in the management of pulmonary metastases from malignant melanoma. Acta Oncol 49(2):192–200. doi:10.3109/02841860903440254
70. Bastiaannet E, Uyl-de Groot CA, Brouwers AH, van der Jagt EJ, Hoekstra OS, Oyen W, Verzijlbergen F, van Ooijen B, Thompson JF, Hoekstra HJ (2012) Cost-effectiveness of adding FDG-PET or CT to the diagnostic work-up of patients with stage III melanoma. Ann Surg 255(4):771–776. doi:10.1097/SLA.0b013e31824a5742
71. Vidal M, Vidal-Sicart S, Torrents A, Perissinotti A, Navales I, Paredes P, Pons F (2012) Accuracy and reproducibility of lymphoscintigraphy for sentinel node detection in patients with cutaneous melanoma. J Nucl Med 53(8):1193–1199. doi:10.2967/jnumed.112.104463
72. Goerres GW, Kamel E, Heidelberg TN, Schwitter MR, Burger C, von Schulthess GK (2002) PET-CT image co-registration in the thorax: influence of respiration. Eur J Nucl Med Mol Imaging 29(3):351–360
73. Osman MM, Cohade C, Nakamoto Y, Marshall LT, Leal JP, Wahl RL (2003) Clinically significant inaccurate localization of lesions with PET/CT: frequency in 300 patients. J Nucl Med 44(2):240–243
74. Metser U, Miller E, Lerman H, Even-Sapir E (2007) Benign nonphysiologic lesions with increased 18F-FDG uptake on PET/CT: characterization and incidence. Am J Roentgenol 189(5):1203–1210. doi:10.2214/ajr.07.2083

75. Liu Y, Ghesani NV, Zuckier LS (2010) Physiology and pathophysiology of incidental findings detected on FDG-PET scintigraphy. Semin Nucl Med 40(4):294–315. doi:10.1053/j.semnuclmed.2010.02.002
76. Kazama T, Swanston N, Podoloff DA, Macapinlac HA (2005) Effect of colony-stimulating factor and conventional- or high-dose chemotherapy on FDG uptake in bone marrow. Eur J Nucl Med Mol Imaging 32(12):1406–1411. doi:10.1007/s00259-005-1890-0
77. Klijanienko J, Petras S, De Bosschere L, Paulmier B, Le Tourneau C, Rodriguez J (2012) False-positive FDG PET/CT uptake in Warthin tumor in head and neck oncological patients confirmed by a fine needle aspiration. Diagn Cytopathol 40(3):282–284. doi:10.1002/dc.21640
78. Finkelstein SE, Carrasquillo JA, Hoffman JM, Galen B, Choyke P, White DE, Rosenberg SA, Sherry RM (2004) A prospective analysis of positron emission tomography and conventional imaging for detection of stage IV metastatic melanoma in patients undergoing metastasectomy. Ann Surg Oncol 11(8):731–738. doi:10.1245/aso.2004.01.023
79. Wagner JD, Schauwecker D, Davidson D, Logan T, Coleman JJ 3rd, Hutchins G, Love C, Wenck S, Daggy J (2005) Inefficacy of F-18 fluorodeoxy-D-glucose-positron emission tomography scans for initial evaluation in early-stage cutaneous melanoma. Cancer 104(3):570–579. doi:10.1002/cncr.21189
80. Cantorias MV, Figueroa SD, Quinn TP, Lever JR, Hoffman TJ, Watkinson LD, Carmack TL, Cutler CS (2009) Development of high-specific-activity (68)Ga-labeled DOTA-rhenium-cyclized alpha-MSH peptide analog to target MC1 receptors overexpressed by melanoma tumors. Nucl Med Biol 36(5):505–513. doi:10.1016/j.nucmedbio.2009.01.017
81. Wei L, Zhang X, Gallazzi F, Miao Y, Jin X, Brechbiel MW, Xu H, Clifford T, Welch MJ, Lewis JS, Quinn TP (2009) Melanoma imaging using (111)In-, (86)Y- and (68)Ga-labeled CHX-A″-Re(Arg11)CCMSH. Nucl Med Biol 36(4):345–354. doi:10.1016/j.nucmedbio.2009.01.007
82. Ren G, Liu S, Liu H, Miao Z, Cheng Z (2010) Radiofluorinated rhenium cyclized alpha-MSH analogues for PET imaging of melanocortin receptor 1. Bioconjug Chem 21(12):2355–2360. doi:10.1021/bc100391a
83. Dimitrakopoulou-Strauss A, Strauss LG, Burger C (2001) Quantitative PET studies in pretreated melanoma patients: a comparison of 6-[18F]fluoro-l-dopa with 18F-FDG and (15)O-water using compartment and non-compartment analysis. J Nucl Med 42(2):248–256
84. de Vries EFJ, Luurtsema G, Brüssermann M, Elsinga PH, Vaalburg W (1999) Fully automated synthesis module for the high yield one-pot preparation of 6-[18F]fluoro-l-DOPA. Appl Radiat Isot 51(4):389–394. doi:10.1016/s0969-8043(99)00057-3
85. Beer AJ, Haubner R, Sarbia M, Goebel M, Luderschmidt S, Grosu AL, Schnell O, Niemeyer M, Kessler H, Wester HJ, Weber WA, Schwaiger M (2006) Positron emission tomography using [18F]Galacto-RGD identifies the level of integrin alpha(v)beta3 expression in man. Clin Cancer Res 12(13):3942–3949. doi:10.1158/1078-0432.ccr-06-0266
86. Yang J, Guo H, Miao Y (2010) Technetium-99m-labeled Arg-Gly-Asp-conjugated alpha-melanocyte stimulating hormone hybrid peptides for human melanoma imaging. Nucl Med Biol 37(8):873–883. doi:10.1016/j.nucmedbio.2010.05.006
87. Cobben DC, Jager PL, Elsinga PH, Maas B, Suurmeijer AJ, Hoekstra HJ (2003) 3′-18F-fluoro-3′-deoxy-l-thymidine: a new tracer for staging metastatic melanoma? J Nucl Med 44(12):1927–1932
88. Ribas A, Benz MR, Allen-Auerbach MS, Radu C, Chmielowski B, Seja E, Williams JL, Gomez-Navarro J, McCarthy T, Czernin J (2010) Imaging of CTLA4 blockade-induced cell replication with (18)F-FLT PET in patients with advanced melanoma treated with tremelimumab. J Nucl Med 51(3):340–346. doi:10.2967/jnumed.109.070946
89. Wilson WR, Hay MP (2011) Targeting hypoxia in cancer therapy. Nat Rev Cancer 11(6):393–410. doi:10.1038/nrc3064
90. Wyss MT, Honer M, Schubiger PA, Ametamey SM (2006) NanoPET imaging of [(18)F]fluoromisonidazole uptake in experimental mouse tumours. Eur J Nucl Med Mol Imaging 33(3):311–318. doi:10.1007/s00259-005-1951-4
91. Rudman SM, Jameson MB, McKeage MJ, Savage P, Jodrell DI, Harries M, Acton G, Erlandsson F, Spicer JF (2011) A phase 1 study of AS1409, a novel antibody-cytokine fusion protein, in patients with malignant melanoma or renal cell carcinoma. Clin Cancer Res 17(7):1998–2005. doi:10.1158/1078-0432.ccr-10-2490
92. Dadachova E, Revskaya E, Sesay MA, Damania H, Boucher R, Sellers RS, Howell RC, Burns L, Thornton GB, Natarajan A, Mirick GR, DeNardo SJ, DeNardo GL,

Casadevall A (2008) Pre-clinical evaluation and efficacy studies of a melanin-binding IgM antibody labeled with 188Re against experimental human metastatic melanoma in nude mice. Cancer Biol Ther 7(7):1116–1127

93. Revskaya E, Jongco AM, Sellers RS, Howell RC, Koba W, Guimaraes AJ, Nosanchuk JD, Casadevall A, Dadachova E (2009) Radioimmunotherapy of experimental human metastatic melanoma with melanin-binding antibodies and in combination with dacarbazine. Clin Cancer Res 15(7):2373–2379. doi:10.1158/1078-0432.ccr-08-2376
94. Povoski SP, Hall NC, Martin EW Jr, Walker MJ (2008) Multimodality approach of perioperative 18F-FDG PET/CT imaging, intraoperative 18F-FDG handheld gamma probe detection, and intraoperative ultrasound for tumor localization and verification of resection of all sites of hypermetabolic activity in a case of occult recurrent metastatic melanoma. World J Surg Oncol 6:1. doi:10.1186/1477-7819-6-1
95. Franc BL, Mari C, Johnson D, Leong SP (2005) The role of a positron- and high-energy gamma photon probe in intraoperative localization of recurrent melanoma. Clin Nucl Med 30(12):787–791
96. Buchbender C, Heusner TA, Lauenstein TC, Bockisch A, Antoch G (2012) Oncologic PET/MRI, part 1: tumors of the brain, head and neck, chest, abdomen, and pelvis. J Nucl Med 53(6):928–938
97. Muller-Horvat C, Radny P, Eigentler TK, Schafer J, Pfannenberg C, Horger M, Khorchidi S, Nagele T, Garbe C, Claussen CD, Schlemmer HP (2006) Prospective comparison of the impact on treatment decisions of whole-body magnetic resonance imaging and computed tomography in patients with metastatic malignant melanoma. Eur J Cancer 42(3):342–350. doi:10.1016/j.ejca.2005.10.008
98. Pfannenberg C, Aschoff P, Schanz S, Eschmann SM, Plathow C, Eigentler TK, Garbe C, Brechtel K, Vonthein R, Bares R, Claussen CD, Schlemmer HP (2007) Prospective comparison of 18F-fluorodeoxyglucose positron emission tomography/computed tomography and whole-body magnetic resonance imaging in staging of advanced malignant melanoma. Eur J Cancer 43(3):557–564. doi:10.1016/j.ejca.2006.11.014
99. Laurent V, Trausch G, Bruot O, Olivier P, Felblinger J, Regent D (2010) Comparative study of two whole-body imaging techniques in the case of melanoma metastases: advantages of multi-contrast MRI examination including a diffusion-weighted sequence in comparison with PET-CT. Eur J Radiol 75(3):376–383. doi:10.1016/j.ejrad.2009.04.059
100. Dellestable P, Granel-Brocard F, Rat AC, Olivier P, Regent D, Schmutz JL (2011) Impact of whole body magnetic resonance imaging (MRI) in the management of melanoma patients, in comparison with positron emission tomography/computed tomography (TEP/CT) and CT. Ann Dermatol Venereol 138(5):377–383. doi:10.1016/j.annder.2011.02.023

Part VI

Emerging Technologies for Marker Validation

Chapter 31

Immune System Functional Pathway Analysis Using Single Cell Network Profiling (SCNP): A Novel Tool in Cancer Immunotherapy

Alessandra Cesano and David Spellmeyer

Abstract

The development of cancer immunotherapies has been ongoing for many years and has shown limited success. Novel biomarkers are needed to identify patients most likely to respond to anticancer immune-therapeutic approaches. Moreover, a systems-level approach is required for comprehensive understanding of the interconnected components, pathways, and cell types associated with an immune response. In this chapter, we describe single cell network profiling (SCNP), a novel method for assessing and measuring immune function/dysfunction at a systems level. SCNP is a multiparametric flow-cytometry-based analysis that can simultaneously measure, at the single cell level, both extracellular surface markers and changes in intracellular signaling proteins in response to extracellular modulators. Measuring changes in signaling proteins following the application of an external modulation informs on the functional capacity of the signaling network which cannot be assessed by the measurement of basal signaling alone. In addition, the simultaneous analysis of multiple pathways in multiple cell subsets can provide insight into the connectivity of both cell signaling networks and immune cell subtypes. The experimental steps associated with an SCNP assay are (1) pre-analytical sample preparation; (2) modulation for functional analysis; (3) staining with antibody cocktail; (4) data acquisition on flow cytometer; and (5) data analysis and metrics. Important considerations for each step of the assay will be discussed, and data demonstrating the utility of SCNP for immune monitoring applications will be summarized.

Key words Single cell network profiling, Multiparametric, Flow cytometry, Signaling pathways, Quantitative, Immunotherapy

1 Introduction

The development of cancer immunotherapies has been ongoing for many years and has shown limited success [1]. Melanoma and renal cell carcinoma are traditionally thought to be "immuno-sensitive" tumors [2, 3], but until recently, interleukin-2 and interferon-α2β were the only approved immunotherapeutic agents for those diseases in the United States with response rates in the single digits [4–7]. In 2011, the FDA-approved ipilimumab, an anti-CTLA-4

Magdalena Thurin and Francesco M. Marincola (eds.), *Molecular Diagnostics for Melanoma: Methods and Protocols*, Methods in Molecular Biology, vol. 1102, DOI 10.1007/978-1-62703-727-3_31, © Springer Science+Business Media New York 2014

monoclonal antibody, for treatment of unresectable, metastatic melanoma [8]. Phase III clinical trials demonstrated that ipilimumab improved overall survival in patients with metastatic melanoma who no longer responded to standard therapy and extended survival in patients with metastatic melanoma who had not received prior therapy [8]. Despite these successes, ipilimumab treatment still benefits only a subset of patients (~30 %) and is associated with significant side effects and cost [9]. Novel biomarkers are therefore needed to identify patients most likely to respond to this drug and other anticancer immune-therapeutic approaches [10]. In this chapter, a new approach to assess and measure immune function/dysfunction at a systems level will be described.

1.1 Systems Immunology: A Network Approach for Characterizing Immune Function

A systems-level approach is required for comprehensive understanding of the interconnected components, pathways, and cell types associated with an immune response. Traditionally and mainly due to technological limitations, reductionist approaches analyzing individual components within the immune system have been used in research. The advent of high-throughput technologies is now ushering in a new era of systems immunology, which aims to understand the complex network of components which create an immune response [11]. Here, we describe a novel technology, single cell network profiling (SCNP), that allows for simultaneous functional measurements of multiple cell subpopulations within complex tissues (such as bone marrow and peripheral blood (PB)) without the need for physical cell separation [12–15]. This enables a more integrated description of immune function than traditional studies which often focus on the behavior of specific cell types physically isolated from heterogeneous tissues such as PB, spleen, or lymph nodes.

1.2 Unique Aspects of Single Cell Network Profiling for Immune Monitoring

SCNP is a multiparametric flow-cytometry-based analysis that can simultaneously measure, at the single cell level, both extracellular surface markers and changes in intracellular signaling proteins in response to extracellular modulators. Measuring changes in signaling proteins following the application of an external modulation informs on the functional capacity of the signaling network which cannot be assessed by the measurement of basal signaling alone [16]. In addition, the simultaneous analysis of multiple pathways in multiple cell subsets can provide insight into the connectivity of both cell signaling networks and immune cell subtypes [17].

The integration of four different parameters makes SCNP technology unique (*see* Fig. 1):

(a) First, the level of resolution provided, i.e., single cell level. In the SCNP assay, the measurements of posttranslational protein changes after exposure to extracellular modulators (such as cytokines, chemokines, and pharmacologic agents) are made at the single cell level since the technology is flow cytometry based.

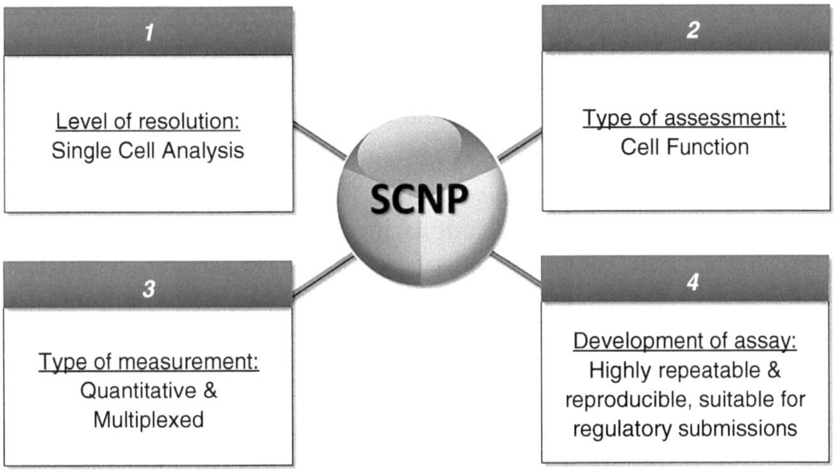

Fig. 1 Four key parameters contribute to the uniqueness of the SCNP platform

(b) Second, the type of assessment performed, i.e., cell function. Unlike the "snapshot" view of cellular signaling provided by measuring the basal or resting phosphorylation state of an intracellular protein, the application of extracellular modulation forces the intracellular signaling network to respond, revealing dynamic information about the way the network processes information. Thus the functional capabilities of key signaling networks can be compared, for instance, between the cells of healthy individuals and diseased patients, allowing detection and characterization of signaling abnormalities associated with disease or in the same patient over time (e.g., disease monitoring), allowing the identification of changes associated with disease progression or with response to therapeutic agents.

(c) Third, the type of measurement performed, i.e., quantitative and multiplexed. Since different modulators can act on the same intracellular pathways and, in heterogeneous tissues, on multiple cell subsets at the same time, the SCNP approach allows measurement in a quantitative fashion and simultaneously of changes in intracellular protein levels in response to different modulators in different cell subpopulations without the need for cell separating/sorting.

(d) Finally but importantly, for such an approach to be useful not only in a research context but also in a clinical one (e.g., development of clinically actionable biomarkers for disease status or response to treatment), it must be highly accurate and reproducible, meeting regulatory standards of analytic validity [18]. This has been recently achieved with coefficients of variations (CV) of functional assays pathway stimulation routinely below

5 % [13]. Achieving this goal requires strict instrument standardization and performance monitoring, rigorous attention to sample quality and reagent qualification, and the introduction of automation and validated methodology [13].

When applied to pathways shown to be important in disease pathology, this method of mapping signaling networks has potential applications in the development of disease profiling, the identification of novel disease targets, predictive tests for therapeutic response and patient selection and overall for improved efficiency of drug development [12–15, 19–27]. Recently, we have published a "map" of the healthy immune signaling network, in which several age-associated signaling nodes were identified in specific subsets of cells within PB mononuclear cell samples from healthy individuals [28]. These studies underscore the potential utility of SCNP for immune monitoring applications as well as biomarker development for immune-mediated diseases.

1.3 Application of SCNP to Immune Profiling in Healthy and Melanoma Subjects

The SCNP assay has been used for immune profiling in both healthy subjects and melanoma patients. We utilized SCNP to perform broad functional characterization of the healthy immune cell signaling network [28]. As expected, many of the immunomodulators included in the study induced cell type-specific responses, highlighting the complexity of the regulation of biological function during immune responses. For a subset of the modulators and specific cell types investigated, differential receptor expression and/or differential activation patterns have been previously reported. In instances where such data is available, the cell type-specific signaling responses were generally consistent with those reports [29–31]. This map can be compared with those generated using samples from patients with immune-based disorders to identify changes in the network architecture that occur under pathological conditions and can be applied to the analysis of samples obtained longitudinally from treated patients to monitor individual responses to therapeutics. We have also demonstrated that some of the variation in healthy immune signaling responses can in fact be attributed to donor demographic characteristics such as age or race [32]. Finally, we have examined CD4+ T cell signaling in the context of CTLA-4 expression, a study which has direct relevance to the ipilimumab mechanism of action. We have shown that signal transduction activities differed between CTLA-4-defined CD4+ subsets, and between healthy and melanoma samples. Further studies are ongoing, which will expand on the biological findings and assess the association between ipilimumab response and signaling differences. These studies demonstrate the utility of SCNP for immune monitoring and point to the promise of using this method for cancer immunotherapy biomarker development.

2 Materials

2.1 Cell Sample Preparation

1. Ficoll-Paque Histopaque (GE Healthcare, Sunnyvale CA).
2. Amine Aqua viability dye to evaluate cell health and sample quality (Invitrogen, Carlsbad CA).
3. Cleaved Poly (ADP-ribose) polymerase 1 (cPARP)-specific antibody (BD, San Jose, CA).

2.2 Signaling Assay

1. 96-well tissue culture treated flat bottom plates (Costar Sigma-Aldrich, St. Louis MO).
2. Foil plate seal (E&K Scientific).
3. Modulators specific to desired assay which are selected based on biological relevance and performance in previously conducted studies (*see* Table 1 for examples).
4. 1.6 % Paraformaldehyde (PFA).
5. 100 % Methanol (MeOH) stored at −20 °C.

2.3 Immuno-staining Assay

1. Fluorescence-activated cell sorter (FACS) buffer: Phosphate-buffered saline (1×, PBS), 10.5 % Bovine serum albumin (BSA) with 0.05 % NaN_3.
2. Wash buffer: 1× PBS, 0.5 % BSA.
3. Antibodies to detect desired target which are selected based on biological relevance and performance in previously conducted studies (*see* Table 2 for examples). Primary antibody cocktails for

Table 1
Examples of modulators for analysis of immune system

Modulator	Concentration	Source
IFNα	1,000 IU/mL	PBL Interferon Source, Piscataway, NJ
IFNγ	250 ng/mL	BD Biosciences, San Jose, CA
IL-4	50 ng/mL	BD Biosciences, San Jose, CA
IL-10	50 ng/mL	BD Biosciences, San Jose, CA
α-IgD	5 μg/mL	BD Biosciences, San Jose, CA
IL-2	50 ng/mL	R&D Systems, Minneapolis, MN
IL-6	50 ng/mL	R&D Systems, Minneapolis, MN
IL-27	50 ng/mL	R&D Systems, Minneapolis, MN
CD40L	0.5 μg/mL	R&D Systems, Minneapolis, MN
R848	5 μg/mL	Invitrogen, San Diego, CA
LPS	1 μg/mL	Sigma Aldrich, St. Louis, MO
PMA	40 nM	Sigma Aldrich, St. Louis, MO

Table 2
Examples of antibodies for analysis of immune system

Antibody	Source
α-CD3 (clone UCHT1)	BD Biosciences, San Jose, CA
α-CD4 (clone RPA-T4)	BD Biosciences, San Jose, CA
α-CD45RA (clone HI100)	BD Biosciences, San Jose, CA
α-CD20 (clone H1)	BD Biosciences, San Jose, CA
α-pNFκB (clone K10-895.12.50)	BD Biosciences, San Jose, CA
α-cPARP (clone F21-852)	BD Biosciences, San Jose, CA
α-pStat1 (clone 4a)	BD Biosciences, San Jose, CA
α-pStat3 (clone 4/p-Stat3)	BD Biosciences, San Jose, CA
α-pStat5 (clone 47)	BD Biosciences, San Jose, CA
α-pStat6 (clone 18/p-Stat6)	BD Biosciences, San Jose, CA
α-pErk (clone 20A)	BD Biosciences, San Jose, CA
α-pAtk (clone D9E)	Cell Signaling Technology, Danvers, MA
α-pS6 (clone 2F9)	Cell Signaling Technology, Danvers, MA
α-CD14 (clone RMO52)	Beckman Coulter, Brea, CA

cell surface markers and intracellular signaling molecules, and secondary antibodies are selected based on biological relevance and performance in previously conducted studies [28, 32].

4. SPHERO™ Rainbow Calibration Particles for calibration of raw fluorescence intensity readouts to control for instrument variability and enable comparison of data between plates and instruments (Spherotech, Lake Forest, IL).

2.4 Data Acquisition and Processing

1. Flow cytometry instruments: BD LSRII or BD FACS Canto II (BD, San Jose, CA).
2. FACS DIVA software (BD Biosciences, San Jose CA) for acquiring flow cytometry data.
3. WinList software (Verity House Software, Topsham, ME) for flow cytometry data analysis.

3 Methods

The experimental steps involved in SCNP assay are summarized below and in Fig. 2.

1. Pre-analytical step: Tissue sample (e.g., PB sample) is obtained from a donor. The sample can be assayed "fresh" (as whole unfractionated blood or after Ficoll separation of mononu-

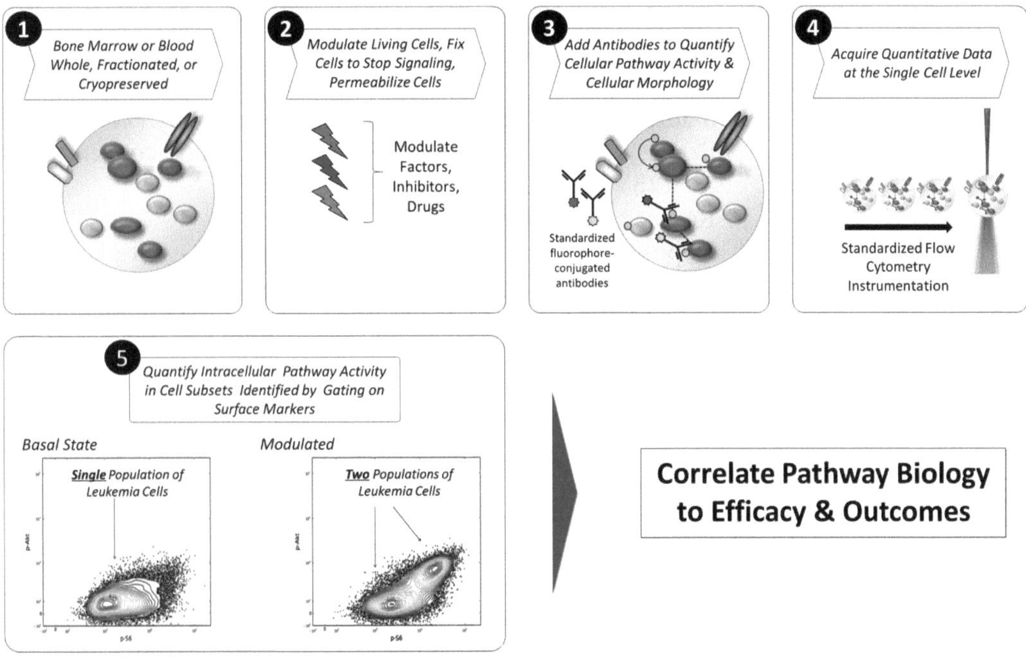

Fig. 2 Schematic of the SCNP assay. The experimental steps associated with an SCNP assay are: (*1*) Pre-analytical sample preparation; (*2*) Modulation for functional analysis; (*3*) Fixation, permeabilization, and staining with antibody cocktail; (*4*) Data acquisition on flow cytometer; and (*5*) Data analysis and metrics

clear cells) or cryopreserved (after Ficoll separation of mononuclear cells). In the latter case, the sample will be thawed and dead cells eliminated by a second Ficoll separation before testing in the SCNP assay.

2. Modulation for functional analysis: Living cells are treated with different modulators chosen to engage the specific intracellular pathways of interest (*see* Table 1); after modulation, cells are fixed and cell membranes permeabilized.
3. Staining with antibody cocktails: Cells are then exposed to a mixture of antibodies, some directed against surface markers (allowing the phenotypic identification of different cell subsets) and some against specific posttranslational modification of intracellular proteins.
4. Data acquisition by flow cytometer: Stained cells are then analyzed by flow cytometry. BD LSRII or BD FACS Canto II instruments measure up to ten parameters (eight fluorochromes and two light scatter parameters) per cell.
5. Data analysis and metrics: In SCNP assay terminology, a "signaling node" is used to refer to a proteomic read out in the presence or absence of a specific modulator. Intracellular pathway activity is then quantified using specific metrics in each cell subset identified by gating on surface markers.

3.1 Thawing of Samples

1. Thaw samples in a 37 °C water bath and underlay with Ficoll to remove dead cells and debris (*see* **Note 1**). Perform automated cell count.
2. Stain cells with Amine Aqua to measure viability (*see* **Note 2**). Perform final automated cell count and adjust concentration to 1.25×10^6 live cells/mL.
3. Rest cells for 1.5 h at 37 °C.
4. Deposit samples (10^5 cells per well) into 96-well plates pre-warmed to 37 °C (*see* **Note 3**). For positive controls, include a row of an established cell lines (e.g., GDM-1, U937, or RS4;11) in each plate (10^5 cells per well). Eight peak SPHERO™ Rainbow Calibration Particles can also be included as a way to normalize instrument variance (*see* **Note 4**).

3.2 Signaling Assay

1. Rest samples for 30 min at 37 °C (unless otherwise specified, all steps in this subheading to occur at 37 °C).
2. Add modulators to samples in 96-well plate (*see* **Note 5**) and incubate for 15 min.
3. Fix cells by incubation with 200 μL pre-warmed 2.4 % PFA per well for 10 min. Centrifuge plate at 1,000 × g for 5 min and aspirate PFA.
4. Permeabilize cells by adding 1 mL 100 % MeOH at −20 °C per well. Seal plates, and incubate overnight at −80 °C.

3.3 Phenotypic Assay

1. Remove cells from 37 °C and put on ice. Add 25 μL primary antibody cocktail (for cell surface markers) to each well (*see* **Note 5**), and incubate on ice for 30 min.
2. Wash cells 2× with 1 mL each ice-cold FACS buffer. Centrifuge plates at 400 × g for 5 min, then aspirate wash buffer.
3. Incubate cells with 2° antibody cocktail in the dark at room temperature for 30 min.
4. Wash plates 2× with FACS buffer, then incubate with 1 mL of 1.6 % PFA for 5 min. Centrifuge, aspirate supernatant, seal plate, and store in dark at 4 °C.

3.4 Stain for Signaling Pathways

1. Remove plates from −80 °C and wash 2× with FACS buffer.
2. Add antibody cocktail to cells in 96-well plate (*see* **Note 5**), and incubate samples at ambient temperature for 1 h in the dark. The antibody cocktail contains both antibody-directed against surface markers (for gating of cell subsets) and against intracellular read outs.
3. If no secondary antibody is needed, wash plates 2× with FACS buffer followed by a wash with 1.6 % PFA. Seal plate and store at 4 °C.
4. If secondary antibody is needed, wash plates 2× with FACS buffer then incubate with 2° antibody at room temperature in the dark for 30 min. Wash 2× with FACS buffer, then 1× wash with 1.6 % PFA. Centrifuge and aspirate PFA, seal plate, and store in dark at 4 °C.

3.5 Acquisition of Data

1. Load fixed, stained cells in 96-well plates onto cytometer and acquire data with FACS Diva software (*see* **Note 6**).
2. Export FCS files and confirm that metadata matches DIVA XML input file. Perform gating on cell populations of interest (*see* **Note 6**).
3. Analysis of data can be done with WinList software.
4. Obtain raw data for Fluorescence Intensity (FI) from instrument (*see* **Note 7**).
5. Convert raw FI to calibrated intensity metrics (ERFs, Equivalent Number of Reference Fluorophores) (*see* **Note 7**).
6. Calculate of metrics used to quantify SCNP assay readouts and interpret functionality and biology of each signaling node (*see* **Note 8**).

4 Notes

1. The SCNP assay can be used with any live cell suspension. For immune system analysis applications, PB samples have been extensively used. Previous studies have shown that different preparations of PB samples are acceptable for the SCNP assay. Specifically, fresh whole PB, fresh Ficoll-fractionated or cryopreserved samples can be used to generate reproducible and accurate data. "Bridging" studies which compare the results of SCNP assay read outs between paired fresh and cryopreserved samples have been previously published [33], and results suggest that SCNP assays developed and validated using cryopreserved PB samples can be applied to fresh samples and integrated prospectively into frontline clinical trials and clinical practice. This sample input flexibility has important implications for the clinical applicability of the SCNP assay. For example, the ability to apply the SCNP technology to fresh whole blood enables pharmacodynamic studies [19], while analysis of cryopreserved Ficoll-fractionated samples allows for development of patient stratification biomarkers using retrospective sample sources [12, 18, 21].
2. Because SCNP is a proteomic, quantitative evaluation of modulated cell function, sample quality is a critical pre-analytical consideration. In SCNP assay, sample quality is evaluated by measuring "cell health" defined as the percentage of live (Amine Aqua negative) and non-apoptotic (cleaved PARP negative) cells (*see* Fig. 3). The Amine Aqua stain employs an amine-reactive fluorescent dye to evaluate cell viability. Cells that are Amine Aqua negative have intact membranes and are considered viable. The cleaved PARP antibody is utilized as a marker of cells undergoing apoptosis. Cells that are cleaved PARP negative are considered non-apoptotic. In multiple

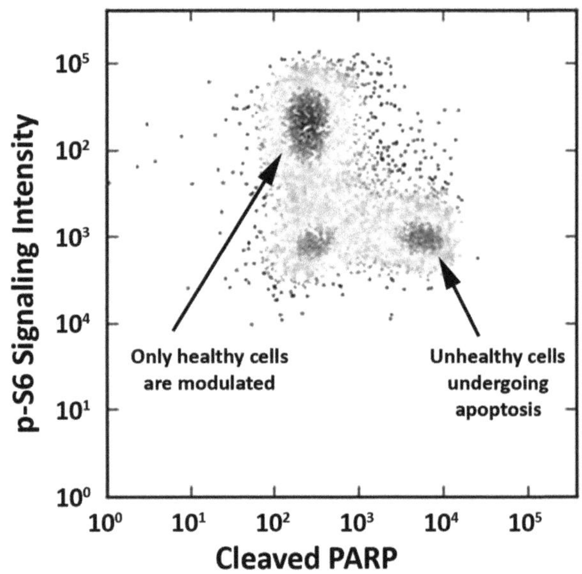

Fig. 3 Association between cell health and intrinsic cell signaling capability. Only "healthy" cells (i.e., Amine Aqua and cleaved PARP negative) are signaling in response to modulation, as demonstrated by increase in p-S6 signaling intensity, while unhealthy cells undergoing apoptosis (cleaved PARP positive) do not show signaling. This analysis of sample quality/cell health is integrated into study design and qualification of samples

studies, we have shown an association between cell health and intrinsic cell signaling capability. Based on these findings, we have implemented procedures to test all samples for quality as part of the SCNP assay (i.e., cell health) to assess their "evaluability" based on pre-defined cutoffs. Therefore, analysis of sample quality/cell health must be integrated into study design and qualification of samples. Based on the above considerations, 48 h is considered the maximum time that can elapse from PB sample collection to SCNP testing (or sample cryopreservation for future inclusion in SCNP assay) [34].

3. The SCNP assay has been optimized for a 96-well plate format. Figure 4 provides a schematic example of a plate layout and emphasizes the high-throughput nature of the SCNP platform. In each plate, experimental samples are tested along with important instrument and laboratory work flow controls (*see* **Note 4**).

   While the multiplexing capability of flow cytometry is limited by the number of available fluorophores, the SCNP multiparametric analysis can expand the array of signaling nodes that are evaluable beyond the number of available fluorophores by maintaining a constant cocktail of surface antibodies while changing the intracellular readout cocktail [13]. Because of the many assay components involved (*see* Fig. 4), software and informatics tools for plate layout design and

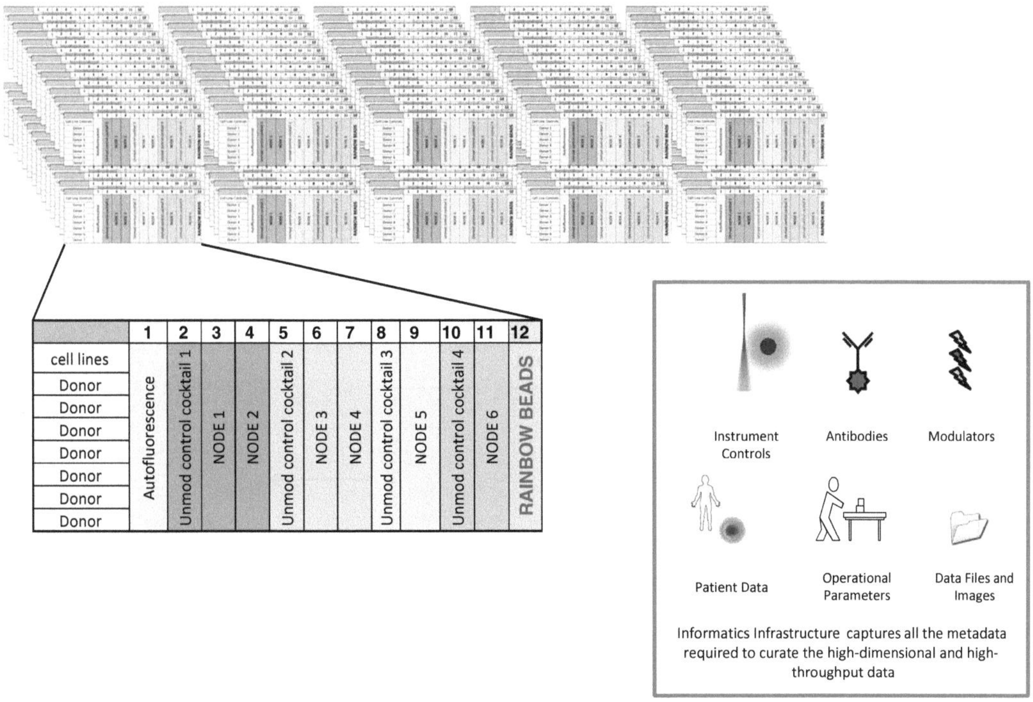

Fig. 4 SCNP platform is scalable in high-throughput cytometry formats. Diagram illustrates a sample plate setup, which includes seven patient samples, control cell lines and calibration particles, six different nodes with unmodulated controls, and an autofluorescence control. Semiautomated system uses Hamilton robotics for high-throughput processing. This flexible plate setup enables SCNP utility in numerous applications, including measurement of multiple kinetic time points, IC_{50} determinations, and high-throughput drug discovery screening

experimental planning have been developed to allow for highly flexible experimental setups while simultaneously ensuring rigorous data curation of experimental data for every well. This informatics infrastructure is a critical aspect of the multiplexing capabilities of the SCNP platform (*see* Fig 4).

4. Three types of controls are used to ensure accuracy and reproducibility in SCNP experiments: Instrument controls, cell line controls, and process controls (*see* Fig. 5).
   (a) Instrument Controls. Linearity verification is performed daily for all fluorescence detectors on each cytometer using eight Peak SPHERO™ Rainbow Calibration Particles (RCP), Spherotech Lake Forest, IL. The slope, intercept, and R squared values obtained from the linear regression are used to standardize, qualify, and monitor the instrument during setup. In addition, RCP are also run in each plate where they are used to calibrate the raw fluorescence intensity readouts to control for instrument variability and allow for comparison of data between plates and instruments. Acceptable CV for the RCP are those below 2 %.

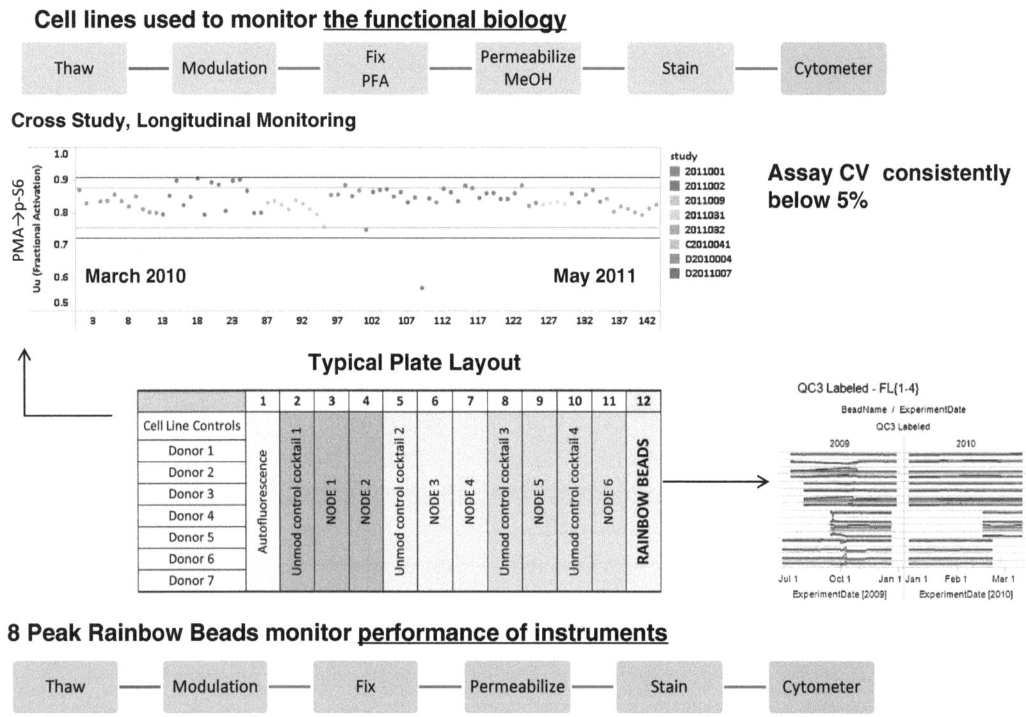

Fig. 5 Summary of assay controls used to monitor performance of SCNP assay. Instrument controls, cell line controls, and process controls are used to ensure accuracy and reproducibility in SCNP experiments. Cell line controls are included on each plate to ensure consistency in assay performance and monitor functional biology. Assay coefficient of variation (CV) is consistently below 5 %, as shown in the cross-study during longitudinal monitoring. Rainbow calibration particles (RCP) are run in each plate to calibrate the raw fluorescence intensity readouts to control for instrument variability and allow for comparison of data between plates and instruments. Acceptable CV of the RCP are below 2 %

(b) *Cell Line Controls.* Multiple cell lines, such as GDM-1, U937, and RS4;11, are included as controls on each plate to ensure consistency in assay performance. In combination, these cell lines provide plate-based controls for all modulator/antibody readout combinations used in a typical study and they are used to identify potential technical variability at the modulation, fixation, and staining steps in the laboratory work flow. Acceptable CVs are below 5 % for each of the nodes examined. Higher variance is usually indicative of either technical issues such as cytometer clogs or an inherent lack of cell line responsiveness to specific modulators or poor signaling due to poor cell health.

(c) *Process Controls.* Several data analysis tools have been developed to facilitate experimental setup and data tracking to ensure verification of data integrity at each step in the sample processing workflow [35]. These tools are used to manage the sample, reagent, and instrument data from initial study design through processing and to un-blinding of clinical data (when applicable). Additionally, a set of internal software tools have been developed to perform high-volume gating, to calculate all metrics employed, and to allow for data analysis, interpretation, and visualization. Together these represent significant process efficiency improvements in SCNP assays.

5. Two groups of measurements are typically performed for each sample: cell surface marker expression and intracellular signaling. Modulators, antibodies, and reagents are selected based on biological relevance and performance in previously conducted studies. The selection of modulators, antibodies, and reagents is customized for each application. We specifically titer each of the antibodies to determine the optimal concentrations for the conditions (modulations and samples) tested. Tables 1 and 2 list the modulators and antibodies, respectively, previously used for an analysis of the immune system [28, 32].
6. Flow cytometry data are acquired using FACS DIVA software on LSRII or CantoII Flow Cytometers. All flow cytometry data are analyzed with WinList software. For all analyses, dead cells and debris are excluded by forward scatter (FSC), side scatter (SSC), Amine Aqua viability dye, and/or cPARP exclusion. PB cell subsets are identified according to an immunophenotypic gating scheme. Importantly, multiple immune cell subsets are examined simultaneously in the same well (*see* Fig. 6).
7. Functional signaling requires appropriate metrics that are different from those used to quantify surface/static markers. For the SCNP assay, functional biology must be accurately represented by transformation of raw instrument readouts. The combination of calibrated instruments, standardized reagents, and rigorous data tracking enabled by the data curation at experiment setup allows for robust biological interpretations. Novel measures of biological function, which can be applied at the single cell level and calibrated to correct for any instrument variance, have been developed. Figure 7a shows the workflow for calculation of the metrics used to quantify the assay readouts. In all cases, the raw instrument fluorescence intensities are converted to calibrated intensity metrics (ERFs, Equivalent Number of Reference Fluorophores) [36–38]. The calibration is applied on a plate-by-plate basis using the rainbow calibration particles as shown in Fig. 4. This correction ensures that data across the plate and between plates are calibrated to the same values, regardless of the instrument used for acquisition.
8. The normalized assay readouts for surface and intracellular markers are measured using many broad classes of calculated metrics that are applied to interpret the functionality and biology of each signaling node (*see* Fig. 7a). Two are used commonly and are described here.

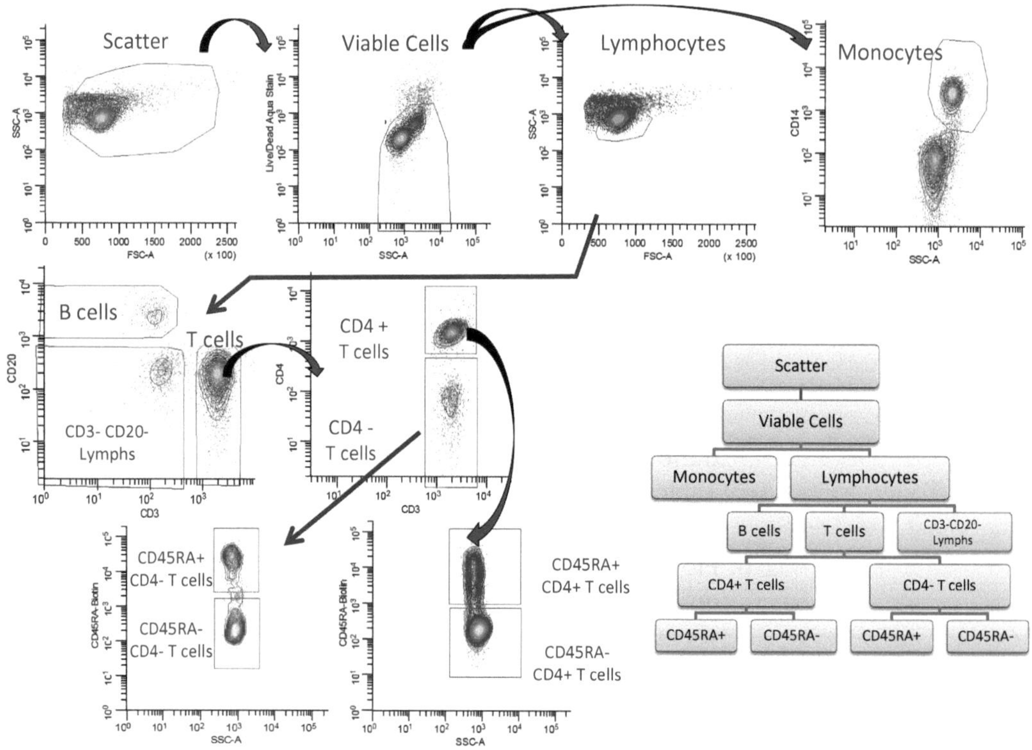

Fig. 6 Immunophenotypic gating scheme for lymphoid cell subsets. Multiple immune subsets are simultaneously examined in the same sample. Gating schemes can be modified to examine specific cell subsets depending on the biological question being addressed

(a) The Fold Metric Class measures the magnitude of the responsiveness of a cell population to modulation relative to the same cell population in the reference well (i.e., unmodulated) by comparing the median fluorescence values of the responsive cell population to that of the reference population on a log2 scale. While this metric is similar to those employed in molecular profiling, we emphasize that this metric is calculated for each of the cell populations of interest, rather than being applied to the whole population. This allows for greater insights into the functional biology of the complex tissues.

(b) The "U" Metric Class measures the fraction or proportion of a cell population that is responsive to modulation. The metric is calculated relative to the same population in the reference well by comparing the overlap of the responsive cellular population relative to the reference population evaluated on a cell-by-cell basis. This class is mathematically equivalent to an AUC metric (which is a scaled Mann–Whitney U metric) and is scaled to range from zero to one. For overlapping populations, the U metric has a value of 0.5. A value different from 0.5 indicates the responsive population has shifted to higher fluorescence (values >0.5) or to lower fluorescence (values <0.5).

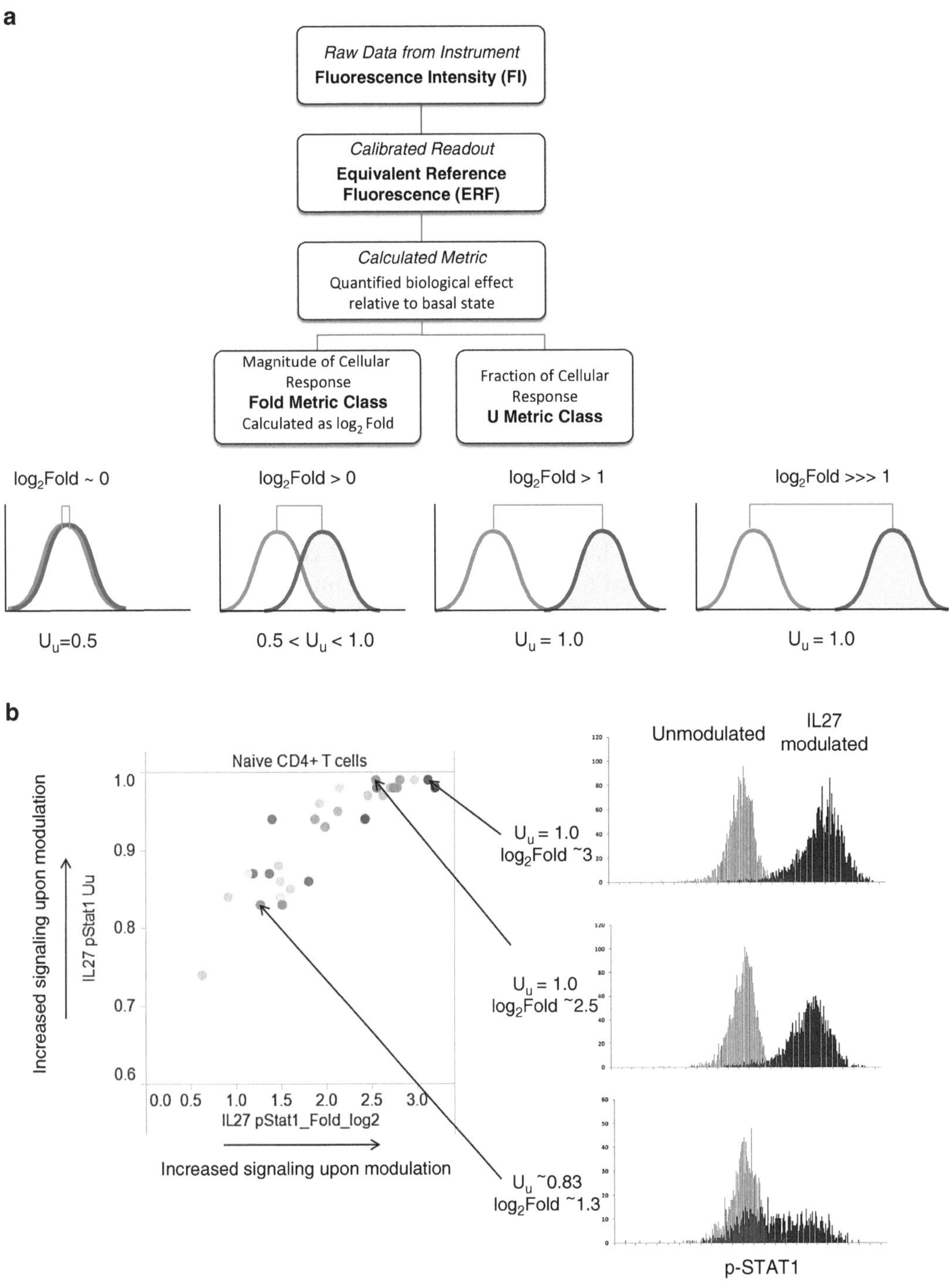

Fig. 7 Data analysis and metrics. (**a**) Functional signaling required appropriate metrics that are different from those used to quantify surface/static markers. (**b**) Example of U_u vs. Log_2Fold metric (color figure online)

This metric has an upper limit of 1.0, which represents the situation in which there is no overlap between the modulated and reference populations.

Figure 7b shows the comparison of the two metrics for IL-27-induced signaling in the naïve CD4+ T Cell population in healthy donors [28]. The scatter plot shows the correlation between the U_u and log2Fold metrics for 30 donors. The histograms show two populations of unmodulated (red) and modulated (blue) for three different donors chosen for illustrative purposes. As the induced signaling increases, both the log2Fold and U_u metrics increase. The bottom histogram shows a relatively broad response of the cells to modulation (blue), resulting in a log2Fold value of ~1.3. The U_u value of 0.83 indicates that approximately 83 % of the responding cells are observed to have a p-STAT1 readout higher than the corresponding unmodulated cells. The middle histogram plot shows population shifts in which the U_u has reached the maximum value of 1.0 (100 % of the modulated cells have a p-STAT1 readout higher than unmodulated cells), while the log2Fold has increased to 2.5. The top histogram shows a sample in which the responsive population shifts to even higher intensity values, which is captured by the increasing log2Fold metric. In this case, the U_u metric does not increase above 1.0.

References

1. Franks HA, Wang Q, Patel PM (2012) New anticancer immunotherapies. Anticancer Res 32:2439–2453
2. Pilla L, Valenti R, Marrari A et al (2006) Vaccination: role in metastatic melanoma. Expert Rev Anticancer Ther 6:1305–1318
3. Sivendran S, Glodny B, Pan M et al (2010) Melanoma immunotherapy. Mt Sinai J Med 77:620–642
4. Zito CR, Kluger HM (2012) Immunotherapy for metastatic melanoma. J Cell Biochem 113:725–734
5. Kirkwood JM, Tarhini AA, Panelli MC et al (2008) Next generation of immunotherapy for melanoma. J Clin Oncol 26:3445–3455
6. Chi M, Dudek AZ (2011) Vaccine therapy for metastatic melanoma: systematic review and meta-analysis of clinical trials. Melanoma Res 21:165–174
7. Homsi J, Grimm JC, Hwu P (2011) Immunotherapy of melanoma: an update. Surg Oncol Clin N Am 20:145–163
8. Hodi FS, O'day SJ, Mcdermott DF et al (2010) Improved survival with ipilimumab in patients with metastatic melanoma. N Engl J Med 363:711–723
9. Weber J (2007) Review: anti-CTLA-4 antibody ipilimumab: case studies of clinical response and immune-related adverse events. Oncologist 12:864–872
10. Yang JC (2011) Melanoma vaccines. Cancer J 17:277–282
11. Schubert C (2011) Systems immunology: complexity captured. Nature 473:113–114
12. Kornblau SM, Minden MD, Rosen DB et al (2010) Dynamic single-cell network profiles in acute myelogenous leukemia are associated with patient response to standard induction therapy. Clin Cancer Res 16:3721–3733
13. Cesano A, Rosen DB, O'meara P et al (2012) Functional pathway analysis in acute myeloid leukemia using single cell network profiling assay: effect of specimen source (bone marrow or peripheral blood) on assay readouts. Cytometry B Clin Cytom 82:158–172
14. Covey TM, Cesano A (2010) Modulated multiparametric phosphoflow cytometry in hematological malignancies: technology and clinical applications. Best Pract Res Clin Haematol 23:319–331
15. Covey TM, Cesano A, Parkinson DR (2010) Single-cell network profiling (SCNP) by flow cytometry in autoimmune disease. Autoimmunity 43:550–559
16. Irish JM, Hovland R, Krutzik PO et al (2004) Single cell profiling of potentiated

phospho-protein networks in cancer cells. Cell 118:217–228
17. Butcher EC, Berg EL, Kunkel EJ (2004) Systems biology in drug discovery. Nat Biotechnol 22:1253–1259
18. Cesano A, Parkinson D (2012) Applications of multiparametric flow cytometry: providing new insights into biology to bridge the gap between research discovery and clinical application. Cytometry A 81:732–733
19. Covey TM, Putta S, Cesano A (2010) Single cell network profiling (SCNP): mapping drug and target interactions. Assay Drug Dev Tech 8:321–343
20. Lacayo NJ, Cesano A, Westfall M, Lackey A et al (2010) Single cell network profiling (SCNP) signatures predict response to induction therapy and relapse risk in pediatric patients with Acute Myeloid Leukemia: Children's Oncology Group (COG) study POG-9421. Blood (ASH Annual Meeting Abstracts) 116, Abstract 954
21. Parkinson DR, Cesano A (2009) Patient-specific classifications of human malignant disease. Curr Opin Mol Ther 11:252–259
22. Rosen DB, Cordeiro JA, Cohen A et al (2012) Assessing signaling pathways associated with in vitro resistance to cytotoxic agents in AML. Leuk Res 36:900–904
23. Rosen DB, Minden MD, Kornblau SM et al (2010) Functional characterization of FLT3 receptor signaling deregulation in acute myeloid leukemia by single cell network profiling (SCNP). PLoS One 5:e13543
24. Rosen DB, Putta S, Covey T et al (2010) Distinct patterns of DNA damage response and apoptosis correlate with Jak/Stat and PI3kinase response profiles in human acute myelogenous leukemia. PLoS One 5:e12405
25. Irish JM, Kotecha N, Nolan GP (2006) Mapping normal and cancer cell signalling networks: towards single-cell proteomics. Nat Rev Cancer 6:146–155
26. Irish JM, Czerwinski DK, Nolan GP et al (2006) Altered B-cell receptor signaling kinetics distinguish human follicular lymphoma B cells from tumor-infiltrating nonmalignant B cells. Blood 108:3135–3142
27. Irish JM, Czerwinski DK, Nolan GP et al (2006) Kinetics of B cell receptor signaling in human B cell subsets mapped by phosphospecific flow cytometry. J Immunol 177:1581–1589
28. Longo DM, Louie B, Putta S et al (2012) Single-cell network profiling of peripheral blood mononuclear cells from healthy donors reveals age- and race-associated differences in immune signaling pathway activation. J Immunol 188:1717–1725
29. Larange A, Antonios D, Pallardy M et al (2009) TLR7 and TLR8 agonists trigger different signaling pathways for human dendritic cell maturation. J Leukoc Biol 85:673–683
30. Hall JC, Rosen A (2010) Type I interferons: crucial participants in disease amplification in autoimmunity. Nat Rev Rheumatol 6:40–49
31. Van Boxel-Dezaire AH, Stark GR (2007) Cell type-specific signaling in response to interferon-gamma. Curr Top Microbiol Immunol 316:119–154
32. Longo DM, Louie B, Mathi K et al (2012) Racial differences in B cell receptor signaling pathway activation. J Transl Med 10:113
33. Cesano A, Gotlib JR, Lacayo NJ et al (2010) Sample cryopreservation does not affect functional read outs in SCNP assays: implications for biomarker development. Blood (ASH Annual Meeting Abstracts) 116:4843
34. Longo D, Louie B, Evensen E et al (2011) Impact of time from blood draw to peripheral blood mononuclear cell (PBMC) processing and cryopreservation on functional pathway activity as measured by single cell network profiling (SCNP) assays. Blood ASH Annual Meeting Abstracts 118:4922
35. Putta S, Spellmeyer D, Evensen E et al (2010) Informatics platform and workflows for robust high throughput single cell network profiling (SCNP). In: ISAC.
36. Purvis N, Stelzer G (1998) Multi-platform, multi-site instrumentation and reagent standardization. Cytometry 33:156–165
37. Shults KE, Miller DT, Davis BH et al (2006) A standardized ZAP-70 assay–lessons learned in the trenches. Cytometry B Clin Cytom 70:276–283
38. Wang L, Gaigalas AK, Marti G et al (2008) Toward quantitative fluorescence measurements with multicolor flow cytometry. Cytometry A 73:279–288

Chapter 32

Quantitative and Spatial Image Analysis of Tumor and Draining Lymph Nodes Using Immunohistochemistry and High-Resolution Multispectral Imaging to Predict Metastasis

Kim R.M. Blenman and Peter P. Lee

Abstract

Immunohistochemistry is an essential tool for clinical and translational research laboratories. It is mostly used as a qualitative measure of morphology and cell types within tissue. We have developed a high-resolution multispectral imaging method to expand the uses of immunohistochemistry by making it quantitative. In this chapter we describe the technology, both hardware and software, that we use for this method and give examples of applications.

Key words Immunoprofiling, Lymph nodes, Immunohistochemistry, Multiplex, Multispectral imaging, Chromogen, GemIdent, Vectra, Nuance, InForm

1 Introduction

Metastasis in melanoma and other cancers is thought to be initially spread through the lymphatic vascular system into draining lymph nodes [1, 2]. Tumor-draining lymph nodes (TDLNs) receive direct afferent drainage from the primary tumor and may be the first step in tumor dissemination to distant sites. For melanoma, sentinel lymph node (SLN) biopsy can help to predict metastasis, treatment, and clinical outcome [1, 2]. It has been suggested that waiting until the presence of palpable nodes to perform elective lymph node dissection may allow the spread of melanoma to regional and distant sites which could result in a decrease in long-term survival [1]. However, the mere presence of SLN metastasis is not an absolute predictor of disease-free or overall survival [2]. Although controversial, what may be a better predictor of metastasis and clinical outcome is the state of the microenvironment, specifically immune cells, within the tumor region and the TDLNs [3–10].

Magdalena Thurin and Francesco M. Marincola (eds.), *Molecular Diagnostics for Melanoma: Methods and Protocols*, Methods in Molecular Biology, vol. 1102, DOI 10.1007/978-1-62703-727-3_32, © Springer Science+Business Media New York 2014

Immune profile changes at sites of immune–cancer interactions, such as the tumor microenvironment and TDLNs, may represent a sensitive predictor of local and distant tumor metastasis [3–5, 9, 11–14]. We generate immune profiles that include complete immunophenotyping and identification of cellular spatial relationships within and between the tumor microenvironment and TDLNs from formalin-fixed paraffin-embedded (FFPE) lymph node and tumor specimens from cancer patients. In this chapter, we present an integrated approach to quantitative analysis of tissue that includes capturing architectural information. This involves multiplexed immunoenzyme labeling by immunohistochemistry (IHC), high-resolution multispectral imaging with automated scanning of the entire tissue section, image analysis to identify each cell by immunophenotype, and assessment of spatial relationships. We give a brief overview of this emerging technology using a variety of tissue preparation techniques, image acquisition hardware, and image analysis software.

1.1 Technology

Traditional conventional images generated *via* light microscopy are limited in their ability to facilitate robust quantitative analysis when assessing multiple analytes on the same microscope slide. This is due to the inherent complexity in the output of the staining including overlapping chromogens, densely populated staining areas, and varied staining intensities within and between chromogens, all of which inhibit the accuracy of cell count and identification. Spectral light microscopy generates quantitative spectral data for each pixel in an image which allows mitigation of these issues with the help of appropriate analysis software. We currently use liquid crystal tunable filter (LCTF)-based multispectral imaging to facilitate quantitative assessment of tumor and immune cell populations within tumor and lymph node samples through brightfield microscopy.

Our experience with quantitative imaging instruments has been with Bacus Laboratories Image Slide Scanner (BLISS) (Bacus Laboratories, Lombard, Il) in the past and currently Vectra (CaliperLS—Perkin Elmer, Woburn, MA) [15, 16]. With each system we performed whole slide imaging and acquired hundreds of sequential low power field images at 40× and thousands of sequential high power field images at 200×. The BLISS system is the first system that we used to acquire quantitative images. It is not a multispectral imaging system but it performs whole slide scanning of up to 2 × 3 inch microscope slides. It uses a matrix array in which it overlays a grid onto the slide and captures high-resolution composite images at the vertices of all grid lines corresponding to the location of the tissue on the slide [17]. The system was used primarily for three-color staining which included two chromogens and a hematoxylin counterstain. As we increased the complexity of our staining up to seven colors, we required a higher complexity system such as multispectral imaging for analysis. The Vectra system is the multispectral LCTF-based system that we currently use and the primary scanning instrument described in this chapter. The LCTF is an optical filter that uses an electronically controlled liquid crystal element to transmit wavelengths of light in the visible and near-infrared ranges. In LCTF-based multispectral imaging, images are acquired at each wavelength by sequentially tuning the filter and exposing the sensor. Multispectral imaging and analysis allows one to measure the expression levels of multiple analytes concurrently and simultaneously measure their spatial relationship to structures within the tissue, various cell populations, or subcompartments within the cell. Multispectral imaging and analysis also allow one to separate overlapping chromogens by spectral unmixing [18–20].

(a) *Spectral Unmixing.* IHC is a key tool used in clinical pathology and basic research. It involves staining of a tissue section with a purified primary antibody followed by a peroxidase- or phosphatase-conjugated secondary antibody and developing the stain with a chromogenic substrate such as 3,3′-diaminobenzidine (DAB). There are various shades of brown, red, blue, and green substrates commercially available. When more than one of these basic color substrates deposits on the same location in the tissue, it is difficult to distinguish each color with the naked eye. In red green blue (RGB) imaging systems as the name implies there are only three colors/signals. RGB imaging systems are limited in their ability to distinguish between similar chromogens or unmix those chromogens if they are colocalized [21]. If n or $n+1$ measurements are required to unmix n signals, the ability to unmix more than three chromogens with an RGB sensor is unlikely since the maximum number of n signals is three. RGB sensors are able to unmix the chromogen DAB (brown) from hematoxylin (blue). However, spectral overlap makes it difficult to unmix colors such as brown from red because of overlap between the spectral profiles [21]. Multispectral imaging does not share this disadvantage. In spectral unmixing, the optical signal from each chromogen is isolated such that each can be measured separately and quantitatively [21]. Specifically, images from a multispectral sensor are arranged in cubes with a wavelength-based spectral profile that can range from the visible to the near-infrared wavelength. This wavelength-based spectral profile is generated for each individual pixel in the cube. Each image cube is a spectral image data set with a spectrum λ at every pixel with Cartesian coordinate x, y that make up lambda planes and subsequently group to make up lambda stacks (*see* Fig. 1) [22]. These distinct spectral profiles allow for accurate unmixing of similarly colored or colocalized chromogens [21].

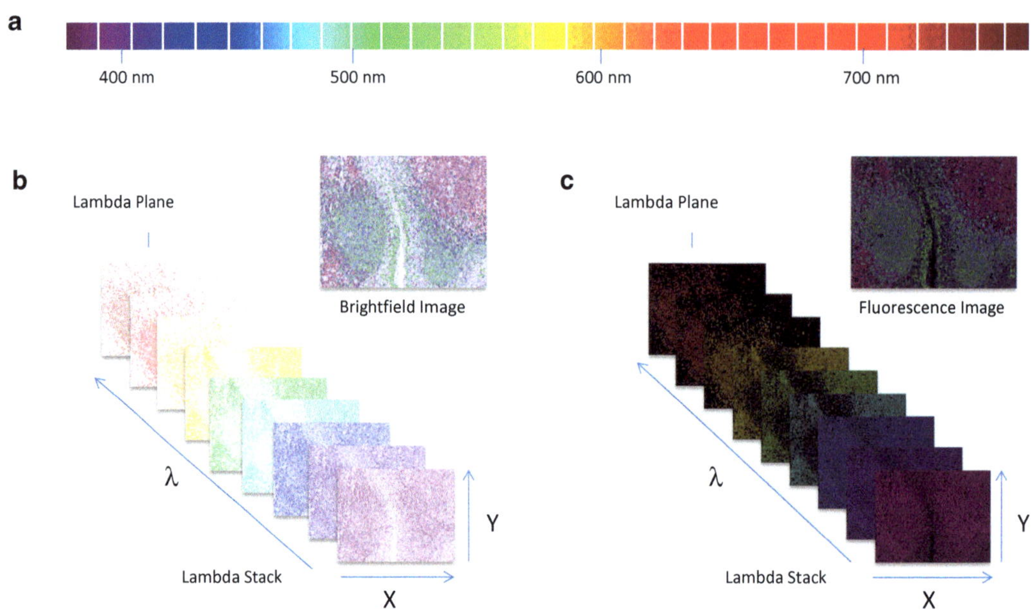

Fig. 1 Spectral imaging lambda stack. (**a**) Wavelength range for multispectral imaging. (**b**, **c**) are examples of the type of lambda stacks that can be expected with spectral imaging

Separating individual chromogen signals from one another, termed linear unmixing (*see* Fig. 1), is generally accomplished through a least-squares fit method [20, 23]. For least-squares fit, the coefficients of linear combinations of the amount of each individual chromogen spectrum are adjusted for the optimal fit that will best reconstitute the full spectrum [20, 23]. Linear unmixing assumes that the total detected signal S for every channel λ can be expressed as a linear combination of contributing chromogens (Chrom$X$) such that $A(X)$ is the contribution of an individual chromogen and R is the reference library of the individual chromogen used for unmixing (*see* Eq. 1) [23].

Equation 1: S is the total detection signal. l is the wavelength channel. Chrom$X$ is the contributing chromagen. AX is the contribution of an individual chromagen. R is the reference library of the individual chromagen used for unmixing.

$$S(1) = A1 \times Chrom1(1) + A2 \times Chrom2(1) + etc\ldots = \mathrm{S}A1 \times Ri(1)$$

Using the known reference library R, the contributions of the chromogens A are determined by calculating the contribution values that most closely match the signals S in the channels. The least-squares fit minimizes the square difference between calculated and measure values by adjusting the fit coefficients as shown in Eq. 2 from Mansfield et al. [20, 23].

Equation 2: *Sij* is the measured spectrum at pixel coordinates *i,j*. *A*, *B*, etc is the reference library used for unmixing. *aij*, *bij*, etc. is the least-squares fit coefficients at pixel coordinates *i,j*.

$$S(\lambda) = A1 \times Chrom1(\lambda) + A2 \times Chrom2(\lambda) + etc\ldots = \sum A1 \times Ri(\lambda)$$

The resulting unmixed images are the foundation for all data analysis of the specified spectral imaging data set [20]. The Vectra imaging system captures images at 20 nm wavelength intervals from 420 to 720 nm. A spectral library is incorporated into the acquisition protocol that allows for unmixing of each of the chromogens into independent channels.

(b) *Digital Imaging -Visualizing Results.* Images are visualized by using a variety of software that allows pseudo-coloring and quantitative analysis of the image. When we used the BLISS imaging system, we used MetaMorph image analysis software. MetaMorph was used to stitch BLISS images together and to record areas occupied by immune cells, tumor, or the entire node. With our current imaging system, Vectra, we use Nuance software, InForm software, and GemIdent (in-house) software. Nuance is used to generate our spectral libraries. Either InForm or GemIdent are used to determine the actual number of cells containing a specific chromogen, to determine the percentages of colocalized chromagens, and to generate Cartesian coordinates for spatial analysis through independently created algorithms. Although InForm and GemIdent are used to generate the same type of data, InForm is capable of performing batch analysis on multiple slides through the creation and incorporation of an analysis algorithm. For all currently used software, each unmixed image which is generated from Nuance's spectral library representing a lambda stack is assigned an arbitrary color corresponding to a single chromogen on the image. These unmixed images are then reassembled into one composite image. The composite image displays the locations and intensities of the chromogens. This information are then converted by the software into the relevant quantitative data.

(c) *Analysis.* Nuance, InForm, and GemIdent require similar basic steps for generation of data. The first step requires transformation of the initial collected RGB image into an image that incorporates data from the previously generated spectral profile at each pixel. This allows for enhancement of key structures in the image for use in combining spectral profiles, generating segmentation images, identifying morphology by pattern including specific cell types, and identifying spatial relationships. Software such as these often have an initial training step where

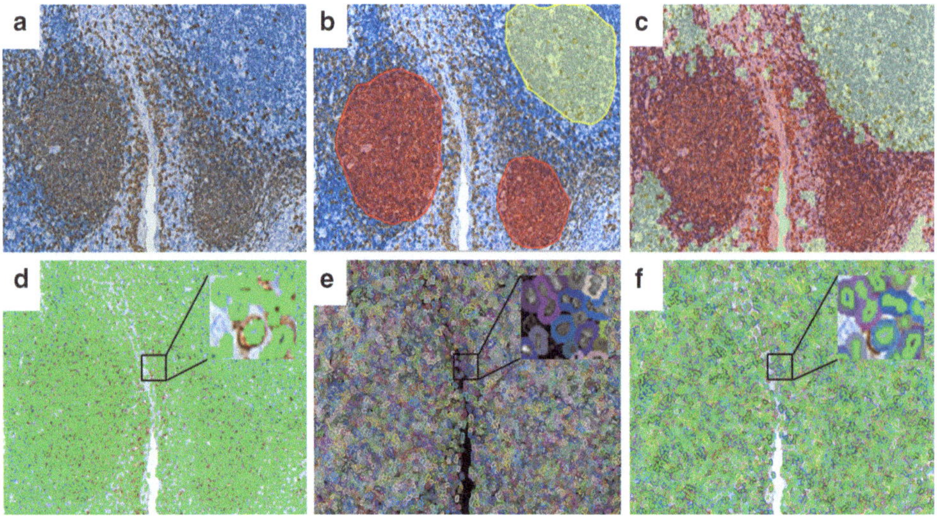

Fig. 2 Example of InForm training with segmentation. Tissue was stained for CD3⁺ T cells with Ferangi Blue chromogen, CD20⁺ B cells with DAB, and hematoxylin counterstain. (**b**, **c**) show tissue segmentation. (**d**–**f**) show cell segmentation. (**a**) RGB image. (**b**) Processing region selected by user for tissue segmentation. The tissue was separated into a B cell region and a T cell region. (**c**) Tissue segmentation map showing the segmented regions generated from (**b**). (**d**) Nuclear segmentation map showing software-defined regions that are positive for hematoxylin staining. (**e**) Cytoplasmic segmentation map showing the software-defined areas that are identified for cytoplasmic staining. (**f**) Combination of the nuclear and cytoplasmic segmentation maps

the user teaches the software to consistently recognize specific components in the images. The software can then segment the cells into components such as cellular (nuclear, cytoplasmic, membrane), regional (follicular, intrafollicular), and cell type (tumor, non-tumor). The information generated from the segmentation is used to generate the desired quantitative results. The MetaMorph software will be briefly discussed in an upcoming section showing an example of how basic quantitation without multispectral imaging can be used to generate data focused on clinical outcome.

Figures 2 and 3 show examples of image analysis using InForm software. Nuclear staining is represented by hematoxylin. Membrane staining is represented by cell membrane markers CD3 for T cells and CD20 for B cells, and each marker is developed with a unique chromogen, Ferangi Blue (blue) and DAB (brown), respectively. The images are unmixed into monochrome images for each individual stain. The samples undergo segmentation to identify nuclear area and cytoplasm/membrane area (*see* Fig. 2). The total number of cells is based on the total number of nuclear structures identified by the software. Therefore, the total number of $CD3^{+}$ T cells or

a

b

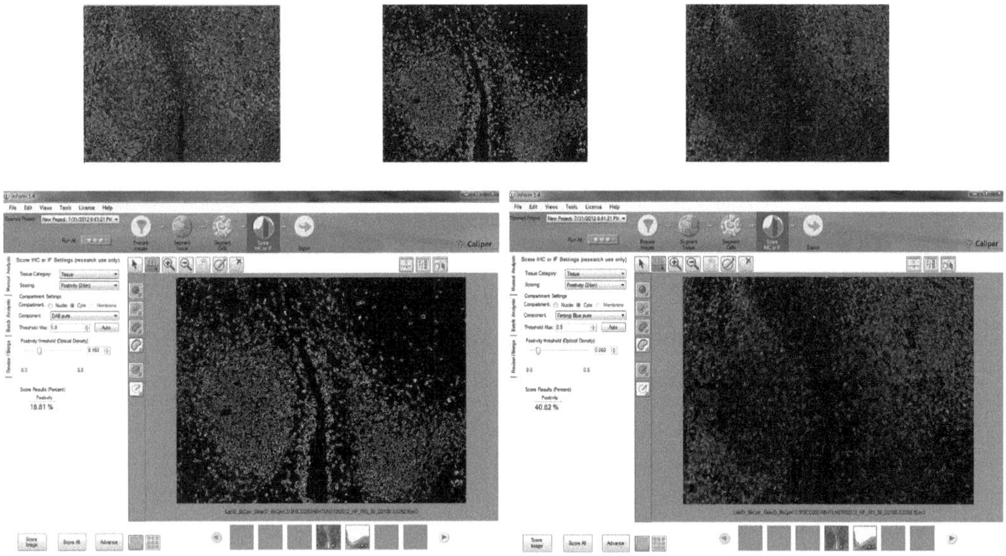

c

Tissue Category	Cell Compartment	Stain Component	Positivity	Tissue Category Area (percent)	Number of Cells	Positivity Threshold
Tissue	Nucleus	HTLN			4995	0.054

Fig. 3 Example of InForm data output. (**a**) Unmixed component images of hematoxylin (*left*), CD20^{+} B cells (*middle*), and CD3^{+} T cells (*right*). (**b**) Percentage of positive cells identified for CD20^{+} B cells (*left*) and CD3^{+} T cells (*right*). (**c**) Total cell count in image based on hematoxylin nuclear staining

CD20^{+} B cells is based on the number of nuclear structures that are enclosed by the respective membrane markers (*see* Fig. 3). Although the whole slide is scanned, the data that is generated is limited to each individual high power field cube. We then generate algorithms based on Cartesian coordinates to link the data from the entire tissue together for identification of spatial relationships. Other groups have used the same or similar systems and have generated similar data [24–27].

Figure 4 shows an example of an image analysis from GemIdent software. Nuclei are stained with hematoxylin. T cells were marked by CD3 and Ferangi Blue substrate, and B cells were marked by CD20 and DAB substrate. For this software, high power field unmixed images labeled with corresponding chromogens generated from the Vectra were uploaded. All of the images are automatically stitched together to regenerate a composite image of the whole slide that was originally scanned. GemIdent software analyzes the whole slide image and the individual cubes. The composite image undergoes a training session in which the user defines and marks the desired phenotypes manually on several representative cubes from the composite image. The software takes the manually generated

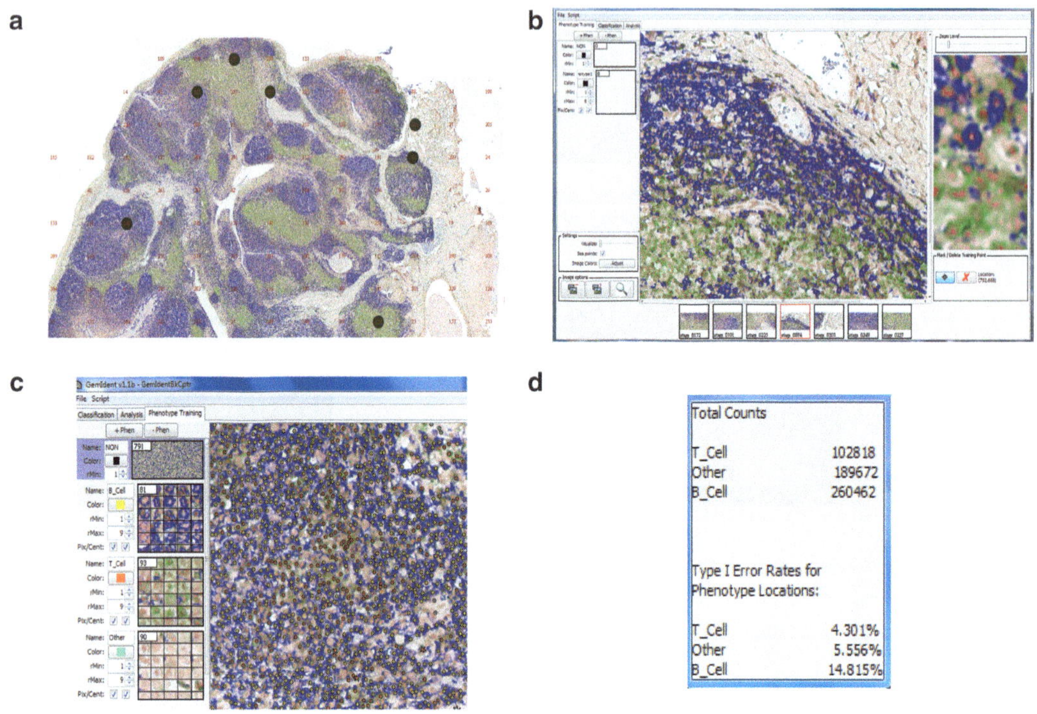

Fig. 4 Example of GemIdent analysis and data output. (**a**) Stitched together composite image of all unmixed image cubes created in Vectra by GemIdent. The numbers represent the cube ID numbers. The *black circles* represent cubes selected for training set. (**b**) Sample view of the selected training cubes. (**c**) Sample view of phenotype training. (**d**) Total counts and type I error rates for composite image A. Type I error rate is the rate at which GemIdent fails to find the phenotype of interest

phenotypes and teaches itself to automatically recognize the phenotypes exactly as the user has defined. The software then applies the phenotype to the entire composite whole slide image. Cell counts and Cartesian coordinates of each phenotype including co-localized phenotypes are generated automatically as the output of the software analysis (*see* Fig. 4). Further analysis can be performed using separate algorithms to identify other types of spatial relationships such as cell clustering (*manuscript in press*).

(d) *Data Management.* Data management is challenging with such high-complexity data. Since the acquired images contain a significant amount of metadata in combination with the image itself, the file sizes can be quite large. A unique folder on a designated hard drive is created for each scanned slide. In our hands, the folder size can routinely be greater than 100 GB per slide. We have used many methods of storage which range from transferring data to external hard drives (least stable method) to transferring multiple copies of the data to multiple network cloud storage systems (most stable method for our purposes). One must consider the data storage aspect of these quantitative analysis systems carefully and devise an actionable plan before one purchases such a system.

1.2 Application

(a) Quantitation of tumor and immune cell populations. We previously used non-multispectral quantitative imaging to study alterations in the immune profile of TDLNs from 77 breast cancer patients [15]. The lymph nodes were analyzed by immunohistochemistry for $CD4^+$ T cells, $CD8^+$ T cells, $CD1a^+$ dendritic cells, and cytokeratin-positive breast tumor cells. The area of the node occupied by each immune cell type and by tumor was determined through BLISS computerized image acquisition and MetaMorph analysis software. Using BLISS we acquired 160–4,130 sequential images at 200× of the entire lymph node section. The number of images depended on the size of the tissue section. The images were stitched together by MetaMorph Imaging Software to regenerate the original whole image. Standardized thresholds of each stain for the cells of interest were identified by using control nodes. These standardized thresholds were then applied with an automated MetaMorph script and MetaMorph log set to record areas occupied by the cells of interest, tumor, and entire node for all samples. Using this method quantitative results were generated focusing on clinical outcome. Specifically we found a threshold percentage of $CD4^+$ T cells and $CD1a^+$ dendritic cells that correlated with longer disease-free survival. An example of the data that we can extract from this quantitative method is shown in Fig. 5 [15].

(b) Identification of spatial relationships between cells. We have used multispectral quantitative imaging to study spatial relationships between cells such as the average distance between cells or the local density of a cell population [16]. We hypothesized that the architectural relationships between immune cell subsets and infiltrating tumor cells within TDLNs may provide additional mechanistic and prognostic information in regard to metastasis. $CD3^+$ T cells stained with Vulcan Fast Red chromogen (red) and $CD20^+$ B cells stained with DAB chromogen (brown) within TDLNs from breast cancer patients and healthy lymph nodes were analyzed. The nucleus was counterstained with hematoxylin (blue). Using Vectra we acquired thousands of sequential image cubes at 200× of the entire lymph node section, which were stitched together and analyzed by GemIdent. We found that even when the proportions of T and B cells were similar, the spatial grouping patterns of these cells differed between healthy and tumor-draining lymph nodes [16]. An example of the data that we can extract from this quantitative method is shown in Fig. 6 [16].

a b

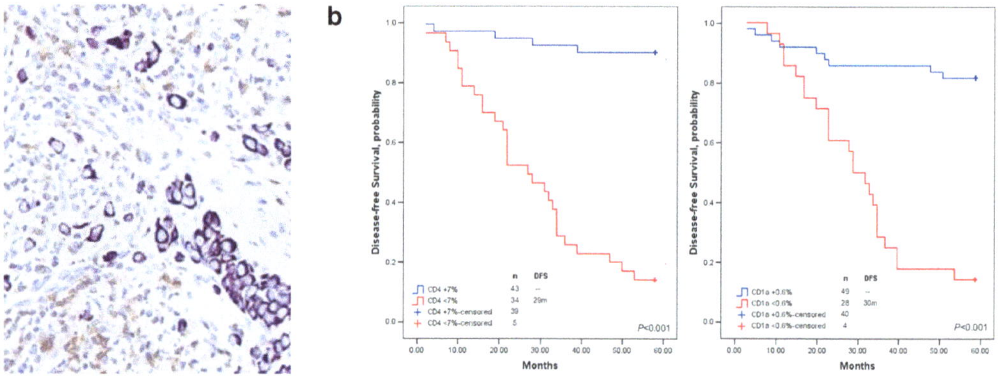

c

Lymph Node Group	Cell Population[a]	Tumor-Free Lymph Node, *n* (%)	Tumor-Involved Lymph Node, *n* (%)	X^2 Test[b] *p*-Value
SLN (*n* = 18)[c]	CD4			<0.001
	<7% (*n* = 7)	0 (0.0)	7 (100.0)	
	≥7% (*n* = 11)	9 (81.8)	2 (18.2)	
	CD1a			0.017
	<0.6% (*n* = 9)	2 (22.2)	7 (77.8)	
	≥0.6% (*n* = 9)	7 (77.8)	2 (22.2)	
ALN (*n* = 75)[d]	CD4			0.298
	<7% (*n* = 34)	21 (61.8)	13 (38.2)	
	≥7% (*n* = 41)	30 (73.2)	11 (26.8)	
	CD1a			0.784
	<0.6% (*n* = 33)	23 (69.7)	10 (30.3)	
	≥0.6% (*n* = 42)	28 (66.7)	14 (33.3)	

[a] Down-regulated immune profile by CD4% or CD1a% nodal surface area thresholds determined from training set analysis.
[b] X^2 test for tumor-free lymph node immune profile CD4 and CD1a thresholds versus tumor-involved lymph node immune profile CD4 and CD1a thresholds.
[c] Nine tumor-involved SLNs from training set series 2 (*n* = 18).
[d] Seven tumor-involved ALNs from training set series 2 (*n* = 27), and 17 tumor-involved from test set (*n* = 48); total 24 of 75 axillary nodes are tumor-involved.

Fig. 5 Non-multispectral quantitative imaging results focused on clinical outcome. (**a**) Image of multiplexed immunoenzyme staining of tumor (*purple*) and immune cells (*brown*). (**b**) Survival analysis data generated from the subsequent quantitative immune profiling data showing that individuals with lower percentages of CD4+ T cells and CD1a+ dendritic cells have significantly poorer clinical outcome. (**c**) Relationship between immune profile and nodal metastases in TDLNs based on separation by quantitative data [reproduced from Kohrt et. al. 2005 PLoS Med]

2 Materials (*See* Note 1)

2.1 Tissue Collection, Fixation, Embedding, and Sectioning

For our studies, we used FFPE human tissues from either archival or fresh leftover pathology specimens. Three to four micron sections were cut from each embedded block and placed on microscope slides by a pathology core facility (*see* **Note 2**).

2.2 Deparaffinization and Rehydration

1. Slide Brite reagent (Biocare, Concord, CA, USA) or Xylene (Sigma Chemical Company, St. Louis, MO) for dewaxing and clearing of slide.
2. Ethanol (Sigma) for rehydration of slide.
3. Milli-Q Water (Millipore, Billerica, MA) for rehydration of slide.
4. Tissue TEK Rack (VWR, Radnor, PA).
5. Slide Holder (Plastic) (VWR, Radnor, PA).

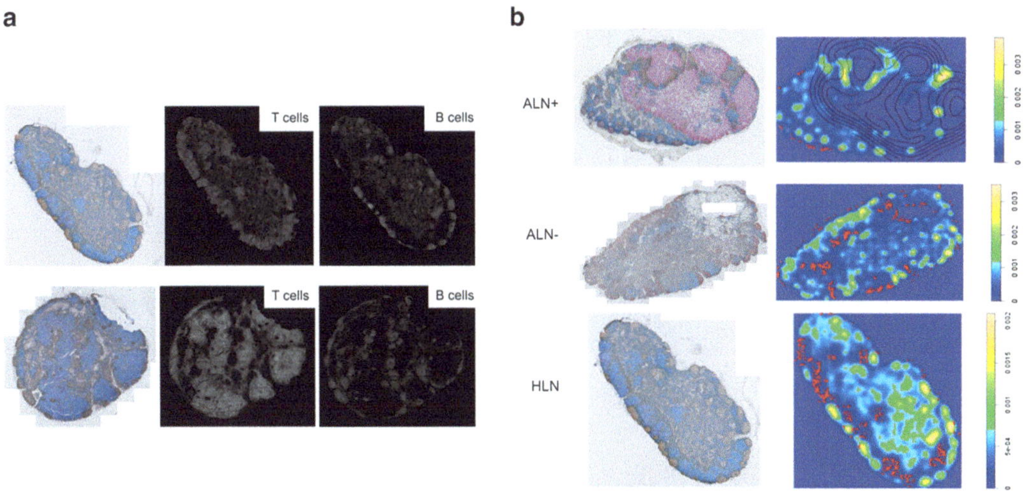

Fig. 6 Identification of spatial relationships between cells via multispectral imaging. (**a**) Maps of T cell and B cell distributions in TDLN whole tissue sections. Row 1 and row 2 are two different lymph nodes. (**b**) Density plots of B cells in ALN^+, ALN^-, and HLN whole tissue sections. ALN-, axillary lymph node negative; ALN+, axillary lymph node positive; HLN, healthy lymph node. [reproduced from Setiadi et al. 2010 PLoS One]

2.3 Multiplexed Immunoenzyme Labeling

1. Pap Pen for creating a barrier around the tissue on the slide (DAKO, Carpinteria, CA).
2. Microcentrifuge Tubes (1.5 ml) and Conical Tubes (15 ml, 50 ml) (Fisher, Pittsburgh, PA).
3. Humidity Slide Moisture Chamber (Newcomer Supply, Middleton, WI).
4. Coplin Jars (Plastic and Glass) and Wheaton Dishes (Glass) (VWR, Radnor, PA, USA).
5. Orbital Shaker (Fisher, Pittsburgh, PA).
6. Biocare Decloaking Chamber or pressure cooker for slides (Biocare, Concord, CA).
7. Peroxidazed I reagent for blocking endogenous peroxidase activity (Biocare, Concord, CA).
8. Tris-buffered saline (modified TBS, 1×, Biocare, Concord, CA).
9. DIVA Antigen Retrieval Solution for unmasking formalin cross-linked epitopes (Biocare, Concord, CA).
10. Background Sniper reagent for reducing nonspecific background staining for IHC (Biocare, Concord, CA).
11. Antibody Diluent (DAKO, Carpinteria, CA).
12. Primary antibodies (*see* Table 1).
13. Alkaline phosphate (AP)- and horse radish peroxidase (HRP)-conjugated secondary antibodies (*see* Table 1).

Table 1
Details of antibodies, chromogens, and mounting medium used

Antibody	Concentration	Antibody supplier	Positive control tissue	Chromogen (or dye)	Enzyme	Chromogen supplier	Chromagen reaction product	Mounting medium
Anti-CD20/ Anti-CD3 Cocktail	RTU	Biocare (Concord, CA, USA)	Tonsil	DAB; Ferangi Blue	HRP; AP	Biocare (Concord, CA, USA)	Brown; Blue	Faramount/ Ecomount
Anti-CD4	1:20	Novacastro; Vector Laboratories, (Burlingame, CA, USA)	Tonsil	DAB	HRP	Dako (Carpinteria, CA, USA)	Brown	Faramount
Anti-CD8	1:25	Dako (Carpinteria, CA, USA)	Tonsil	DAB	HRP	Dako (Carpinteria, CA, USA)	Brown	Faramount
Anti-CD1a	1:100	Dako (Carpinteria, CA, USA)	Skin	DAB	HRP	Dako (Carpinteria, CA, USA)	Brown	Faramount
Anti-Cytokeratin	1:25; 1:200	Biocare (Concord, CA, USA)	Skin or Adenocarcinoma	Vulcan Fast Red; VIP	AP; HRP	Biocare (Concord, CA, USA); Vector Laboratories, (Burlingame, CA, USA)	Fuchsia/ Magenta; Purple	Faramount/ Ecomount
				Hematoxylin		Biocare (Concord, CA, USA); Innogenex (San Ramon, CA, USA)	Purplish-Blue	Faramount/ Ecomount

14. Substrates for stain development (*see* Table 1).
15. Milli-Q Water (Millipore, Billerica, MA).
16. CAT Hematoxylin for histological nuclear staining (Biocare, Concord, CA).
17. Ecomount (Biocare, Concord, CA) or Faramount (DAKO, Carpinteria, CA) Mounting Medium for permanent slide mounting.
18. Slide Staining Rack (Glass) (VWR, Radnor, PA).
19. SHUR/Dry Slide Dryer (Triangle Biomedical Science Inc, Durham, NC).
20. Glass Coverslips (VWR, Radnor, PA).
21. Brightfield Microscope (Fisher, Pittsburgh, PA).

2.4 Image Acquisition and Analysis

1. BLISS (Bacus Laboratories/Olympus, Lombard, IL).
2. Vectra Intelligent Imaging System (CaliperLS/Perkin Elmer, Hopkinton, MA).
3. MetaMorph Imaging Analysis Software (Molecular Devices, Sunnyvale, CA).
4. InForm Software (CaliperLS/Perkin Elmer, Hopkinton, MA).
5. Nuance Software (CaliperLS/Perkin Elmer, Hopkinton, MA).
6. GemIdent Software (custom in-house software) [28].

3 Methods (*See* Notes 1 *and* 2)

3.1 Deparaffinization and Rehydration (Total Time: ≥30 Min)

1. Load slides into plastic slide rack.
2. Place slide rack into Tissue Tek containers and deparaffinize by incubating in Slide Brite or Xylene 3×, at room temperature for 3–10 min each.
3. Place slide rack into Tissue Tek containers and rehydrate by incubating in reducing concentrations of ethanol and ending in water at room temperature as follows: In seven Tissue Tek containers prepare two containers with 100 % ethanol, two containers with 95 % ethanol, one container with 70 % ethanol, one container with 50 %, and one container with Milli-Q water. In the order listed above incubate the slide rack in each of the Tissue Tek containers with the ethanols for 3 min each and in Milli-Q water for 5 min (*see* **Note 3**).

3.2 Antigen Retrieval (Total Time: ≥50 Min)

1. Use the Pap Pen to draw a circle around the tissue. This ensures that subsequent small-volume reagents that are added to the slide can be confined to the tissue region.

2. Block excess of endogenous peroxidase by incubating in Peroxidazed I for 5–10 min.
3. Wash the slides in 1× TBS.
4. Transfer slides to a coplin jar containing DIVA antigen retrieval solution. Place coplin jar in the decloaking chamber, and set the temperature and time according to the optimal conditions for antigen epitope exposure for the primary antibody of interest (*see* **Note 4**).
5. Remove the coplin jar from the decloaking chamber and place at room temperature undisturbed for at least 10 min.
6. Pour off half the DIVA antigen retrieval solution from the coplin jar and replace with water. Repeat several times to slowly bring the tissue temperature down to room temperature.

3.3 Immunostaining (Total Time: ≥2½ h) (See Note 5*)*

1. Prepare cocktails of primary antibodies in antibody diluent. Incubate 100–200 μl of the antibody cocktail at the optimized dilution at room temperature for a minimum of 60 min or overnight at 4 °C (*see* **Notes 6–8**).
2. Wash the slide in 1× TBS.
3. Prepare the relevant cocktails of secondary antibodies conjugated to unique corresponding enzymes such as HRP and AP. Incubate 100–200 μl of the antibody cocktail at the optimized dilution at room temperature for a minimum of 20 min (*see* **Note 9**).
4. Wash the slide in 1× TBS.
5. Incubate the slide in 100–200 μl of chromogen A substrate corresponding to its specific enzyme-conjugated secondary antibody of interest (e.g., Ferangi Blue for AP) at room temperature for the desired development time (*see* **Note 9**).
6. Wash the slide in Milli-Q water to stop the enzyme-catalytic reaction.
7. Wash the slide in 1× TBS.
8. Incubate the slide in 100–200 μl of chromogen B of interest (e.g., DAB for HRP) at room temperature for the desired development time.
9. Wash the slide in Milli-Q water to stop the enzyme-catalytic reaction.
10. Counterstain with nuclear stain of your choice (e.g., hematoxylin) at room temperature for the desired development time.
11. Wash the slide in Milli-Q water.
12. Air-dry the slide or bake in slide oven at 60 °C for 10 min.

13. Coverslip with mounting medium (e.g., Ecomount) (*see* **Note 10**).

3.4 Multispectral Imaging Using Vectra

We use Vectra to scan our slides and the Nuance software to generate the previously described spectral libraries required for unmixing of the images for analysis in the InForm and GemIdent software.

1. *Imaging using Vectra*. We routinely do automated scanning of slides in a batch format. The details (please refer to user's manual) of the actual procedure for the process are too numerous to add here. Instead we give a top-level view of the process highlighting only the key points.
2. *Generate the spectral library using the Nuance software* (*see* Fig. 7). Scan representative slides of the tissue of interest with single stains of each of the chromogens of interest. The spectral profiles of each of these single stains are used to unmix images that contain multiple stains in order to quantitate each

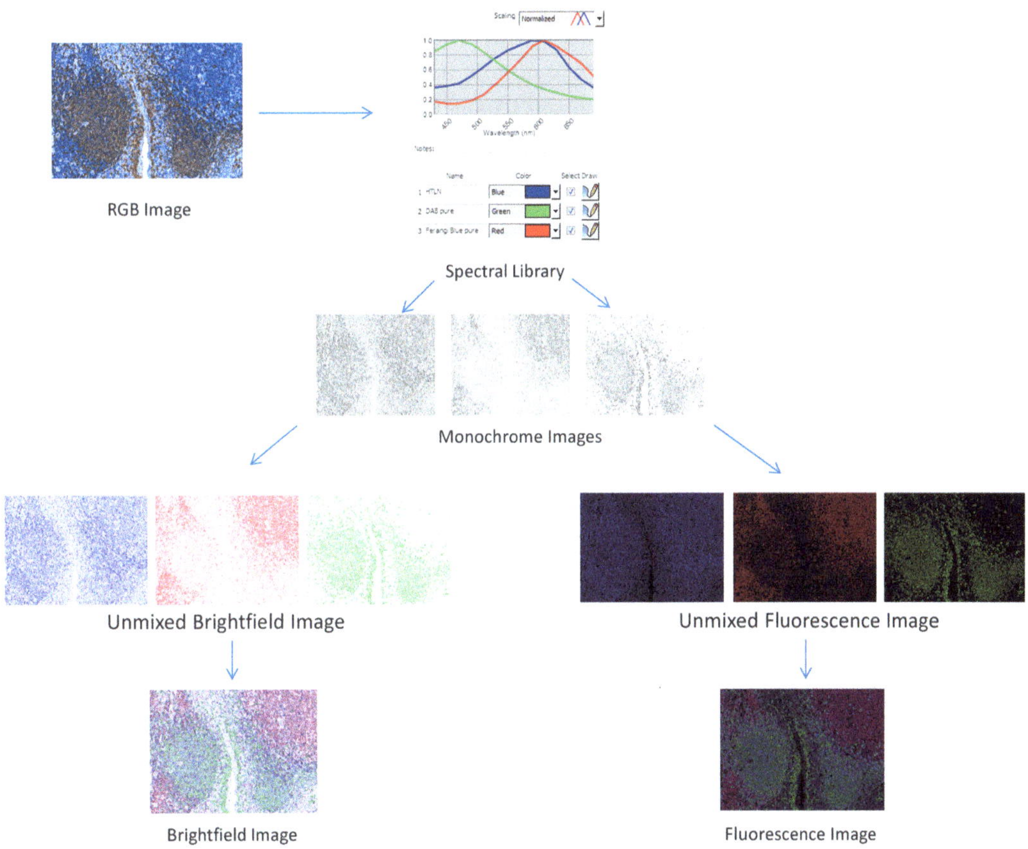

Fig. 7 Spectral unmixing via Nuance. The spectral library is used during acquisition and analysis for GemIdent and InForm

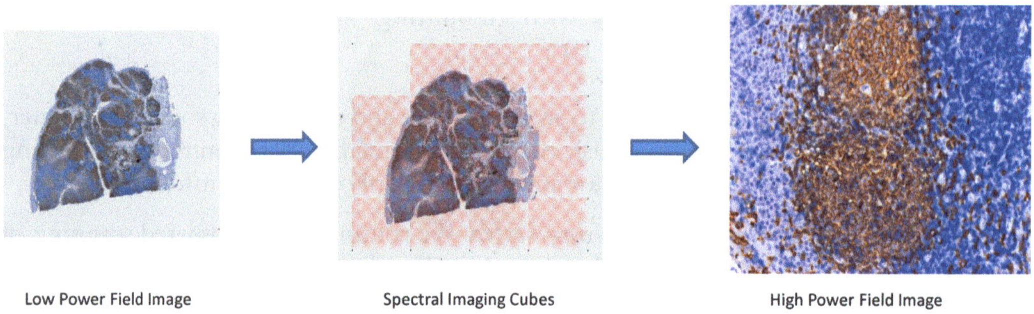

Fig. 8 Scanning of an image with Vectra. Low power field images of tissue area of interest are collected. Spectral imaging cubes are subsequently identified and selected for high power field imaging

target antigen separately. This process has been used by several other groups with the same or similar systems [29–33] (*see* **Note 11**).

3. *Generate the Tissue Finding and High Power Field algorithms using the InForm software* (*see* Fig. 8). The Tissue Finding algorithm helps the instrument differentiate between glass and tissue. In essence, as the name specifies, it finds the tissue on the slide. The High Power Field algorithm tells the instrument from which areas of the tissue one desires to take the 200× high power field images. Most users prefer to choose areas with specific cell types such as "tumor." In this case they will design the High Power Field algorithm to only scan areas that contain tumor.
4. *Batch Scanning using the Vectra software.* Use one representative slide to prepare the slide set for batch processing. Take the representative slide through autoexposure, autofocusing, setting of home Z, and brightfield reference collection. Use the software to mark the area on the slide where most of the tissue from all of the slides in the slide set is located. Insert both the Tissue Finding and High Power Field algorithms into the software. Adjust other optimization parameters in the low and high power field imaging settings as desired to obtain optimal images. These collected parameters will be automatically used for the slide set.

3.5 Image Analysis

1. *Image analysis.* We routinely use both InForm and GemIdent software for quantitative analysis. Again, the details (please refer to user's manual) of the actual procedure for the process are too numerous to add here. Instead we give a top-level view of the process highlighting only the key points.
2. *InForm image training* (*see* Fig. 2). The purpose of this process is to generate an analysis algorithm by manually training the software to recognize the structures/phenotypes of interest to be analyzed based on the type of analysis desired. The types of analysis that can be done are scoring, tissue

segmentation, cell segmentation, and object counting. This can be done by selecting "New Project" and selecting the desired analysis method. Each image cube is loaded in manually and analyzed separately (*see* **Notes 12** and **13**).

3. *InForm batch processing*. Once one is satisfied with the accuracy of the identification of the desired structures/phenotypes of interest, one can use the created analysis algorithm to analyze all subsequent images automatically through batch processing. This is done by selecting the batch processing tab, inserting the algorithm, selecting the images to be analyzed, and designating the location for data export.
4. *InForm data output* (*see* Fig. 3). The information that is automatically generated by checking the appropriate box in the View Editor are Cartesian coordinates of each cell, ODs of chromagens for each cell, cell counts, etc. This data can be exported and converted into a spreadsheet format.
5. *GemIdent image training* (*see* Fig. 4). The purpose of this process is the same as for InForm but with a slightly different format. Load unmixed Tiff files from Vectra into GemIdent. Select chromogens to be analyzed. The image cubes for the entire scanned tissue section will automatically be stitched together. Manually select several cubes that are representative of the entire image for training. Create phenotypes such as T cells and B cells. Click directly on the nucleus of a cell to select it for a specific cell phenotype. On that same cell highlight the "NON" phenotype, and click on several area of the membrane of the cell to define the boundaries of the cell. This will help to ensure accurate cell count and spatial analysis of the specific cell phenotype. Select 10–12 cells per image for each cell phenotype (*see* **Note 14**).
6. *GemIdent classification* (*see* Fig. 4). Once one has selected the appropriate number of representative cells, one can now teach the software to recognize the phenotypes by clicking on Classify Trained. After completion click on Find Centers. The number of cells in each created phenotype will appear. If the data is unsatisfactory, retrain and reclassify until the desired result is achieved. If the data is satisfactory, do a full classification on the whole tissue by first highlighting all of the cubes on the tissue. Then select for analysis "Those Clicked On" and "Classify, Centers, and Sanity Check."
7. *GemIdent output* (*see* Fig. 4). Cell counts for each created phenotype and Cartesian coordinates are automatically exported to a text file in the results folder.

4 Notes

1. We perform high-complexity multiplexed immunoenzyme labeling of up to seven colors. There have been a limited number of articles on how to perform such high-complexity labeling [34, 35]. A successful protocol depends not only on the antibodies (primary and secondary) and chromogens but also on all of the steps involved in the multiplexed staining.
2. The protocol must start out with a good tissue section. It is suggested that the tissue be optimally fixed in 10 % neutral buffered formalin and then immediately paraffin embedded [36].
3. It is critical that the tissue section slides are completely deparaffinized before labeling is attempted [36]. Inadequately deparaffinized slides will result in weak or no staining. To resolve inadequate deparaffinization, either increase the incubation time or increase the number of deparaffinization steps.
4. The optimal fixation and antigen retrieval method for one target antigen may not work or be compatible for another target antigen that one is interested in assessing concurrently.
5. For brightfield chromogen stains, optimize antibody concentrations with single stains first before mixing combinations together in order to determine the optimal concentration for positive signal with minimal to no background. Also, the optimal temperature and incubation time will need to be determined empirically by testing various combinations.
6. For immunostaining, it is best to prepare cocktails of primary antibodies that have been raised in different host species. This limits the potential of cross-reactivity.
7. When possible choose antibodies that have already been optimized for IHC. Antibodies that work for western blotting, flow cytometry, or immunofluorescence on cryopreserved tissue do not necessarily work on FFPE tissue. When testing an antibody for the first time, it is most efficient to test it out on a tissue that is known to be positive for the target antigen of interest.
8. For consistently successful quantitative IHC, choose high-quality stable antibodies and chromogens. As combinations are put together, carefully assess the output for cross-reactivity between antibodies, and ensure that no chromogen blocks the view of a subsequent chromogen to the same location [20].
9. Not all combinations of chromagens work well together or in the same order with every primary antibody that is used. Some primary antibody–chromogen combinations could block or interact chemically with other primary antibody–chromagen

combinations. For example, we have observed that prolonged exposure of DAB to Vulcan Fast Red changes the color of DAB from brown to reddish brown. We have also observed that co-localization of light chromagens with dark chromagens such as DAB or NBT-BCIP (nitro-blue tetrazolium chloride plus 5-bromo-4-chloro-3′-indolyphosphate p-toluidine) are difficult to visualize under a standard brightfield microscope.

10. Some chromagens are soluble in organic solutions, and some are soluble in water. Ensure that the mounting medium that is used for coverslipping is compatible with all chromagens used in the multiplexed assay. It is also best to allow the mounting medium to completely cure before scanning the slide.
11. To generate the best spectral libraries for unmixing and analysis, it is important to have at minimum a single stain control for each of the chromogens of interest. It has been suggested that the controls for the library be expanded to include all possible combinations of the markers of interest to confirm accurate labeling, identify any cross talk, and identify any location blockages by a single label.
12. For InForm training, select not only the nicely stained areas of the slide but also areas with artifacts such as air bubbles, folds in tissue, poorly stained areas, and dust/lint. This allows the software to better identify the cell phenotypes of interest.
13. For InForm, cell segmentation is based on nuclear staining. Therefore, in order to get accurate cell counts it is critical that the nuclear counterstain that is used is dark enough to be read by the software.
14. For GemIdent, the number of training examples required for an accurate classification is dependent on the quality of the staining and the degree of homogeneity in the phenotypes' color and morphological features. This number generally ranges between 50 and 200 training points per phenotype. Run times will vary on the size of the tissue as well as the complexity of the image.

Acknowledgment

This work was supported by the US National Institute of Health National Cancer Institute grant R01 CA127947-03 and the US Department of Defense Era of Hope grant W81XWH-12-1-0366.

References

1. Morton DL, Thompson JF, Cochran AJ, Mozzillo N, Elashoff R, Essner R et al (2006) Sentinel-node biopsy or nodal observation in melanoma. N Engl J Med 355:1307–1317
2. Parrett B, Fadaki L, Rhee JY, Leong SPL (2011) The biology and clinical relevance of sentinel lymph nodes in melanoma. In: Murph PM (ed) Melanoma in the clinic—diagnosis. Management and complications of malignancy. InTech, Rijeka, Croatia, pp 225–238
3. Burton AL, Roach BA, Mays MP, Chen AF, Ginter BA, Vierling AM et al (2011) Prognostic significance of tumor infiltrating lymphocytes in melanoma. Am Surg 77:188–192
4. Taylor RC, Patel A, Panageas KS, Busam KJ, Brady MS (2007) Tumor-infiltrating lymphocytes predict sentinel lymph node positivity in patients with cutaneous melanoma. J Clin Oncol 25:869–875
5. Mandala M, Imberti GL, Piazzalunga D, Belfiglio M, Labianca R, Barberis M et al (2009) Clinical and histopathological risk factors to predict sentinel lymph node positivity, disease-free and overall survival in clinical stages I-II AJCC skin melanoma: outcome analysis from a single-institution prospectively collected database. Eur J Cancer 45:2537–2545
6. Kruper LL, Spitz FR, Czerniecki BJ, Fraker DL, Blackwood-Chirchir A, Ming ME et al (2006) Predicting sentinel node status in AJCC stage I/II primary cutaneous melanoma. Cancer 107:2436–2445
7. Azimi F, Scolyer RA, Rumcheva P, Moncrieff M, Murali R, McCarthy SW et al (2012) Tumor-infiltrating lymphocyte grade is an independent predictor of sentinel lymph node status and survival in patients with cutaneous melanoma. J Clin Oncol 30:2678–2683
8. Mihm MC Jr, Clemente CG, Cascinelli N (1996) Tumor infiltrating lymphocytes in lymph node melanoma metastases: a histopathologic prognostic indicator and an expression of local immune response. Lab Invest 74:43–47
9. Oble DA, Loewe R, Yu P, Mihm MC Jr (2009) Focus on TILs: prognostic significance of tumor infiltrating lymphocytes in human melanoma. Cancer Immun 9:3
10. Rao UN, Lee SJ, Luo W, Mihm MC Jr, Kirkwood JM (2010) Presence of tumor-infiltrating lymphocytes and a dominant nodule within primary melanoma are prognostic factors for relapse-free survival of patients with thick (t4) primary melanoma: pathologic analysis of the e1690 and e1694 intergroup trials. Am J Clin Pathol 133:646–653
11. Hussein MR, Elsers DA, Fadel SA, Omar AE (2006) Immunohistological characterisation of tumour infiltrating lymphocytes in melanocytic skin lesions. J Clin Pathol 59: 316–324
12. Laghi L, Bianchi P, Miranda E, Balladore E, Pacetti V, Grizzi F et al (2009) CD3+ cells at the invasive margin of deeply invading (pT3-T4) colorectal cancer and risk of post-surgical metastasis: a longitudinal study. Lancet Oncol 10:877–884
13. Galon J, Costes A, Sanchez-Cabo F, Kirilovsky A, Mlecnik B, Lagorce-Pages C et al (2006) Type, density, and location of immune cells within human colorectal tumors predict clinical outcome. Science 313:1960–1964
14. Camus M, Tosolini M, Mlecnik B, Pages F, Kirilovsky A, Berger A et al (2009) Coordination of intratumoral immune reaction and human colorectal cancer recurrence. Cancer Res 69:2685–2693
15. Kohrt HE, Nouri N, Nowels K, Johnson D, Holmes S, Lee PP (2005) Profile of immune cells in axillary lymph nodes predicts disease-free survival in breast cancer. PLoS Med 2:e284
16. Setiadi AF, Ray NC, Kohrt HE, Kapelner A, Carcamo-Cavazos V, Levic EB et al (2010) Quantitative, architectural analysis of immune cell subsets in tumor-draining lymph nodes from breast cancer patients and healthy lymph nodes. PLoS One 5:e12420
17. Manley S, Mucci NR, De Marzo AM, Rubin MA (2001) Relational database structure to manage high-density tissue microarray data and images for pathology studies focusing on clinical outcome: the prostate specialized program of research excellence model. Am J Pathol 159:837–843
18. Levenson RM (2006) Spectral imaging perspective on cytomics. Cytometry A 69:592–600
19. Levenson RM, Mansfield JR (2006) Multispectral imaging in biology and medicine: slices of life. Cytometry A 69:748–758
20. Mansfield, J.R., Hoyt, C., and Levenson, R.M. (2008) Visualization of microscopy-based spectral imaging data from multi-label tissue sections. Curr Protoc Mol Biol Chapter 14, Unit 14 19.
21. Taylor CR, Levenson RM (2006) Quantification of immunohistochemistry–issues concerning methods, utility and semi-

quantitative assessment II. Histopathology 49:411–424
22. Garini Y, Young IT, McNamara G (2006) Spectral imaging: principles and applications. Cytometry A 69:735–747
23. Zimmermann T (2005) Spectral imaging and linear unmixing in light microscopy. Adv Biochem Eng Biotechnol 95:245–265
24. Fiore C, Bailey D, Conlon N, Wu X, Martin N, Fiorentino M et al (2012) Utility of multispectral imaging in automated quantitative scoring of immunohistochemistry. J Clin Pathol 65: 496–502
25. Feldman MD (2008) Beyond morphology: whole slide imaging, computer-aided detection, and other techniques. Arch Pathol Lab Med 132:758–763
26. Grunkin M, Raundahl J, Foged NT (2011) Practical considerations of image analysis and quantification of signal transduction IHC staining. Methods Mol Biol 717:143–154
27. Fiorentino M, Zadra G, Palescandolo E, Fedele G, Bailey D, Fiore C et al (2008) Overexpression of fatty acid synthase is associated with palmitoylation of Wnt1 and cytoplasmic stabilization of beta-catenin in prostate cancer. Lab Invest 88:1340–1348
28. Holmes S, Kapelner A, Lee PP (2009) An interactive java statistical image segmentation system: GemIdent. J Stat Softw 30
29. Snyder EL, Bailey D, Shipitsin M, Polyak K, Loda M (2009) Identification of CD44v6(+)/ CD24- breast carcinoma cells in primary human tumors by quantum dot-conjugated antibodies. Lab Invest 89:857–866
30. O'Donnell RK, Feldman M, Mick R, Muschel RJ (2008) Immunohistochemical method identifies lymphovascular invasion in a majority of oral squamous cell carcinomas and discriminates between blood and lymphatic vessel invasion. J Histochem Cytochem 56:803–810
31. Isse K, Lesniak A, Grama K, Roysam B, Minervini MI, Demetris AJ (2012) Digital transplantation pathology: combining whole slide imaging, multiplex staining and automated image analysis. Am J Transplant 12: 27–37
32. Gilbert CM, Parwani A (2010) The use of multispectral imaging to distinguish reactive urothelium from neoplastic urothelium. J Pathol Inform 1:23
33. Tholouli E, Sweeney E, Barrow E, Clay V, Hoyland JA, Byers RJ (2008) Quantum dots light up pathology. J Pathol 216:275–285
34. van der Loos CM (2010) Chromogens in multiple immunohistochemical staining used for visual assessment and spectral imaging: the colorful future. The J Histotechnol 33:31–40
35. van der Loos CM (2008) Multiple immunoenzyme staining: methods and visualizations for the observation with spectral imaging. J Histochem Cytochem 56:313–328
36. Robertson D, Savage K, Reis-Filho JS, Isacke CM (2008) Multiple immunofluorescence labelling of formalin-fixed paraffin-embedded (FFPE) tissue. BMC Cell Biol 9:13

Chapter 33

COLD-PCR Enriches Low-Level Variant DNA Sequences and Increases the Sensitivity of Genetic Testing

Elena Castellanos-Rizaldos, Coren A. Milbury, Minakshi Guha, and G. Mike Makrigiorgos

Abstract

Detection of low-level mutations is important for cancer biomarker and therapy targets discovery, but reliable detection remains a technical challenge. The newly developed method of CO-amplification at Lower Denaturation temperature PCR (COLD-PCR) helps to circumvent this issue. This PCR-based technology preferentially enriches minor known or unknown variants present in samples with a high background of wild type DNA which often hampers the accurate identification of these minority alleles. This is a simple process that consists of lowering the temperature at the denaturation step during the PCR-cycling protocol (critical denaturation temperature, T_c) and inducing DNA heteroduplexing during an intermediate step. COLD-PCR in its simplest forms does not need additional reagents or specific instrumentation and thus, can easily replace conventional PCR and at the same time improve the mutation detection sensitivity limit of downstream technologies. COLD-PCR can be applied in two basic formats: fast-COLD-PCR that can enrich T_m-reducing mutations and full-COLD-PCR that can enrich all mutations, though it requires an intermediate cross-hybridization step that lengthens the thermocycling program. An improved version of full-COLD-PCR (*i*mproved and *c*omplete *e*nrichment, ice-COLD-PCR) has also been described. Finally, most recently, we developed yet another form of COLD-PCR, temperature-tolerant-COLD-PCR, which gradually increases the denaturation temperature during the COLD-PCR reaction, enriching diverse targets using a single cycling program. This report describes practical considerations for application of fast-, full-, ice-, and temperature-tolerant-COLD-PCR for enrichment of mutations prior to downstream screening.

Key words Coamplification at lower denaturation temperature (COLD-PCR), Mutation detection, Low-level mutations, Cancer, Diagnosis, Prognosis, Therapy targets

1 Introduction

In the era of personalized medicine, the detection of rare DNA variants in biological specimens is important as it may influence certain clinical decisions in the fields of cancer, prenatal diagnosis, or infectious diseases [1–5]. As commonly applied, PCR does not contain an inherent selectivity towards variant (mutant) alleles, thus both variant and wild type alleles are amplified with similar

Magdalena Thurin and Francesco M. Marincola (eds.), *Molecular Diagnostics for Melanoma: Methods and Protocols*, Methods in Molecular Biology, vol. 1102, DOI 10.1007/978-1-62703-727-3_33, © Springer Science+Business Media New York 2014

efficiencies according to their original concentrations. The burden of identifying a low-level mutation falls on downstream assays, such as Sanger sequencing, pyrosequencing, matrix-assisted laser desorption/ionization time-of-flight (MALDI-TOF), restriction fragment length polymorphism (RFLP), denaturing high-performance liquid chromatography (dHPLC), and others.

We recently developed CO-amplification at Lower Denaturation temperature (COLD-PCR) [6], a new form of PCR that preferentially amplifies rare variants in the presence of a high background of wild type DNA, regardless of mutation type or position in the target of interest. The use of COLD-PCR during the amplification step from genomic DNA increases the sensitivity of detection of these low-level mutations prior to using downstream detection technologies such as Sanger sequencing, pyrosequencing, next-generation sequencing, mutation scanning, and mutation genotyping [7].

COLD-PCR enriches low-level mutations within the region of interest by reducing the denaturation temperature during PCR. There are several assays currently available that have the ability to enrich mutations during the process of PCR. For example, peptide nucleic acid (PNA)-based assays [8] can inhibit wild type DNA amplification by forming a PCR clamp or by preventing the primer from annealing to the wild type allele, thus preferentially amplifying the mutated allele. Alternatively, the Fluorescent Amplicon Generation (FLAG) assay [9] employs a highly thermostable restriction enzyme *Psp*GI in the PCR reaction that continuously digests the wild type allele leaving the mutant allele to be amplified during the course of PCR. In each of these two examples, and several others, the disadvantage is that they are designed to enrich only known mutations and therefore low-level unknown mutations remain undetectable [10]. COLD-PCR uniquely enables enrichment of unknown low-level mutations, irrespective of their type or position on the amplicon.

The principle of COLD-PCR is illustrated in Fig. 1. A single-base alteration anywhere along the sequence results in a small variation of the melting temperature of the amplicon (T_m) between 0.2 and 1.5 °C in 200 bp length amplicons [11, 12]. The temperature below the T_m has been defined as *critical denaturation temperature* (T_c). Amplicons differing by a single nucleotide result in variable PCR amplification efficiencies when the PCR denaturation temperature is set to the T_c. This important observation can be used during PCR for the selective amplification of minority alleles differing by one or more nucleotides at any position of a given sequence.

COLD-PCR can be applied in two formats, full-COLD-PCR and fast-COLD-PCR, depending on whether it is important to identify all possible mutations or to achieve the highest degree of mutation enrichment. The detailed methodological approach of full- and fast-COLD-PCR is presented in Fig. 1a, b, respectively.

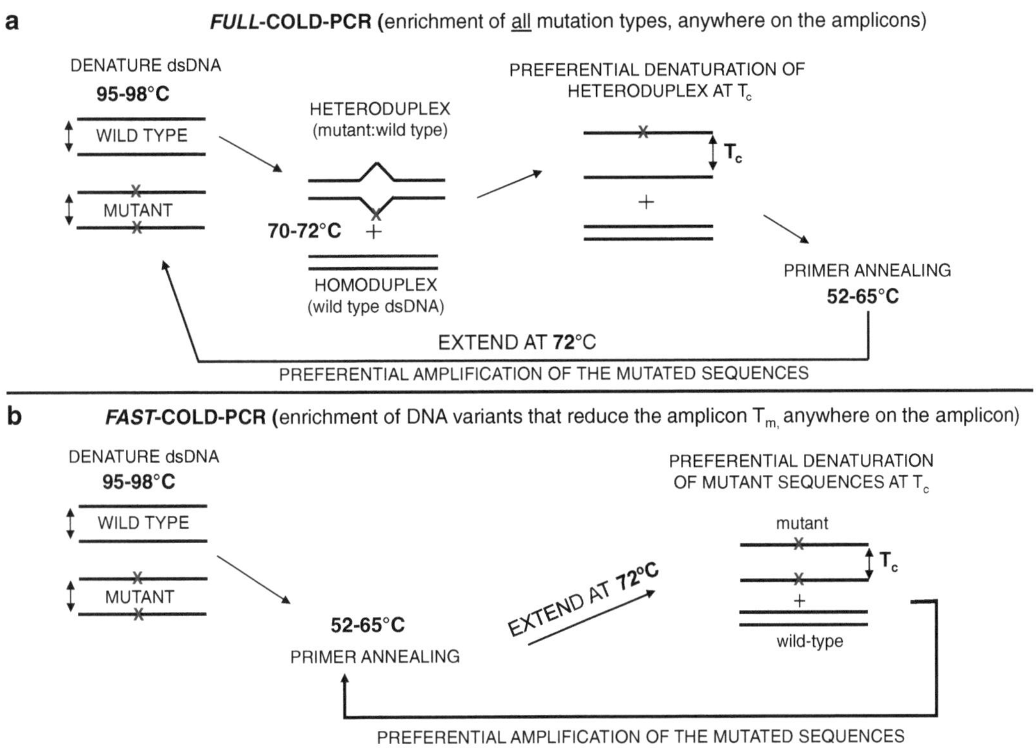

Fig. 1 *COLD-PCR protocol schematic* [6]. The two main forms of COLD-PCR reported full-COLD-PCR (*panel* **a**) and fast-COLD-PCR (*panel* **b**) are described. (**a**) *Full-COLD-PCR*: after denaturation (95.0–98.0 °C), single strands of DNA are re-annealed and cross-hybridized at 70.0–72.0 °C. Cross-hybridization of mutated DNA strand with the wild type DNA strand forms a mismatch-containing structure (heteroduplex), which is more unstable and denatures at a lower melting temperature than a fully matched structure (wild type: wild type, homoduplex). The next step in PCR cycle is to go to the Critical Denaturation Temperature (T_c) to denature most of these heteroduplexed structures. Then primer annealing and extension occur, which favors the amplification of mutated alleles. (**b**) *Fast-COLD-PCR* is simpler and faster to use than full-COLD-PCR, but is only applicable to mutations that decrease the melting temperature of the mutant amplicon compared to the wild type amplicon. Instead of the standard denaturation temperature, the critical temperature (T_c) preferentially denatures mutated alleles, followed by primer annealing and extension. This process preferentially allows the amplification of the T_m decreasing mutated alleles

In full-COLD-PCR (Fig. 1a), an intermediate hybridization step (70.0–72.0 °C) is used during the PCR cycling to allow heteroduplex formation (cross-hybridization of mutant and wild type alleles). These DNA heteroduplexes are less stable than homoduplexes resulting in lower denaturation temperatures. Therefore, when the denaturation temperature is set at the T_c, the majority of heteroduplex molecules denature and amplify over subsequent PCR cycles, whereas most homoduplex molecules remain double-stranded, reducing the amplification efficiency of the most abundant allele (wild type). By using the T_c instead of the regular denaturation temperature (95.0–98.0 °C) throughout the course of PCR, DNA variants at any position in the interrogated amplicon are enriched during COLD-PCR amplification. In fast-COLD-PCR (Fig. 1b) the heteroduplex formation step is not necessary and setting the denaturation temperature at the T_c will favor the amplification of homoduplex molecules that contain T_m-reducing mutants (G:C > A:T or G:C > T:A). The process of full-COLD-PCR is somewhat longer than conventional PCR due to the incorporation of a cross-hybridization step to enable formation of heteroduplexes that may result in modest enrichment levels. The enrichment obtained by full-COLD-PCR is generally less than the one obtained with fast-COLD-PCR, because the formation of heteroduplexes is only efficient over the last 10–15 cycles prior to the reaction reaching saturation. To improve on this aspect, a new form of COLD-PCR was developed, ice-COLD-PCR, that provides improved and complete enrichment of all mutation types [13]. Briefly, ice-COLD-PCR incorporates a single-strand, wild type-specific oligonucleotide (reference sequence, added in excess within the reaction), which enables formation of heteroduplexes even in early PCR cycles. This reference sequence contains a 3′ modification (phosphate group) that helps to prevent polymerase extension during PCR amplification, and is somewhat shorter on both sides relative to the PCR amplicon so that primers do not bind to it. The thermocycling program is similar to that of *full-COLD-PCR*; an excess of wild type oligonucleotides incorporated in the reaction binds to other wild type alleles in the sample and at the T_c the mutant allele heteroduplex preferentially denatures and amplifies during PCR, while the wild type allele amplification is inhibited. However, it is important to notice that for all of these COLD-PCR forms a strict control of the T_c is required to attain optimal enrichment. More recently, we reported on a novel form of COLD-PCR, temperature-tolerant (TT) COLD-PCR that circumvents the T_c stringency and allows the amplification of different targets applying one set of cycling conditions [14]. This method includes a gradual increase of the T_c, a step-up protocol that spans a 1.5–3.0 °C window in small temperature increments (e.g., 0.3 °C) favoring the enrichment of mutations whose denaturation temperature is gradually reached during the reaction. This protocol has been adapted for every form of COLD-PCR, fast-, full-, and ice-COLD-PCR, allowing all mutation types to be enriched during the cycling protocol.

2 Materials

2.1 COLD-PCR Reagents and Equipment

1. Wild type genomic DNA samples, such as reference human male genomic DNA (Promega, Madison, WI, USA).
2. Genomic DNA that will be interrogated, purified from tissue, plasma, FFPE, or other sources.

3. Standard PCR oligonucleotides (from vendors such as Integrated DNA Technologies, Inc., Coralville, IA, USA). For full- and ice-COLD-PCR formats, the T_m of these primers must be such that they do not generate amplicons at the temperature used for heteroduplex formation (usually 70.0 °C).
4. Polymerase system (such as GoTaq Flexi DNA Polymerase system, Promega, Inc.; HF-2 *Taq* polymerase, BD-Clontech, Inc.; Jumpstart *Taq* polymerase, Sigma-Aldrich; or Phusion high fidelity polymerase, Finnzymes Inc.).
5. Deoxyribonucleotide triphosphate (dNTP) mix.
6. Fluorescent dye (such as LCGreenPlus+, Idaho Technologies, Inc. or SYBR Green, Invitrogen, Inc.). PCR in real time is not required for COLD-PCR, but can be helpful to identifying the T_c.
7. A Smart Cycler II real-time thermocycler (Cepheid, Inc.) is used at our laboratory; however, other real-time or standard PCR thermocyclers with high temperature precision and reproducibility may be used.
8. Optionally, Light Scanner HR96 system (Idaho Technologies, Inc.) can be utilized for high resolution melt (HRM) analysis, to prescreen the samples before Sanger sequencing. Any real-time PCR thermocyclers that incorporates the HRM option can also be employed.
9. If ice-COLD-PCR is used: a 3′-phosphorylated oligonucleotide complementary to the wild type strand is required. Other 3′ end modifications that prevent polymerase extension can be used as well. Also, a maximum overlap of the reference sequence with the priming region should be no more than ~5 bp, so that the primers do not bind to it.

3 Methods

3.1 Procedure: Identification of the Critical Denaturation Temperature

The T_c should be determined experimentally for each COLD-PCR amplicon.

1. Perform real-time melting analysis in the same instrument and reagents that will be used for COLD-PCR. In our laboratory, this is done in the presence of LCGreenPlus+ dye on a Smart Cycler II real-time PCR thermocycler, to determine the T_m of a wild type amplicon first or the T_m of the hybridized duplexes in ice-COLD-PCR (*see* Subheading 3.6), *see* also **Note 1**. A good initial approximation to the T_c is then given by the empirical formula $T_c = T_m - 1.0$.
2. To fine-tune the choice of T_c, a series of denaturation temperatures at 0.5 °C decrements below the amplicon T_m should be evaluated. The appropriate T_c will be the lowest temperature

that reproducibly yields a high-quality PCR product and provides good enrichment. The optimal T_c value may be dependent on the amplicon size (typically, amplicons smaller than 200 bp are required), GC content, and reagents composition (*see* **Note 2**).

3. For the TT-COLD-PCR approach, the determination of the exact T_c is not necessary, but the T_m of the amplicon still has to be derived experimentally to establish the appropriate cycling protocol.

3.2 COLD-PCR Reagent Conditions and Concentrations

Use the same standard reagent conditions in COLD-PCR or TT-COLD-PCR reactions as used in conventional PCR. The use of a fluorescence dye (such as LCGreen+) allows the PCR to be monitored in real time. Although any polymerase system can be employed, the use of a high fidelity enzyme such as Phusion™ high fidelity DNA polymerase with reported error rates of 4.2×10^{-7} is recommended. Final reaction concentrations usually applied in our laboratory are as follows:

1. 1X Phusion™ Buffer that contains 1.5 mmol/L $MgCl_2$ (or other 1× PCR Buffer with the incorporation of 1.5–4 mmol/L $MgCl_2$).
2. dNTP mix: 0.2 mmol/L (each).
3. Primers (upstream and downstream): 0.1–0.5 μmol/L (each).
4. LCGreenPlus+dye: 0.1–1×.
5. Phusion™ DNA polymerase: 0.5 U (or any DNA polymerase system).
6. Template DNA: If the template is genomic DNA, 10–100 ng is used as input. If the template is a PCR product from a first PCR reaction; 1:1,000–1:10,000 dilution is usually used as input template for the COLD-PCR reaction.
7. Balance to 25.0 μl with DNAse, RNAse-free water.
8. If ice-COLD-PCR is performed: Oligonucleotide reference sequence: ~25 nmol/L.

3.3 PCR Thermocycling Conditions

COLD-PCR thermocycling conditions should be designed as either fast-, full-, or ice-COLD-PCR depending upon the type of mutation enrichment that is desired, as discussed in more detail below (*see* Subheading 3.5). If multiple amplicons in independent reactions need to be tested under the same cycling conditions, or when the exact T_c is unknown, the temperature-tolerant (TT)-COLD-PCR approach would be appropriate. Thermocycling protocols for all COLD-PCR formats are presented below.

1. *Fast-COLD-PCR thermocycling protocol*: Initial denaturation: 98.0 °C for 30 s, then ~5 cycles conventional PCR when using

a preamplified PCR product as a template (if genomic DNA template is used, perform conventional PCR until 3 cycles before the real-time PCR threshold, C_T-3 cycles) as follows: 98.0 °C for 10 s, annealing at 52.0–65.0 °C for 20 s and extension at 72.0 °C for 10 s. Then, automatically switch to COLD-PCR conditions, 25–35 cycles of denaturation at critical denaturation temperature (T_c) for 10 s, annealing at 52.0–65.0 °C for 20 s, and extension at 72.0 °C for 10 s (*see* **Notes 3** and **4**).

2. *Full-COLD-PCR thermocycling protocol*: Initial denaturation: 98.0 °C for 30 s, followed by ~5 cycles conventional when using a preamplified PCR template (if genomic DNA template is used, 25 cycles or $\approx C_T$) at 98.0 °C for 10 s, annealing at 52.0–65.0 °C for 20 s and extension at 72.0 °C for 10 s. Then, 25–35 cycles of denaturation at 98.0 °C for 10 s, heteroduplex formation (cross-hybridization) at 70.0–72.0 °C for 30 s, T_c for 10 s, annealing at 52.0–65.0 °C for 20 s, and extension at 72.0 °C for 10 s (*see* **Notes 4** and **5**).
3. *ice-COLD-PCR thermocycling protocol*: The protocol is similar to full-COLD-PCR (refer to above protocol). There is a cross-hybridization step at 70.0 °C where both the mutant and wild type alleles bind to the reference sequences, forming either a homoduplex or heteroduplex (*see* **Notes 4**, **6**, and **7**).
4. *Temperature-tolerant (TT)-COLD-PCR thermocycling protocol*: A single cycling protocol will amplify and simultaneously enrich DNA variants on various amplicons. Fast-, full-, and ice-COLD-PCR formats can be adapted to this protocol. The lowest T_m for all the amplicons that will be analyzed is the minimum T_m (T_{mmin}) (*see* **Note 8**).
   - *Fast-TT-COLD-PCR*: Initial denaturation: 98.0 °C for 30 s, followed by ~5 cycles when using a preamplified PCR template (if genomic DNA template is used, C_T-3 cycles) at 98.0 °C for 10 s, annealing at 52.0–65.0 °C for 20 s, and extension at 72.0 °C for 10 s. Then, 5–10 cycles of denaturation at the first critical denaturation temperature (T_{c1} normally, $T_{c1} = T_{mmin} - 2$ °C) for 20 s, annealing at 52.0–65.0 °C for 20 s, and extension at 72.0 °C for 10 s, followed by 5–10 cycles of denaturation at the second critical denaturation temperature (T_{c2}, $T_{c2} = T_{c1}$ +0.3 °C) for 20 s, annealing at 52.0–65.0 °C for 20 s, and extension at 72.0 °C for 10 s, repeated successively until a 1.5–2.0 °C temperature window is covered.
   - *Full-TT-COLD-PCR*: Initial denaturation: 98.0 °C for 30 s, followed by ~5 cycles when using a preamplified PCR template (if genomic DNA template is used, 25 cycles or $\approx C_T$) at 98.0 °C for 10 s, annealing at 52.0–65.0 °C for

20 s, and extension at 72.0 °C for 10 s. Then, 5–10 cycles of denaturation at 98.0 °C for 10 s, heteroduplex formation (cross-hybridization) at 70.0–72.0 °C for 30 s, first critical denaturation temperature (T_{c1} normally, $T_{c1} = T_{mmin} - 2.0$ °C) for 10 s, annealing at 52.0–65.0 °C for 20 s, and extension at 72.0 °C for 10 s. This is followed by consecutive 5–10 cycles for the next critical denaturation temperature (T_{c2}, $T_{c2} = T_{c1} + 0.3$ °C), repeated in consecutively until a 1.5–2.0 °C temperature window is spanned.

- *ice-TT-COLD-PCR*: Follow the same protocol as for TT-full-COLD-PCR.

3.4 Guidelines for the Design of COLD-PCR Amplicons and Primers

1. Choose a target PCR amplicon that possesses preferentially a single melting domain. The amplicon melting profile can be predicted by using DNA melting prediction software tools such as uMELT developed by the Wittwer lab (http://www.dna.utah.edu/umelt/um.php). If the target amplicons have multiple melting domains, the amplicon should be split and primers should be designed to amplify single melting domains. The presence of a single melting domain can also be tested experimentally by doing a real-time PCR in the presence of an intercalating dye, followed by melting analysis.
2. Enrichment of mutations via COLD-PCR is more efficient for amplicons smaller than 200 bp, as single base variations will have a larger effect on the T_m [11, 12].
3. The degree of enrichment obtained with COLD-PCR will be variable depending on amplicon size, DNA sequence, mutation location, type of DNA variation, and experimental conditions; however, in all cases the use of COLD-PCR followed by downstream detection methods is expected to improve the current limit of detection for minority alleles. In difficult cases such as A>T mutations in the vicinity of GC-rich sequences, the use of LNA-assisted ice-COLD-PCR [13] can provide satisfactory enrichment.
4. We have demonstrated mutation enrichment by ~1 order of magnitude (range, 6–22-fold) for mutant alleles in amplicons ~100–200 bp in length, and enrichment of up to ~2 orders of magnitude for shorter amplicons <100 bp [6, 15–17]. For deletions and/or insertions of 3 bp or more, the enrichment can be greater than 2 orders of magnitude [6].
5. Primer design guidelines for COLD-PCR are the same as for conventional PCR; however, the T_m for each primer should not be higher than 65.0 °C for full-COLD-PCR or ice-COLD-PCR because it may affect the formation of heteroduplex molecules during the hybridization step (if primers anneal at

70.0 °C, polymerase may extend and cause problems). In the event the target region has a high melting temperature, the heteroduplex formation step can be performed at temperatures slightly higher than 70.0 °C (for instance, at 72.0 °C).

3.5 Guidelines for the Selection of Full-, Fast-, Ice-, or Temperature-Tolerant-COLD- PCR

1. Whether to perform full-, fast-, ice-, or temperature-tolerant (TT)-COLD-PCR depends on the DNA variant likely to be present, the number of targets of interest and the desired mutation enrichment. For enriching insertions, deletions, and single base substitutions that result in either a comparable T_m or increase the T_m, full-COLD-PCR or ice-COLD-PCR [13] should be applied. For example, T:A→A:T, C:G→G:C will result in a comparable T_m, while T:A→G:C and T:A→C:G will increase the T_m. Conversely, for insertions, deletions, and single base substitutions (such as G:C→A:T or G:C→T:A) that lower the amplicon melting temperature, fast-COLD-PCR will be suitable to achieve better enrichment. Getting experience with fast-COLD-PCR is highly recommended for first-time users of COLD-PCR, as it is simple and results in substantial mutation enrichment with minimal effort involved.
2. If multiple targets need to be screened or if the exact T_c has not yet been determined, a temperature-tolerant approach in a full-, fast-, or ice-COLD-PCR format is advisable. TT-COLD-PCR allows the interrogation of multiple genomic regions by using a single cycling protocol.

3.6 Guidelines for the Determination of T_m and T_c of the Amplicon

1. The establishment of the amplicon T_m can be done by a melt curve analysis after real-time PCR amplification performed on wild type DNA under conventional conditions in the presence of an intercalating dye. Differences in the T_m values may be observed between instruments, buffer compositions, or reagent concentrations. Every time there is a change, T_m values should be redetermined (Fig. 2).
2. Ice-COLD-PCR: In this case, the T_m of the reference sequence will differ from that of the amplicon as it is shorter in length. The experimental determination of the T_m is done by using primers that generate an amplicon (wild type) of the same length and sequence as the reference sequence. Then, the T_m determination for the hybridized duplexes is by conventional PCR followed by a melt curve analysis of the RS amplicon duplex.
3. To fine-tune and define the optimal T_c of a target amplicon, test samples containing 10 % dilutions of DNA with known mutations (typically from commercial cell lines or clinical samples) in wild type DNA background can be used. This enables the assessment of the mutation abundance before and after COLD-PCR, in addition to the mutation enrichment (*see* **Note 9**).

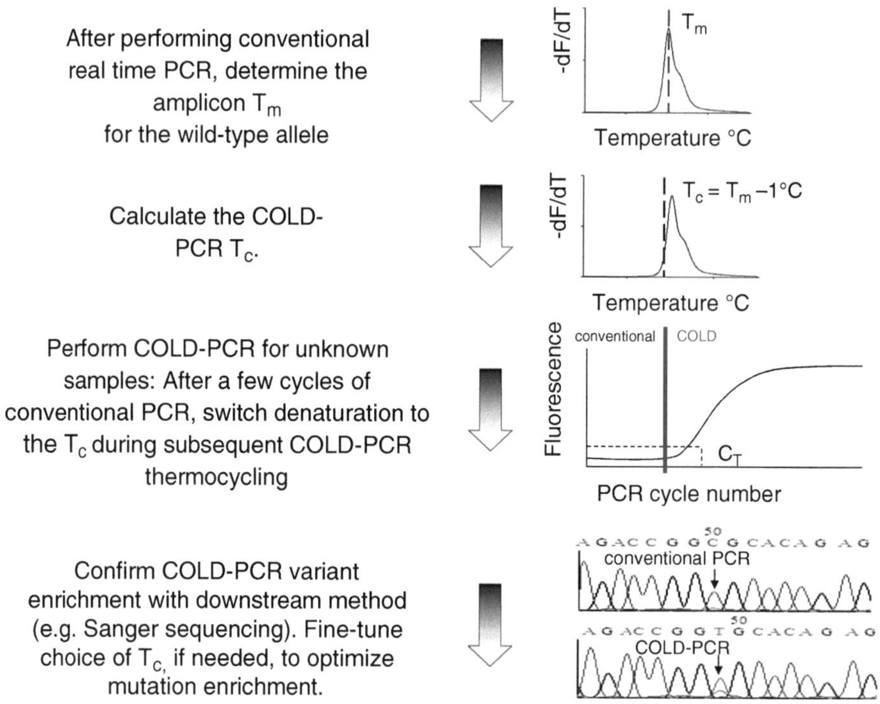

Fig. 2 A general overview of the optimization process for COLD-PCR is presented. The T_m is the amplicon melting temperature, as determined by –dF/dT plots (the negative derivative of fluorescence over temperature) and it is obtained by a post-real-time PCR melt curve analysis of the wild type amplicon; the T_c is the critical denaturation temperature employed in COLD-PCR. The C_T is the threshold cycle of the PCR amplification curve, for real-time PCR-based embodiments

4. As described in Subheading 3.3, fine-tuning of the T_c for fast-, full-, or ice-COLD-PCR should be performed as follows: (1) amplification of 10 % mutant dilution under conventional denaturation conditions (~95.0–98.0 °C), (2) change the denaturation temperature to a T_c of 0.5 °C below the amplicon T_m, (3) T_c = amplicon T_m − 1.0 °C, and (4) T_c = amplicon T_m − 1.5 °C. Next, evaluation of mutant enrichment according to the temperature gradient above can be predetermined by post-PCR high resolution melt (HRM) curve analysis and further confirmed by Sanger sequencing (*see* **Note 10**).
5. Alternatively the enriched mutant fraction can be determined using a restriction fragment length polymorphism (RFLP) assay that differentiates between mutant and wild type alleles, followed by gel, dHPLC, or capillary electrophoresis, if an appropriate restriction endonuclease is available [18].
6. The optimal T_c should be selected on the basis of the lowest denaturation temperature capable of still generating a reproducible PCR amplicon. To date, we have observed that for the majority of amplicons tested, $T_c = T_m - 1.0$ °C. The Ferrari/

Cremonesi group has reported a PCR-gradient-based approach to determine the optimal T_c (*see* **Note 11**), which is not dependent on real-time PCR [19, 20]. This can be used for non-real-time PCR thermocyclers.

3.7 Guidelines for the Determination of the Temperature Window for Temperature Tolerant COLD-PCR

1. The first step is to determine the melting temperatures (T_m) of the amplicons that will be screened, as previously described (Subheading 3.6).
2. TT-fast, TT-full-, or TT-ice-COLD-PCR protocols can be applied depending on the type of variant that is to be detected (*see* Subheading 3.5).
3. Typically, temperature windows spanning 1.5–2 °C can be applied, although larger temperature windows in bigger temperature increments during cycling are also possible [14]. This temperature range can be adapted in a step-wise manner, with consecutive steps of 5–10 cycles at each step, incrementing 0.3 °C in each step. The first T_c of the cycling protocol should be ≥1.5–2 °C below the lowest melting temperature of the amplicons tested [minimum T_m, $T_c = T_{mmin} - (1.0–2.0\ °C)$] (Fig. 3).
4. Additionally, if amplicons with higher T_ms have to be evaluated by using the same cycling conditions, but in different wells of a single thermocycler, variable DMSO/formamide/other organic solvent concentrations can be added within each reaction (1–5 % of the total reaction volume in order to lower the amplicon T_m) so that their final T_m is within the temperature range selected.

3.8 Selecting the Proper Thermocycler

1. When applying fast-, full-, or ice-COLD-PCR formats, the degree of mutant enrichment is highly dependent upon a precise T_c. A variance of ~0.5 °C in T_c may result in either failed amplification or poor enrichment (*see* **Note 12**). It is important that the selected thermocycler is highly precise in temperature such that there is little well-to-well variation. The SmartCycler II (Cepheid, Inc.) is excellent for optimization of thermocycling conditions because each well is individually controlled and calibrated.
2. Air-cooled thermocyclers, such as the centrifugal Rotor-Gene Q (Qiagen, Inc.) and the rotary glass capillary systems such as the LightCycler 480 (Roche, Inc.) and the LightScanner 32 (Idaho Technologies, Inc.) can also be used. In some of them, the anticipated well-to-well variation is as little as 0.01–0.05 °C. Some of these systems provide high temperature precision, real-time monitoring, high-throughput sample processing, as well as post-PCR high resolution melting (HRM). The HRM platform is valuable in its ability to detect quickly and effortlessly the presence of a low-level mutant, as well as offer a potential indication of mutation enrichment based upon the

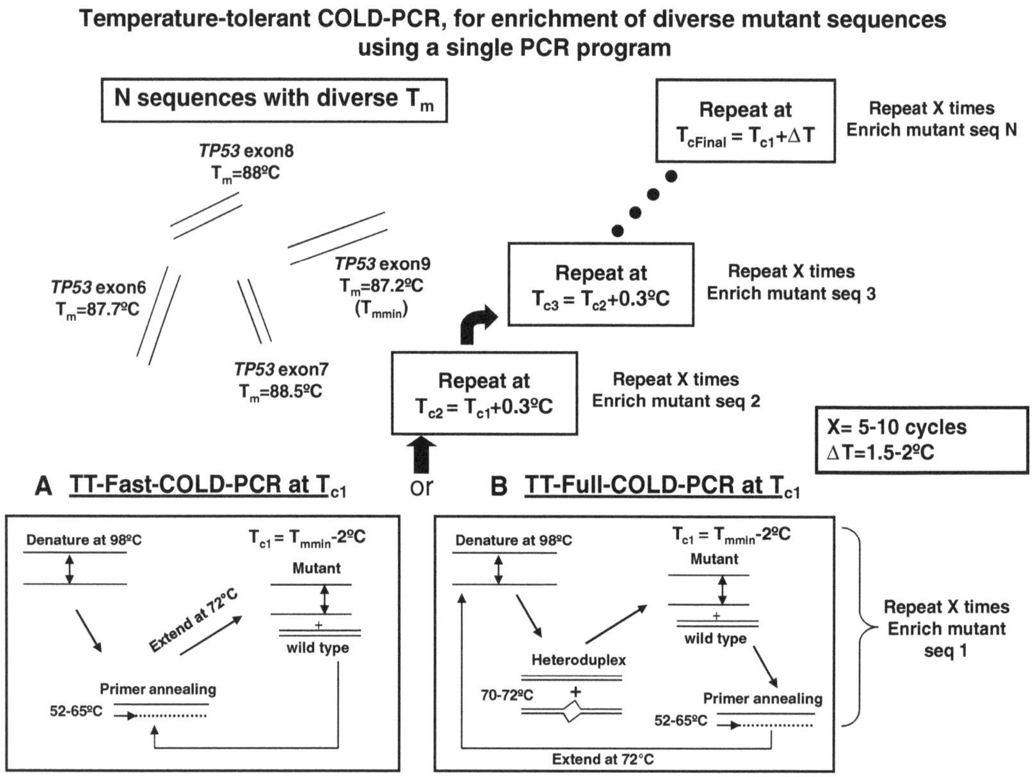

Fig. 3 *Temperature tolerant COLD-PCR.* Temperature tolerant (TT)-COLD-PCR protocol adapted to the two main forms of COLD-PCR, (**a**) fast- and (**b**) full-COLD-PCR for enrichment and amplification of multiple sequences under the same cycling protocol. TT-COLD-PCR (fast- or full-) is a step-up protocol where the different temperature steps are repeated 5–10 cycles each and the critical denaturation temperature is incremented by 0.3 °C at each step. The final temperature window that encompasses the different T_c of the targets of interest range from 1.5 to 3.0 °C, depending upon instrument limitations, polymerase system, or the formation of primer dimers. Adapted from Castellanos-Rizaldos et al. [14]

differential melt curve profiles relative to wild type control samples.

3. When the temperature tolerant approach is the protocol of choice, the temperature fluctuations observed between wells or different platforms do not severely affect the overall enrichment, so this relaxes somewhat the requirement for temperature stringency.

3.9 Assays Downstream of COLD-PCR

After COLD-PCR enrichment, several methods can be used to detect enriched minority alleles. Some of these downstream applications include:

1. *Sanger sequencing*: use this approach for both known and unknown mutation scanning and to determine the approximate degree of enrichment. It is broadly available; however, the

sensitivity is limited to detecting ~20 % mutant in a wild type background [21]. This mutation sensitivity limit can increase by 5–100-fold if one or two successive rounds of COLD-PCR are applied instead of conventional PCR [15, 18, 22].

2. *Pyrosequencing*: use this approach for scanning both known and unknown mutations. The detection sensitivity is around 5–10 % mutant alleles into wild type background [23]. COLD-PCR followed by pyrosequencing can identify mutations down to 0.5–1 % mutant in wild type DNA dilution, with mutation enrichments of 5–35-fold [6].
3. *MALDI-TOF genotyping*: use for high-throughput detection of known mutation; the detection sensitivity is around ~5–10 % mutant into wild type DNA [24]. The combination of fast-COLD-PCR with MALDI-TOF can increase this sensitivity by reliably detecting somatic mutations down to 0.1–0.5 % in wild type DNA background and provides mutation enrichments by 10–100-fold [7].
4. *TaqMan genotyping*: use for genotyping and quantifying known mutations; the sensitivity limit for mutation detection under conventional Taqman-PCR conditions is around 10 % mutant into wild type DNA [25–27]. The combination of this method with COLD-PCR improves the detection limit to 0.8 % of mutant DNA into wild type DNA under fast-COLD-PCR conditions in TaqMan format; and 0.1 % after two rounds of COLD-PCR-TaqMan [7]. The use of locked-nucleic acids/PNA modifications in the Taqman probe improves the mutation enrichment further (unpublished data).
5. *High Resolution Melting*: use for high-throughput and fast mutation scanning showing altered melting profiles compared to a wild type sequence [28]. Mutation detection limit is highly amplicon-dependent; however, COLD-PCR improves readily the detection limit, and most importantly, enables sequencing of the identified DNA variant. The application of COLD-PCR prior to HRM analysis instead of PCR under standard cycling conditions can accurately identify mutant mixtures as little as 0.1 % mutant DNA into wild type DNA [29].
6. *Next-generation sequencing* (*NGS*): high performance technology use for mutation detection; the reported sensitivity in this case is about ~2 % [15]. The enrichment of low abundance mutations by COLD-PCR before NGS, improves the sensitivity by allowing the detection of 0.02 % mutant alleles into wild type DNA background [15].

4 Notes

1. The amplicon T_m may differ when different PCR reagents are used (buffer composition and buffer batch, polymerase system, etc.), fluorescent dye type and concentration. Therefore, T_m values have to be derived experimentally in each case. It is important to keep track of the buffer lot number, as manufacturers occasionally change PCR buffer composition without warning. If the buffer changes, the optimal T_c has to be redetermined. It is important to consider that the efficiency of enrichment may be affected if an amplicon contains multiple melting domains and some mutant variants may not even enrich if they are located in the sequence between two melting regions.
2. We have observed that $T_c = T_m - 1.0$ °C is typically optimal for fast-COLD-PCR. However, this may vary depending on the amplicon and those that contain a high GC content normally present a T_c equivalent to the T_m of the amplicon—(0.5–0.8)°C.
3. Fast-COLD-PCR can be applied in two formats, either in a nested format from a larger PCR amplicon or directly from genomic DNA. In a nested fast-COLD-PCR reaction, a preliminary conventional PCR is performed. The PCR product generated is diluted (1:1,000–1:10,000) and subsequently used as a template for the fast-COLD-PCR reaction. Amplifying directly from genomic DNA is advantageous due to its simplicity; however, the reaction often reaches saturation before enough COLD-PCR cycles are applied. Thus the mutation enrichment can be smaller when amplifying directly from genomic DNA. One important consideration during the thermocycling protocol is when to begin the COLD-PCR cycling as the timing may determine the degree of enrichment achieved. In the nested format, ~5–10 cycles of amplification at a standard denaturation temperature are appropriate before beginning the COLD-PCR cycles. When amplifying directly from genomic DNA, amplification using the T_c should start ~3 cycles before the threshold cycle number (C_T) to accumulate a sufficient amount of DNA template. The C_T can be determined from the amplification profiles via real-time thermocycling or the PCR thermocycling program can be manually set to start the COLD-PCR cycles at a set C_T. Some real-time thermocyclers can be programmed such that specific cycling conditions automatically begin or end according to the C_T of the reaction, thus accommodating for sample-to-sample variation.
4. The number of initial cycles of conventional PCR is important. COLD-PCR cycling, using a certain T_c, must be initiated before the amplification growth curve reaches the reaction C_T.

5. Full-COLD-PCR can be applied similar to fast-COLD-PCR in a nested approach or, alternatively, directly from genomic DNA. Following conventional cycles, the PCR product is denatured at 98.0 °C then cross-hybridized at 70.0 °C for 30 s. We have found 70.0 °C is the ideal temperature for cross-hybridization; however, this hybridization temperature may be increased to 72.0 °C in case that the primers anneal at 70.0 °C (especially in those genomic regions where GC content is high). If this is the case, primer annealing and extension can occur during this step.
6. It is imperative to confirm the quality and purity of the 3′-modification on the oligonucleotide reference sequence for ice-COLD-PCR. If the reference sequence is not properly purified, it will be extended by the polymerase, resulting in wild type template amplification and therefore jeopardizing the mutation enrichment.
7. ice-COLD-PCR can be applied in a nested format as fast- or full-COLD-PCR. If this is the case, enough regular PCR cycles should precede ice-COLD-PCR conditions in order to generate heteroduplexed structures.
8. Temperature tolerant (TT)-COLD-PCR: In this case, the temperature window used may be as broad as 1.5–3.0 °C using finer T_c gradient, however, the number of cycles that can be performed is limited to the instrument, primer dimmer formation, polymerase inactivation, or reaction saturation. During TT-COLD-PCR, mutant enrichment will occur simultaneously for all amplicons, as long as their T_c falls within the T_c range examined, in individual tubes under the same cycling conditions.
9. Evaluation of mutant (or variant) DNA serial dilutions is important to allow the user to confirm both the successful amplification of the mutant fraction and enrichment of mid-, low-, and extremely low abundances of the mutant fraction.
10. If enrichment is not detected, confirm the empirical amplicon T_m and ensure that reagents and concentrations have not been altered.
11. Lower T_c can be evaluated in an attempt to increase mutation enrichment; however, if the T_c is too low, PCR will likely fail to amplify or will not be reproducible. The gradient approach described by Ferrari/Cremonesi [19, 20] is another alternative.
12. Well-to-well variation in thermocycling equipment can result in enrichment variability. Always ensure that the thermocycler is properly calibrated and shows consistent results.

Acknowledgment

This work was supported by the Innovative Molecular Analysis Technologies Program of the NCI, grants CA-111994 and CA-151164 (G.M.M.). The contents of this manuscript do not necessarily represent the official views of the National Cancer Institute or the National Institutes of Health.

References

1. Kobayashi S, Boggon TJ, Dayaram T, Janne PA, Kocher O, Meyerson M, Johnson BE, Eck MJ, Tenen DG, Halmos B (2005) EGFR mutation and resistance of non-small-cell lung cancer to gefitinib. N Engl J Med 352:786–792
2. Sjoholm MIL, Hoffmann G, Lindgren S, Dillner J, Carlson J (2005) Comparison of archival plasma and formalin-fixed paraffin-embedded tissue for genotyping in hepatocellular carcinoma. Cancer Epidemiol Biomarkers Prev 14:251–255
3. Barcellos LF, Klitz W, Field LL, Tobias R, Bowcock AM, Wilson R, Nelson MP, Nagatomi J, Thomson G (1997) Association mapping of disease loci, by use of a pooled DNA genomic screen. Am J Hum Genet 61:734–747
4. Kimura T, Holland WS, Kawaguchi T, Williamson SK, Chansky K, Crowley JJ, Doroshow JH, Lenz H-J, Gandara DR, Gumerlock PH (2004) Mutant DNA in plasma of lung cancer patients: potential for monitoring response to therapy. Ann N Y Acad Sci 1022:55–60
5. Li J, Berbeco R, Distel RJ, Janne PA, Wang L, Makrigiorgos GM (2007) s-RT-MELT for rapid mutation scanning using enzymatic selection and real time DNA-melting: new potential for multiplex genetic analysis. Nucleic Acids Res 35:e84
6. Li J, Wang L, Mamon H, Kulke MH, Berbeco R, Makrigiorgos GM (2008) Replacing PCR with COLD-PCR enriches variant DNA sequences and redefines the sensitivity of genetic testing. Nat Med 14:579–584
7. Milbury CA, Li J, Liu P, Makrigiorgos GM (2011) COLD-PCR: improving the sensitivity of molecular diagnostics assays. Expert Rev Mol Diagn 11:159–169
8. Dabritz J, Hanfler J, Preston R, Stieler J, Oettle H (2005) Detection of Ki-ras mutations in tissue and plasma samples of patients with pancreatic cancer using PNA-mediated PCR clamping and hybridisation probes. Br J Cancer 92: 405–412
9. Amicarelli G, Shehi E, Makrigiorgos GM, Adlerstein D (2007) FLAG assay as a novel method for real-time signal generation during PCR: application to detection and genotyping of KRAS codon 12 mutations. Nucleic Acids Res 35:e131
10. Milbury CA, Li J, Makrigiorgos GM (2009) PCR-based methods for the enrichment of minority alleles and mutations. Clin Chem 55:632–640
11. Lipsky RH, Mazzanti CM, Rudolph JG, Xu K, Vyas G, Bozak D, Radel MQ, Goldman D (2001) DNA melting analysis for detection of single nucleotide polymorphisms. Clin Chem 47:635–644
12. Liew M, Pryor R, Palais R, Meadows C, Erali M, Lyon E, Wittwer C (2004) Genotyping of single-nucleotide polymorphisms by high-resolution melting of small amplicons. Clin Chem 50:1156–1164
13. Milbury CA, Li J, Makrigiorgos GM (2011) Ice-COLD-PCR enables rapid amplification and robust enrichment for low-abundance unknown DNA mutations. Nucleic Acids Res 39:e2
14. Castellanos-Rizaldos E, Liu P, Milbury CA, Guha M, Brisci A, Cremonesi L, Ferrari M, Mamon H, Makrigiorgos GM (2012) Temperature-tolerant COLD-PCR reduces temperature stringency and enables robust mutation enrichment. Clin Chem 58: 1130–1138
15. Milbury CA, Correll M, Quackenbush J, Rubio R, Makrigiorgos GM (2012) COLD-PCR enrichment of rare cancer mutations prior to targeted amplicon resequencing. Clin Chem 58:580–589
16. Pritchard CC, Akagi L, Reddy PL, Joseph L, Tait JF (2010) COLD-PCR enhanced melting curve analysis improves diagnostic accuracy for KRAS mutations in colorectal carcinoma. BMC Clin Pathol 10:6
17. Kristensen LS, Daugaard IL, Christensen M, Hamilton-Dutoit S, Hager H, Hansen LL (2010) Increased sensitivity of KRAS mutation detection by high-resolution melting analysis of COLD-PCR products. Hum Mutat 31:1366–1373
18. Li J, Milbury CA, Li C, Makrigiorgos GM (2009) Two-round coamplification at lower

denaturation temperature-PCR (COLD-PCR)-based sanger sequencing identifies a novel spectrum of low-level mutations in lung adenocarcinoma. Hum Mutat 30:1583–1590
19. Brisci A, Damin F, Pietra D, Galbiati S, Boggi S, Casetti I, Rumi E, Chiari M, Cazzola M, Ferrari M et al (2012) COLD-PCR and innovative microarray substrates for detecting and genotyping MPL Exon 10 W515 substitutions. Clin Chem
20. Galbiati S, Brisci A, Lalatta F, Seia M, Makrigiorgos GM, Ferrari M, Cremonesi L (2011) Full COLD-PCR protocol for noninvasive prenatal diagnosis of genetic diseases. Clin Chem 57:136–138
21. Vogelstein B, Kinzler KW (1999) Digital PCR. Proc Natl Acad Sci U S A 96:9236–9241
22. Luthra R, Zuo Z (2009) COLD-PCR finds hot application in mutation analysis. Clin Chem 55:2077–2078
23. Ogino S, Kawasaki T, Brahmandam M, Yan L, Cantor M, Namgyal C, Mino-Kenudson M, Lauwers GY, Loda M, Fuchs CS (2005) Sensitive sequencing method for KRAS mutation detection by Pyrosequencing. J Mol Diagn 7:413–421
24. Wood LD, Parsons DW, Jones S, Lin J, Sjoblom T, Leary RJ, Shen D, Boca SM, Barber T, Ptak J et al (2007) The genomic landscapes of human breast and colorectal cancers. Science 318: 1108–1113
25. Wilkening S, Hemminki K, Thirumaran RK, Bermejo JL, Bonn S, Forsti A, Kumar R (2005) Determination of allele frequency in pooled DNA: comparison of three PCR-based methods. Biotechniques 39:853–858
26. De La Vega FM, Lazaruk KD, Rhodes MD, Wenz MH (2005) Assessment of two flexible and compatible SNP genotyping platforms: TaqMan® SNP Genotyping Assays and the SNPlex(TM) Genotyping System. Mutat Res 573:111–135
27. Li J, Wang L, Janne PA, Makrigiorgos GM (2009) Coamplification at lower denaturation temperature-PCR increases mutation-detection selectivity of TaqMan-based real-time PCR. Clin Chem 55:748–756
28. Erali M, Voelkerding KV, Wittwer CT (2008) High resolution melting applications for clinical laboratory medicine. Exp Mol Pathol 85:50–58
29. Milbury CA, Li J, Makrigiorgos GM (2009) COLD-PCR-enhanced high-resolution melting enables rapid and selective identification of low-level unknown mutations. Clin Chem 55:2130–2143

Chapter 34

Isolation of Circulating MicroRNAs from Microvesicles Found in Human Plasma

John F. Quackenbush, Pamela B. Cassidy, Lawrence M. Pfeffer, Kenneth M. Boucher, Jason E. Hawkes, Susan R. Pfeffer, Levy Kopelovich, and Sancy A. Leachman

Abstract

Intact miRNAs can be isolated from the circulation in significant quantities despite the presence of extremely high levels of RNase activity. The remarkable stability of circulating miRNAs makes them excellent candidates for biomarkers in diagnostic applications as well as therapeutic targets in a variety of disease states including melanoma. Circulating RNA molecules are resistant to degradation by RNases because they are encapsulated in membrane-bound microvesicles. We describe a convenient method for the use of ExoQuick, a proprietary resin developed by Systems Biosciences (Mountain View, CA), whereby microvesicles can be purified under gentle conditions using readily available laboratory equipment. This protocol allows for isolation all microvesicles, regardless of their origin, and provides a convenient method for identifying potential cancer-specific biomarkers from biological fluids including serum and plasma.

Key words MicroRNA, Microvesicles, Plasma, Serum, ExoQuick

1 Introduction

MicroRNAs (miRNAs) are highly conserved small, noncoding regulatory RNA molecules 18–22 nucleotides in length. They regulate mRNA stability and protein translation by directing RNA-induced silencing complexes (RISCs) to the 3′ UTR of target mRNA transcripts [1, 2]. MicroRNAs play a pivotal role in development, cell signaling, proliferation, and differentiation by regulating the expression of networks of genes necessary for cell function [3, 4]. Globally, miRNA-induced gene silencing regulates the precise timing of cellular events through the synchronous inhibition of genes that are functionally interdependent [5].

John F. Quackenbush and Pamela B. Cassidy have contributed equally to this work

Magdalena Thurin and Francesco M. Marincola (eds.), *Molecular Diagnostics for Melanoma: Methods and Protocols*, Methods in Molecular Biology, vol. 1102, DOI 10.1007/978-1-62703-727-3_34, © Springer Science+Business Media New York 2014

Significantly, aberrant expression of miRNAs has been found for nearly all types of human cancer [6–9], and the alterations are reflected in the biology of the tumors [10].

Intact miRNAs can be isolated from the circulation in significant quantities despite the presence of extremely high levels of RNase activity [11]. The remarkable stability of circulating miRNAs makes them excellent candidates for biomarkers in diagnostic applications as well as therapeutic targets in a variety of disease states including melanoma. Indeed, differentially expressed circulating miRNA has now been demonstrated for many forms of cancer [12], and a recent study has shown that a panel of five miRNAs can be used to estimate risk of recurrence in stage II melanoma patients [13].

There is clear evidence that circulating RNA molecules are resistant to degradation by RNases because they are encapsulated in membrane-bound microvesicles. Microvesicles are 50–100 nm in diameter and originate from either multi-vesicular bodies within the cell or directly from the plasma membrane. The former are often called exosomes, while the later are often called shedding vesicles or microparticles. The physical properties of the two classes of microvesicles differ only slightly (e.g., size, density, and cholesterol content) and since purification protocols invariably exploit these properties, preparations usually contain a mixture of exosomes and shedding vesicles [14]. Both exosomes and shedding vesicles have been shown to be actively secreted by many different cell types including cancer cells [15], and an online database called Exocarta, catalogs the RNAs, proteins, and lipids that have been identified in microvesicles [16].

Until recently, common methods for isolating microvesicles involved ultracentrifugation, size exclusion chromatography, and antibody capture; however, these techniques are labor intensive, require specialized equipment and often result in poor recovery [17, 18]. The use of ExoQuick, a proprietary resin developed by Systems Biosciences (Mountain View, CA), facilitates the purification of microvesicles under gentle conditions using readily available laboratory equipment. ExoQuick precipitation has been shown to result in much higher recovery and purity of microvesicles from ascites when compared to the other isolation methods [17]. This protocol isolates all microvesicles, regardless of their origin, and provides a convenient method for identifying potential cancer-specific biomarkers from biological fluids.

It is estimated that 5–10 % of all malignant melanomas occur in familial clusters [19]; and 20–40 % of these pedigrees carry germline mutations in either the *CDKN2A* locus or *CDK4* gene. The remainder of familial melanoma kindreds harbors no known melanoma-associated germline mutations. Familial and sporadic melanomas share similar histopathologies, prognostic factors, and survival rates [20], although familial melanoma patients develop tumors at an earlier age and are prone to develop multiple primary melanomas. We propose that these facts are consistent with the hypothesis that the genetic alterations driving familial and sporadic melanomas are the same. Our laboratory has a large archive of citrate plasma obtained from familial melanoma patients and their family members, including spouse controls, as well as samples collected from cases of sporadic melanoma. Thus our plasma archive is a valuable tool for the identification of biomarkers of melanoma predisposition in both high-risk and general populations, including miRNAs contained in circulating microvesicles. In order to explore this possibility, we have developed and optimized a simple and reproducible protocol for the isolation and quantification of miRNA contained in microvesicles derived from very small amounts of archived human plasma. This present study is the starting point for an on-going study of biomarkers of melanoma.

2 Materials

2.1 Preparation of Platelet-Poor Plasma

1. Acid-citrate-dextrose (ACD) Vacutainer Sodium citrate, yellow topped blood collection tubes (Becton, Dickinson).
2. Screw capped cryo-vials with washers (Fisherbrand, 2 mL).

2.2 Removal of Clotting Factors and Isolation of Exosomes

1. Pacific Hemostasis Thromboplastin D to initiate blood coagulation (Thermo Scientific).
2. ExoQuick Exosome Precipitation Solution (Systems Bioscience Mountain View, CA).

2.3 Isolation of Exosomal RNA

1. miRNeasy Mini Kit for purification of microRNA and total RNA (Qiagen Sciences).
2. Microtube Pestle 1.5 mL for microcentrifuge tubes (USA Scientific).
3. Chloroform (Fisher Chemicals).
4. 100 % Ethanol (Pharmco Products, Inc., Brookfield CT).
5. Amicon Ultra YM-3, 0.5 mL Centrifugal Filters 3 kDa MWCO for nucleic acid concentration (Millipore).
6. P1000 pipette model with compatible filter tips (Gilson).
7. Synthetic RNA used as positive experimental control miRNAs (Dharmacon, Thermo Scientific):

   Cel-miR-39, 5′ UCACCGGGUGUAAAUCAGCUUG 3′

   Cel-miR-54, 5′ UACCCGUAAUCUUCAUAAUCCGAG 3′

2.4 Determining the Integrity and Quantity of Exosomal RNA

1. Agilent 2100 Bioanalyzer Instrument (Agilent Technologies, Santa Clara, CA).
2. Agilent RNA 6000 Pico Kit (Agilent Technologies, Santa Clara, CA).
3. RNA 6000 ladder standards as a reference for data analysis (Agilent Technologies, Santa Clara, CA).

2.5 Determining Relative Abundance of Exosomal miRNA by qPCR

1. miScript RT kit for reverse transcription (RT) of total RNA for miRNA detection and quantification. Buffers are supplied with the miScript RT kit for cDNA synthesis to enable miRNA quantification using individual primer assay (Qiagen Sciences, Germantown MD).
2. Custom Synthetic Oligos (Operon Technologies and IDT Technologies) for real-time PCR with the miScript SYBR Green PCR kit (*see* **Note 1**):

   mir21 5′-TAGCTTATCAGACTGATGTTGA-3′

   mir29a 5′-CGGTAGCACCATCTGAAATCGGTTA-3′

   Let7a 5′-GGGTGAGGTAGTAGGTTGTATAGTT-3′

   Let7g 5′-TGAGGTAGTAGTTTGTACAGTT-3′

   mir30d 5′-TGTAAACATCCCCGACTGGAAG-3′

   mir92a 5′-AGGTTGGGATCGGTTGCAATGCT-3′
3. miScript SYBR Green PCR Kit with universal primer (Qiagen Sciences, Germantown MD).
4. RotorGene-Q qPCR instrument or any comparable instrument may be used.
5. Tris–EDTA (TE) Buffer, 10 mM Tris–HCl (pH 8.0), 1 mM EDTA (Ambion/LifeTechnologies).

3 Methods

3.1 Preparation of Platelet-Poor Plasma

1. Collect whole blood in yellow top sodium citrate tubes (*see* **Note 2**). Heparin blood collection tubes are not suitable; however, other types of tubes may be used (*see* **Note 3**).
2. Invert tubes five times, place on ice and process within 1 h of the blood draw.
3. Centrifuge at 4 °C and 1,400 × g for 10 min.
4. Make note of plasma packed cell volumes and signs of hemolysis (*see* **Note 4**).
5. Remove upper layer (plasma) and store at −80 °C in 500 μL aliquots in screw capped cryo-vials.
6. Thaw plasma and centrifuge at 3,000 × g, at room temperature for 15 min, to completely remove of any contaminating cells (*see* **Note 5**).
7. Transfer supernatant to a clean 1.5 mL tube. Discard precipitate.

3.2 Removal of Clotting Factors from Plasma

1. Reconstitute Thromboplastin D with 4 mL of RNase-free water. This material is stable for 2 weeks at 4 °C.
2. Forcibly inject 200 μL of Thromboplastin D solution into each plasma sample. Invert tubes a few times and incubate at 37 °C for 15 min.
3. Centrifuge at room temperature at 8,000 × g for 15 min.

4. Transfer supernatant to a clean 1.5 mL tube. Discard precipitate.

3.3 Isolation of Exosomes

1. Add 140 μL of ExoQuick solution, mix by inverting and place overnight at 4 °C.
2. Centrifuge at 1,500 × g at room temperature for 15 min.
3. Carefully remove supernatant by aspiration.
4. Centrifuge again and remove any remaining liquid by aspiration.

3.4 Isolation of Exosomal RNA

1. Aliquot a quantity of Qiazol (700 μL per sample) sufficient to process all of the samples. Add 0.05 fmol/mL of Cel39 and Cel54 synthetics RNAs to Qiazol solution as a normalizing control (*see* **Note 6**).
2. Add exactly 700 μL of the Qiazol solution to each pellet. Resuspend pellets using a combination of smashing the pellet with a disposable plastic pestle and pipetting up and down with a P1000 pipet with a filter tip.
3. Allow suspensions incubate at room temperature for 5 min.
4. Add 140 μL of chloroform and shake tubes vigorously for 15 s.
5. Allow suspension sit at room temperature for 5 min. This step promotes the dissociation of nucleic acid–protein complexes.
6. Centrifuge at 12,000 × *g* at 4 °C for 15 min.
7. Remove 280 μL of the upper aqueous phase and transfer to a new tube (*see* **Note 7**).
8. Add 420 μL of 100 % ethanol (1.5 volumes), mix thoroughly by pipetting up and down and immediately load the entire 700 μL on a miRNeasy MinElute spin column with 1.5 mL collection tube (*see* Subheading 2.3, **item 1**).
9. Centrifuge at 8,000 × *g* at room temperature for 15 s.
10. Remove flow-through from collection tube by aspirating if reusing the collection tube (*see* **Note 8**).
11. Add 700 μL RNeasy buffer RWT (included in kit) to the column and centrifuge at 8,000 × *g* at room temperature for 15 s.
12. Add 500 μL RNeasy buffer RPE to the column and centrifuge at 8,000 × *g* at RT for 15 s.
13. Add 500 μL RNeasy buffer RPE to the column and centrifuge at 8,000 × *g* at room temperature for 15 s.
14. Place column in a new tube and centrifuge at 12,000 × *g* for 2 min to dry the membrane.
15. Place column in a new collection tube, add 120 μL of RNase-free water to the center of the membrane and let the column incubate for 2 min.
16. Centrifuge at 8,000 × *g* at room temperature for 15 s.

17. Add an additional 300 μL of RNase-free water to the flow-through, and load the resulting solution onto an Amicon Ultra YM-3 filter, and centrifuge at 14,000 × *g* at room temperature for 45 min (*see* **Note 9**).
18. Invert the in a new collection tube and centrifuge at 8,000 × *g* at room temperature for 2 min to recover the RNA.
19. Determine the volume of each sample and adjust to exactly 20 μL with RNase-free water (*see* **Note 10**).

3.5 Determining the Quality and Quantity of Exosomal RNA

1. Run 2 μL of each sample on the Agilent Bioanalyzer Pico Chip according to manufactures recommendations (*see* **Note 11**). RNA analysis is based on chip technology and electrophoretical separation of miRNAs. Figure 1 shows intense band in the size range of small noncoding RNA (16–35 nucleotides). RNA concentration is estimated by this method to be 1.308 ng/μL.

3.6 Reverse Transcription Synthesis of Exosomal cDNA for miRNA Detection

1. miScript RT mix is an optimized solution of poly(A) polymerase and reverse transcriptase. Unlike mRNAs, miRNAs are not polyadenylated. Using the miScript RT protocol, polyadenylation is followed by RT which is primed by an oligo-dT primer linked to a universal tag. This tag serves as the compliment to the reverse primer used in the qPCR assay described below.

   Prepare the miScript Reaction using the following amounts of reagents for each sample:

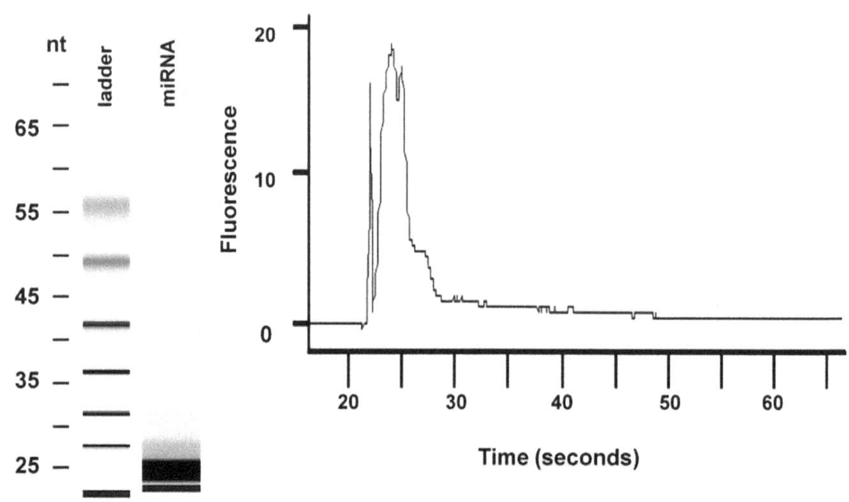

Fig. 1 Agilent RNA 6000 Pico Chip analysis. This is the typical pattern observed for exosomal RNA recovered using this protocol (14–36 nucleotides) and it shows that miRNA is of high quality and quantity. RNA concentration is estimated by this method to be 1.308 ng/μL. Two distinct 18s and 28s ribosomal bands, which are the hallmarks of total eukaryotic cellular RNA are absent and there is a broad, but intense band in the size range of small noncoding RNA

miScript RT Buffer 5 ×[a]	2 μL
miScript Enzyme Mix[a]	0.5 μL
RNase-free H_2O	5.5 μL
Exosomal RNA (1:10 dilution)[b]	2 μL

[a](*see* **Note 12**)

[b](*see* **Note 13** for a very important comment on RNA input)

2. Incubate at 37 °C for 60 min followed by 95 °C for 5 min.
3. Dilute cDNA to 100 μL by adding 90 μL of TE Buffer.

3.7 Determining the Relative Abundance of Exosomal miRNAs by qPCR

1. Use Qiagen miScript SYBR with universal primer master mix according manufacturers recommendations.
2. Real-time PCR detection of specific miRNA is performed using miScript SYBR PCR assay. Forward primer should be added for a final concentration of 0.3 μM (*see* **Note 1**). The reverse primer is included in the master mix.
3. Use the following PCR conditions:

   Initial activation: 95 °C for 5 min.

   Cycling: 40× (95 °C, 10 s; 58 °C, 10 s; 72 °C, 10 s).

   Melt: 72–95 °C raising 1 °C each step and waiting 5 s between each step.
4. Determine fold change using the delta–delta *Ct* method [21]. Cel-39 and Cel-54 spike-ins are used as normalizing technical control miRNAs.

4 Notes

1. Sanger miRBase database (www.mirbase.org) was used to obtain the sequence for all mature (completely processed) miRNAs. Forward primers were essentially the DNA equivalent of the mature miRNA. Primers were designed for a target temperature of 60 °C as determined by IDT Oligo Analyzer (http://www.idtdna.com/analyzer/Applications/OligoAnalyzer/). Some miRNA target sequences required addition or subtraction of bases at the 5′end to approach this target temperature. All primers were validated using a four point standard curve (10, 1, 0.1, and 0.01 ng) of Stratagene Reference Human Total RNA. Primers passed with an efficiency of 1.8–2.0 and single melting peaks. QPCR was carried out on a Qiagen RotorGene-Q instrument; however, other comparable instruments may also be used. The reverse primer is included in the miScript SYBR Green PCR Kit listed in the Materials Subheading 2.5, **item 2**.

2. We have large archives of citrate plasma from melanoma patients, people who are at a high risk of developing melanoma and healthy volunteers. This protocol was optimized to utilize these blood products. When we initially compared RNA yields from unclotted plasma vs. serum using this protocol, we got consistently higher and more reproducible yields from serum. This was presumably due to the presence of clotting factors in the plasma, which interferes with the exosome precipitation by the Exoquick resin. By adding the thromboplastin D step, we found obtained much more reproducible and higher yields when using citrate plasma.
3. We have found that this protocol works well with lavender-topped EDTA plasma tubes, tan-topped SST serum tubes, and red-topped serum tubes. However, we have not performed a detailed statistical analysis of miRNA levels in serum and plasma samples drawn from the same patient, therefore we highly recommended that only one type of tube be used for all samples in an experiment. We have also determined, however, that this protocol *does not* work with green-topped heparin tubes. Heparin is a known inhibitor of PCR and has a molecular weight greater than molecular weight cut-off of the Amicon Ultra YM-3 columns used in Subheading 3.4, **step 18**. Thus heparin likely gets concentrated during this step and interferes with downstream analyses.
4. Since our goal is to compare miRNA between patient samples, it is important that the citrate plasma tubes be filled completely to the 8.5 mL level. This ensures that the volume of plasma used in each analysis is consistent. It is also important to compare samples with similar packed cell volumes (hematocrit) and to exclude (or at the very least make note of) samples with high amounts of hemolysis [22], which are indicated by pink-colored plasma.
5. This step was added to ensure the complete removal of any contaminating cells. In order to demonstrate that our protocol achieves this, we performed the experiment described in Fig. 2. We added various amounts (0; 10,000; 50,000; and 200,000) of mouse melanocyte cells to 500 μL of human plasma and then processed RNA following the stated protocol. We were unable to detect mouse transcripts in the isolated RNA when mouse cells were added directly to the plasma, however mouse transcripts were easily detected when the mouse cells were added directly into the Qiazol solution used for the RNA purification (positive control).
6. We have adopted the strategy of using spike-in *C. elegans* miRNAs as normalizing controls as previously suggested by Mitchell et al. [23]. Since there are no known control microRNAs in exosomes, this approach seems to be the most reasonable way

Mouse cells added (number)	0	10^4	$5X10^4$	$2X10^5$	$2X10^5$
Cells added to	-	Plasma	Plasma	Plasma	Qiazol
RNA recovered(ng)	98	81	97	79	720
Mouse transcripts?	No	No	No	No	Yes (Ct 22)
Delta Ct (mir21-cel39)	4.3	4.1	4.2	4.0	3.7
Delta Ct (mir92b-cel39)	5.1	5.8	5.6	5.5	5.5

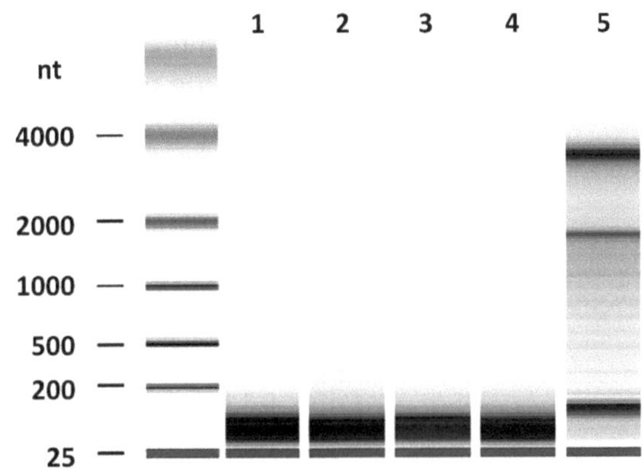

Fig. 2 Exoquick precipitation for removal of cells and their RNAs from plasma by using current protocol. Mouse melanocytes were added either directly into plasma from a healthy human volunteer before exosome isolation (*lanes 2–4*) or into the RNA extraction buffer (Qiazol, positive control, *lane 5*). Plasma without cells added served as the negative control (*lane 1*). Agilent Bioanalyzer results are shown below for each sample. In *lane 1* the negative control sample contains only small RNAs, while in *lane 5*, analysis of the positive control sample shows strong bands corresponding to the 28s and 18s ribosomal RNAs that are associated with cellular RNA. RNAs from samples isolated from plasma to which melanocytes were added (*lanes 2–4*) are identical to the negative control, indicating that there was no contamination from cellular RNA. RNA was also analyzed by qPCR. Both human miR21 and miR92b were detected at nearly identical levels in samples where mouse cells were added to plasma; however mouse mRNA transcripts from both GPx1 and GADPH (which can arise *only* from the added cells) were detected only in the positive control

to normalize microRNA levels. By adding the spike-in miRNA directly into enough Qiazol to process every sample in the study and carefully adding 700 μL of this to each sample we have a direct way to compare one sample to the next.

7. We have adopted the strategy of removing 280 μL of the aqueous phase. While this results in the loss of a small amount of RNA, it also minimizes the risk of contamination with proteins from the interphase layer and yields a higher-purity RNA product.

8. For **steps 10–14**, it is important to minimize salts coming in contact with the outside of the spin column because during the elution step this could contaminate the RNA solution. This can be accomplished by carefully aspirating the flow-through from the bottom of the collection tube. Do not simply pour out the flow-through and reuse the collection tube. Another option is to use a clean collection tube for each wash. Qiagen sells bulk collection tubes (cat # 19201).
9. The Amicon Ultra filter serves two very important functions. First, it effectively removes residual contaminants (salts and phenol) which carryover from the Qiagen miRNeasy protocol. These contaminants interfere with downstream steps such as PCR or ligation reactions. Second, the Amicon Ultra filter is a convenient way to concentrate the RNA sample. This column has a reservoir of 15 μL which insures the sample will not go dry under the stated conditions.
10. It is important to carefully measure the volume of each sample after concentration and adjust the volume so it is the same for each sample. Variations in volume are a potential source for error in the experiment and when we expect to find only two- to threefold difference in miRNA levels it is important to make sure the volumes are identical.
11. The Agilent Bioanalyzer and the Pico RNA chip are used to assess integrity and quantity of RNA in these samples (*see* Fig. 1). RNA analysis is based on chip technology and electrophoretical separation of miRNAs. Data are translated into gel-like images of band and electropherograms. Software automatically compares the unknown sample to the RNA ladder fragments to determine the concentration of the sample and identify RNA peaks. We do not recommend determining quantity and quality using the Nanodrop instrument as the RNA concentrations obtained using this protocol are below the limits of detection for this instrument.
12. If one prepares a single solution containing these reagents in sufficient quantities for all of the reactions in a single experiment, it is much more convenient, reduces cross contamination and improves uniformity of results. Then 18 μL can be dispensed into one PCR tube for each sample and miRNA can be added to each sample separately.
13. In order to insure that the qPCR analysis itself is linear, we analyzed serial dilutions of single cDNA preparations and found that results for qPCR reaction were linear over an 800-fold range for the four miRNAs analyzed in this work (cel39, mir21, mir29a, mir30d, mir92a, and let7g; data not shown). When we varied RNA inputs into RT reactions (1.8, 3.6, 7.2, and 14.4 ng), qPCR analysis of the resulting cDNAs showed that the RT reaction appears to become nonlinear for all of the

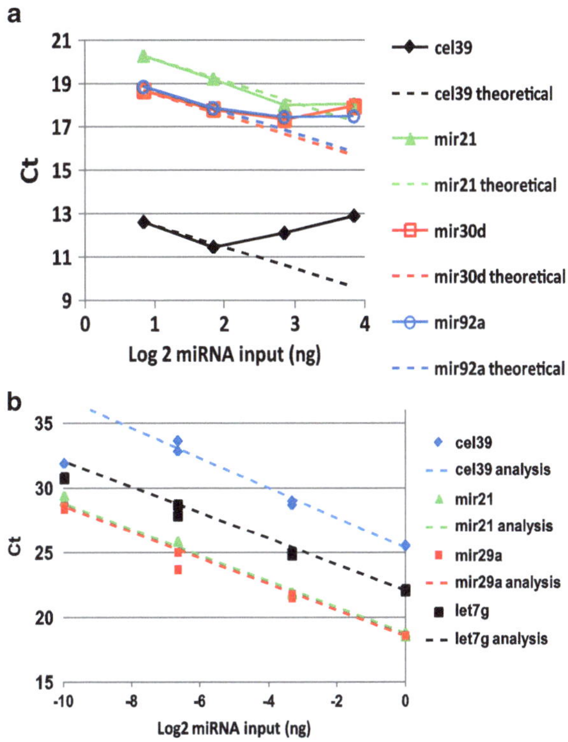

Fig. 3 Analysis of qPCR and RT performance using miScript RT. (**a**) Results from qPRC analysis of cDNAs generated in miScript RT reactions with varying inputs of RNA isolated from circulating exosomes deviate significantly from theoretical values. After we first demonstrated that analysis of serial dilutions of cDNA generated in a *single* RT reaction were linear with the expected efficiency (data not shown), we examined the performance of the RT reaction itself. QPCR analysis of a series of cDNAs generated in *separate* (1.8, 3.6, 7.2, and 14.4 ng RNA input) reactions showed that the amount of cDNA generated by RT reactions deviates from the theoretical values above input of 3.6 ng RNA for all of the miRNAs except mir21. Theoretical values were determined by using the relationship $Ct = mx + b$, where x is the log 2 of the RNA input and Ct is the result of the qPCR analysis. The slope m is equal to −1 (which would be expected if the RT and qPCR reactions were 100 % efficient). The y-intercept was calculated by substituting the experimental Ct values for the lowest miRNA input into the equation and solving for b; using these values the theoretical line was generated. (**b**) RT reaction of 0.001–1 ng miRNA is linear. Data points represent individual analyses of each cDNA for each miRNA transcript. *Lines* were generated by linear regression analysis of all of the data points for qPCR analysis of each miRNA

miRNAs except miR21 after an input of 3.6 ng (Fig. 3a). In other words, doubling the RNA input from 3.6 to 7.2 ng does not give the corresponding decrease in threshold cycle (Ct) of the qPCR reaction. This effect was most severe for the most abundant miRNA, the housekeeping miRNA Cel 39.

Table 1
Linear regression analysis of RT reactions of miRNA (0.001–1 ng input)

	R^2	Slope
cel39[a]	0.987089	-1.15821
mir21	0.996976	-1.07016
mir29a	0.982676	-0.97368
let7g	0.99290	-0.88975

[a]The result for the lowest input was omitted for the analysis of the cel39 data

These results suggest that either: (1) there is an inhibitor in the miRNA preparation that affected only the RT reaction or (2) that we were somehow exceeding the maximum capacity of the miScript reaction. Qiagen recommends a maximum input of 1 μg of total cellular RNA into their MiScript RT reaction. Total cellular RNA is composed largely of 18s and 28s ribosomal RNA, which are 2 and 5 kb in length, respectively. Small noncoding RNAs which we isolate in the circulation are in the size range of 14–36 bases in length. Using this information we estimate that one microgram of total cellular RNA has the same number of *molecules* as 3.7–10 ng of samples such as those we have prepared here, which are composed primarily of miRNAs. Thus, it is likely that in the experiment shown in Fig. 3a, the reactions with highest RNA input have exceeded the capacity of the MiScript reaction mixture. With this in mind, we then went on to define the optimal range of inputs for the MiScript reaction of RNA isolated using our protocol. We demonstrate the range of linear results for the RT reaction in Fig. 3b, where we decreased the amount of cel39 miRNA by 100-fold from that shown in Fig. 3a, and prepared serial dilutions (1, 0.1, 0.01, and 0.001 ng) of plasma-derived miRNA for use in 10 μL RT reactions. We then analyzed the cDNA products of the four reactions. We demonstrate that all points (except the lowest concentration of cel39) are in the linear range and the net efficiencies of the RT and qPCR reactions are very high (as reflected in the slope which should be −1.0 if both reactions are 100 % efficient, Table 1). These results highlight the remarkably high yield of miRNAs obtained using this protocol.

Acknowledgment

This work was supported by a subcontract with the NCI number N201143, the Tom C. Mathews Familial Melanoma Research Clinic, the Huntsman Cancer Foundation, and the Cancer Center Support Grant for the University of Utah 5P30CA042014-23.

References

1. Bartel DP (2009) MicroRNAs: target recognition and regulatory functions. Cell 136: 215–233
2. Bartel DP, Chen CZ (2004) Micromanagers of gene expression: the potentially widespread influence of metazoan microRNAs. Nat Rev Genet 5:396–400
3. Pillai RS (2005) MicroRNA function: multiple mechanisms for a tiny RNA? RNA 11: 1753–1761
4. Bushati N, Cohen SM (2007) microRNA functions. Annu Rev Cell Dev Biol 23:175–205
5. Sayed D, Abdellatif M (2011) MicroRNAs in development and disease. Physiol Rev 91: 827–887
6. Lee YS, Dutta A (2009) MicroRNAs in cancer. Annu Rev Pathol 4:199–227
7. Erson AE, Petty EM (2008) MicroRNAs in development and disease. Clin Genet 74: 296–306
8. Ruan K, Fang X, Ouyang G (2009) MicroRNAs: novel regulators in the hallmarks of human cancer. Cancer Lett 285:116–126
9. Calin GA, Croce CM (2006) MicroRNA signatures in human cancers. Nat Rev Cancer 6:857–866
10. Iorio MV, Croce CM (2012) MicroRNA dysregulation in cancer: diagnostics, monitoring and therapeutics. A comprehensive review. EMBO Mol Med 4:143–159
11. Kottel RH, Hoch SO, Parsons RG, Hoch JA (1978) Serum ribonuclease activity in cancer patients. Br J Cancer 38:280–286
12. Reid G, Kirschner MB, van Zandwijk N (2011) Circulating microRNAs: association with disease and potential use as biomarkers. Crit Rev Oncol Hematol 80:193–208
13. Friedman EB, Shang S, Vega-Saenz de Miera E, Fog JU, Teilum MW, Ma MW, Berman RS, Shapiro RL, Pavlick AC, Hernando E, Baker A, Shao Y, Osman I (2012) Serum microRNAs as biomarkers for recurrence in melanoma. J Transl Med 10:155
14. Cocucci E, Racchetti G, Meldolesi J (2009) Shedding microvesicles: artefacts no more. Trends Cell Biol 19:43–51
15. Meckes DG Jr, Raab-Traub N (2011) Microvesicles and viral infection. J Virol 85: 12844–12854
16. Mathivanan S, Fahner CJ, Reid GE, Simpson RJ (2012) ExoCarta 2012: database of exosomal proteins, RNA and lipids. Nucleic Acids Res 40:D1241–D1244
17. Taylor DD, Zacharias W, Gercel-Taylor C (2011) Exosome isolation for proteomic analyses and RNA profiling. Methods Mol Biol 728:235–246
18. Thery C, Amigorena S, Raposo G, Clayton A (2006) Isolation and characterization of exosomes from cell culture supernatants and biological fluids. Curr Protoc Cell Biol. Chapter 3, Unit 3. 22
19. Florell SR, Boucher KM, Garibotti G, Astle J, Kerber R, Mineau G, Wiggins C, Noyes RD, Tsodikov A, Cannon-Albright LA, Zone JJ, Samlowski WE, Leachman SA (2005) Population-based analysis of prognostic factors and survival in familial melanoma. J Clin Oncol 23:7168–7177
20. Pho L, Grossman D, Leachman SA (2006) Melanoma genetics: a review of genetic factors and clinical phenotypes in familial melanoma. Curr Opin Oncol 18:173–179
21. Livak KJ, Schmittgen TD (2001) Analysis of relative gene expression data using real-time quantitative PCR and the 2(−Delta Delta C(T)) Method. Methods 25:402–408
22. Pritchard CC, Kroh E, Wood B, Arroyo JD, Dougherty KJ, Miyaji MM, Tait JF, Tewari M (2012) Blood cell origin of circulating microRNAs: a cautionary note for cancer biomarker studies. Cancer Prev Res (Phila) 5:492–497
23. Mitchell PS, Parkin RK, Kroh EM, Fritz BR, Wyman SK, Pogosova-Agadjanyan EL, Peterson A, Noteboom J, O'Briant KC, Allen A, Lin DW, Urban N, Drescher CW, Knudsen BS, Stirewalt DL, Gentleman R, Vessella RL, Nelson PS, Martin DB, Tewari M (2008) Circulating microRNAs as stable blood-based markers for cancer detection. Proc Natl Acad Sci U S A 105:10513–10518

Chapter 35

Detection of Circulating Tumor Cells by Photoacoustic Flowmetry

Ryan M. Weight and John A. Viator

Abstract

Detection of circulating tumor cells (CTCs) in human blood and lymph systems has the potential to aid clinical decision making in the treatment of cancer (Cristofanilli et al. New Engl J Med 351:781–791, 2004; Check Cap Today 19:1.76–1.86, 2005; Braun and Naume J Clin Oncol 8:1623–1626, 2005). The presence of CTCs may signify the onset of metastasis, indicate relapse, or may be used to monitor disease progression. We built and tested a photoacoustic flowmetry system for detecting circulating melanoma cells (CMCs) by exploiting the broadband absorption spectrum of melanin within CMCs. The device was tested on cultured melanoma cells in saline suspension, melanoma cells spiked in human blood, and in a Stage IV melanoma patient. The device showed a detection threshold of a single pigmented melanoma cell from culture. Results show the potential to assay blood samples from healthy and metastatic patients for the presence of cancerous melanoma providing a method for cancer screening.

Key words Cancer detection, Laser-induced ultrasound, Melanoma, Photoacoustic, PBMC

1 Introduction

The use of photoacoustics, or laser-induced ultrasound, to detect CTCs in human blood samples presents a new approach to cancer diagnostics. Photoacoustics occurs when the optical energy of a photon is transduced into a mechanical disturbance, resulting in an acoustic wave [1–5]. The photoacoustic effect is obtained from *transient thermoelastic expansion*, in which laser energy is deposited into a confined region of matter such that rapid heating occurs followed by rapid expansion. This expansion causes a mechanical fluctuation in the medium manifested as an acoustic wave detectable by pressure sensors.

In order to create photoacoustic waves using thermoelastic expansion, the targeted CTC must have some intrinsic optical absorber. While most cells are colorless in the visible wavelengths of light, melanocytes produce melanin, a broadband optical absorber.

Magdalena Thurin and Francesco M. Marincola (eds.), *Molecular Diagnostics for Melanoma: Methods and Protocols*, Methods in Molecular Biology, vol. 1102, DOI 10.1007/978-1-62703-727-3_35, © Springer Science+Business Media New York 2014

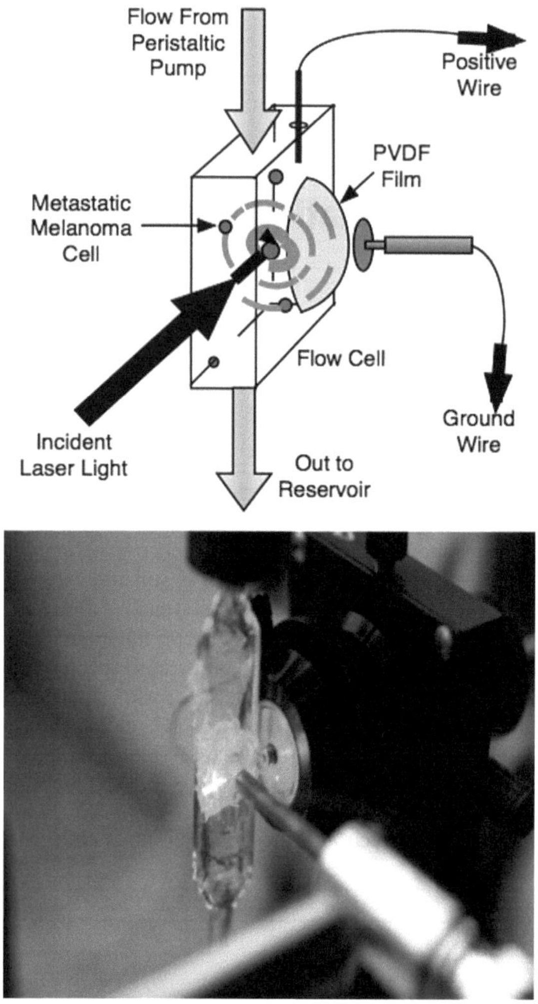

Fig. 1 Photoacoustic apparatus. (*Top*) Schematic of photoacoustic apparatus detecting human melanoma cells [8]. (*Bottom*) Photograph of photoacoustic device

Melanoma cells are derived from melanocytes with as many as 95 % of such cells containing melanin. Preliminary work in the photoacoustic detection of pigmented CTCs has proven successful, identifying small concentrations of cultured human melanoma cells in vitro using the endogenous absorption enabled by the melanosomes [5].

A depiction of the detection apparatus is given in Fig. 1. The schematic represents melanoma cells interacting with laser energy thus propagating a pressure wave. The *photoacoustic waveforms* generated by the presence of melanoma within suspension are detected using a piezoelectric copolymer film used to transduce mechanical acoustic energy to a voltage waveform.

2 Materials

2.1 Detection Apparatus

1. Spectrocell customized flow cell as described in Subheading 3.1, **step 1** (Oreland, PA).
2. 100 % silicone sealant (DAP, Inc., Baltimore, MD).
3. Masterflex L/S Economy Drive peristaltic pump (Cole-Parmer Instr., Vernon Hills, IL).
4. L/S 14 platinum-cured silicon tubing attached to each end of flow chamber and integrated into peristaltic pump. This tubing will serve to connect the reservoir to the flow chamber (Cole-Parmer Instr., Vernon Hills, IL).
5. Copper wire for positive lead (Consolidated, Inc., Franklin Park, IL).
6. Copper plate for negative lead/ground (Small Parts, Inc., Miami Lakes, FL).
7. Micro-coaxial cable (Microstock, Inc., West Point, PA).
8. 31-221-VP BNC connector (Jameco Electronics, Belmont, CA).
9. RG 58 coaxial cable (Pomona Electronics, Everett, WA).
10. Q-switched, frequency tripled Nd:YAG laser (Quantel, LES ULIS cedex, France) housed in a Vibrant Integrated Tunable Laser System (Opotek, Carlsbad, CA) (*see* **Note 3**).
11. Zap-It Laser Alignment Paper (Kentek Corp., Pittsfield, NH).

2.2 Acoustic Wave Detection and Data Acquisition

1. 100 μm polyvinylidene diflouride (PVDF) copolymer film (Ktech Corp., Albuquerque, NM).
2. SR445A 350 MHz Amplifier (Stanford Research Systems, Sunnyvale, CA).
3. TDS 2024 200 MHz Oscilloscope (Tektronix, Beaverton, OR) triggered by a Photodiode (Thorlabs, Newton, NJ).
4. Cylindrical lens (LJ1014L2-B, Thorlabs, Newton, NJ).
5. Two Plano-Convex lenses, 100 and 50 mm focal length (LA1509 and LA1131, Thorlabs, Newton, NJ).

2.3 Peripheral Blood Mononuclear Cell Layer Isolation

1. Histopaque 1077 (Sigma-Aldrich, Inc., St. Louis, MO) for cell separation.
2. Dulbeccos Phosphate-Buffered Saline (PBS) (Invitrogen Corp., Grand Island, NY) for cell washing (*see* **Note 4**).

3 Methods

3.1 Detection Apparatus

The detection apparatus encompasses the excitation chamber, acoustic detection mechanism, signal propagation, and the flow system.

1. The flow chamber is where laser excitation and acoustic wave propagation and detection occurs. The flow chamber is custom designed by Spectrocell and consists of a 1 mm × 10 mm horizontal aperture with a vertical height of 45 mm for a total fluid volume of 0.9 ml. The top and bottom of the flow chamber are tapered to cylindrical ports with an inner diameter of 2.7 mm and an outer diameter of 4.95 mm. These ports serve to connect the chamber to the pump tubing.
2. A cylindrical hole measuring 5 mm in diameter is cut into one side of the flow chamber where a piezoelectric film is affixed.
3. The piezoelectric film is employed as the acoustic wave detector. The film is cut to a diameter slightly larger than the 5 mm diameter aperture on the 10 mm side of the flow cell and is affixed to the outside of the flow cell using a small beaded ring of silicone applied using a syringe and 20 gauge needle.
4. Copper electrodes are used for both positive signal detection and grounding. The positive electrode is a stripped 0.6 mm diameter copper wire approximately 17 mm in length inserted directly under the PVDF film (Subheading 3.4, **step 4**). The electrode is sealed with 100 % silicon sealant. It extends the horizontal length of the flow cell and leaves an external lead.
5. The negative electrode, or ground, consists of a thin, 4 mm diameter copper plate soldered to a 3.5 mm diameter bare micro-coaxial cable that measures 13 mm in length. The cable is in turn soldered to a 31-221-VP BNC connector which connects to a grounded RG 58 coaxial cable. The BNC connector screws into a cut 50.8 mm diameter cast acrylic housing applying the flat copper plate flush against the external side of the PVDF film, thus providing a ground to one side of the piezoelectric film.
6. Pulsed laser light from a Q-switched, Nd:YAG laser at 420 nm and 5 ns pulse is focused into the 1 mm side of the flow chamber at a height equal to that of the detection aperture (Fig. 1).
7. The output beam should be focused to around 1 mm point that will pass through the center of the solute within the flow chamber. This can be accomplished using a cylindrical lens in series with two plano-convex lenses to collimate the beam.
8. The energy input into the system should range from 10.0 to 20.0 mJ after collimating the beam with an optimal radiant energy of 15 mJ.
9. Alignment and spot size should be measured using laser alignment paper set at the entry point of the beam into the flow chamber using a single 5 ns pulse (*see* **Notes 1–2**).

3.2 Acoustic Wave Detection and Data Acquisition

1. When pigmented cells are irradiated in a fluid medium, they become point sources of acoustic energy that propagate in all directions. So the effect of irradiating these cells in buffered saline is that of a compression wave or moving band of high pressure. When such an acoustic wave strikes a surface of the PVDF film, that copolymer layer is disturbed and consequently forms a charge on the conducting surface of the film. The exterior of the film is grounded by a copper plate electrode therefore conferring a positive charge to the interior surface of the PVDF film as shown in Fig. 2 (Top).
2. The transduced voltage sensed at the positive electrode immersed in saline solution is amplified by 125 times.
3. Voltage signals are displayed by an oscilloscope triggered by a photodiode upon each laser firing. Strong photoacoustic signals should resemble the waveform shown in Fig. 2 (Bottom).

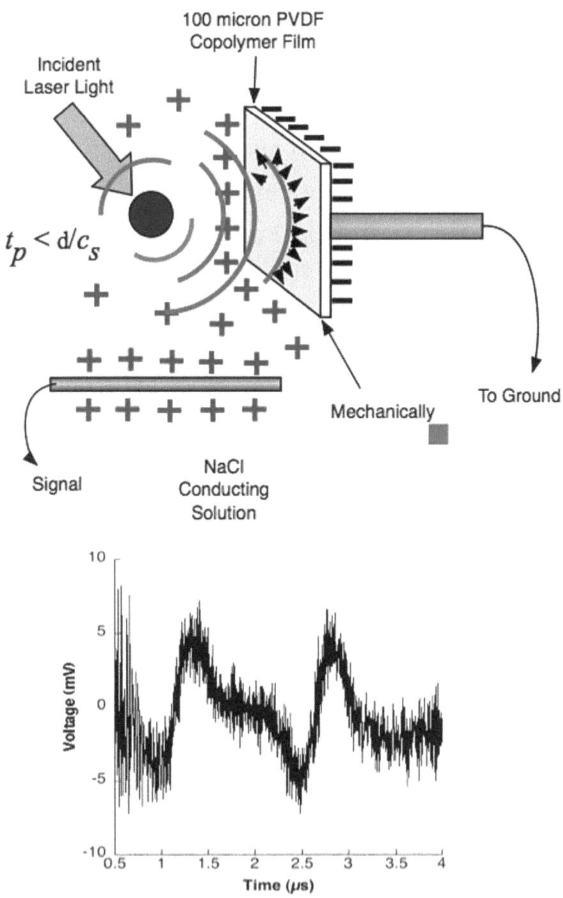

Fig. 2 (*Top*) Schematic showing the photoacoustic mechanism as it applies to this system. The figure represents the interior of detection chamber. Single chromophore excitation. Equation for pulse time noted. (*Bottom*) A typical Photoacoustic waveform is depicted

3.3 Peripheral Blood Mononuclear Cell Layer Isolation

1. Obtain whole sample of blood in pink top (ETDA) Vacutainer or 30 ml syringe with 1–2 ml of heparin. Be sure that blood is drawn slowly to avoid RBC lysis.
2. Place 3 ml of Histopaque 1077 in 15 ml conicals (or 15 ml Histopaque in 30 ml conicals).
3. Carefully and slowly layer 4–5 ml of blood onto Histopaque layer for 15 ml conical (30 ml of blood for 50 ml conical). Do not allow blood to break the surface of the Histopaque layer. This is very important!
4. Spin down samples in centrifuge at 300 × g for 30 min with no brake.
5. Carefully pipette off the peripheral blood mononuclear cell (PBMC) layer directly above the Histopaque layer using transfer pipette. Place the PBMCs into a new clean 15 or 50 ml conical. Refer to Fig. 3.
6. Fill the conicals containing pipetted PBMCs with PBS buffer until full. Mix well by inverting tubes multiple times or shaking gently.
7. Centrifuge the PBS/PBMC mixture at 200 × g for 10 min with no brake.
8. Carefully pipette off supernatant leaving cell pellet intact.
9. Add 2 ml of Promega Cell Lysis Solution to each 15 ml conical (6 ml for 50 ml conical) (*see* **Notes 5** and **6**).
10. Mix cell pellet evenly into solution using pipette.
11. Let solution sit for 10 min. Agitate solution at least once to assure proper RBC lysis.
12. Centrifuge at 150 × *g* for 8 min with no brake.
13. Pipette off supernatant leaving intact cell pellet.
14. Wash again with PBS solution in same manner as before.
15. Centrifuge at 150 × *g* for 8 min with no brake.

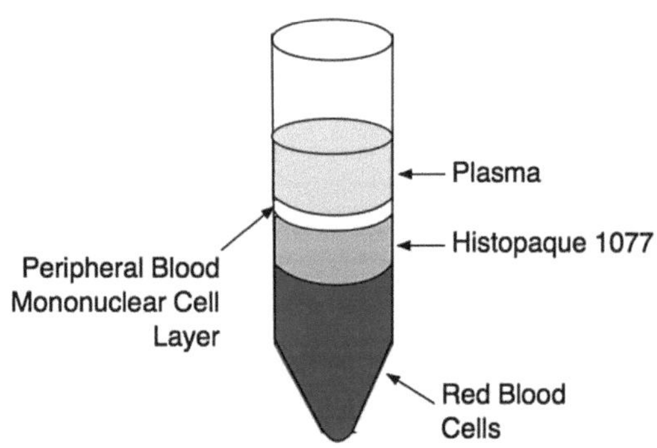

Fig. 3 Centrifuge gradient

16. Pipette off supernatant.
17. Resuspend cells in 1.8 % Saline. 5 ml of 1.8 % saline is a good volume. Choose volume based on number of cells per ml of desired solution.

3.4 Setup Preparation and Flow Cell Construction

1. Clean flow chamber with KOH bath. Rinse with DI water and dry with compressed Nitrogen.
2. Prepare 100 μm PVDF using razor blade. Cut a square sample and trim corners. Make just large enough to overlap detection aperture by about 0.5–1 mm.
3. Line cut out portion of flow chamber with silicone using 3 ml syringe and medium gauge needle. Lay positive wire so that bare end is in the detection aperture.
4. Place PVDF over wire and silicone. Be sure that the wire cladding remains within the PVDF circumference so that it does not short circuit the PVDF.
5. Reseal with additional silicone around wire lead.

3.5 Sample Processing Technique

1. Connect flow cell to tubing so that the system is run under negative pump pressure.
2. Tune the laser to an output of 18.25 mJ out of OPO at 450 nm.
3. Introduce sample to reservoir (*see* **Notes** 7 and **8**).
4. Lock flow cell into place and take sample. Ensure that circuit is closed by connecting "table" ground to external surface of coaxial cable at the point of positive lead connect.
5. Optimal flow rates are between 1 and 4 ml/min (*see* **Note 9**).
6. When finished with sample, drain flow chamber by emptying reservoir and inverting flow cell allowing solution to clear. Refer to Fig. 4 for overview of setup.

3.6 Cleaning Between Samples and Clearing System

1. Introduce saline solution to reservoir effectively filling the reservoir.
2. Release flow chamber and hold it upright (or induce vertical flow).
3. Set pump setting to 20 ml/min and allow entire solution to clear through system while flow chamber remains upright.
4. Allow air bubbles to wash flow chamber using solution remaining in flow chamber by keeping cell held upright. Tap the flow chamber if necessary to remove particles that may become settled in detection aperture.
5. Invert flow chamber to clear remaining solution entirely and cease flow.

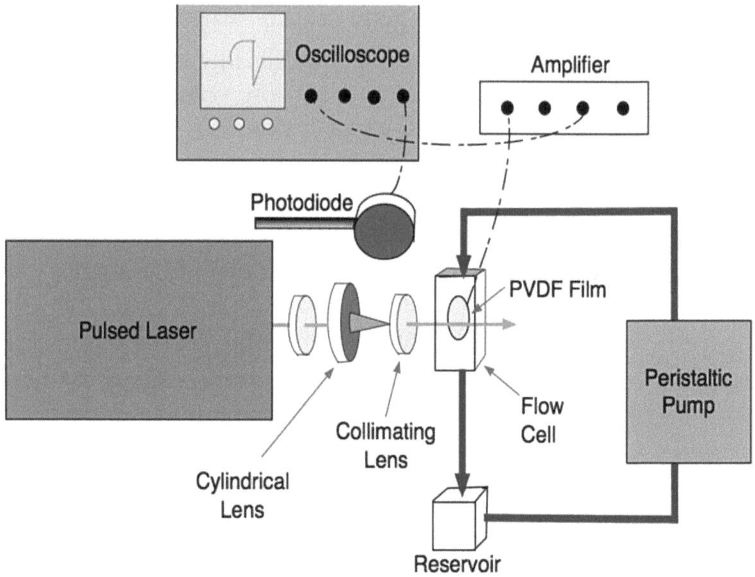

Fig. 4 Schematic of photoacoustic system for CTC detection

4 Notes

1. A tradeoff exists between radiant energy and sufficient radiant exposure. One must possess a radiant beam large enough to encompass the entire detection chamber, and thus all the cells, while providing enough energy for sufficient signal strength. The laser beam exiting the output port of the Vibrant takes the form of an ellipse. Ideally, the beam should be focused into the flow chamber as accurately as possible so that the beam profile takes on a circular shape of approximately 1 mm in diameter to cleanly enter the 1 mm wall of the flow chamber.
2. A substantial amount of focus must be placed on the alignment of the beam entering the flow chamber. Calibration is crucial to ensure that the beam captures the entire flow chamber and thus the entire specimen. Lenses need to be adjusted in holders that allow for translational manipulations on the order of microns. In addition the flow chamber should be clamped into the same position with each measurement by using notches, markings, or both. Care must be taken to secure the detection apparatus so that the beam enters the excitation field at the exact same point for each sample. This path should center in front of the PVDF film.
3. It is recommended that the laser is outfitted with an optical parametric oscillator which allows for the output of variable wavelengths ranging from 410 to 710 nm. These wavelengths may be tuned by the operator to maximize photoacoustic response.

4. Avoid PBS made from tablets as it will induce a PA response. Only use PBS from concentrated solution or made with individual components.
5. It is important to note when isolating the PBMCs, agranular and granular WBCs may be isolated using repeated washing with Promega Cell Lysis Solution without use of Histopaque. If Histopaque is used, only agranulocytes are obtained which decreases the pyro-electric effect or "white noise" created by excitation of nuclear material contained within cytoplasmic granules.
6. When washing cell block isolate Promega washes may be repeated indefinitely until no visual red blood cells remain. However, each additional wash reduces the resulting quantity of isolated PBMCs.
7. Fill flow cell by circulating solution at a flow rate of about 4 ml/min. Hold flow chamber upright to ensure proper and complete filling. If air bubbles become trapped in the aperture simply hold the flow chamber upright and apply a jostling force to dislodge the trapped air. Remember, air does not conduct a photoacoustic signal and must be removed from the system. Increasing the flow rate may help as well.
8. If flow chamber leaks, apply additional silicone to plug the leak. Make sure that the system is an entirely closed circuit and well grounded.
9. Lower flow rates reduce noise in the system and allow for cells to maintain excitation for longer periods of time at low concentrations. 1 ml/min will place a particle within the beam path for approximately 1.8–2.0 s.

Acknowledgments

We acknowledge the support of the Department of Biological Engineering and the Christopher S. Bond Life Sciences Center at the University of Missouri.

References

1. Viator JA, Jacques SL, Prahl SA (1999) Depth profiling of absorbing soft materials using photoacoustic methods. J Sel Top Quantum Electron 5:989–996
2. Viator J, Choi B, Ambrose M, Spanier J, Nelson J (2003) *In vivo* port wine stain depth determination using a photoacoustic probe. Appl Optics 42:3215–3224
3. Viator J, Komadina J, Svaasand L, Aguilar G, Choi B, Nelson J (2004) A comparative study of photoacoustic and reflectance methods for determination of epidermal melanin content. J Investig Dermatol 122:1432–1439
4. Viator J, Jacques S, (2005) Depth limitations for photoacoustic imaging of burn injury, *in vivo ASME Proceedings.*
5. Weight R, Dale P, Caldwell C, Lisle A, Viator J (2006) Photoacoustic detection of metastatic melanoma cells in the human circulatory system. Opt Lett 31:2998–3000

Part VII

Marker Validation Requirements for Clinical Applicability

Chapter 36

Statistical Design and Evaluation of Biomarker Studies

Kevin K. Dobbin

Abstract

We review biostatistical aspects of biomarker studies, including design and analysis issues, covering the range of settings required for translational research—from early exploratory studies through clinical trials.

Key words Translational research, Experimental design, Sample size, Power

1 Introduction

Biomarker development and validation is a long process involving many individual experiments and studies as steps along the way. The ultimate objective of that process should be used to guide it to a successful conclusion. Typically, the ultimate objective is to develop a biomarker that will be clinically useful for decision making. The marker has predictive or prognostic value, or can serve as a surrogate biomarker for a clinical outcome in phase III trials. This chapter focuses on biostatistical issues in the developmental process for prognostic and predictive biomarkers.

Table 1 shows a purely predictive and a purely prognostic marker, and a marker that is a mix of the two. For the prognostic marker, marker positive individuals have a 20 % better survival probability, regardless of treatment; for the predictive marker, marker positive individuals have a 40 % better survival probability under treatment, but the exact same survival probability under control; for the prognostic and predictive marker, survival for marker positive patients is 20 % greater under control, but 30 % greater under treatment—the treatment provides more of a survival boost for marker positive individuals. Examples of predictive biomarkers include biomarkers for response to anti-cytotoxic T-lymphocyte antigen 4 (CTLA-4) therapies, or response or resistance to BRAF-targeted therapies discussed in Part II of this volume. A review by Rothberg et al. [1] found promising prognostic tissue biomarkers

Magdalena Thurin and Francesco M. Marincola (eds.), *Molecular Diagnostics for Melanoma: Methods and Protocols*, Methods in Molecular Biology, vol. 1102, DOI 10.1007/978-1-62703-727-3_36, © Springer Science+Business Media New York 2014

Table 1
Survival percentages conceptual examples for different marker types

	Prognostic marker (%)		Predictive marker (%)		Prognostic and predictive (%)	
Treated	70	90	40	80	70	100
Control	40	60	40	40	40	60
	Marker –	Marker +	Marker –	Marker +	Marker –	Marker +

for early stage melanoma patients including melanoma cell adhesion molecule (MCAM)/MUC18, matrix metalloproteinase-2, Ki-67, proliferating cell nuclear antigen, and p16/INK4A.

Purely prognostic biomarkers run the danger of providing patients with predictions of a fate which cannot be altered. Their clinical utility is only realized if (1) there are multiple treatments alternatives available and (2) the prognostic signal is so strong that it offsets any potential survival disadvantage or toxic side effects. Many biomarker studies have focused on prognostic markers because they are the proverbial low hanging fruit—they are easier to study than predictive markers. But the potential utility of predictive markers is more straightforward. In general, a predictive marker is the more clinically useful type (*see*, e.g., ref. 2).

The ultimate clinical context should be clarified as soon as possible in the biomarker development process. Many biomarkers may be biologically interesting, but have no potential clinical utility. Attempts should arguably not be made to move these markers to the clinic until there is a use for them. Often, researchers want to know how good a biomarker has to perform to be clinically useful. There is no hard and fast biostatistical rule. The answer depends very much on the clinical context. A biomarker needs to be good enough to impact treatment decisions made by doctors and patients. These may be complex decisions involving drug toxicities, side effects, quality of life, and other factors.

Unfocused biomarker studies with no clear clinical objectives have plagued biomarker development [3]. Many biomarker studies in early developmental phases are carried out under uncontrolled conditions and reported in ways that make it difficult to assess the scientific evidence for their potential value. Often multiple exploratory comparisons are carried out, but only the most interesting finding reported. This inflates the nominal p-value. For example, if ten independent biomarkers were studied for their association with survival using a Cox model, then even if none are survival-related there is a greater than 65 % probability of a false positive at significance level 0.10, and greater than 40 % chance of a false positive at significance level 0.05. Thus, reporting the lowest p-value alone turns the idea of statistical significance on its head. Publication bias results when this phenomenon happens across several studies.

Surrogate biomarkers are traditionally defined as biomarkers that can be substituted in place of the primary endpoint in a phase III clinical trial [4]. Just as tumor shrinkage is often an adequate endpoint for a phase II study, but inadequate for a phase III study, so many biomarkers useful for phase II may have little hope of ever being a surrogate biomarker in a phase III study. Surrogacy requires both that the surrogate is predictive of the clinical outcome, and that the surrogate fully captures the effect an intervention under study may have on the clinical outcome (*see* refs. 5, 6). Statistically, this very difficult to prove [7], typically requiring meta-analysis of multiple studies in similar populations. Very few surrogate biomarkers for phase III research exist [8].

This chapter discusses design and analysis of biomarker studies, focusing on biostatistical issues, and is organized as follows. Subheading 2 discusses biomarker studies on specimens without accompanying clinical data. Subheading 3 addresses studies of stored specimens with accompanying clinical data. Subheading 4 discusses prospective studies.

2 Biomarker Studies on Cell Lines, Animals, and Stored Patient Samples Without Clinical Data

Cell lines and animal models are used in the early developmental stages of a biomarker. Because of the potential for both biological and assay performance changes when moving from cell lines and animals to human specimens, hypotheses generated from these studies require further validation. The biomarker may be more or less concentrated in human specimens, resulting in a stronger or weaker biological signal. Alternatively, the assay performance may differ by specimen type, resulting in higher or lower noise levels. Any statistical conclusions from cell lines and animal models remain tentative regarding clinical performance.

Stored patient samples lacking clinical outcome data can be useful to assess assay analytic performance using reference and calibration standards. Assay accuracy, precision, specificity, robustness, linearity, dynamic range, and timing can be assessed.

Stored samples without extensive clinical data can be used to validate a biomarker's reproducibility before its use in a clinical trial. When evaluating reproducibility in anticipation of a phase III clinical trial, the way in which the biomarker will be used in the trial is important. The National Cancer Institute has developed terminology which is useful for distinguishing among uses: integral, integrated, and correlative. An integral test is a test that must be performed for the trial to proceed; an example is a test to establish patient eligibility for the phase III trial. An integrated test is a preplanned test that is performed on patients during a trial, where the trial objective is to identify or validate the test for future use; an example is a prospective validation study of a predictive biomarker in a randomized clinical trial. Clinical Laboratory Improvement Amendments (CLIA) certification is required by federal agencies such as the Centers for Medicare and Medicaid Services. But CLIA certification is not enough to assure that the biomarker reproducibility is adequate for use as an integral or integrated marker. Further proof of the reproducibility may be required. Such reproducibility studies can be conducted on stored patient samples. Ideally, the samples will have enough information about processing, handling, and patient characteristics accompanying them to assure that they are representative of the patients to be included in the planned trial and of the specimens to be assayed.

The most common reproducibility measure for binary assays (i.e., assays with just two outcomes, such as responders vs. nonresponders to interferons) is Cohen's kappa. The most common reproducibility measure (e.g., ref. 9) for continuous assays (e.g., an assay that measures expression level of a gene) is the intraclass correlation coefficient (ICC). If we let variance between individuals be noted as σ_b^2, and measurement error variance by σ_e^2, then the ICC is defined as (*see*, e.g., ref. 10):

$$\mathrm{ICC} = \frac{\sigma_b^2}{\sigma_b^2 + \sigma_e^2} \quad (1)$$

For an ideally reproducible biomarker, all of the variation between individuals is attributable to biological variation, and none to measurement error. A perfectly reproducible biomarker assay has ICC = 1. Usually, the reproducibility is lower, such as in the 0.70–0.90 range. Assay reproducibility studies need to be large enough that the statistical conclusions from them are robust and can be generalized to a future phase III clinical trial. If a gold-standard exists against which the assay result can be compared, then the area under the receiver operating characteristic (ROC) curve, called the AUC, is often used. Figure 1 shows the confidence interval widths for Cohen's kappa and the ICC resulting from typical reproducibility studies. The figure shows that there is generally a lot of uncertainty for sample sizes less than 100. For example, if $n = 30$ patients are measured twice to assess reproducibility using the ICC, then the confidence interval width for an assay with true ICC 0.70 is expected to be 0.40; a 95 % interval might go from 0.52 to 0.92, for example. As a result, reproducibility studies near phase III clinical trial implementation can require large sample sizes, larger than intuition may suggest. If multiple laboratories or technicians are involved, then sample size requirements will increase even more.

The samples used for a reproducibility study should not represent a wider range of disease severity than is encountered in the clinic. For example, if the biomarker will be useful only for

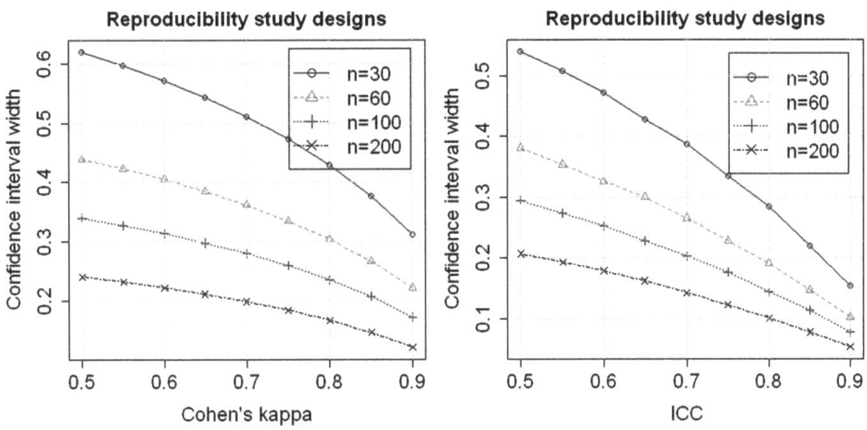

Fig. 1 Confidence interval (95 %) widths for reproducibility measures. Sample sizes of n = 30, 60, 100, and 200 biological specimens, with two replicate measurements per sample. *Left* is the expected confidence interval width for Cohen's Kappa statistic for a binary (i.e., two categories, such as good and poor prognosis) outcome. *Right* is the intraclass correlation coefficient for a continuous outcome. *Left* calculated using Shoukri (2004, p. 96) and *right* using Monte Carlo simulation and an exact confidence interval procedure (Burdick et al., 2005)

making clinical decisions about patients with Stage I melanoma, then no higher stages should be included in the reproducibility study; similarly, if the eligibility criteria for the study require patients with stage III melanoma, no lower or higher stages should be included. Including a wider range of stages will be expected to increase the biological variation among the samples. In Eq. 1 above, this would mean artificially inflating the σ_b^2 term. This will bias the ICC estimate towards one—making the reproducibility look better than it really is. The result can be a very biased and deceptive reproducibility measurement that will not hold up in the planned clinical trial.

3 Retrospective Studies on Stored, Clinically Annotated Samples

Banked, clinically annotated specimens can potentially be a very valuable resource for biomarker development and validation. But in order to realize this potential they must meet many criteria. The target population must be represented in a reasonably unbiased way. The therapeutic treatments received by patients must be similar to the therapeutic treatments currently under study. If the study involves validation of a predictive biomarker, then the samples must be from a randomized study of the therapy response being predicted; as shown in Table 1, a randomized study is needed to estimate the relationship between biomarker and outcome in both treated and untreated patients. In addition to the specimens being of high quality, and processing and storage being properly performed, the documentation accompanying the specimens needs to be high quality. The level of quality required is not achieved by simple careful data entry from medical records; in general, there must be a thorough quality control process in place, a common data elements (CDE) dictionary, a manual of operations (MOO), and documented regular reviews of the database for quality and concordance. These are the types of quality control processes commonly found in industrial plants, but unfortunately very uncommon in banked tumor samples. The exception may be clinical trials specimen banks.

Any study utilizing banked, clinically annotated specimens should either be a validation study of an existing biomarker, or have a careful statistical validation as part of the experimental design and analysis plan. In particular, all technical issues with instrumentation, reagents, quantitation, etc. should have been definitively settled before this point. If these issues have not been settled, then the resulting assay may be a house of cards that quickly falls apart, thus wasting precious patient material.

The validation phase of biomarker development should be seen as a sharp break from any previous assay development phases. It is easy for assay developers to not appreciate the importance of this break and to inadvertently introduce bias into the study by continuing to "tweak" the assay. There should be a mechanism for preventing this from happening. A validation study of a biomarker requires that all aspects of the biomarker assay be "nailed down" a priori, and that none be "tuned" to the new dataset. In particular, any cutpoints should be predefined and not developed from the data collected. The data should additionally be blinded, so that those producing the biomarker assay measurements do not have access to data on the clinical endpoint which is being used to assess the marker. One way to ensure this blinding is to enlist an honest broker who is the only one with access to the codes that link the clinical data to the individual specimens. The two are only joined when the assay measurements have been submitted.

The purpose of a biomarker validation study is to assess the marker's association with the clinical endpoint of interest. The clinical endpoint serves as the (best available) gold standard against which to judge the marker's performance. Because this step of the biomarker development is near clinical implementation, the study should be designed to provide accurate and unbiased estimates of positive predictive value, negative predictive value, sensitivity, and specificity. A receiver operating characteristic curve may also be useful as a descriptive graph, but because it does not take prevalence into account can potentially be misleading if there is imbalance between the classes or outcome groups.

Sometimes, it is not feasible to have a pure validation study. For example, particularly with a complex biomarker combining multiple biological features together, such as a gene expression signature, previous studies may have been relatively small so that the signature could undergo significant improvement with a larger sample size. In this case, statistical resampling methods can be used to produce unbiased estimates of biomarker performance. But implementing these methods requires a Ph.D.-trained Statistician or Biostatistician because there is a great risk of inadvertently introducing bias into the data analysis. The results from such a study will need further validation.

Simon et al. [11] suggest that the level of evidence from a set of well-designed studies of stored samples with clinical outcome data can rise to a level nearly equivalent the level of a gold-standard prospective clinical trial. An example cited there is the finding that patients with advanced colorectal cancers whose tumors exhibit K-RAS mutations do not benefit from monoclonal antibodies directed against epidermal growth factor receptor [12, 13]. If widely accepted, this "prospective-retrospective" approach could greatly speed up the translation of new biomarkers into clinical use. This validation approach requires very high quality data and tightly controlled processes such as are usually only found in the context of clinical trial specimens.

It is critical in biomarker studies to establish that the biomarker is adding evidence to already existing prognostic factors. Statistical methods for evaluating this are based on multivariate analyses that include the biomarker and other prognostic factors. But such multivariate analyses are often unrealistic because they include patients whose range of prognoses is far outside the actual range in which the biomarker information would be likely to have an impact. A preferable approach is to restrict the selection criteria for patients used in the biomarker study to only those who are close enough to clinical equipoise that the marker information would be used. This thinking should produce more homogeneous patient sets for biomarker studies. Homogeneous patient sets are much better than heterogeneous patient sets because trends seen in heterogeneous multivariate analyses may not hold up in the clinically relevant subgroup. Hence, multivariate analyses are no substitute for a homogeneous patient cohort.

4 Clinical Trials

Biomarkers for safety or efficacy can be useful in phase I and II clinical trials [14, 15]. In phase I studies, a biomarker may be used to make critical dose-escalation decisions or to make preliminary tentative assessments of efficacy. In phase II studies, the biomarker may be used as a critical enrollment criterion for the trial. For example, a study of T cell therapies may use biomarkers to restrict to a subpopulation likely to benefit from the intervention. Alternatively, in phase II studies biomarkers can be used for more tentative pharmacodynamic or pharmacokinetic assessments.

The level of statistical evidence required for an integral biomarker being used in a critical way should be higher than for a biomarker that is being used in a secondary correlative analysis.

Biomarkers can be incorporated into a phase III trial protocol. Biomarker studies using stored patient samples from a phase III trial are treated above in Subheading 3. The statistical issues with correlative biomarker studies incorporated into a protocol are similar to the use of banked clinical trial specimens discussed in Subheading 3 above. But there is a logistical problem with correlative studies in protocols. Biotechnology is changing very rapidly, but a phase III trial typically takes several years to complete; the chances that technology may improve in that timeframe, or that another more promising technology or biomarker will emerge, are fairly high. Thus there is a big timing problem with these types of studies. It is likely that the question addressed by the biomarker study will be a moot one by the time the clinical trial data is analyzed. Often, a viable alternative is to bank specimens for later study during the trial, so that if a better marker is developed between the trial start and the analysis time, it can be used instead.

Now we turn to phase III trial designs. First we discuss stratified designs. A stratified design is shown in Fig. 2. In a stratified design, the biomarker is measured for all patients. Patients are stratified into typically two groups by biomarker status, and each group is randomized to the treatment or control arm. The advantage of this design is that it enables one to evaluate both the predictive and prognostic value of the biomarker. Freidlin et al. [16] give several examples of this type of design being used in cancer trials. An important advantage of this design is that it can be viewed as ethical even if the biomarker is completely useless, because no treatment decisions are being made based on biomarker status. All decisions are made randomly. From the patient's and doctor's perspective, the trial is identical to any randomized study. Hence if the biomarker's value is in doubt, this design may be preferred. Some disadvantages of this design are that it may require a large sample size, may be expensive to evaluate all individuals for marker status, and measuring the biomarker up front may be logistically difficult. This last point can be ameliorated by recognizing that randomization can precede biomarker measurement, and subsequently a stratified analysis is performed using marker status as the stratification factor. This approach could be troublesome if problems arose in the assay, such as a significant proportion of patients for whom biomarker status could not be assessed, or if the lag-time between registration and assaying created analytic issues.

Enrichment designs use the biomarker in order to select patients. Typically, the subgroup selected is the one for which there is clinical equipoise. The subgroup or subgroups not selected are those who are thought to be unlikely to benefit from the intervention, and/or those who are thought will almost surely benefit from

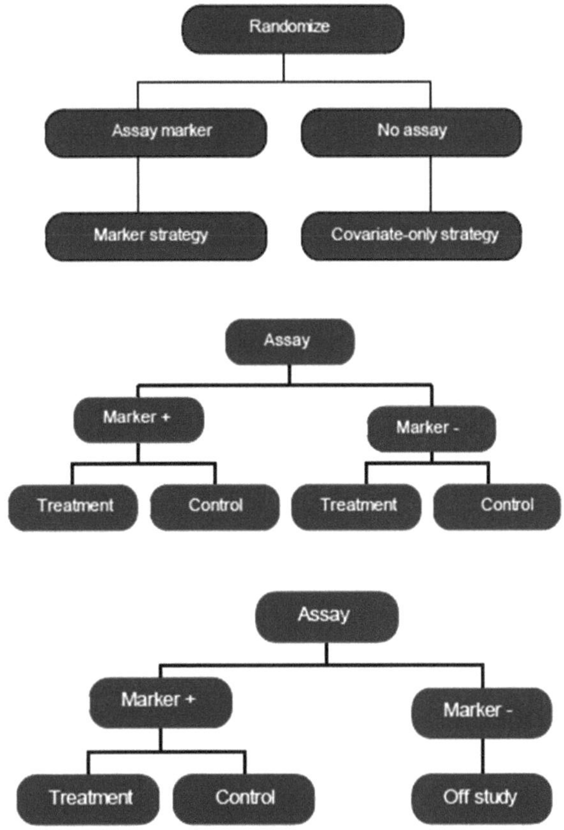

Fig. 2 Phase III biomarker trial design. Marker strategy design, marker stratified design, and enrichment design (*top to bottom*)

the intervention. Examples include the use of HER2 to select patients likely to respond to Herceptin therapy [17], and the middle range of OncotypeDX scores to select patients whose probability of benefiting from adjuvant chemotherapy is uncertain [18].

A marker strategy design is also shown in Fig. 2. In this design, patients are randomized to have their treatment guided by either standard clinical covariates only or by a biomarker-based strategy that may include standard clinical covariates. This design reduces assay cost compared to the stratified design because the biomarker only needs to be measured in half of the patients—namely, those randomized to the biomarker-strategy arm. A statistical problem with this design is that, because one is comparing strategies, rather than treatments, there will be some patients who would receive the same treatment in the biomarker-strategy arm as they would have received in the clinical-covariates-only arm. If the "Identical guidance" group is large in Fig. 3, then the biomarker-guided therapy is a minor modification on the existing covariate-only-guided therapy and is probably not useful. But there may be a relatively small subgroup of patients for whom the biomarker-guided therapy is

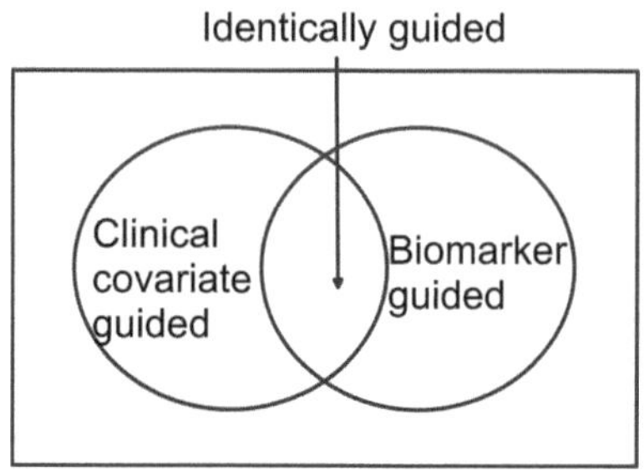

Fig. 3 Biomarker-strategy design

preferable. There will be very small power to identify the effect in this subgroup. For example, if the two therapy recommendations agree 80 % of the time, then the sample size in the subgroup the two differ on is $n/5$. If the trial enrolled 1,000 patients, there would only be 200 to detect the difference between the treatment strategies in the relevant subgroup. A way around this is the modified marker strategy design (e.g., ref. 2), which only randomizes patients for whom the biomarker-guided therapy decision differs from the clinical-covariates-only-guided therapy decision. This design is being used in the MINDACT trial in Europe [19]. Advantages of this approach are that it gives information both on which subset of patients will benefit from the biomarker measurement (if any), as well as on the size of the benefit, and that not all patients need to be randomized. Disadvantages are that the biomarker must be measured on all patients, and that the clinical-covariates-only-guided therapy strategy must be widely accepted and relatively static.

Acknowledgment

This work was supported by the Distinguished Cancer Scholars grant program of the Georgia Research Alliance.

References

1. Rothberg BEG, Bracken MB, Rimm DL (2009) Tissue biomarkers for prognosis in cutaneous melanoma: a systematic review and meta-analysis. J Natl Cancer Inst 101:452–474
2. Simon R (2010) Clinical trial designs evaluating the medical utility of prognostic and predictive biomarkers in oncology. Per Med 7:33–47
3. McShane LM, Altman DG, Sauerbrei W, Taube SE, Gion M, Clark GM (2005) Reporting recommendations for tumor marker prognostic studies (REMARK). J Natl Cancer Inst 97:1180–1184
4. Prentice RL (1989) Surrogate endpoints in clinical trials: discussion, definition and operational criteria. Stat Med 8(4):431–440
5. Friedman LM, Furberg CD, DeMets DL (2010) Fundamentals of clinical trials, 4th edn. Springer, New York
6. Cook TD, DeMets DL (2008) Introduction to statistical methods for clinical trials. Chapman and Hall, New York
7. Fleming TR, DeMets DL (1996) Surrogate end points in clinical trials: are we being misled? Fleming TR and DeMets DL. Ann Intern Med 125(7):605–613

8. Buyse M, Sargent DJ, Grothey A, Matheson A, de Gramont A (2010) Biomarkers and surrogate end points: the challenge of statistical validation. Nat Rev Clin Oncol 7:309–317
9. Dobbin KK, Beer DG, Meyerson M, Yeatman TJ, Gerald WL, Jacobson JW, Conley B, Buetow KH, Heiskanen M, Simon RM, Minna JD, Girard L, Misek DE, Taylor JMG, Hanash S, Naoki K, Hayes DN, Ladd-Acosta C, Enkemann SA, Viale A, Giordano TJ (2005) Interlaboratory comparability study of cancer gene expression analysis using oligonucleotide microarrays. Clin Cancer Res 11:565–572
10. Shoukri MM (2004) Measures of interobserver agreement. Chapman and Hall, Boca Raton
11. Simon RM, Paik S, Hayes DF (2009) Use of archived specimens to evaluate prognostic and predictive biomarkers. J Natl Cancer Inst USA 101(21):1446–1452
12. Amado RG, Wolf M, Peeters M, Van Cutsem E, Siena S, Freeman DJ, Juan T, Sikorski R, Suggs S, Radinsky R, Patterson SD, Chang DD (2008) Wild-type KRAS is required for panitumumab efficacy in patients with metastatic colorectal cancer. J Clin Oncol 26:1626–1634
13. Karapetis CD, Khambata-Ford S, Jonker DJ, O'Callaghan CJ, Tu D, Tebbutt NC, Simes RJ, Chalchal H, Shapiro JD, Robitaille S, Price TJ, Shepherd L, Au HJ, Langer C, Moore MJ, Zalcberg JR (2008) K-RAS mutations and benefit from cetuximab in advanced colorectal cancer. N Engl J Med 359:1757–1765
14. Dancey JE, Dobbin KK, Groshen S, Jessup JM, Hruszkewicz AH, Koehler M, Parchment R, Ratain MJ, Shankar LK, Stadler WM, True LD, Gravell A, Grever MR, Biomarkers Task Force of the NCI Investigational Drug Steering Committee (2010) Guidelines for the development and incorporation of biomarker studies in early clinical trials of novel agents. Clin Cancer Res 16(6):1745–1755
15. McShane LM, Hunsberger S, Adjei AA (2009) Effective incorporation of biomarkers in phase II trials. Clin Cancer Res 15(6):1898–1905
16. Freidlin B, McShane LM, Korn EL (2009) Randomized clinical trials with biomarkers: design issues. J Natl Cancer Inst 102:152–160
17. Vogel CL, Cobleigh MA, Tripathy D, Gutheil JC, Harris LN, Fehrenbacher L, Slamon DJ, Murphy M, Novotny WF, Burchmore M, Shak S, Stewart SJ, Press M (2002) Efficacy and safety of trastuzumumab as a single agent in first-line treatment of HER2-overexpressing metastatic breast cancer. J Clin Oncol 20(3): 716–726
18. Sparano JA (2006) TAILORx: trial assigning individualized options for treatment (Rx). Clin Breast Cancer 7(4):347–350
19. Cardoso F, Van't Veer L, Rutgers E, Loi S, Mook S, Piccart-Gebhart MJ (2008) Clinical application of the 70-gene profile: the MINDACT trial. J Clin Oncol 26(5): 729–735

Chapter 37

Tissue Resources for Clinical Use and Marker Studies in Melanoma

Jonathan L. Curry, Michael A. Davies, Tiffany L. Calderone, Katherine Nathanson, Victor G. Prieto, and Jeffrey E. Gershenwald

Abstract

The adequate procurement and preservation of high-quality tissue specimens from patients with melanoma is a critical clinical issue as patients' tumor samples are now used not only for pathological diagnosis but are also necessary to determine the molecular signature of the tumor to stratify patients who may benefit from targeted melanoma therapy. Tissue resources available for physicians and investigators include formalin-fixed paraffin-embedded (FFPE) tissue and frozen tissue, either preserved in optimal cutting temperature (OCT) media or snap frozen. Properly preserved tissue may be used to evaluate melanoma biomarkers by immunohistochemistry (IHC) with tissue microarray (TMA) technology, to perform genetic and genomic analyses, and for other types of translational research in melanoma.

Key words Frozen section, Prognostic markers, Therapy targets, Eligibility criteria, Tissue preservation, Tissue microarray analysis

1 Introduction

Recent insights into the genetic aberrations and other molecular underpinnings of melanoma, in addition to an improved understanding of the role of the immune system, have ushered in a new and exciting era of rapidly evolving targeted [1, 2] and immune-based treatments for this disease. The use of tissue in contemporary translational melanoma investigation is essential to identify biomarkers that improve treatments and personalize the management of patients [3]. Examples of overarching themes in this arena include tissue-based research initiatives that: (1) enhance prognostic assessment, (2) predict response to a specific therapy, (3) predict resistance to a specific therapy, or (4) elucidate mechanisms of resistance—all of which are critical to improve treatments for patients with melanoma. In this chapter, we focus our attention on the tissue resources that may be employed for such efforts.

Magdalena Thurin and Francesco M. Marincola (eds.), *Molecular Diagnostics for Melanoma: Methods and Protocols*, Methods in Molecular Biology, vol. 1102, DOI 10.1007/978-1-62703-727-3_37, © Springer Science+Business Media New York 2014

1.1 Use of Tissue in the Era of Targeted Therapy in Melanoma

Focused profiling has demonstrated that oncogenic driver mutations in *BRAF* and *NRAS* are present in ~70 % of patients with cutaneous melanoma, while other genetic events have been identified in other melanoma subtypes (i.e., *KIT*, *GNαQ*, and *GNα11*). Vemurafenib, a small molecule inhibitor that potently and selectively inhibits the most common mutation that occurs in melanoma (BRAF V600E), improved clinical responses rates, progression-free survival, and overall survival compared to chemotherapy in a randomized phase III clinical trial of metastatic melanoma patients whose tumors harbored this mutation [4]. On the other hand, vemurafenib, and other mutant-selective BRAF inhibitors (i.e., dabrafenib), appear to cause increased growth of melanomas that do not have activating *BRAF* mutations [5–7]. Thus, the currently approved use of vemurafenib is limited to patients with mutations that result in amino acid substitutions at the V600 residue of the BRAF protein. As a result of these findings, as well as the demonstration of activity of other targeted therapies in molecularly defined subpopulations (e.g., imatinib in metastatic melanoma patients with *KIT* mutations), molecular testing is becoming part of the standard evaluation for any patient with metastatic disease, as well as in patients with unresectable, clinically localized disease [8]. As molecular testing rapidly evolves from testing of single genes to panel-based testing using massively parallel sequencing, the need for high-quality tissue specimens has become a critical clinical issue. Molecular testing platforms vary significantly in their sensitivity for mutation detection; thus, characterization of specimens being analyzed (i.e., percent tumor cells, presence of necrosis, amount of melanin pigment) is critical to the interpretation of testing results. The type of specimens collected, and the amount of DNA and/or RNA isolated from them, is crucial to determine what types of molecular testing can be done, based on the requirements of the different testing platforms.

In addition to clinical testing implications, the development of the BRAF inhibitors has demonstrated in multiple ways the essential role played by tissue-based research. Although there are multiple examples demonstrating the critical nature of pretreatment molecular testing for patient selection, generally less attention is paid to the pharmacodynamic effects of agents. However, in the initial study of imatinib in patients with metastatic melanoma, biopsies were taken both pretreatment and again 2 weeks later. This study demonstrated a direct effect of imatinib on the pattern of expression of five known imatinib targets: ABL, BCR-ABL, KIT, and PDGF receptors alpha and beta [9]. The viable tumor in the posttreatment biopsies showed a marked decrease in the percentage and intensity of expression of the targets, thus suggesting that the "sensitive" melanoma cells were killed by the therapy, whereas the "resistant" cells were able to survive, similar to the effects of antibiotics on bacteria. In a more recent study, a phase I trial of vemurafenib, a cohort of 15 patients also agreed to allow tumor biopsies to be performed both pretreatment and after approximately 1–2 weeks of therapy. The specimens were analyzed for the expression of phosphorylated (active) ERK (P-ERK), a downstream effector of the BRAF-MEK-ERK pathway that vemurafenib is designed to inhibit. This analysis demonstrated a nearly linear relationship in these patients between the degree of P-ERK inhibition that was achieved with vemurafenib treatment, and the degree of tumor shrinkage that was achieved clinically [10]. Thus, this analysis demonstrated not only the importance of selecting the correct patients, but also that the dose of medication that the patients received and that reached the tumor was critical to the antitumor activity, which has significant implications for the management and adjustment of dosing in patients.

Although vemurafenib and other structurally unrelated V600 mutant-selective BRAF inhibitors achieve clinical responses in ~50 % of patients, the duration of these responses can be quite transient, lasting on average 5–6 months [4, 11]. A growing number of studies have been reported describing the molecular changes that are detected in samples of tumor tissue at the time of disease progression. Although there is no universal agreement, these studies have reported that many of the progressing lesions demonstrate reactivation of the BRAF-MEK-ERK pathway, as exemplified by recovery of P-ERK expression [12, 13]. Tissue-based analyses have demonstrated multiple mechanisms by which this reactivation can occur, including alternative splicing of *BRAF*, copy-number gain of *BRAF*, and acquired mutations in *NRAS* or *MEK1* [14–17]. Laboratory experiments performed on cell lines established from these progressing lesions demonstrated that the resistance to the selective BRAF inhibitors was maintained in vitro, allowing for functional testing of various strategies to overcome this resistance. One strategy that emerged from these studies was to combine a selective BRAF inhibitor with an MEK inhibitor. A randomized phase II study has now demonstrated that combined treatment with trametinib (an MEK inhibitor) and dabrafenib (a BRAF inhibitor) compared to treatment with dabrafenib alone in BRAF-mutant melanoma patients who have not previously been treated with a BRAF inhibitor results in significant improvements in clinical response rate (76 vs. 54 %), progression-free survival (median 9.4 vs. 5.8 months), and the duration of clinical responses (median 10.5 vs. 5.6 months) [18]. This combination also achieved clinical responses in ~20 % of patients who had previously developed disease progression on selective BRAF inhibitors [19]. Analyses of patient-derived specimens are ongoing to better understand the heterogeneity of the responses to this combination regimen and to characterize resistance mechanisms in order to develop other rational therapeutic approaches [2, 20].

In summary, the development of the BRAF inhibitors demonstrates the marked and rapid clinical impact that tissue-based research can have on patient care and outcomes. As the pattern of metastases in melanoma often allows for repeated biopsies to be performed safely, there is a tremendous opportunity to use tissue-based research approaches to rapidly develop rational, more effective treatments for patients. However, the types and quality of the research that can be performed critically depend upon the amount and quality of the tissue samples that are obtained for research. The amount of DNA needed for genetic and genomic analyses can vary widely depending on the type. Additional DNA always is needed beyond the amount for the actual technique for quality control purposes, so it is crucial to account for that extra amount in any planned investigation. It also is important to recognize that although technologies, such as Ion Torrent (Life Technologies™), can be used to perform massively parallel sequencing on as little as 10 ng of DNA, they can be particularly error-prone when using low quantities of DNA. The data obtained from massively parallel sequencing are more reliable with large amounts of DNA, usually 250–500 ng. For techniques such as array-based comparative genomic hybridization or whole exome sequencing, 1 μg (1,000 ng) of DNA is generally needed. Massively parallel sequencing has the advantage that it is more sensitive than other techniques, generally requiring approximately 20 % tumor to detect mutations, so that macrodissection may not need to be done, depending on specific tumor architecture. Such endeavors therefore require careful planning before tissue specimens are collected to ensure that the methods used will yield analytes that are both sufficient and appropriate for the planned analyses. Considerations include the sensitivity of the analytical platform to determine the level of tumor purity that will be required, as well as the amount of material needed for different assays. Thus, translational research using tissue specimens critically depends upon close communication and collaboration between scientists and physicians to maximize opportunities to advance our understanding of melanoma tumor biology and care of patients [2, 20].

1.2 Fresh Frozen Tissue for Clinical Use

Tissue samples, both tumor and normal, may be obtained in various ways: fine needle aspiration (FNA), image-guided core needle biopsy, punch biopsy, skin ellipse, and other surgical excision specimens. It should be stressed that core biopsy—whether collected as freshly frozen or FFPE—is superior to fine needle aspiration (FNA), since it usually provides more tissue for analysis (*see* **Notes 1** and **2**) [21]. FNAs can be used for targeted mutation analysis, specifically *BRAF* V600E mutations, but are currently not particularly useful for larger research studies. Preferred sizes for punch biopsies of cutaneous and subcutaneous lesions are 4–6 mm when feasible. A single punch biopsy, skin ellipse, or other surgical excision specimen-containing high-quality tumor is generally sufficient for most targeted research purposes at a single point in time.

Of great importance is the establishment of standard operating procedures (SOPs) to optimally archive biospecimens for research use, a principal goal of which is to maximize tissue preservation for contemporary or possible future molecular-based translational studies that include extraction of DNA, RNA, and protein (the latter of which is particularly important for assessment of phosphoprotein expression and cell-signal pathways). Strategies to collect and archive FFPE tissue are well documented elsewhere [22, 23]. FFPE tissue, although generally the most widely collected and most commonly employed for clinical DNA-based mutational testing, will not be further discussed since it is such a common fixture in all CLIA (Clinical Laboratory Improvement Amendments) certified clinical pathology laboratories.

Optimal Cutting Temperature (OCT) compound is especially useful for embedding frozen tissue, and since the tissue is *not* fixed in formalin when this procedure is used, it improves RNA and DNA recovery and quality. A key advantage of the OCT approach is that it facilitates histological evaluation of all samples prior to molecular analyte preparation. A frozen section H&E obtained from an OCT-embedded specimen, albeit of lesser quality than that from permanent (i.e., FFPE) H&E sections, enables histological assessment pertaining to the presence, quality and quantity of tumor. This consideration is particularly important since fibrosis, necrosis, hemorrhage, melanin pigmentation, and significant lymphocytic infiltrate can all "contaminate" melanoma tumor specimens and may adversely impact the yield and quality of analytes (e.g., secondary to fibrosis, necrosis, hemorrhage) or the extent to which the expression profiles are related to the tumor (e.g., from heavy lymphocytic infiltrates or melanin pigmentation). OCT also prevents tissue from desiccation and crumbling, acts as an insulator from thermal change and limits ice crystal formation (*see* **Note 3**). If tissue samples are obtained by core (punch or needle) biopsies, each core should be embedded in OCT as separate blocks.

Controlled snap freezing (in isopentane (2-methylbutane) prechilled in liquid nitrogen) is a viable alternative when OCT processing is not feasible, and is a preferred approach by some investigators. During surgery, fresh tissue may be acquired by the transfer of the surgical specimen from the operating room to the pathology department in a tumor container *without* formalin fixative. Once it arrives in the pathology department, the tissue specimen may be sectioned (tissue cores may also be obtained with a punch biopsy instrument) and snap frozen; this processing should be performed as a coordinated effort with the clinical/research pathology team so that diagnostic material is not compromised. Alternatively, this process can also sometimes be coordinated so that it is performed in the operating room once the specimen has been removed, which may achieve further reduction in ischemic time. If necessary, to obtain H&E sections of the specimen, it is possible to later transfer the frozen tissue to OCT without thawing the tissue and then obtain frozen sections.

Fresh-tissue samples should be frozen as soon as possible. If they cannot be frozen immediately, the tissue should be refrigerated and frozen as soon as possible. Time is critical as the longer a specimen is at room temperature the greater the opportunity for RNAses and proteases to degrade their respective macromolecules, especially important if the downstream application will depend on RNA or proteins. RNA integrity is reduced in direct proportion to delayed tissue processing in freshly harvested tissues [24]. Ischemia time affects the expression of proteins, which is more enhanced at room temperature and mainly leads to a decrease of signal intensity of a resected specimen [25]. Snap-frozen tissue samples should be transferred to either liquid nitrogen (preferred) or to a −80 °C freezer. Tissue samples processed in OCT should be transferred as soon as possible to a −80 °C freezer. Frozen tissue samples should be transported on dry ice in a closed but non-sealed Styrofoam or other ultralow temperature container (*see* **Note 4**). Frozen tissue samples should be securely stored long-term either in liquid nitrogen or in at −80 °C or colder. If future uses of the tissue are unknown, storing the tissue in the vapor phase of liquid nitrogen will help to ensure long-term viability. Storage equipment may include: small (2″ × 3″) plastic, zip-top bags; mega-cassettes (for example, with each tissue or cryomold wrapped in aluminum foil); cryoboxes; and plastic or metal storage freezer racks (e.g., for cryovial and cryomold storage). The freezer should be on an electrical emergency power line and be alarmed and centrally monitored. We use both a digital (usually wired to unit) and an analog (a thermometer probe in the interior that is independently connected to the alarm system) alarm approach for operational redundancy. Time intervals between collection and freezing should be documented, and is particularly helpful for troubleshooting since preservation of protein and other molecular analyte expression may vary over time.

1.3 Labeling and Quality Assurance for Fresh Frozen Samples

Accurate labeling is essential. Ideally, labels should include a specimen ID that is guaranteed to be unique across all samples and linked to a complete sample description by electronic means—specific procedures for labeling specimens which may include use of unique sample IDs and/or barcodes should be standardized and clearly be defined in the protocol to ensure accuracy and uniformity. The label must *not* include patient-identifying information and must be compliant with the Health Insurance Portability and Accountability Act (HIPAA) and any institutional and other State and Federal regulations. The type of label media, and ink used must be selected with care for appropriate resistance to chemicals, temperature extremes, storage media, and transport conditions.

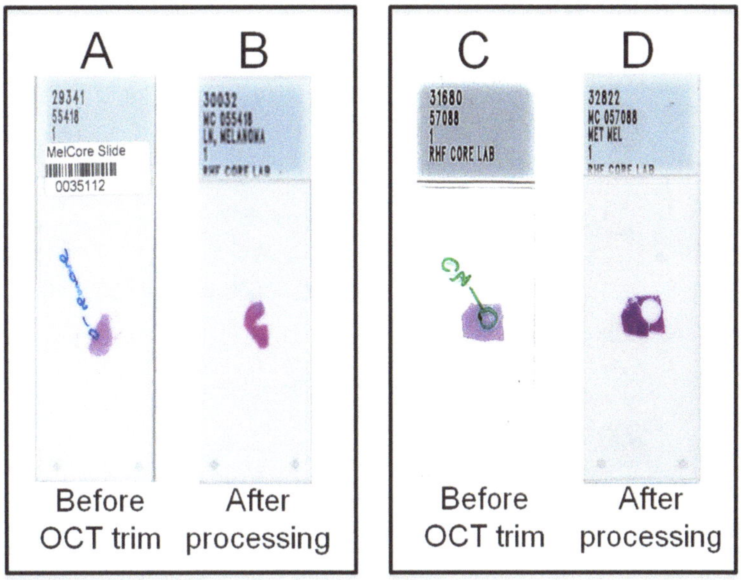

Fig. 1 H&E-based "trimming" of OCT specimens. Examples of H&E-stained OCT tumor sections before (*A* and *C*) and following (*B* and *D*) trimming of OCT blocks to maximize tumor cell nuclei and to remove areas of necrosis. Note that circled areas (*A* and *C*) were identified for trimming

To assess the quality of collected frozen tissue, an H&E-stained, cryostat section should be prepared from the frozen OCT block to confirm the presence of tumor and identify potential contaminants and/or other potential confounding material. Histological features that should ideally be recorded include assessment of percent tumor cells, preservation of tumor morphology, presence of any confounding material, such as necrotic, fibrotic, and/or hemorrhagic regions, amount of melanin pigment, and/or inflammatory infiltrate. The H&E slide may be used as a guide to isolate or "macrodissect" desirable portions of the sample for molecular analyses (i.e., viable tumor and adjacent normal tissue) and remove areas that may confound subsequent analyses and/or analyte preparation (e.g., areas of fibrosis, necrosis, hemorrhage, and excessive melanin pigment) (*see* Fig. 1).

1.4 Tissue Microarray Technology

Tissue microarrays (TMAs) offer an efficient, effective laboratory tool to analyze dozens of formalin-fixed, paraffin-embedded (FFPE) tissue samples on a single microscope slide and provide a very valuable research tool for immunohistochemical (IHC) screening of known or putative cancer biomarkers. TMAs are assembled by obtaining tissue cores containing 0.6–2.0 mm diameter samples of patient tumors from donor FFPE tissue blocks and placing these cores in predrilled holes of recipient (master) paraffin blocks. These master blocks are arrayed to a grid that is linked to pathological and clinical data (*see* Fig. 2) [26]. Manual or automated tissue arrayers provide precise, reproducible quality transfer

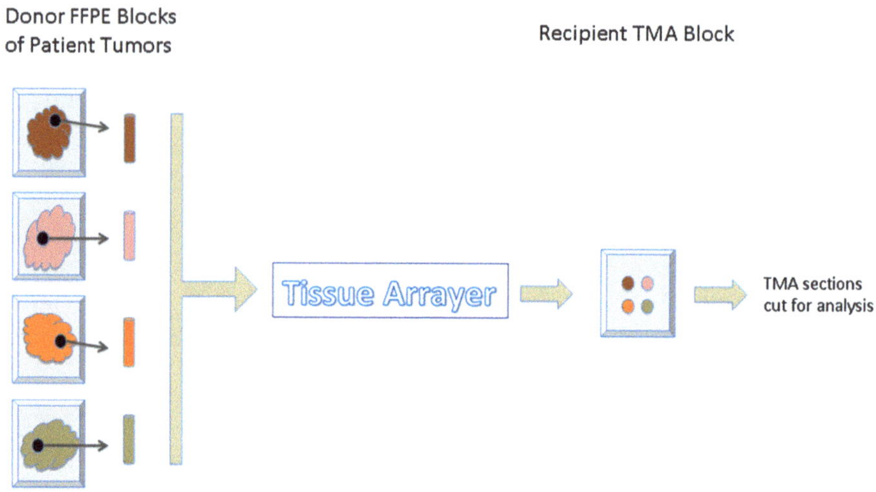

Fig. 2 Diagram of assembled TMA. Tissue cores of patient's tumors obtained from formalin-fixed paraffin-embedded (FFPE) donor blocks are placed in recipient TMA block by a tissue arrayer. This process can place dozens of donor tissue cores in one TMA block that can be cut and evaluated on a single microscopic slide

of tissue cores or histospots from donor blocks to the master TMA blocks. One TMA block may provide up to 500 or more (depending on the diameter of tissue cores and how frequently the TMA block is refaced) 5-μm thick, FFPE sections available for high-throughput profiling, enabling on each slide the equivalent of over 100 assays (depending on the core size) [27].

Traditional IHC evaluation of hundreds of tumor samples by whole slide sections requires that they be stained in batches and requires days to complete. Each batch is de facto exposed to inherent variables during the course of the processing and staining procedures. In contrast, TMAs allow evaluation of tissue samples in a single, consistent IHC procedure, and can usually be completed in one day. TMAs also conserve tissue samples and preserve much of the tissue within each block since only small cores of tumor tissue are used for analysis. In summary, when compared with IHC evaluation of a whole slide section of tissue, TMAs save valuable time, reagents, and cost in analyzing biomarkers, and in addition control for many inherent immunohistochemical variables of tissue-based research efforts.

The accuracy of TMAs in elucidating underlying biology has been raised as a concern since protein expression in cancer may be heterogeneous and TMAs by their design examine only a fraction of any given tumor. However, several groups have demonstrated significant correlation in IHC results obtained from TMA histospots or whole-tissue sections [27–29]. Increasing the number of tissue cores from donor FFPE tumor block on the array has been shown to reduce error rate of negative IHC results that may result from tumor heterogeneity. In general, two 0.6 mm histospots (i.e., two 0.6-mm tissue cores from a single donor FFPE tumor block) adequately represent IHC staining of entire histological section in most tumors [26–28]. However, fibroblastic tumors may require three 0.6 mm tissue cores from a donor FFPE tumor block to achieve a concordance of 91–96 % when compared to whole-tissue sections; four 0.6 mm tissue cores may be necessary for some melanocytic tumors to reach a concordance of 96.6 % [30, 31]. In some cases, use of multiple cores may significantly reduce the number of available sections. It is also important to note that the layout of the cores on the block should be arranged so as to make the block asynchronous in both (i.e., *x* and *y*) axes to minimize confusion in orienting the block.

In summary, TMAs provide a way of efficiently analyzing multiple tumor samples while also preserving tissue. Although some tumors show heterogeneous immunogenicity, use of more than one core per sample markedly improves the correlation of immunohistochemical results between TMAs and whole-tissue sections. Although details of individual studies employing TMAs in the melanoma biomarker arena are beyond the scope of this chapter, the interested reader is directed to recent studies that have successfully employed TMAs, many of which were constructed as institutional or inter-institutional initiatives through the NIH-funded SPORE (Specialized Program of Research Excellence) programs that have focused research efforts in melanoma. Recent relevant studies that have utilized TMAs to evaluate the prognostic significance of biomarkers in melanoma include the following: (1) phosphorylated STAT3 (p-STAT3) expression in patients with stage IV melanoma did not convey risk for CNS metastasis [32]; (2) NEDD9 protein expression was shown to be significantly upregulated in metastatic melanoma compared to melanocytic nevi [33]; (3) detection of mitosis and melanoma cells in G2 phase of the cell cycle with histone H3K79me3T80ph defined a subset of primary melanomas with risk for metastasis [34]; (4) confirmation of expression of imatinib targets in melanoma patients, particularly those with acral-lentiginous melanoma [9, 26]; (5) expression of galectin 3 in melanoma lesions and its possible relationship to sun exposure[35]; and (6) decreased expression of retinoid receptors in primary and metastatic melanoma, and its possible correlation with impaired prognosis [36].

2 Materials

2.1 General Materials

Safety glasses or face shield, disposable latex gloves, laboratory coat, protective shoes.

2.2 Labeling and Storage

1. Laser Cryo-Labels (we use 1.42″ × 0.55″ removable Laser Labels), Histoprep Marker, permanent ink pen (e.g., Sharpie©), #2 pencil (*see* **Note 5**).
2. Cryovials, racks for cryovials.

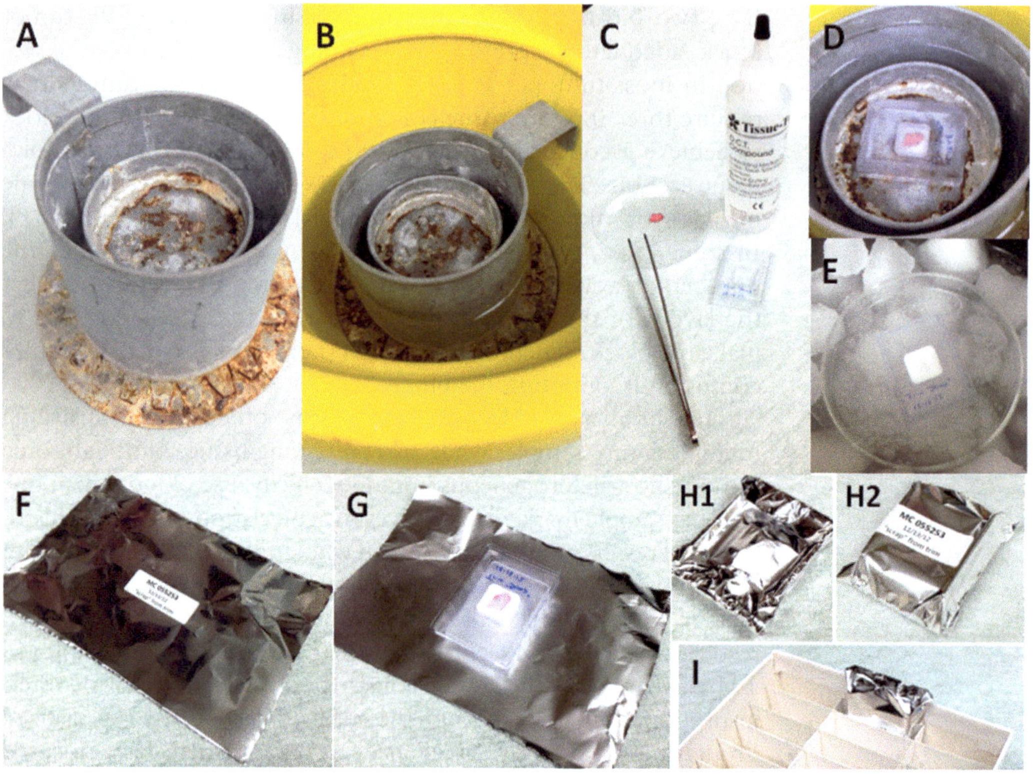

Fig. 3 Frozen tissue preparation. (**a**) Example of liquid nitrogen cryomold freezing stand (LN_2 Stand). (**b**) LN_2 stand in ice bucket with liquid nitrogen. (**c**) Examples of: OCT compound; labeled cryomold; and prepped tissue ready for freezing (not on ice; for demonstration purposes only). (**d**) Process of rapid freezing of tissue in OCT (partially hardened) using LN_2 stand. (**e**) Process of rapid freezing of tissue in OCT (fully hardened) using slurry method (*see* **Note 15**). (**f**) Example of labeled aluminum foil OCT archival sample wrapper. (**g**) Example of frozen OCT sample just prior to wrapping. (**h**) Examples of wrapped sample (**1**) backside and (**2**) front side. (**i**) Example of wrapped labeled sample placed in archival cryobox

3. Tissue-Tek® OCT™ compound, cryomold, Parafilm®, heavy-duty aluminum foil.
4. Cryo/freezer boxes (5″ × 5″ × 2″, 9 × 9 grid usually works best) (Fisher Scientific). For cryomold storage, we convert a 9 × 9 (81 cell) grid insert by removing dividers to form a 3 × 9 grid: remove the 1st two dividers, leave a divider, then remove another two dividers, leave a divider, then remove the last two dividers) (*see* Fig. 3i).
5. Liquid nitrogen freezer or permanent Dewar storage space, and/or −80 °C freezer.

2.3 Preparing Biospecimen for Cryo-Storage

1. Liquid nitrogen (LN_2) in approved LN_2 transport carrier (*see* **Notes 6–7**). Alternatively, 100 % isopropanol/dry ice slurry (slurry method) in a non-leaking ice bucket or other ultralow temperature container may also be employed in clinical pathology laboratories (*see* **Note 8**).

2. Freezer/cryo-gloves.
3. Liquid nitrogen cryomold freezing stand (LN_2Stand) in ice bucket—outside the clinical pathology laboratory, we use a custom-built double metal cylinder/can welded together with an outside top-edge handle. The interior solid can is 2″ shorter and about half the diameter of the outer open-top can and provides a horizontal metal-disc surface with a raised lip to hold the cryomold (*see* Fig. 3a) Liquid nitrogen is placed into the outer ring between the two cylinders and between the outer cylinder and ice bucket (*see* Fig. 3b).
4. Disposable, preferably sterile, scalpels or scalpel blades (note—autoclaved single-edge razor blades can also be used).
5. Forceps, disposable petri dish, glass petri dish (to autoclave unwrapped single-edge razor blades or when slurry method is used), Kimwipes©, Bunsen burner.
6. PBS, isopropyl alcohol, Tissue-Tek® OCT compound.

3 Methods

3.1 Initial Specimen Preparation

1. Employ universal precautions consistent with regulatory requirements at all times.
2. Preprepare labels when possible; we find that printed cryo-labels work best. When hand-preparing labels, markers that support cryo-temperatures are recommended (i.e., alcohol-based permanent markers may smudge or fade and will not stay if using slurry method for freezing).
3. Remove any excess blood from the tissue using paper towel, gauze, or equivalent. If necessary, rinse in sterile PBS and blot dry (*see* **Notes 9–13**).
4. Tissue should be cut on a dissection board or similar set-up using a clean/sterile razor blade or scissors (*see* **Note 9**). For the tissue to "fit" in either cryovials or cryomolds, at least one of the tissue dimensions should be no greater than the maximum thickness of 0.5 cm. When sterile technique is required/desired, we often place the tissue in a sterile Petri dish and trim with sterile blades (if possible, perform in a laminar air flow hood).
5. Use separate forceps for each specimen to minimize the possibility of cross-contamination.
6. Discard any unused tissue according to procedures for disposal of human biological waste material.
7. Discard the blade(s) according to procedures for disposal of biohazard sharps.
8. If possible, weigh sectioned specimen prior to freezing (see also below).

9. When possible, the following should also be recorded:
   (a) Time (in minutes) before tissue has been frozen.
   (b) Freezing temperature and/or conditions employed.

3.2 OCT Embedding

1. Pre-procedure preparation:
   (a) Prepare foil wrappers—cut heavy-duty aluminum foil into rectangles (approximately 5″ × 3″).
   (b) Label cryomolds with printed cryolabel and/or permanent marker, and prepare (preferably print) sticker labels for foil wrappers. Labels should include: study ID, sample ID, tissue type/description, and date. Place cryomolds on a flat surface in a manner that will allow for easy identification of planned contents.
2. When sample is available, fill the bottom of each cryomold with a thin layer (less than 1 mm) of OCT by slowly and carefully filling the mold. It is important to avoid formation of bubbles and creation of uneven surfaces. If necessary, carefully tapping the bottom of the cryomold on a flat hard surface facilitates distribution of OCT.
3. If possible, weigh and record each section of the specimen prior to placing it in a cryomold.
4. If possible, prechill the prepared cryomold (**step 2**). This can be done by: (a) setting on ice for 2–5 min or (b) partially freezing the cryomold just prior to transferring specimen (**step 5**) by holding cryomold over the liquid nitrogen with forceps until OCT starts to become cloudy. Do not let the OCT fully harden at this time.
5. Using forceps, transfer the specimen to the prechilled OCT-filled cryomold.
6. Cover the exposed tissue with OCT; ensure the top surface of the OCT compound completely covers the tissue and is level. If the tissue section is taller than the cassette, the OCT can be layered (*see* **Note 14**).
7. The OCT can be hardened by placing the filled cryomold flatly on the interior metal-disc surface of the Liq N2 Stand (*see* Fig. 3a, d) that has been acclimated in liquid nitrogen (*see* Fig. 3b). Avoid allowing the cryomold to come in direct contact with the liquid nitrogen (*see* **Notes 7–15**). Specimen(s) are sufficiently frozen when the OCT has become completely white and firm. One may use the Slurry Method as an alternative approach to OCT processing (*see* Fig. 3e) (*see* **Note 8**).
8. While the OCT is hardening, adhere the appropriate sample label to a precut foil wrap in the center of the foil (*see* Fig. 3f).

9. After the OCT has hardened (i.e., has become firm and solid white in appearance), place the cryomold face down onto the non-labeled side of the appropriately pre-labeled foil wrap (Fig 3g). Fold the long side of aluminum wrap over the long edges to the back of the cryomold. Tuck short ends over short edges to the back of the cryomold (i.e., similar to wrapping a gift). After completing these folding maneuvers (*see* Fig. 3h1), the label should be positioned in the middle of the front of the wrapped OCT tissue (*see* Fig. 3h2).
10. Place samples on dry ice in a Styrofoam container or other suitable device with lid until transferred to −80 °C freezer for storage.
11. The wrapped OCT specimen is then placed into the 3×9 divided (27 cell) 5″×5″×2″ cryo-storage box (*see* Fig. 3i) and stored in a −80 °C freezer rack. We also suggest that the rack, box and grid position of the OCT specimen be documented in the study database.

3.3 Snap Freezing

1. Pre-procedure preparation: label 1.8 ml or similar cryovials using a permanent cryomarker (i.e., ethanol and freezer-resistant).
2. To determine specimen section weight: record weight of the empty vial, add tissue, and then reweigh. Subtract weights to determine the weight of the specimen and record.
3. Place individual specimen section in a 1.8 ml cryovials using forceps. Use separate forceps for each specimen to minimize the possibility of cross-contamination.
4. Tightly secure the cap and submerge in liquid nitrogen for "snap freezing" (*see* **Notes 5–8**).
5. Place samples on dry ice in Styrofoam container or other suitable device with lid until transferred to −80 ° freezer for storage.
6. The snap-frozen specimen-containing cryovial is then placed in a 9×9 (i.e., 81 cell) 5″×5″×2″ cryo-storage box and stored at −80 °C or colder in freezer racks. We also suggest that the rack, box, and grid position of the snap-frozen specimen be notated in the study database.
7. If cryostat sections will be performed on snap-frozen tissue samples (and not embedded in OCT), mount tissue samples to gum tragacanth to ensure desired tissue specimen orientation (e.g., skin punch tissue specimens) and snap-freeze. Wrap labeled snap-frozen tissue samples in Parafilm® then cover in aluminum foil and store at −80 °C [37].

4 Notes

1. While both core biopsies and FNA biopsies are commonly employed for diagnostic purposes, core biopsies usually provide more tissue and are preferred for research purposes. The minimum size for fresh/frozen tissue collection is generally 0.25 cubic cm, which is generally achieved with approximately four passes of a 14-gauge needle. In the diagnostic setting, the collection of 2–4 fresh/frozen cores for research is recommended, in addition to two cores for diagnosis. The fraction of cores that will contain viable tumor will decrease if/as the tumor shrinks in response to therapy. Therefore, fewer cores may be obtainable as lesions become smaller. If a previous biopsy site is noted in the specimen to be sampled, if at all possible, biopsies should not be taken from near that site. Core biopsies may alter the biology of adjacent tissue—e.g., they introduce inflammatory material from wound reaction and biomolecules involved in wound healing—which can be problematic if a subsequent core taken from that tissue is used. Notably, many genes involved in wound healing are also noted to be involved in cancer progression [38].
2. If possible, representative adjacent normal tissue should be collected in addition to the tumor tissue. Normal tissue should be maximally distant from the tumor, although clear definitions of what constitutes normal control tissue in the context of primary melanoma research (e.g., is normal skin a good normal control?) are not well established. Nonetheless, if normal skin is to be collected, it should be collected as far from the primary site as practical. Collection of germline DNA (i.e., extracted from peripheral blood mononuclear cells (PBMC)) should be considered in all protocols that include the collection of tumor tissue for DNA isolation, as defining truly "normal" tissue for melanoma research is indeed challenging.
3. Do not slow-freeze. Samples in cryovial or OCT/cryomolds should be snap frozen. Slow freezing promotes the formation of ice crystals, which can damage nucleic acids (e.g., RNA) in the specimen. The slower a sample freezes, the larger the ice crystals that may form. Older models of cryostats that require significant specimen freeze time should be avoided whenever possible.
4. Containers used to transport samples with dry ice needs ventilation so there is no buildup of the CO_2 within the container.
5. If a pen is used to label cryovials or other receptacles that will be stored in freezing conditions, ensure that the pen is waterproof/solvent-proof and can withstand long-term freezing conditions. For cryovials, if no cryomarker is available, pencil

may work on the writing surface and withstand long-term LN_2 conditions; it is advisable to confirm this functionality in advance of specimen processing.

6. Use freezer gloves and a face shield while working with liquid nitrogen. Take precautions to avoid accidental spillage or spattering of liquid nitrogen.
7. Do not place the specimen directly in liquid nitrogen. If the tissue is frozen too quickly, it may shatter, potentially causing difficulty with H&Es and IHC.
8. If liquid nitrogen is not available, the slurry method can be used by making an isopropanol/dry ice slurry. It is best to use crushed dry ice mixed with 100 % isopropanol until the ice is moistened throughout, but not so much as to have a layer of pure isopropanol over the ice. The slurry should be ready to use once the isopropanol stops forming new bubbles. It is not recommended to simply use dry ice for freezing.
9. Instruments should be changed or thoroughly cleaned between dissection of normal and tumor tissue to prevent cross-contamination—even a tiny amount of cross-contamination can interfere with analyte preparation and potentially adversely confound results.
10. If RNA analyte preparation is planned, use a sterile RNAse-free container. Rinse tissue in DEPC-treated water or RNAse-free PBS. We do not recommend RNAlater® particularly with cutaneous/subcutaneous tissue as the RNAlater® makes the connective tissue more rigid, and causes the homogenization process to be less efficient, giving lower yields with greater degradation of RNA.
11. Do not add serum to the specimen.
12. Do not directly touch the biopsy/specimen without sterile gloves.
13. Use sterile or disposable equipment for both dissection and snap freezing.
14. When tissue is taller than cryomold, the OCT can be layered in steps until the tissue is completely covered. Add OCT only up to the top of the tissue insert section of the cryomold. Partially freeze/harden the tissue in OCT—the OCT will become cloudy/white on the edges. Before the OCT that is next to the tissue becomes cloudy, remove from liquid nitrogen (or dry ice/alcohol slurry) and add another layer of OCT onto the partially hardened previous layer of OCT and reexpose to cold (until it gets cloudy) and repeat if necessary. Once the tissue is completed covered by OCT, let it freeze completely.
15. Alternative approach: OCT preparation without Liq N2 Stand—use of a petri dish to freeze OCT/tissue in cryomold: Carefully position a Petri dish at the surface of the liquid nitrogen using

forceps or the isopropanol/dry ice slurry (*see* Fig. 2e); allow the petri dish to stabilize with the liquid nitrogen or slurry; place the filled cryomold in the Petri dish and freeze until the OCT media is completely hard.

Acknowledgments

This work was supported by NIH grant P50 CA093459 University of Texas MD Anderson Cancer Center SPORE in Melanoma and an NIH/SAIC Cancer Genome Atlas Project for melanoma contract, also awarded to MD Anderson.

References

1. Davies MA, Gershenwald JE (2010) Targeted therapy for melanoma: a primer. Surg Oncol Clin N Am 20:165–180
2. Wilson M, Zhao F, Letrero R et al (2012) Somatic mutation status of melanomas and effect on clinical outcome in patients on ECOG 2603. Society for Melanoma Research 2012 Congress, Hollywood, CA
3. Becker D, Mihm MC, Hewitt SM et al (2006) Markers and tissue resources for melanoma: meeting report. Cancer Res 66:10652–10657
4. Chapman PB, Hauschild A, Robert C et al (2011) Improved survival with vemurafenib in melanoma with BRAF V600E mutation. N Engl J Med 364:2507–2516
5. Heidorn SJ, Milagre C, Whittaker S et al (2010) Kinase-Dead BRAF and Oncogenic RAS Cooperate to Drive Tumor Progression through CRAF. Cell 140:209–221
6. Poulikakos PI, Zhang C, Bollag G et al (2010) RAF inhibitors transactivate RAF dimers and ERK signalling in cells with wild-type BRAF. Nature 464:427–430
7. Halaban R, Zhang W, Bacchiocchi A et al (2010) PLX4032, a selective BRAF(V600E) kinase inhibitor, activates the ERK pathway and enhances cell migration and proliferation of BRAF melanoma cells. Pigment Cell Melanoma Res 23:190–200
8. Woodman SE, Lazar AJ, Aldape KD et al (2012) New strategies in melanoma: molecular testing in advanced disease. Clin Cancer Res 18:1195–1200
9. Ivan D, Niveiro M, Diwan AH et al (2006) Analysis of protein tyrosine kinases expression in the melanoma metastases of patients treated with Imatinib Mesylate (STI571, Gleevec). J Cutan Pathol 33:280–285
10. Bollag G, Hirth P, Tsai J et al (2010) Clinical efficacy of a RAF inhibitor needs broad target blockade in BRAF-mutant melanoma. Nature 467:596–599
11. Hauschild A, Grob JJ, Demidov LV et al (2012) Dabrafenib in BRAF-mutated metastatic melanoma: a multicentre, open-label, phase 3 randomised controlled trial. Lancet 380:358–365
12. McArthur GA, Ribas A, Chapman PB et al (2011) Molecular analyses from a phase I trial of vemurafenib to study mechanism of action (MOA) and resistance in repeated biopsies from BRAF mutation-positive metastatic melanoma patients. J Clin Oncol. 29: abstract 8502
13. Sosman JA, Pavlick AC, Schuchter LM et al (2012) Analysis of molecular mechanisms of response and resistance to vemurafenib (vem) in BRAF V600E melanoma. J Clin Oncol 30:8503
14. Nazarian R, Shi H, Wang Q et al (2010) Melanomas acquire resistance to B-RAF (V600E) inhibition by RTK or N-RAS upregulation. Nature 468:973–977
15. Villanueva J, Vultur A, Lee JT et al (2010) Acquired resistance to BRAF inhibitors mediated by a RAF kinase switch in melanoma can Be overcome by cotargeting MEK and IGF-1R/PI3K. Cancer Cell 18:683–695
16. Poulikakos PI, Persaud Y, Janakiraman M et al (2011) RAF inhibitor resistance is mediated by dimerization of aberrantly spliced BRAF (V600E). Nature 480:387–390
17. Montagut C, Sharma SV, Shioda T et al (2008) Elevated CRAF as a potential mechanism of acquired resistance to BRAF inhibition in melanoma. Cancer Res 68:4853–4861
18. Flaherty KT, Infante JR, Daud A et al (2012) Combined BRAF and MEK inhibition in melanoma with BRAF V600 mutations. N Engl J Med 367:1694–1703

19. Flaherty KT, Infante JR, Falchook GS et al (2011) Phase I/II expansion cohort of BRAF inhibitor GSK2118436+MEK inhibitor GSK1120212 in patients with BRAF mutant metastatic melanoma who progressed on a prior BRAF inhibitor. Pigment Cell Mel Res 24:1022
20. Daud A, Sosman J, Weber J et al (2012) Mutation and copy number analysis in melanoma biopsies from a Phase I/II study evaluating the combination of dabrafenib and trametinib. Society for Melanoma Research 2012 Congress, Hollywood, CA
21. Singh B (2007) Initial pathology assessment prior to preoperative therapy. Preoperative therapy in invasive breast cancer: reviewing the state of the science and exploring new research directions. Bethesda, Maryland
22. Hewitt SM, Lewis FA, Cao Y et al (2008) Tissue handling and specimen preparation in surgical pathology: issues concerning the recovery of nucleic acids from formalin-fixed, paraffin-embedded tissue. Arch Pathol Lab Med 132:1929–1935
23. Leyland-Jones BR, Ambrosone CB, Bartlett J et al (2008) Recommendations for collection and handling of specimens from group breast cancer clinical trials. J Clin Oncol 26: 5638–5644
24. Ibberson D, Benes V, Muckenthaler MU et al (2009) RNA degradation compromises the reliability of microRNA expression profiling. BMC Biotechnol 9:102
25. Gundisch S, Hauck S, Sarioglu H et al (2012) Variability of protein and phosphoprotein levels in clinical tissue specimens during the preanalytical phase. J Proteome Res 11: 5748–5762
26. Shen SS, Zhang PS, Eton O et al (2003) Analysis of protein tyrosine kinase expression in melanocytic lesions by tissue array. J Cutan Pathol 30:539–547
27. Camp RL, Neumeister V, Rimm DL (2008) A decade of tissue microarrays: progress in the discovery and validation of cancer biomarkers. J Clin Oncol 26:5630–5637
28. Camp RL, Charette LA, Rimm DL (2000) Validation of tissue microarray technology in breast carcinoma. Lab Invest 80:1943–1949
29. Torhorst J, Bucher C, Kononen J et al (2001) Tissue microarrays for rapid linking of molecular changes to clinical endpoints. Am J Pathol 159:2249–2256
30. Hoos A, Urist MJ, Stojadinovic A et al (2001) Validation of tissue microarrays for immunohistochemical profiling of cancer specimens using the example of human fibroblastic tumors. Am J Pathol 158:1245–1251
31. Pacifico MD, Grover R, Richman P et al (2004) Validation of tissue microarray for the immunohistochemical profiling of melanoma. Melanoma Res 14:39–42
32. Lee I, Fox PS, Ferguson SD et al (2012) The expression of p-STAT3 in stage IV melanoma: risk of CNS metastasis and survival. Oncotarget 3:336–344
33. Kim M, Gans JD, Nogueira C et al (2006) Comparative oncogenomics identifies NEDD9 as a melanoma metastasis gene. Cell 125: 1269–1281
34. Martinez DR, Richards HW, Lin Q et al (2012) H3K79me3T80ph is a novel histone dual modification and a mitotic indicator in melanoma. J Skin Cancer 2012:823534
35. Prieto VG, Mourad-Zeidan AA, Melnikova V et al (2006) Galectin-3 expression is associated with tumor progression and pattern of sun exposure in melanoma. Clin Cancer Res 12: 6709–6715
36. Chakravarti N, Lotan R, Diwan AH et al (2007) Decreased expression of retinoid receptors in melanoma: entailment in tumorigenesis and prognosis. Clin Cancer Res 13: 4817–4824
37. Curry JL, Qin JZ, Bonish B et al (2003) Innate immune-related receptors in normal and psoriatic skin. Arch Pathol Lab Med 127:178–186
38. Riss J, Khanna C, Koo S et al (2006) Cancers as wounds that do not heal: differences and similarities between renal regeneration/repair and renal cell carcinoma. Cancer Res 66: 7216–7224

INDEX

A

B

Magdalena Thurin and Francesco M. Marincola (eds.), *Molecular Diagnostics for Melanoma: Methods and Protocols*, Methods in Molecular Biology, vol. 1102, DOI 10.1007/978-1-62703-727-3, © Springer Science+Business Media New York 2014

C

D

E

F

L

M

N

O

P

Q

R

S

T

U

V

W

MIX
Papier aus verantwortungsvollen Quellen
Paper from responsible sources
FSC® C105338

If you have any concerns about our products,
you can contact us on
ProductSafety@springernature.com

In case Publisher is established outside the EU,
the EU authorized representative is:
Springer Nature Customer Service Center GmbH
Europaplatz 3, 69115 Heidelberg, Germany

Printed by Libri Plureos GmbH
in Hamburg, Germany